Monographs on Pathology of Laboratory Animals

Sponsored by the
International Life Sciences Institute

The following volumes have appeared so far

Endocrine System
1983. 346 figures. XV, 366 pages. ISBN 3-540-11677-X

Respiratory System
1985. 279 figures. XV, 240 pages. ISBN 3-540-13521-9

Digestive System
1985. 352 figures. XVIII, 386 pages. ISBN 3-540-15815-4

Urinary System
1986. 362 figures. XVIII, 405 pages. ISBN 3-540-16591-6

Genital System
1987. 340 figures. XVII, 304 pages. ISBN 3-540-17604-7

Nervous System
1988. 242 figures. XVI, 233 pages. ISBN 3-540-19416-9

The following volumes are in preparation

Hemopoietic System
Musculoskeletal System
Cardiovascular System
Special Sense

T. C. Jones U. Mohr R. D. Hunt (Eds.)

Integument and Mammary Glands

With 468 Figures and 34 Tables

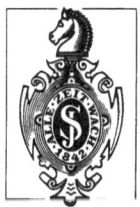

Springer-Verlag Berlin Heidelberg GmbH

Thomas Carlyle Jones, D.V.M., D.Sc.
Professor of Comparative Pathology, Emeritus
Harvard Medical School
New England Regional Primate Research Center
One Pine Hill Drive, Southborough, MA 01772, USA

Ulrich Mohr, M.D.
Professor of Experimental Pathology
Medizinische Hochschule Hannover
Institut für Experimentelle Pathologie
Konstanty-Gutschow-Strasse 8
3000 Hannover 61, Federal Republic of Germany

Ronald Duncan Hunt, D.V.M.
Professor of Comparative Pathology
Harvard Medical School
New England Regional Primate Research Center
One Pine Hill Drive, Southborough, MA 01772, USA

ISBN 978-3-642-83751-7   ISBN 978-3-642-83749-4 (eBook)
DOI 10.1007/978-3-642-83749-4

Library of Congress Cataloging-in-Publication Data.
Integument and mammary glands/T.C.Jones, U.Mohr, R.D.Hunt (eds.).
p.cm. – (Monographs on pathology of laboratory animals)
Includes bibliographies and index.
                    (U.S.: alk. paper)
1.Skin-Cancer-Animal models. 2.Breast-Cancer-Animal models.
3.Skin-Diseases-Animal models. 4.Breast-Diseases-Animal models.
5.Laboratory animals-Diseases. 6.Rodents-Diseases. I.Jones, Thomas Carlyle.
II.Mohr, U. (Ulrich) III.Hunt, Ronald Duncan. IV.Series.
RC280.S5I55 1989 616.99'477'0724-dc20 89-11364

Softcover reprint of the hardcover 1st edition 1989

2123/3140-543210 – Printed on acid-free paper

Foreword

The International Life Sciences Institute (ILSI) was established in 1978 to stimulate and support scientific research and educational programs related to nutrition, toxicology, and food safety, and to encourage cooperation in these programs among scientists in universities, industry, and government agencies to assist in the resolution of health and safety issues.

To supplement and enhance these efforts, ILSI has made a major commitment to supporting programs to harmonize toxicologic testing, to advance a more uniform interpretation of bioassay results worldwide, to promote a common understanding of lesion classifications, and to encourage wide discussion of these topics among scientists. The *Monographs on the Pathology of Laboratory Animals* are designed to facilitate communication among those involved in the safety testing of foods, drugs, and chemicals. The complete set will cover all organ systems and is intended for use by pathologists, toxicologists, and others concerned with evaluating toxicity and carcinogenicity studies. The international nature of the project – as reflected in the composition of the editorial board and the diversity of the authors and editors – strengthens our expectations that understanding and cooperation will be improved worldwide through the series.

Alex Malaspina
President
International Life Sciences Institute

Preface

This book, on the integumentary system, is the seventh volume of a set prepared under the sponsorship of the International Life Sciences Institute (ILSI). One aim of this set on the pathology of laboratory animals is to provide information which will be useful to pathologists, especially those involved in studies on the safety of foods, drugs, chemicals, and other substances in the environment. It is expected that this and future volumes will contribute to better communication, on an international basis, among people in government, industry, and academia who are involved in protection of the public health.

The arrangement of this volume is based, in part, upon the philosophy that the first step toward understanding a pathologic lesion is its precise and unambiguous identification. The microscopic and ultrastructural features of a lesion that are particularly useful to the pathologist for definitive diagnosis, therefore, are considered foremost. Diagnostic terms preferred by the author and editors are used as the subject heading for each pathologic lesion. Synonyms are listed although most are not preferred and some may have been used erroneously in prior publications. The problems arising in differential diagnosis of similar lesions are considered in detail. The biologic significance of each pathologic lesion is considered under such headings as etiology, natural history, pathogenesis, and frequency of occurrence under natural or experimental conditions.

Comparison of information available on similar lesions in man and other species is valuable as a means to gain broader understanding of the processes involved. Knowledge of this nature is needed to form a scientific basis for safety evaluations and experimental pathology. References to pertinent literature are provided in close juxtaposition to the text in order to support conclusions in the text and lead toward additional information. Illustrations are an especially important means of nonverbal communication, especially among pathologists, and therefore constitute important features of each volume.

The subject under each heading is covered in concise terms and is expected to stand alone but, in some instances, it is important to refer to other parts of the volume. A comprehensive index is provided to enhance the use of each volume as a reference.

Some omissions are inevitable and we solicit comments from our colleagues to identify parts which need strengthening or correcting. We have endeavored to include important lesions which a pathologist might encounter in studies involving the rat, mouse, or hamster. Newly recognized lesions or better understanding of old ones may make revised editions necessary in the future.

The editors wish to express their deep gratitude to all of the individuals who have helped with this enterprise. We are indebted to each author and member of the Editorial Board whose name appears elsewhere in the volume. We are especially grateful to the Officers and Board of Trustees of the International Life Sciences Institute for their support and understanding. Several people have worked directly on important details in this venture. These include Mrs. Nina Murray, Executive Secretary; Mrs. Ann Balliett, Editorial Assistant; Mrs. June Armstrong, Medical Illustrator; and Mrs. Katie A. Parker, Secretary. Ms. Sharon K. Coleman, ILSI Coordinator for External Affairs, Mrs. Karen A. Taylor, ILSI Manager of Publications, and Ms. Sharon Senzik, Associate Director, ILSI Research Foundation, were helpful on many occasions.

We are particularly grateful to Dr. Dietrich Götze and his staff at Springer-Verlag for the quality of the published product.

March 1989

THE EDITORS

T. C. Jones
U. Mohr
R. D. Hunt

Table of Contents

List of Contributors

Anton M. Allen, D.V.M., Ph.D.
Chief, Comparative Pathology Section
Veterinary Resources Branch, DRS, NIH
Bethesda, Maryland, USA

Miriam R. Anver, D.V.M., Ph.D.
Senior Pathologist, Clement Associates, Inc.
Fairfax, Virginia, USA

Reza I. Bashey, Ph.D.
Department of Medicine, Jefferson Medical College
Philadelphia, Pennsylvania, USA

Gary A. Boorman, D.V.M., Ph.D.
Chief, Chemical Pathology Branch
National Institute of Environmental Health Sciences
Research Triangle Park, North Carolina, USA

Douglas L. Coleman, Ph.D.
Senior Staff Scientist, The Jackson Laboratory
Bar Harbor, Maine, USA

Gerald L. Coleman, D.V.M.
Central Research, Pfizer Inc.
Groton, Connecticut, USA

John G. Compton, Ph.D.
The Jackson Laboratory
Bar Harbor, Maine, USA

L.H.J.C. Danse, M.Sc., Ph.D.
Laboratory for Pathology
National Institute of Public Health & Environment Hygiene
Bilthoven, The Netherlands

Deborah E. Devor, B.S.
Laboratory of Comparative Carcinogenesis
Division of Cancer Etiology, NCI, NIH
Frederick, Maryland, USA

Robert W. Dunstan, D.V.M., M.S.
The Jackson Laboratory
Bar Harbor, Maine, USA

Pierre Duprat, D.V.M., Ph.D.
Director of Pathology, Safety Assessment
Merck Sharp & Dohme-Chibret
Riom, Cedex, France

Michael R. Elwell, D.V.M., Ph.D.
Chemical Pathology Branch
National Institute of Environmental Health Sciences
Research Triangle Park, North Carolina, USA

Scot L. Eustis, D. V. M., Ph. D.
Chemical Pathology Branch
National Institute of Environmental Health Sciences
Research Triangle Park, North Carolina, USA

Chris Fisher, Ph. D.
Department of Biological Structure, School of Medicine
University of Washington
Seattle, Washington, USA

Peter C. Greaves, MD, ChB, MRCPath.
Safety of Medicines Department
ICI Pharmaceuticals, Mereside, Alderley Park
Macclesfield, Cheshire, United Kingdom

Barry A. Gusterson, Ph. D., MRCPath.
Institute of Cancer Research, The Royal Marsden Hospital
Sutton, Surrey, United Kingdom

Laura Hart Elcock, D. V. M., Ph. D.
Mobay Chemical Corporation
Stilwell, Kansas, USA

Ryohei Hasegawa, M. D.
Department of Pathology, National Institute of Hygienic Sciences
Tokyo, Japan

Masao Hirose, M. D.
Department of Pathology, Nagoya City University Medical School
Nagoya, Japan

Karen A. Holbrook, Ph. D.
Department of Biological Structure, School of Medicine
University of Washington
Seattle, Washington, USA

Michael J. Imber, M. D., Ph. D.
Dermatopathology Unit, Massachusetts General Hospital
Boston, Massachusetts, USA

Sergio A. Jimenez, M. D.
Department of Medicine, Jefferson Medical College
Philadelphia, Pennsylvania, USA

Jun Kanno, M. D.
Pathology/Faculty of Medicine
Tokyo Medical and Dental University
Tokyo, Japan

David G. Keyes, B. S., M. T.
Health and Environmental Sciences
The Dow Chemical Company
Midland, Michigan, USA

Albert M. Kligman, M. D., Ph. D.
Department of Dermatology University of Pennsylvania
Philadelphia, Pennsylvania, USA

Lorraine H. Kligman, Ph. D.
Department of Dermatology University of Pennsylvania
Philadelphia, Pennsylvania, USA

Richard J. Kociba, D. V. M., Ph. D.
Health and Environmental Sciences, The Dow Chemical Company
Midland, Michigan, USA

Moritz A. Konerding, M. D.
Central Animal Laboratory and Institute of Anatomy
University Medical Centre
Essen, Federal Republic of Germany

Stephen G. Lake, D. V. M.
Mobay Chemical Corporation
Stilwell, Kansas, USA

Annabel G. Liebelt, Ph. D.
Registry of Experimental Cancers
National Cancer Institute-National Institutes of Health
Bethesda, Maryland, USA

Allan Lock, D. V. M., M. A.
Chief, Pathology Unit, Comparative Pathology Section
Veterinary Resources Branch, DRS, NIH
Bethesda, Maryland, USA

Akihiko Maekawa, M. D.
Department of Pathology, National Institute of Hygienic Sciences
Tokyo, Japan

Josephine Medado, Research Assistant
Department of Pathology, Michigan Cancer Foundation
Detroit, Michigan, USA

Klaus Militzer, D. V. M.
Central Animal Laboratory and Institute of Anatomy
University Medical Centre
Essen, Federal Republic of Germany

Yoshifumi Miyakawa, D. V. M.
Senior Researcher, Toxicology Research Laboratories
Japan Tobacco Inc., Kanagawa, Japan

Paul Monaghan, Ph. D.
Institute of Cancer Research, Haddow Laboratories
Sutton, Surrey, United Kingdom

Robert E. Mueller, Ph. D.
Supervisor, Pathology Services, Mobay Chemical Corporation
Stilwell, Kansas, USA

Sabine Rehm, Dr. med. vet.
Laboratory of Comparative Carcinogenesis
National Cancer Institute-National Institutes of Health
Frederick, Maryland, USA

Adrianne E. Rogers, M. D.
Department of Pathology, Boston University School of Medicine
Boston, Massachusetts, USA

P. J. M. Roholl, Ph. D.
TNO Institute for Experimental Gerontology
Rijswijk, 2280 HU, The Netherlands

Irma H. Russo, M. D.
Department of Pathology, Michigan Cancer Foundation
Detroit, Michigan, USA

Jose Russo, M. D.
Department of Pathology, Michigan Cancer Foundation
Detroit, Michigan, USA

Hidetaka Sato, M. D.
Department of Pathology, National Institute of Hygienic Sciences
Tokyo, Japan

Barry P. Stuart, D. V. M., Ph. D.
Mobay Chemical Corporation
Stilwell, Kansas, USA

Janos Sugar, M. D., D. MsC.
Director, Professor of Tumor Pathology
Research Institute of Oncopathology
Budapest, Hungary

John P. Sundberg, D. V. M., Ph. D.
The Jackson Laboratory
Bar Harbor, Maine, USA

Eva Szabo, M. D.
Research Institute of Oncopathology
National Oncological Institute
Budapest, Hungary

Michihito Takahashi, M. D.
Department of Pathology, National Institute of Hygienic Sciences
Tokyo, Japan

Muneesh Tewari
Research Assistant, Department of Pathology
Michigan Cancer Foundation
Detroit, Michigan, USA

Vladimir S. Turusov, M. D., D. Sci., Professor
All-Union Cancer Research Centre
Moscow, USSR

Matthew J. van Zwieten, D. V. M., Ph. D.
Division of Safety Assessment
Merck Sharp and Dohme Research Laboratories
West Point, Pennsylvania, USA

Michael J. Warburton, B. Sc., Ph. D.
Senior Lecturer, Department of Histopathology
St. George's Hospital Medical School
London, United Kingdom

Jerrold M. Ward, D. V. M., Ph. D.
Laboratory of Comparative Carcinogenesis
National Cancer Institute-National Institutes of Health
Frederick, Maryland, USA

David M. Williams
Pathologist, Health and Environmental Sciences
The Dow Chemical Company
Midland, Michigan, USA

Chris Zurcher, M. D., Ph. D.
TNO Institute for Experimental Gerontology
Rijswijk, The Netherlands

The Integument

New Approaches and Diagnostic Techniques in Dermatopathology

Michael J. Imber

Introduction

A variety of specialized techniques are available to aid the interpretation and diagnosis of human cutaneous diseases. Neoplastic or inflammatory skin disorders may be evaluated by application of electron microscopy, immunoperoxidase, immunofluorescence, and most recently, nucleic acid hybridization probe analysis (Murphy et al. 1982; Beutner et al. 1987; Kahn et al. 1986; Fenoglio-Preiser and Willman 1987). This chapter will review the microscopic features and differential diagnoses of a number of human cutaneous lesions in which application of one or more special diagnostic techniques may contribute to establishing a correct diagnosis.

Electron Microscopic Demonstration of Characteristic Cytoplasmic Inclusions

Melanocytic Nevi (Melanin Macroglobules). Aberrant formation of giant melanosomes may occur in both proliferative and physiologic disorders of melanocytes (Jimbow et al. 1973). These spherical, deeply pigmented cytoplasmic inclusions are often visible by light microscopy (Fig. 1). They may be observed in melanocytes or keratinocytes. The café-au-lait macules of von Recklinghausen's neurofibromatosis contain melanin macroglobules in approximately 90% of cases (Crowe and Schull 1953; Benedict et al. 1968; Johnson and Charneco 1970). Ultrastructural examination reveals amorphous globular aggregates of electron dense material measuring up to

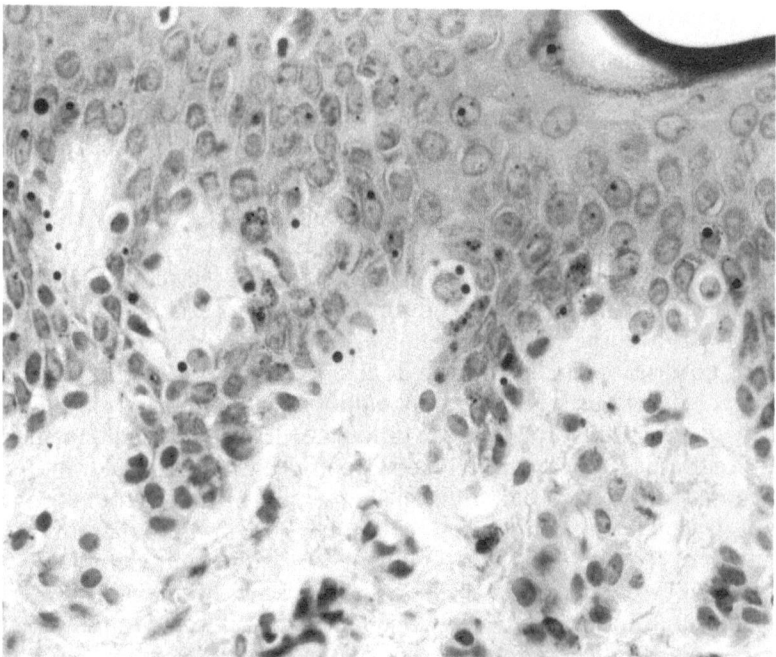

Fig. 1. Dysplastic nevus. Melanin macroglobules are present within the cytoplasm of nevomelanocytes and keratinocytes. H and E, ×500

4 Michael J. Imber

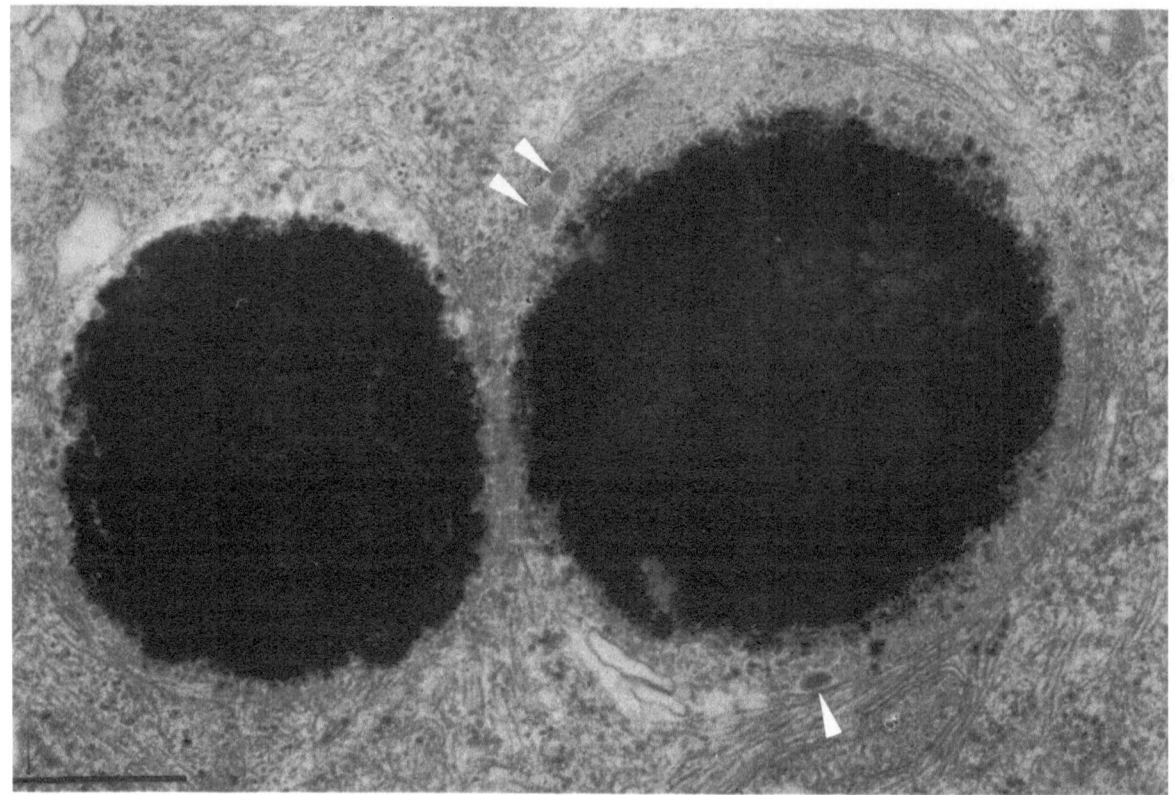

Fig. 2. Melanin macroglobules. Giant melanin macroglobules (or macromelanosomes) are present within the cytoplasm of a melanocyte from a café-au-lait macule. Normal melanosomes are also present *(arrowheads)*. TEM, × 12000

6.0 μm in diameter (Fig. 2). These structures may also be observed in congenital melanocytic nevi, dysplastic nevi, and common acquired nevi.

Histiocytosis X (Birbeck Granules). Proliferative disorders of the dendritic Langerhans' cell comprise the histiocytosis X spectrum of neoplasms (Favara and Jaffe 1987). These include Letterer-Siwe disease, a frequently fatal disorder affecting infants, and eosinophilic granuloma, a benign, localized disease usually seen in adults. Each of these disorders features a cell population with cytologic, ultrastructural, and immunohistochemical properties of epidermal Langerhans' cells, bone-marrow-derived dendritic cells which function in cutaneous antigen presentation (Beckstead et al. 1984).

The histiocytosis X cell displays a characteristic, longitudinal nuclear groove by light microscopy (Fig. 3). Electron microscopy reveals the presence of elongate membranous organelles, the Birbeck granules, within the cytoplasm or arising from the cell membrane (Fig. 4) (Nezelof et al. 1973). The Birbeck granules have an anistropic internal

structure and may resemble a tennis racket in some planes of section. More recently, immunohistochemical techniques have demonstrated the presence of the T6 (CD1) antigen on both epidermal Langerhans' cells and histiocytosis X cells (Murphy et al. 1983; Fox and Berman 1983).

Merkel Cell Tumor (Neurosecretory Granules). This uncommon malignant neoplasm typically is seen as a dermal nodule on the face of elderly individuals (Toker 1972; Tang and Toker 1978). Light microscopy reveals a monomorphous population of small to intermediate size cells arrayed in a trabecular or organoid pattern (Fig. 5). The tumor cells contain nuclei with evenly dispersed, finely granular chromatin, scant cytoplasm, and a high mitotic count. The Merkel cell tumor is also known as the primary cutaneous neuroendocrine carcinoma. Characteristic, membrane-delimited, electron-dense, neurosecretory-type granules may be observed in the cytoplasm of tumor cells by electron microscopy (Fig. 6). The presence of these inclusions distinguish the Merkel cell tumor from histologically similar entities, including

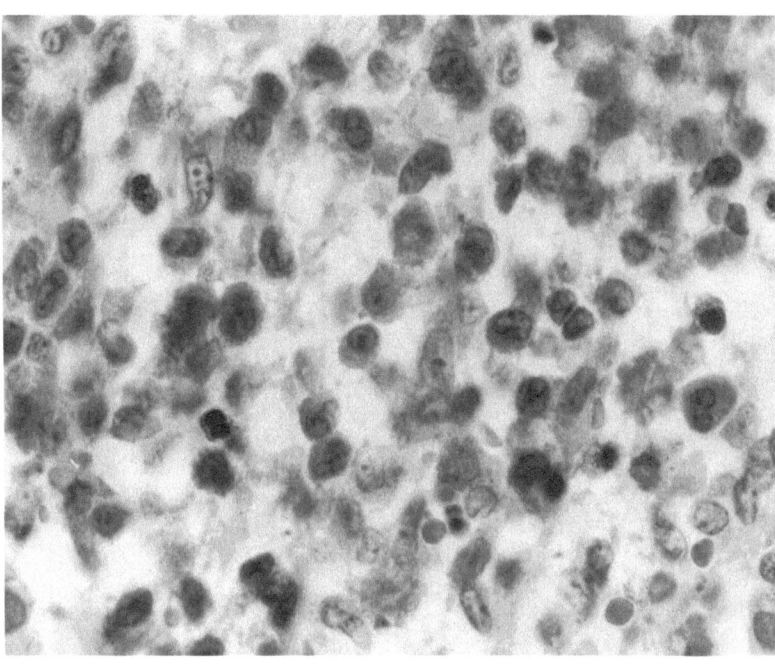

Fig. 3. Eosinophilic granuloma. A polymorphous cellular infiltrate contains numerous histiocytic cells, many of which contain characteristic longitudinal nuclear furrows. H and E, ×450

poorly differentiated carcinomas and lymphomas (Sidhu et al. 1980).

Immunohistochemical Demonstration of Cytoplasmic Antigens in Tumor Diagnosis

Atypical Fibroxanthoma. The atypical fibroxanthoma is an uncommon solitary cutaneous tumor often occurring on sun-exposed skin, which may be a superficial, cutaneous variant of the malignant fibrous histiocytoma (Enzinger 1979; Leong and Milios 1987). The tumor is composed of fascicles of cytologically atypical, pleomorphic spindle cells and admixed, multinucleate giant cells (Fig. 7). There may be a very high mitotic rate. The histologic differential diagnosis of an anaplastic dermal spindle cell neoplasm includes malignant melanoma and squamous cell carcinoma in addition to atypical fibroxanthoma. Immunohistochemical demonstration of intermediate filament proteins by the immunoperoxidase method allows discrimination of tumor types based on patterns of cytoplasmic antigen expression characteristic of different cell lineages. The atypical fibroxanthoma displays positive immunoreactivity for vimentin, an intermediate filament protein characteristic of the fibrohistiocytic lineage (Fig. 8). This tumor is negative for cytokerat-

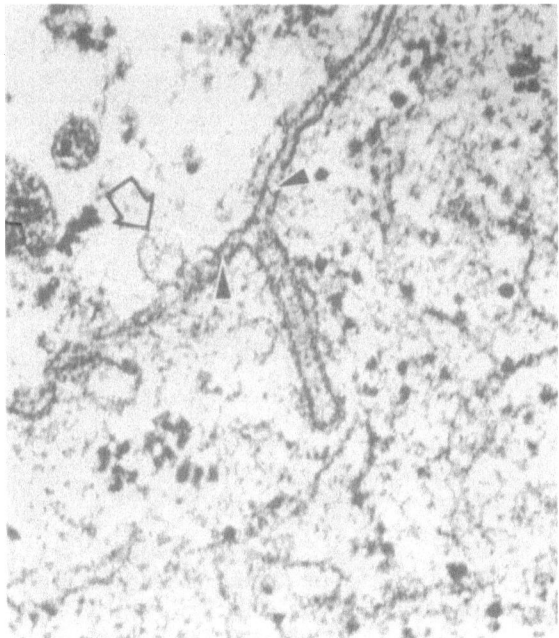

Fig. 4. Birbeck granule. It appears as an elongate cytoplasmic organelle *(arrowheads)*, arising from the plasma membrane in this case of histiocytosis X. TEM, ×20000

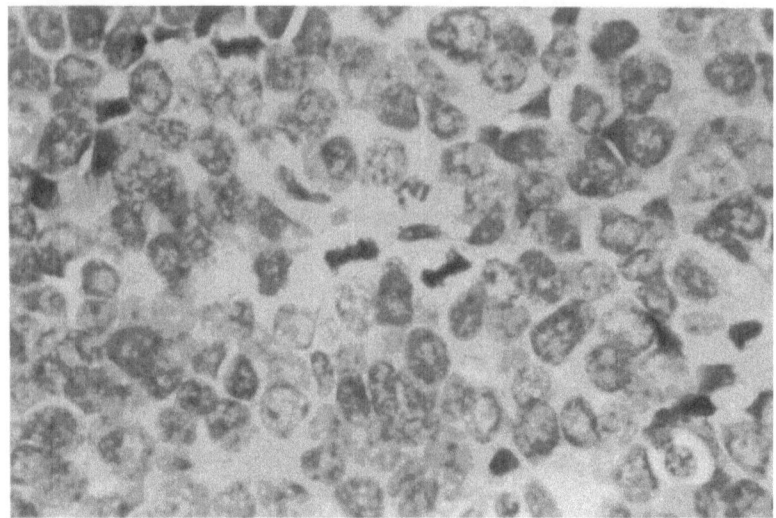

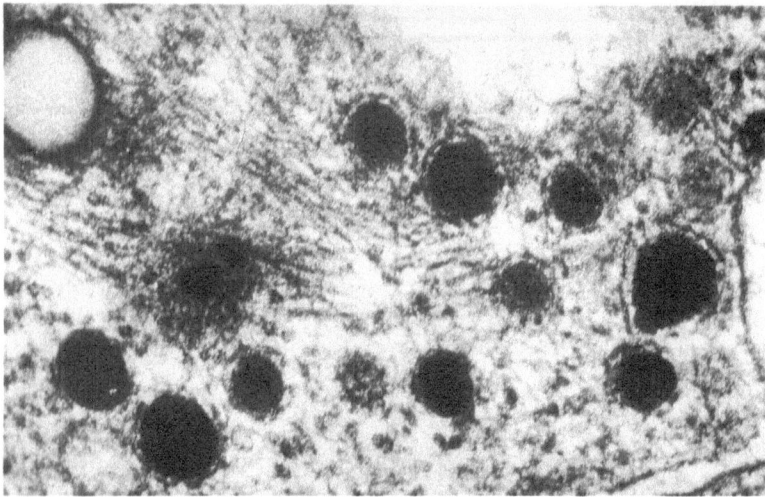

Fig. 5 *(above)*. Merkel cell tumor. There is a monomorphous population of intermediate-sized cells with numerous mitotic figures and uniformly dispersed nuclear chromatin. H and E, ×450

Fig. 6 *(below)*. Neurosecretory granules. The cytoplasm of the Merkel cell tumor contains numerous, electron-dense, membrane-delimited inclusions. TEM, ×10000

Fig. 7 *(upper left)*. Atypical fibroxanthoma. Note pattern of interweaving fascicles of spindle cells with numerous mitotic figures and occasional cytologically bizarre nuclei. H and E, ×200

Fig. 8 *(lower left)*. Atypical fibroxanthoma. Same case as in Fig. 7. The cytoplasm displays positive vimentin immunoreactivity. Anti-vimentin, ×200

Fig. 9 *(upper right)*. Metastatic malignant melanoma. This ▶ lymph node contains expansile aggregates of "balloon cells" with abundant finely granular or clear cytoplasm and minimally anaplastic nuclei. H and E, ×313

Fig. 10 *(lower right)*. Metastatic malignant melanoma. Same case as in Fig. 9. The cytoplasm of the atypical "balloon cells" is strongly positive for S100 protein. IMPOX, anti-S100, ×313

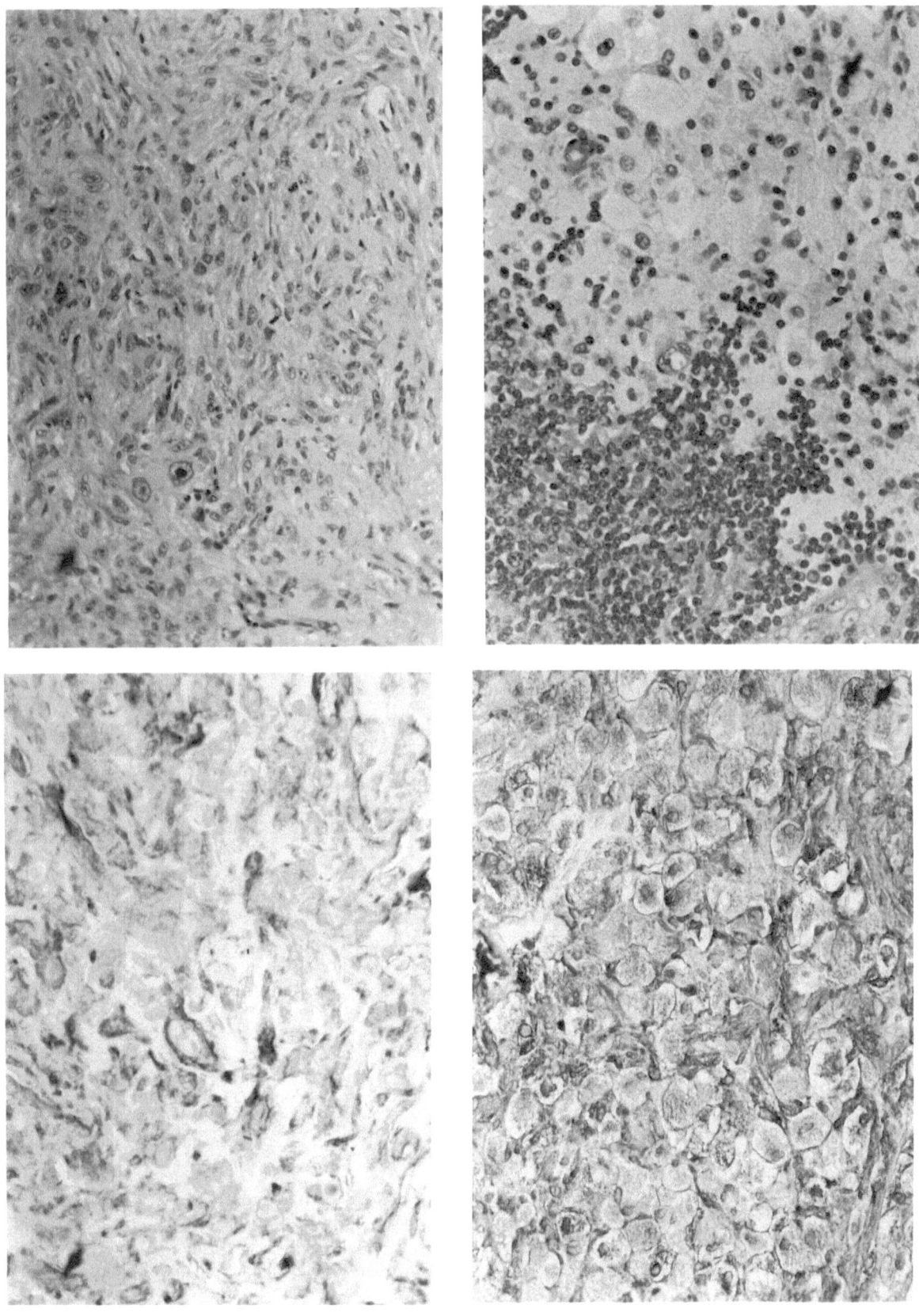

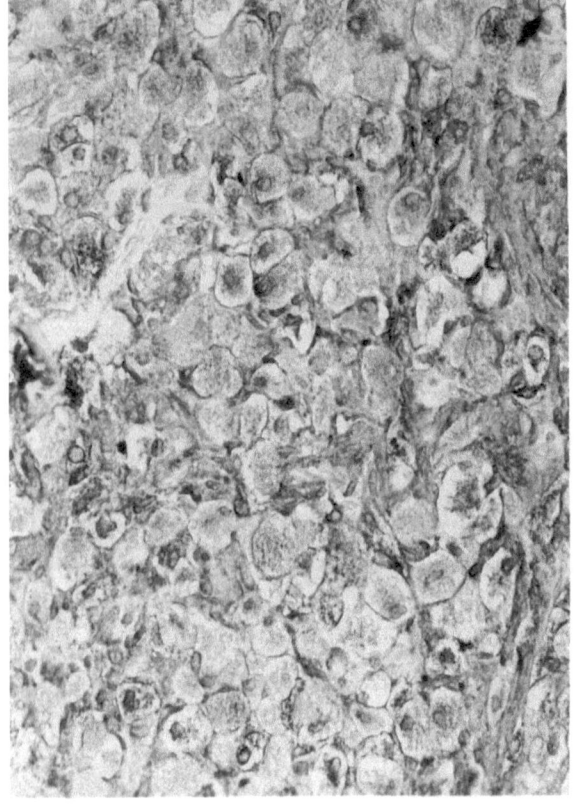

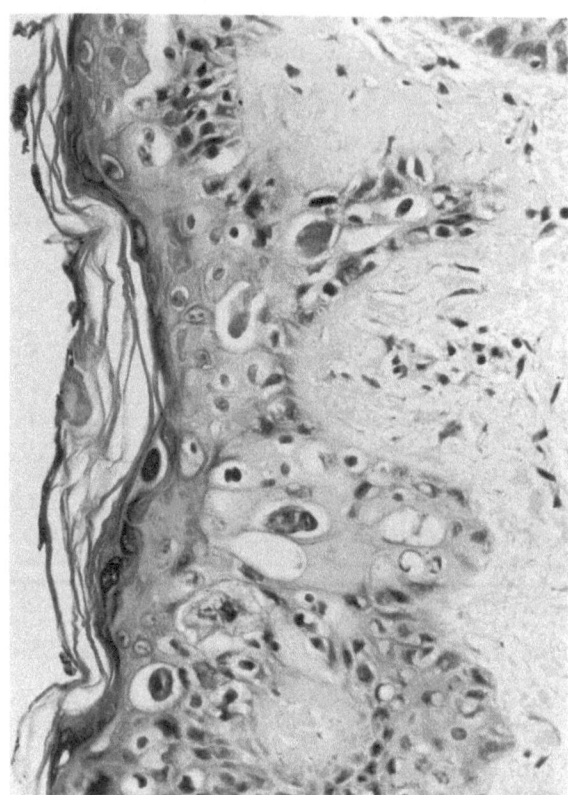

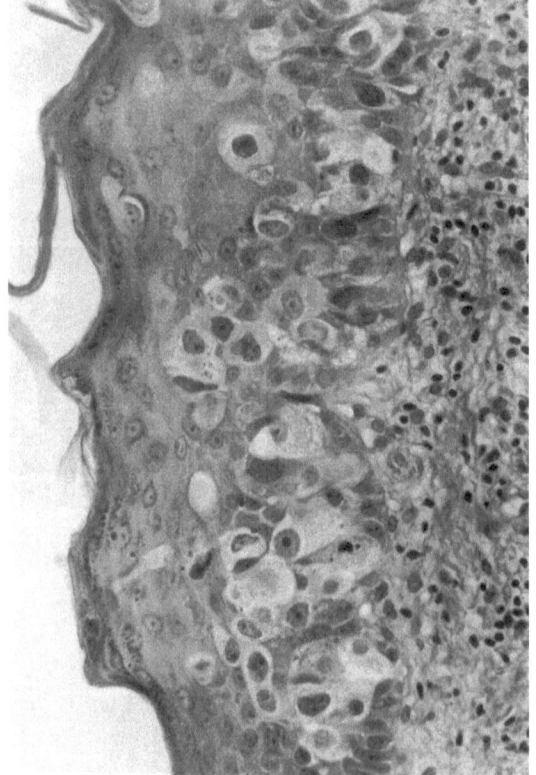

Fig. 11 *(upper left)*. Bowen's squamous cell carcinoma in situ. Extremely bizarre-appearing cells are interspersed singly and in small clusters throughout the epidermis. H and E, ×313

Fig. 12 *(lower left)*. Bowen's squamous cell carcinoma in situ. Same case as in Fig. 11. The intraepidermal anaplastic cells are strongly positive for cytoplasmic keratin. The cytologically normal-appearing keratinocytes also stain positively for keratin, but less intensely. IMPOX, anti-keratin, ×313

Fig. 13 *(upper right)*. Paget's disease of the nipple. Cytologically atypical clear cells with prominent nucleoli and finely vacuolated cytoplasm are interspersed singly and in small clusters throughout the epidermis. H and E, ×313

in intermediate filaments and the cytoplasmic S100 protein, markers which are positive, in squamous cell carcinoma and malignant melanoma respectively (Cochran and Wen 1985; Loeffel et al. 1985).

Malignant Melanoma. Immunohistochemical techniques are often used to establish the histologic type of a metastatic tumor when no primary tumor has been identified (Gatter et al. 1985; Hagen et al. 1986). Malignant melanoma may appear clinically as a metastatic tumor if a primary cutaneous melanoma has previously been excised or has undergone inflammatory regression. An unusual histologic variant of melanoma is the balloon cell melanoma. The tumor cells contain abundant clear or finely granular cytoplasm, minimal nuclear anaplastic features, and often no observable melanin pigment (Fig. 9). The histologic differential diagnosis of such a metastatic clear cell neoplasm includes carcinomas of renal, ovarian, or eccrine origin, as well as malignant melanoma. The demonstration of positive immunohistochemical staining for cytoplasmic S100 antigen supports the diagnosis of metastatic balloon cell melanoma over other clear cell tumor types (Fig. 10) (Kahn et al. 1984).

Bowen's Squamous Cell Carcinoma In Situ. The observation of cytologically malignant cells distributed singly and in small clusters within the epidermis is an important differential diagnostic problem in dermatopathology (Guldhammer and Nørgaard 1986). Bowen's disease is a variant of primary cutaneous squamous cell carcinoma in situ which often is seen as a psoriasiform patch on skin not usually exposed to sun (Callen and Headington 1980). Histologically, this lesion is characterized by the presence of individual, extremely bizarre-appearing keratinocytes dispersed within a dysplastic epidermis (Fig. 11). The immunohistochemical demonstration of strongly keratin-positive-staining cytoplasm within the anaplastic cells reflects the keratinocytic lineage of this neoplasm (Fig. 12).
The pattern of intraepidermal malignant cell spread may also be observed in primary cutaneous malignant melanoma, in which the tumor cell cytoplasm stains positively for S100 protein and negatively for keratin (Shah et al. 1987). Paget's disease of the nipple is a cutaneous manifestation of underlying ductal carcinoma characterized by intraepidermal spread of adenocarcinoma cells (Fig. 13). Paget's cells have negative cytoplasmic staining for S100 protein but may be

reactive for certain specific cytokeratin proteins. Other markers, including carcinoembryonic antigen and gross cystic disease fluid protein, are usually positive.

Immunofluorescence Demonstration of Immunoglobulin Deposition in Cutaneous Blistering Disorders

Pemiphigus. The pemphigus group of cutaneous blistering disorders features epidermal separation secondary to the deposition of autoantibody to antigens present in the epidermal interkeratinocytic space. The demonstration of immunoglobulin deposits by direct immunofluorescence study of human skin and the demonstration of circulating autoantibodies by indirect techniques permit the accurate diagnosis of these disorders and their discrimination from histologically similar but biologically distinct disorders. The variant pemphigus foliaceus is characterized by epidermal separation in the upper stratum spinosum of the epidermis, usually involving the granular layer (Fig. 14) (Stanley et al. 1984). Direct immunofluorescence studies of skin obtained adjacent to lesions reveal IgG deposits within the intercellular space of the epidermis (Fig. 15). Indirect immunofluorescence studies using patient's serum demonstrate the presence of circulating IgG reactive with antigens of the epidermal intercellular substance of the upper stratum spinosum.
The related autoimmune blistering disorder, pemphigus vulgaris, is distinguished by epidermal separation occurring above the basal keratinocyte layer. A similar pattern of IgG deposition is observed in both forms of pemphigus by direct immunofluorescence. The biochemical mechanisms of acantholysis and blister formation have been elucidated in pemphigus vulgaris (Peterson and Wuepper 1984; Farb et al. 1978; Hashimoto et al. 1983). The binding of autoantibody to antigens in the intercellular space stimulates the local release of keratinocyte-derived plasminogen activator. The active serine protease plasmin is subsequently generated in the intercellular space and mediates proteolytic digestion of the interkeratinocytic spinous process, leading to blister formation. A similar mechanism may exist in pemphigus foliaceus (Stanley et al. 1986).

Dermatitis Herpetiformis. The intensely pruritic blistering disorder, dermatitis herpetiformis, has a subepidermal pattern of cutaneous separation. Early lesions reveal the accumulation of neutro-

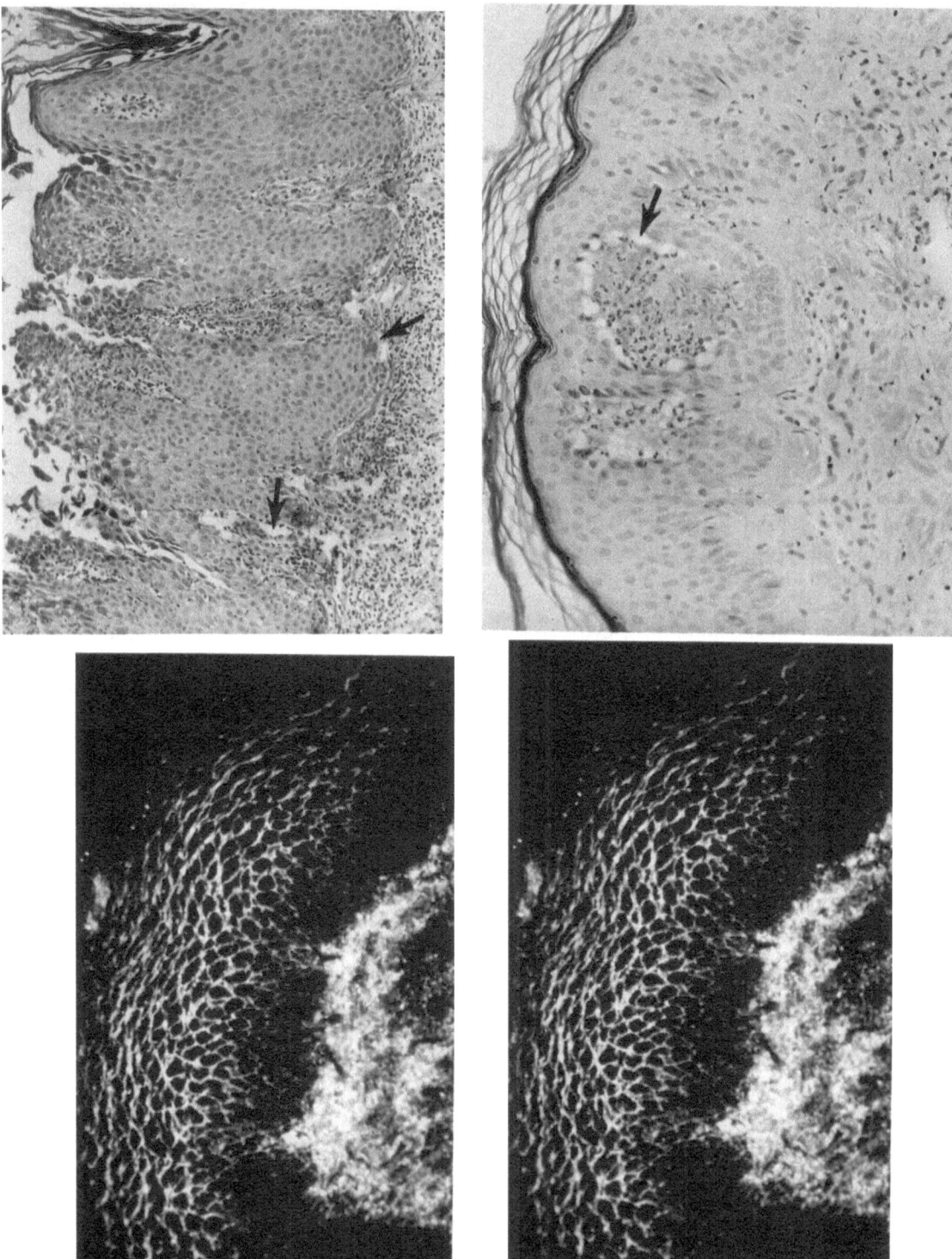

Fig. 14 *(upper left).* Pemphigus foliaceus. Note superficial intraepidermal cleavage at the level of the granular cell layer with acanthotic epidermal hyperplasia *(arrows).* H and E, × 200

Fig. 15 *(lower left).* Pemphigus foliaceus. Note deposition of IgG throughout the suprabasalar intercellular space of the epidermis. DIF, anti-IgG, × 200

Fig. 16 *(upper right).* Dermatitis herpetiformis. A subepidermal separation is present along the dermal-epidermal junction overlying dermal papillae *(arrow).* Neutrophilic microabscesses are present within the adjacent papillae. H and E, × 200

Fig. 17 *(lower right).* Dermatitis herpetiformis. Note coarse granular deposition of IgA within the tips of dermal papillae in perilesional, normal-appearing skin. DIF, anti-Iga, × 170

phils within dermal papillae (Fig. 16). Direct immunofluorescence examination of clinically normal or perilesional skin reveals granular deposits of IgA within dermal papillae in association with anchoring fibrils (Fig. 17).

The presence of coexistent villous atrophy of the small intestine may be demonstrated in almost all patients with dermatitis herpetiformis (Lane et al. 1983). Elimination of dietary gluten will usually lead to remission of skin symptoms as well as intestinal malabsorption, if present. The demonstration of granular IgA deposition in dermatitis herpetiformis is important because in the immunohistologically similar disorder, linear IgA bullous dermatosis, linear deposition of IgA is seen along the basement membrane zone (Yaoita 1978). Linear IgA disease is unrelated to intestinal villous atrophy, and its clinical course is unaffected by dietary gluten.

Bullous Pemphigoid. This acquired, immune-mediated bullous disease occurs in older individuals who develop tense vesicles and bullae on intertriginous skin and extremities (Imber et al. 1987). Characteristic subepidermal separation is evident in biopsy specimens of skin from the edge of a fresh blister (Fig. 18). The blister roof is formed by relatively normal-appearing, intact epidermis. The blister floor is formed by papillary dermis with preservation of its normal festooned morphology. An infiltrate containing neutrophils and eosinophils is usually present in perilesional skin. Linear deposition of IgG and C3 is demonstrable by direct immunofluorescence study of perilesional skin, corresponding to the deposition of immunoreactants in the lamina lucida of the basement membrane zone (Fig. 19). Circulating basement membrane zone-specific antibodies may sometimes be observed by indirect immunofluorescence study.

A protein component of the basal keratinocyte hemidesmosome is the antigenic target of bullous pemphigoid autoantibodies (Westgate et al. 1985). The formation of immune complexes within the lamina lucida leads to complement fixation and activation. Subsequent neutrophil infiltration and degranulation in response to complement-derived chemotactic factors mediate lysis of the epidermal basement membrane zone at the level of the lamina lucida. The presence of an intact lamina densa overlying the blister floor may contribute to the preservation of the normal papillary dermal morphology observed by light microscopy.

Epidermolysis Bullosa Acquisita. This rare, acquired, autoimmune bullous disorder shares overlapping light microscopic and immunohistologic features with bullous pemphigoid but is biologically distinct. Cutaneous blisters form secondary to minor trauma and heal with scarring. Biopsy examination reveals subepidermal separation, and direct immunofluorescence study of perilesional skin demonstrates linear deposition of IgG and C3 in a pattern identical with bullous pemphigoid. Circulating autoantibodies to basement membrane zone antigens may be demonstrated by indirect techniques in almost half of afflicted individuals.

Epidermolysis bullosa acquisita may be distinguished from bullous pemphigoid by two methods. Immunoelectron microscopy of lesional skin reveals deposition of electron-dense immune complexes in the sublamina densa region of the basement membrane zone, as opposed to the lamina lucida, the site of deposits in bullous pemphigoid (Fig. 20). Indirect immunofluorescence study of circulating autoantibody may be performed using normal human skin, artefactually split along the basement membrane zone by hypertonic saline. The osmotically induced separation occurs along the lamina densa, separating the respective antigenic targets of the bullous pemphigoid (lamina lucida), and epidermolysis bullosa acquisita (sublamina densa) antibodies (Woodley et al. 1984; Gammon et al. 1984). Indirect immunofluorescence study of bullous pemphigoid serum reveals antibody deposition along the roof of the osmotically induced substrate blister, while epidermolysis bullosa acquisita serum will preferentially stain the substrate blister floor (Fig. 21).

In Situ Hybridization for the Analysis of Specific Gene Expression

Rana pipiens (Ranatensin). Molecular probes for specific cellular DNA or messenger RNA sequences are rapidly being developed as research and diagnostic tools in surgical pathology. Diagnostic applications of hybridization probes include demonstration of activated oncogenes, viral DNA sequences, and cell-lineage-specific mRNA sequences. An example of a research application is the demonstration of ranatensin gene expression in the poison glands of frog skin by in situ hybridization with a riboprobe for ranatensin mRNA (Fig. 22) (Geller et al. 1970; Yasuhara et al. 1979).

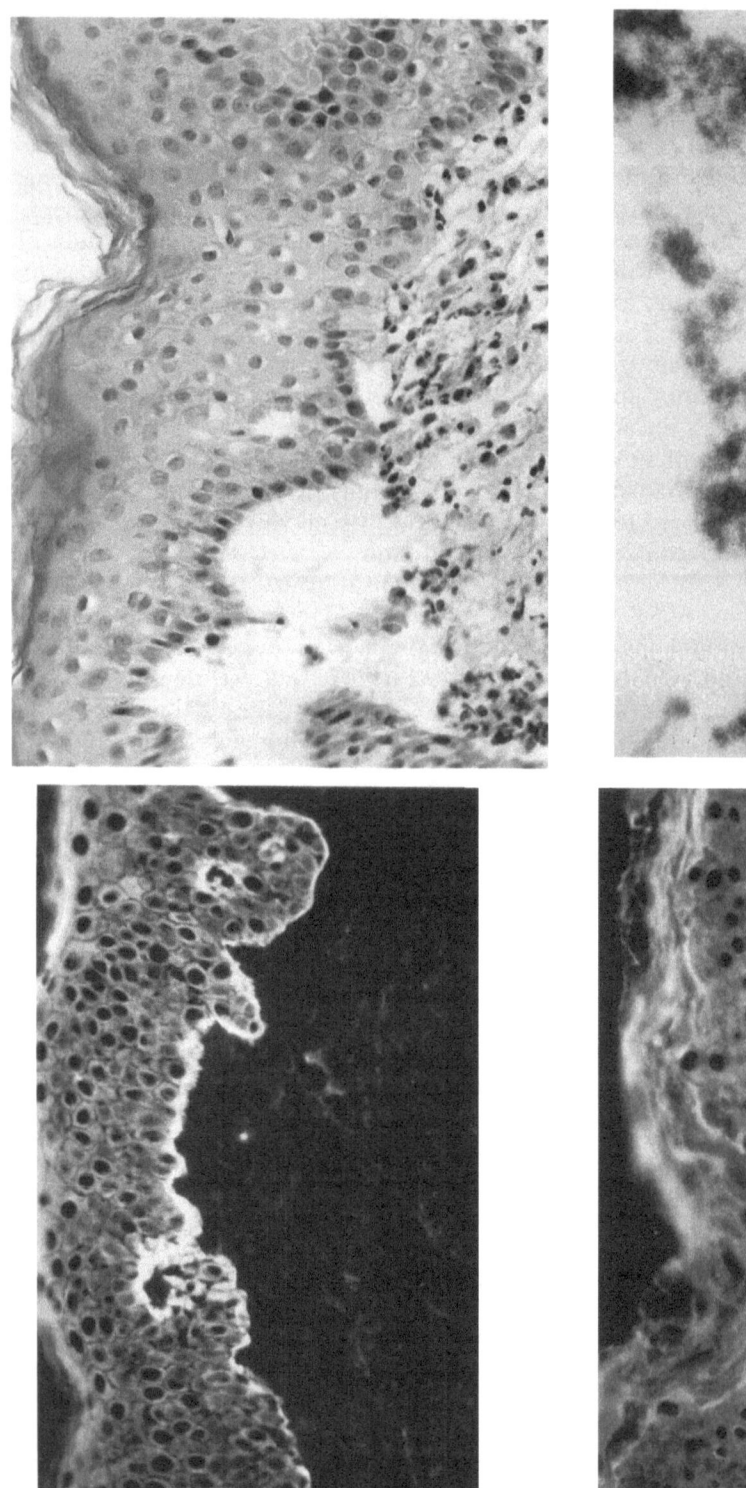

Fig. 18 *(upper left)*. Bullous pemphigoid. Note subepidermal separation. The epidermis forming the blister roof appears normal. The underlying papillary dermal infiltrate includes neutrophils and eosinophils. H and E, ×313

Fig. 19 *(lower left)*. Bullous pemphigoid. Note linear deposition of IgG along the basement membrane zone of perilesional skin. DIF, anti-IgG, ×313

Fig. 20 *(upper right)*. Epidermolysis bullosa acquisita. There are dense, amorphous IgG-containing deposits present within the sublamina densa region of the basement membrane zone. ImmunoEM, ×400

Fig. 21 *(lower right)*. Epidermolysis bullosa acquisita. There is preferential staining at the base of an osmotically induced blister along the basement membrane zone. IIF, anti-IgG, NaCl-split skin substrate, ×400

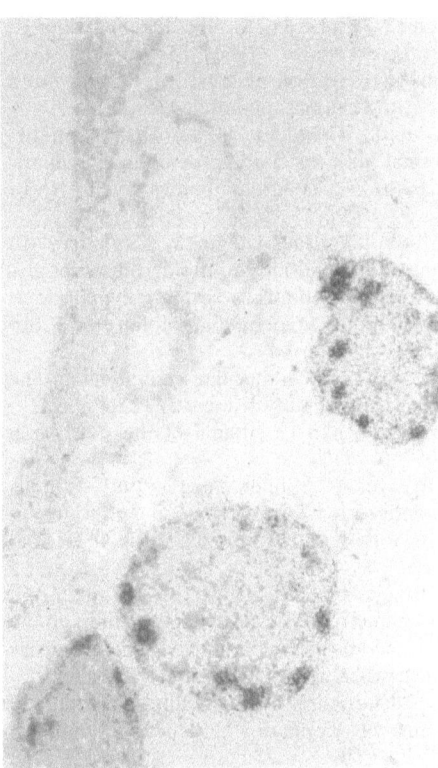

Fig. 22. Normal frog skin. S-labeled riboprobe to ranatensin localizes to the poison glands of normal *Rana pipiens* skin. ISH, ranatensin riboprobe, × 600

Acknowledgments. I would like to thank the following individuals for contributing illustrations used in this chapter: George F. Murphy, M.D., Department of Dermatology, University of Pennsylvania, Philadelphia, PA (Figs. 4, 6 and 21); Dr. Thomas B. Fitzpatrick, Department of Dermatology, Massachusetts General Hospital, Harvard Medical School, Boston, MA (Fig. 2); Dr. Eliot Spindel and Dr. Mary Sunday, Department of Medicine, Brigham and Women's Hospital, Harvard Medical School, Boston, MA (Fig. 22).

References

Beckstead JH, Wood GS, Turner RR (1984) Histiocytosis X cells and Langerhans cells: enzyme histochemical and immunologic similarities. Hum Pathol 15: 826–833

Benedict PII, Szabo G, Fitzpatrick TB et al. (1968) Melanotic macules in Albright's syndrome and in neurofibromatosis. JAMA 205: 618–626

Beutner EH, Chorzelski TP, Jablonska S (1987) Clinical significance of immunofluorescence tests of sera and skin in bullous diseases: a cooperative study. In: Beutner EH, Chorzelski TP, Kumar V (eds). Immunopathology of the skin, 3rd edn. Wiley, New York, pp 177–205

Callen JP, Headington J (1980) Bowen's and non-Bowen's squamous intraepidermal neoplasia of the skin. Relationship to internal pregnancy. Arch Dermatol 116: 422–426

Cochran AJ, Wen DR (1985) S-100 protein as a marker for melanocytic and other tumours. Pathology 17: 340–345

Crowe FW, Schull WJ (1953) Diagnostic importance of café-au-lait spot in neurofibromatosis. Arch Intern Med 91: 758–766

Enzinger FM (1979) Question: are atypical fibroxanthoma and malignant fibrous histiocytoma related pathologic processes? Am J Dermatopathol 1: 185

Farb RM, Dykes R, Lazarus GS (1978) Anti-epidermal-cell-surface pemphigus antibody detaches viable epidermal cells from culture by activation of proteinase. Proc Natl Acad Sci USA 75: 459–463

Favara BE, Jaffe R (1987) Pathology of Langerhans cell histiocytosis. Hematol Oncol Clin North Am 1: 75–97

Fenoglio-Preiser CM, Willman CL (1987) Molecular biology and the pathologist-general principles and applications. Arch Pathol Lab Med 111: 601–619

Fox JL, Berman B (1983) T6-antigen-bearing cells in eosinophilic granuloma of bone. JAMA 249: 3071–3072

Gammon WR, Briggaman RA, Inman AO III, Queen LL, Wheeler CE (1984) Differentiating antilamina lucida and anti-sublamina densa anti-BMZ antibodies by indirect immunofluorescence on 1.0 M sodium chloride-separated skin. J Invest Dermatol 82: 139–144

Gatter KC, Ralfkiser E, Skinner J, Brown D, Heryet A, Pulford KA, Hou-Jensen K, Mason DY (1985) An immunocytochemical study of malignant melanoma and its differential diagnosis from other malignant tumours. J Clin Pathol 38: 1353–1357

Geller RG, Govier WC, Pisano JJ, Tanimura T, Van Clineschmidt B (1970) The action of ranatensin, a new polypeptide from amphibian skin, on the blood pressure of experimental animals. Br J Pharmacol 40: 605–616

Guldhammer B, Nørgaard T (1986) The differential diagnosis of intraepidermal malignant lesions using immunohistochemistry. Am J Dermatopathol 8: 295–301

Hagen EC, Vennegoor C, Schlingemann RO, Van der Velde EA, Ruiter DJ (1986) Correlation of histopathological characteristics with staining patterns in human melanoma assessed by (monoclonal) antibodies reactive on paraffin sections. Histopathology 10: 689–700

Hashimoto K, Shafran KM, Webber PS, Lazarus GS, Singer KH (1983) Anti-cell surface pemphigus autoantibody stimulates plasminogen activator activity of human epidermal cells. J Exp Med 157: 259–272

Imber MJ, Murphy GF, Jordon RE (1987) The immunopathology of bullous pemphigoid. Clin Dermatol 5: 81–92

Jimbow K, Szabo G, Fitzpatrick TB (1973) Ultrastructure of giant pigment granules (macromelanosomes) in the cutaneous pigmented macules of neurofibromatosis. J Invest Dermatol 61: 300–309

Johnson BL, Charneco DR (1970) Café-au-lait spots in neurofibromatosis and in normal individuals. Arch Dermatol 102: 442–446

14   Michael J. Imber

Kahn HJ, Baumal R, Marks A (1984) The value of immunohistochemical studies using antibody to S100 protein in dermatopathology. Int J Dermatol 23: 38-44

Kahn H, Baumal R, From L (1986) Role of immunohistochemistry in the diagnosis of undifferentiated tumors involving the skin. J Am Acad Dermatol 14: 1063-72

Lane AT, Huff JC, Zone JJ, Weston WL (1983) Class-specific antibodies to gluten in dermatitis herpetiformis. J Invest Dermatol 80: 402-405

Leong AS, Milios J (1987) Atypical fibroxanthoma of the skin: a clinicopathological and immunohistochemical study and a discussion of its histogenesis. Histopathology 11: 463-475

Loeffel SC, Gillespie GY, Mirmiran SA, Miller EW, Golden P, Askin FB, Siegal GP (1985) Cellular immunolocalization of S100 protein within fixed tissue sections by monoclonal antibodies. Arch Pathol Lab Med 109: 117-122

Murphy GF, Dickersin GR, Harrist TJ, Mihm MC (1982) The role of diagnostic electron microscopy in dermatology. In: Moschella S (ed) Dermatology update. Elsevier, New York, pp 355-384

Murphy GF, Harrist TJ, Bhan AK, Mihm MC Jr (1983) Distribution of cell surface antigens in histiocytosis X cells. Quantitative immunoelectron microscopy using monoclonal antibodies. Lab Invest 48: 90-97

Nezelof C, Basset F, Rousseau MF (1973) Histiocytosis X: histogenetic arguments for a Langerhans cell origin. Biomedicine 18: 365-371

Peterson LL, Wuepper KD (1984) Isolation and purification of a pemphigus vulgaris antigen from human epidermis. J Clin Invest 73: 1113-1120

Shah KD, Tabibzadeh SS, Gerber MA (1987) Immunohistochemical distinction of Paget's disease from Bowen's disease and superficial spreading melanoma with the use of monoclonal cytokeratin antibodies. Am J Clin Pathol 88: 689-695

Sidhu GS, Feiner N, Flotte TJ, Mullins JD, Schaefler K, Schultenover SJ, Feiner H (1980) Merkel cell neoplasms: histology, electron microscopy, biology and histogenesis. Am J Dermatopathol 2: 101-119

Stanley JR, Koulu L, Thivolet C (1984) Distinction between epidermal antigens binding pemphigus vulgaris and pemphigus foliaceus autoantibodies. J Clin Invest 74: 313-320

Stanley JR, Koulu L, Klaus-Kovtun V, Steinberg MS (1986) A monoclonal antibody to the desmosomal glycoprotein desmoglein 1 binds the same polypeptide as human autoantibodies in pemphigus foliaceus. J Immunol 136: 1227-1230

Tang CK, Toker C (1978) Trabecular carcinoma of the skin: an ultra structural study. Cancer 42: 2311-2321

Toker C (1972) Trabecular carcinoma of the skin. Arch Dermatol 105: 107-110

Westgate GE, Weaver AC, Couchman JR (1985) Bullous pemphigoid antigen localization suggests an intracellular association with hemidesmosomes. J Invest Dermatol 84: 218-224

Woodley DT, Briggaman RA, O'Keefe EJ, Inman AO, Queen LL, Gammon WR (1984) Identification of the skin basement-membrane autoantigen in epidermolysis bullosa acquisita. N Engl J Med 310: 1007-1013

Yaoita H (1978) Identifiction of IgA binding structures in skin of patients with dermatitis herpetiformis. J Invest Dermatol 71: 213-216

Yasuhara T, Ishikawa O, Nakajima T, Araki K, Tachibana S (1979) The studies on the active peptide on smooth muscle in the skin of Rana rugosa. II. The structure of ranatensin-R, the new ranatensin analogue, and granuliberi-R, the new mast cell degranulating peptide. Chem Pharm Bull (Tokyo) 27: 492-498

Squamous Cell Papilloma, Skin, Rat

Masao Hirose

Synonyms. Prickle cell papilloma; squamous papilloma; papilloma; fibroepithelioma.

Gross Appearance

Papilloma of the skin appears as single or multiple small verrucous papules at the site of application of a carcinogen or irradiation. These papules are usually a few millimeters in diameter and rarely exceed 1 cm in diameter. The surface of the tumors may be covered by a keratin mass, and as the tumors grow bigger, their surface can become ulcerated or crusted. Papillomas never adhere to the deeper layer. Small papillomas of less than 3 mm in diameter often undergo spontaneous regression.

Microscopic Features

Squamous cell papillomas are characterized by the papillary proliferation of the squamous epithelium with complex fine or dense stromal connective tissue (Figs. 23 and 24). In the latter case, the tumors may be called fibroepitheliomas. The epithelium is thickened with an obvious grade of maturity from basal cells to spinous and granular cells. Pronounced hyperkeratosis with or without parakeratosis is present. The cells are arranged regularly, and cellular and structural atypia is slight; mitoses are frequent, especially in the basal cell layers. Keratin pearls may be seen in the tissue. The tumors may proliferate downward to subcutaneous tissue, but the basement membrane is well preserved. Infiltration of lymphocytes and polymorphonuclear cells into the stromal tissue or epithelial layer is usually observed. Focal atypical changes or focal invasion (Fig. 25) in big papillomas (0.5–1 cm diameter) is an indication of malignant transformation.

Ultrastructure

We have found no report on the ultrastructure of squamous cell papillomas in the rat. The diagnostic significance of ultrastructural findings is unknown.

Differential Diagnosis

Papillary hyperplasia is a lesion preceding papilloma. The cells composing papillomas and papillary hyperplasia are essentially the same, but papillomas have multibranched stalks, whereas papillary hyperplasias have single, unbranched stalks. Keratoacanthomas can be distinguished by the downward cystic growth of squamous epithelium with pronounced hyperkeratosis. Epidermal inclusion cysts are not neoplasms. They are found in the subcutis and are lined by nonhyperplastic mature squamous epithelium with adnexa and a central keratin mass. Benign basal cell tumors and sebaceous gland tumors may differentiate toward squamous epithelium. Papillomas are composed entirely of squamous epithelium with supporting stroma.

Biologic Features

Squamous cell papillomas arise from the interfollicular epidermis and do not develop from hair follicles (Cherry and Glucksmann 1971; Ghadially 1961; Howell 1962; Zackheim 1964a). They are considered to represent an intermediate stage in the progression from hyperplasia to squamous cell carcinoma. Focal atypical change or invasion, which is an indication of malignant transformation, can be seen in tumors of 0.5–1 cm in diameter (Zackheim 1964a, 1973). However, the frequency of malignant transformation of squamous cell papillomas is not known. Squamous cell papillomas can be in-

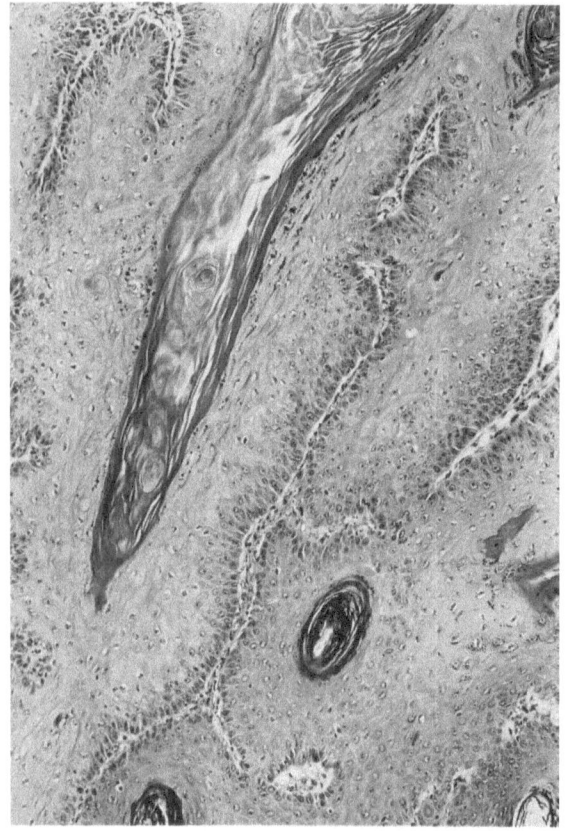

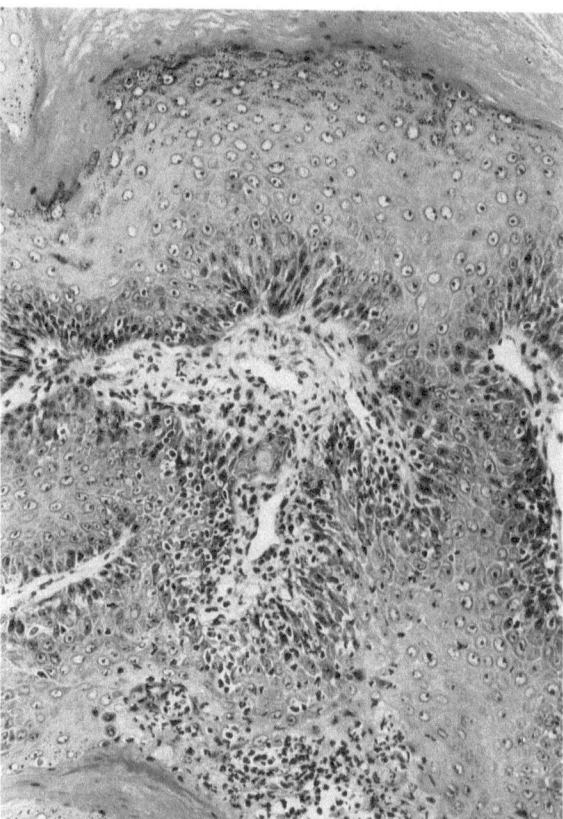

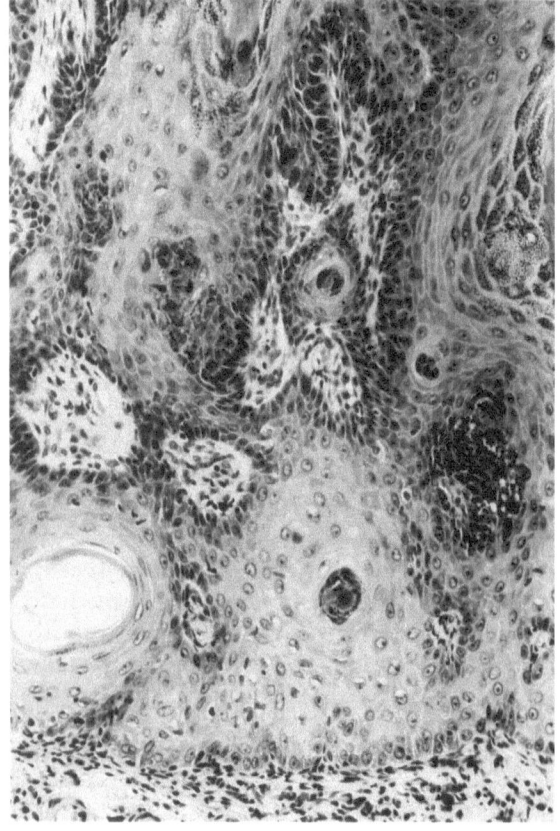

Fig. 23 *(upper left).* Squamous cell papilloma, skin, rat. Mature squamous epithelium has undergone papillary proliferation with fine stromal connective tissue. Maturation from the basal layer to the keratinous layer is clearly visible. The cells are arranged regularly. No invasive growth into the stroma is seen. H and E, ×85

Fig. 24 *(lower left).* Squamous cell papilloma, skin, rat. The cells are arranged regularly except in the basal layer, but no invasive growth is seen. H and E, ×85

Fig. 25 *(upper right).* Part of a squamous cell papilloma with atypical basal nuclei and early signs of invasion in the *center* of the figure. Focal invasion is poorly demarcated because the basement membrane is not preserved. H and E, ×85

Table 1. Incidences of spontaneous squamous tumors in the skin from various strains of rats

Strain	Sex	Experimental period	No. of rats	Incidence of (%)		Reference
				Papilloma	Squamous cell carcinoma	
ACI	M	up to 169 wk	55	1 (1.8)	0	Maekawa and Odashima
	F		209	0	0	1975
BN/Bi	M	up to 44 mo	74	4 (5.4)	0	Burek and Hollander 1977
	F	54 mo	236	0	1 (0.4)	
F344	M	up to 110 wk	1794	12 (0.7)	11 (0.6)	Goodman et al. 1979
	F		1754	3 (0.2)	6 (0.3)	
F344	M	up to 104 wk	1727	29 (1.7)	15 (0.9)	Haseman et al. 1985
	F		1772	5 (0.3)	9 (0.5)	
F344	M	up to 130 wk	296	1 (0.3)	0	Maekawa et al. 1983a
	F		297	0	2 (0.7)	
SD	M	up to 540 days	179	0	0	Prejean et al. 1973
	F		181	1 (0.6)	0	
SD	M, F	up to 104 wk	258	3 (1.2)	2 (0.8)	MacKenzie and Garner 1973
Wistar	M	up to 122 wk	98	1 (1.0)	0	Maekawa et al. 1983b
	F		88	0	0	
Wistar	M	up to 24 mo	279	0	0	Crain 1958
	F		368	0	0	

wk, week; mo, month; M, male; F, female.

duced by direct irradiation of the skin (Albert et al. 1969) or by single or repeated topical applications of a carcinogen such as 7,12-dimethyl-benz[a]anthracene (DMBA) (Cherry and Glucksmann 1971; Glucksmann and Cherry 1971; Howell 1962; Rasmussen et al. 1983; Schweizer et al. 1982; Zackheim 1964a), 3-methylcholanthrene (3-MC) (Howell 1962; Rasmussen et al. 1983; Zackheim et al. 1959), anthramine (Zackheim et al. 1959; Lennox 1955), some azo dyes (Fare 1966), nitrosamines (Hirose et al. 1979; Zabezhinski et al. 1985), and benzo(a)pyrene (Arffmann and Hjoorne 1979), or by continuous topical treatment with the skin tumor promoter 12-O-tetradecanoylphorbol-13-acetate (TPA) after a single application of DMBA (Schweizer et al. 1982). Intragastric administration of DMBA and other carcinogens also induced papillomas in the squamous gastric mucosa (forestomach) (Fukushima and Ito 1985), although at low incidence (Meranze et al. 1969). DMBA is more effective than 3-MC or anthramine for induction of squamous cell papillomas and carcinomas of rat skin (Rasmussen et al. 1983; Zackheim 1964b; Zackheim 1973).

Spontaneous squamous cell papillomas accounted for only 0%, 1.8% of all the tumors in aged male and female Wistar, F344, SD, ACI, and female BN/Bi rats, but for 5.4% of those in male BN/Bi rats (Table 1). These incidences are simi-

lar to those of other histological types of spontaneous skin tumors.

Comparison with Other Species

The most common histologic types of skin tumors induced in mice by a single topical application of DMBA followed by repeated application of TPA or by continuous topical application of other carcinogens are papillomas and squamous cell carcinomas. Their inductions in mice are much more rapid than in rats given similar treatment (Schweizer et al. 1982). In mice, hair follicles and interfollicular regions participate in the formation of squamous papillomas and carcinomas and the growth rate of the papillomas varies with the hair cycle. In rats, hair follicles and the interfollicular regions of the epidermis are not as closely interrelated as in mice and react more independently of one another and give rise to different tumor types (Cherry and Glucksmann 1971). Squamous cell papillomas can be induced in the hamster, rabbit (Stenback 1980), hedgehog (Ghadially 1960) duck (Rigdon 1952), and non-human primates such as rhesus monkeys and galagos (Palotay et al. 1976) by topical treatment with DMBA. In humans, the lesions that are histologically similar to chemically induced squamous cell papillomas are varying papilloma-virus-induced types of verruca and the papillomatous type of seborrheic keratosis (seborrheic verruca): These lesions, however, differ in behavior from chemically induced papillomas in rats. Squamous cell papillomas of rats have the potential to develop into squamous cell carcinomas, but seborrheic keratosis and verrucas rarely undergo malignant transformation. HPV-6, a virus inducing condyloma acuminatum which develops in the moist skin of the genitoanal region in humans, produces a lesion that is similar to the papillomas of rats. According to a follow-up study, about 5.6% of the condyloma acuminatum in human subjects develops into anaplastic genital lesions (Mehregan 1986). Squamous cell papillomas of rats induced by virus have not been reported.

References

Albert RE, Phillips ME, Bennett P, Burns F, Heimbach R (1969) The morphology and growth characteristics of radiation-induced epithelial skin tumors in the rat. Cancer Res 29: 658-668

Arffmann E, Hjøorne N (1979) Influence of surface lipids on skin carcinogenesis in rats. Acta Pathol Microbiol Immunol Scand [A] 87: 143-149

Burek JD, Hollander CF (1977) Incidence patterns of spontaneous tumors in BN/Bi rats. JNCI 58: 99-105

Cherry CP, Glucksmann A (1971) The influence of carcinogenic dosage and of sex on the induction of epitheliomas and sarcomas in the dorsal skin of rats. Br J Cancer 25: 544-564

Crain RC (1958) Spontaneous tumors in the Rochester strain of the Wistar rat. Am J Pathol 34: 311-335

Fare G (1966) Rat skin carcinogenesis by topical applications of some azo dyes. Cancer Res 26: 2406-2408

Fukushima S, Ito N (1985) Papilloma, forestomach, rat. In: Jones TC, Mohr U, Hunt RD (eds) ILSI monograph on pathology of laboratory animals, digestive system. Springer, Berlin Heidelberg New York, pp 289-292

Ghadially FN (1960) Carcinogenesis in the skin of the hedgehog. Br J Cancer 14: 212-215

Ghadially FN (1961) The role of the hair follicle in the origin and evolution of some cutaneous neoplasms of man and experimental animals. Cancer 14: 801-816

Glucksmann A, Cherry CI (1971) The effect of variation in carcinogenic dosage on the induction of tumours in the dorsal and vulval skin of female rats. Br J Cancer 25: 735-745

Goodman DG, Ward JM, Squire RA, Chu KC, Linhart MS (1979) Neoplastic and nonneoplastic lesions in aging F344 rats. Toxicol Appl Pharmacol 48: 237-248

Haseman JK, Huff JE, Rao GN, Arnold JE, Boorman GA, McConnell EE (1985) Neoplasms observed in untreated and corn oil gavage control groups of F344/N rats and (C57BL/6N x C3H/HeN)F1(B6 C3F1) mice. JNCI 75: 975-984

Hirose M, Maekawa A, Kamiya S, Odashima S (1979) Carcinogenic effect of N-ethyl- and N-amyl-N-nitrosourethanes on female Donryu rats. Gann 70: 653-662

Howell JS (1962) Skin tumors in the rat produced by 9,10-dimethyl-1,2-benzanthracene and methylcholanthrene. Br J Cancer 16: 101-109

Lennox B (1955) The production of a variety of skin tumours in rats with 2-anthramine and a comparison with the effects in mice. Br J Cancer 9: 631-639

MacKenzie WF, Garner FM (1973) Comparison of neoplasms in six sources of rats. JNCI 50: 1243-1257

Maekawa A, Odashima S (1975) Spontaneous tumors in ACI/N rats. JNCI 55: 1437-1445

Maekawa A, Kurokawa Y, Takahashi M, Kokubo T, Ogiu T, Onodera H, Tanigawa H, Ohno Y, Furukawa F, Hayashi Y (1983a) Spontaneous tumors in F-344/DuCrj rats. Gann 74: 365-372

Maekawa A, Onodera H, Tanigawa H, Furuta K, Kodama Y, Horiuchi S, Hayashi Y (1983b) Neoplastic and non-neoplastic lesions in aging Slc: Wistar rats. J Toxicol Sci 8: 279-290

Mehregan AH (1986) Pinkus' guide to dermatohistopathology 4th edn. Appleton-Century-Crofts, Norwalk, pp 443-460

Meranze DR, Gruenstein M, Shimkin MB (1969) Effect of age and sex on the development of neoplasms in Wistar rats receiving a single intragastric instillation of 7,12-dimethylbenz(a)anthracene. Int J Cancer 4: 480-486

Palotay JL, Adachi K, Dobson RL, Pinto JS (1976) Carcinogen induced cutaneous neoplasms in nonhuman primates. JNCI 57: 1269-1274

Prejean JD, Peckham JC, Casey AE, Griswold DP, Weisburger EK, Weisburger JH (1973) Spontaneous tumors in Sprague-Dawley rats and Swiss mice. Cancer Res 33: 2768-2773

Rasmussen KS, Glenthoj A, Arffmann E (1983) Skin carcinogenesis in rats by 3-methylcholanthrene and 7,12-dimethylbenz(a)anthracene. Influence of dose and frequency on tumour response and its histological type. Acta Pathol Microbiol Immunol Scand [A] 91: 445-455

Rigdon RH (1952) Tumors produced by methylcholanthrene in the duck. Papilloma, squamous-cell carcinoma, and hemangioma. Arch Pathol Lab Med 54: 368-377

Schweizer J, Loehrke H, Hesse B, Goerttler K (1982) 7,12-dimethylbenz(a)anthracene/12-0-tetradecanoylphorbol-13- acetate-mediated skin tumor initiation and promotion in male Sprague-Dawley rats. Carcinogenesis 3: 785-789

Stenbäck F (1980) Skin carcinogenesis as a model system: observations on species, strain and tissue sensitivity to 7,12-dimethylbenz(a)anthracene with or without promotion from croton oil. Acta Pharmacol Toxicol (Copenh) 46: 89-97

Zabezhinski MA, Pliss GB, Okulov VB, Petrov AS (1985) Skin tumours induced by local and systemic action of N-nitroso-compounds in rats. Arch Geschwulstforsch 55: 117-122

Zackheim HS (1964a) Evolution of squamous cell carcinoma in the rat. Arch Pathol Lab Med 77: 434-444

Zackheim HS (1964b) Comparative cutaneous carcinogenesis in the rat. Differential response to the application of anthramine, methylcholanthrene, and dimethylbenzanthracene. Oncology 17: 236–246

Zackheim HS (1973) Tumours of the skin. In: Turusov VS (ed) Pathology of tumours in laboratory animals, vol 1.

Tumours of the rat (pt 1). IARC, Lyon, pp 1–21 (IARC Sci Publ no 5

Zackheim HS, Simpson WL, Langs L (1959) Basal cell epitheliomas and other skin tumors produced in rats and mice by anthramine and methylcholanthrene. J Invest Dermatol 33: 385–402

Squamous Cell Papilloma, Skin, Mouse

Ryohei Hasegawa, Hidetaka Sato, and Yoshifumi Miyakawa

Synonyms. Epidermoid papilloma, fibroepithelioma, fibroepithelial papilloma, sessile papilloma.

Gross Appearance

The tumor appears as an outgrowth from the skin surface in the form of a wart, 1–10 mm in diameter. The apical surface of the tumor can be keratinized and has either small protuberances or a cauliflower-shaped, uneven, knobby surface; fusion with adjacent papules is common. Large tumors have a dark-brown to black color due to bleeding or imbibition into the keratinized layers of dark substances (Fig. 26). The surrounding skin is even and mobile in relation to the underlying tissues (Bogovsky 1979).

Squamous cell papillomas are of two easily distinguishable types: pedunculated and flat. Pedunculated papillomas have a relatively thin stalk and may become very large. Flat (or sessile) papillomas are less protuberant; their height is less than their diameter at the base.

Microscopic Features

A squamous cell papilloma consists of three well-defined layers of tissue: an inner layer of connective tissue or stroma, an intermediate layer of hyperplastic stratified squamous cell epithelium, and a peripheral layer of keratinized epithelial cells forming a confluent keratin mass.

The stroma consists of connective tissue fibers and cells and carries blood vessels to the tips of the excrescences. The dermis at the base of the papilloma is usually thickened and indurated. In small tumors the stroma is sparse and contains few cells. In large tumors, various degrees of fibrotic induration of the stroma may be observed (Figs. 27 and 28).

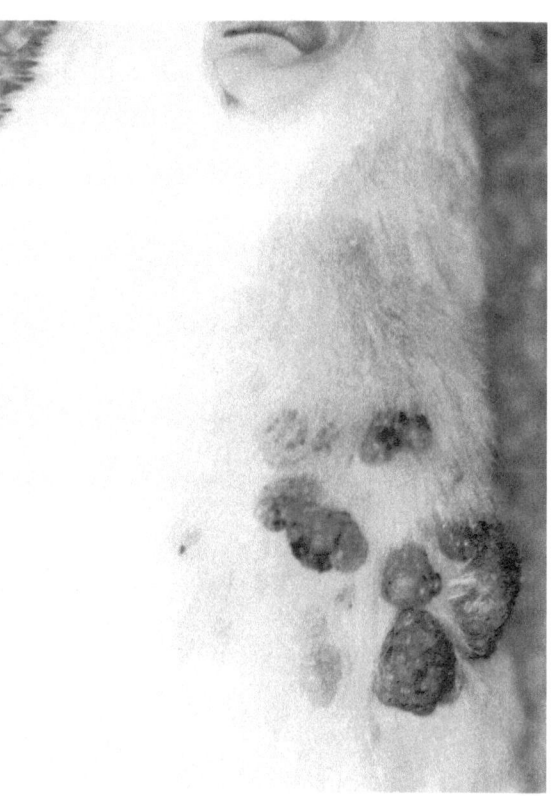

Fig. 26. Gross appearance of squamous cell papillomas. Most tumors are pedunculated. ICR mouse painted with DMBA followed by TPA

The thickness of the relatively regular epithelial layer of the papilloma is variable and may considerably exceed that of the epidermis surrounding the tumor. The basal portions of the epithelium consist of dark-staining, fusiform or columnar cells. The epithelial layer is apparently demarcated from the underlying dermis (Fig. 29). Mitotic figures are usually common.

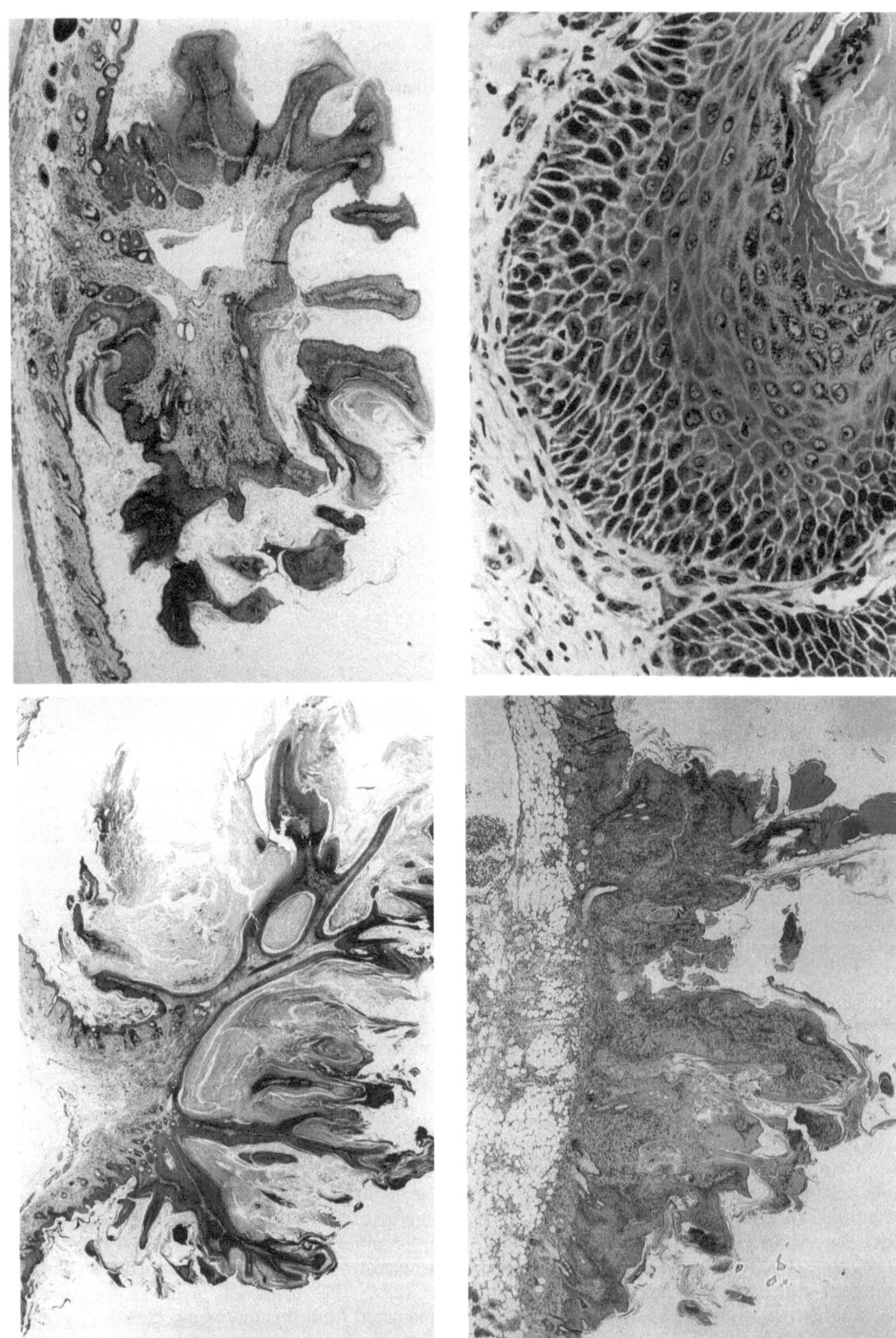

The cells of the outer layers contain keratohyalin, which increases towards the surface. Parakeratotic cells are often present. The size and shape of cells may differ to a certain extent, but the predominantly oval or round nuclei are fairly constant in size. The cells have one or two distinct nucleoli. The peripheral keratinized layer may reach a considerable thickness. A mild to moderate inflammatory infiltrate, mostly lymphocytic but with some polymorphs, is usually present in the underlying dermis. This inflammatory infiltrate often invades the acanthotic epidermis. Mast cells are usually numerous in the dermis underneath tumors. Sometimes at the base of papillomas, cystic epidermoid or acanthotic downgrowths can be observed.

Pedunculated Squamous Cell Papillomas. The tumor is composed essentially of papillary of fingerlike processes with the base at the usually narrow stalk. The stroma forms several long branches which are covered by hyperplastic squamous cell epithelium. Keratin may completely fill the space between the fingerlike projections of the tumor.

Flat Squamous Cell Papillomas. The tumor covers a fairly large area of the skin without apparent stalk formation. The stroma is more delicate. Keratinized epithelium fills the spaces between the outgrowing, relatively short projections and forms a confluent, common, keratinized mass on the apex of tumor (Fig. 30). The type of tumor that was termed "sessile papilloma" (Shubik et al. 1953) is a flat papilloma that contains only one large stromal outgrowth and is covered by hyperplastic and hyperkeratotic epidermis. The stromas of sessile papillomas are not demarcated from the underlying dermis. In some flat papillomas, hyperplastic sebaceous glands can be found.

Ultrastructure

Stratified squamous cell epithelium of the tumor is structurally similar to the normal epidermis. Desmosomes are observed as frequently as in normal squamous epithelium. The desmosomes are occasionally incompletely developed, but are usually not observed in the cytoplasm. The epidermis is clearly demarcated from underlying connective tissue by the basement membrane. The space between adjacent squamous cells is usually wide and contains many cell processes (Figs. 31 and 32).

Differential Diagnosis

Warty growths appearing as small, nodular lesions on the epidermal surface may include not only epidermal tumors but also tumors of skin appendages, connective tissue, and melanocytes. Epidermal tumors can be histologically distinguished from melanomas with little or no difficulty. Among the tumors of epidermal or epithelial orgin, however, it is occasionally difficult to distinguish squamous cell papilloma from keratoacanthoma or squamous cell carcinoma.
In the early stage of progression, keratoacanthoma grossly resembles a flat papilloma, but later it is usually seen as a cup-shaped or saucer-shaped mass of keratin surrounded by thick epithelium. Carcinoma can arise from a pre-existing papilloma or keratoacanthoma or without any apparent connection with a benign tumor or ulcer.
Growth of undifferentiated epithelial cells into the stroma or dermis is a distinguishing feature of squamous cell carcinoma (see p. 25).
In some flat papillomas, hyperplastic sebaceous glands can be found. It is sometimes difficult to decide whether the agglomeration of sebaceous glands represents a simple hyperplasia associated with the papilloma or a true sebaceous adenoma (Rice and Anderson 1986).

Biologie Features

Occurrence. The development of a skin tumor can easily be followed throughout the animal's life.

◄ **Fig. 27** *(upper left).* Pedunculated squamous cell papilloma, skin, ICR mouse. The tumor consists of three well-defined layers of tissue and the papillary processes with a narrow stalk. DMBA followed by TPA; H and E, × 30

Fig. 28 *(lower left).* Pedunculated squamous cell papilloma, skin, SENCAR mouse. Marked keratinized epithelium with keratin masses filling the spaces between the epithelial projections. DMBA followed by PTA; H and E, × 15

Fig. 29 *(upper right).* Higher magnification of Fig. 27. The epithelium of the tumor consists of well-differentiated cells. H and E, × 300

Fig. 30 *(lower right).* Flat squamous cell papilloma, skin, BALB/c mouse. Note papillary growth without apparent stalk formation. DMBA followed by TPA; H and E, × 30

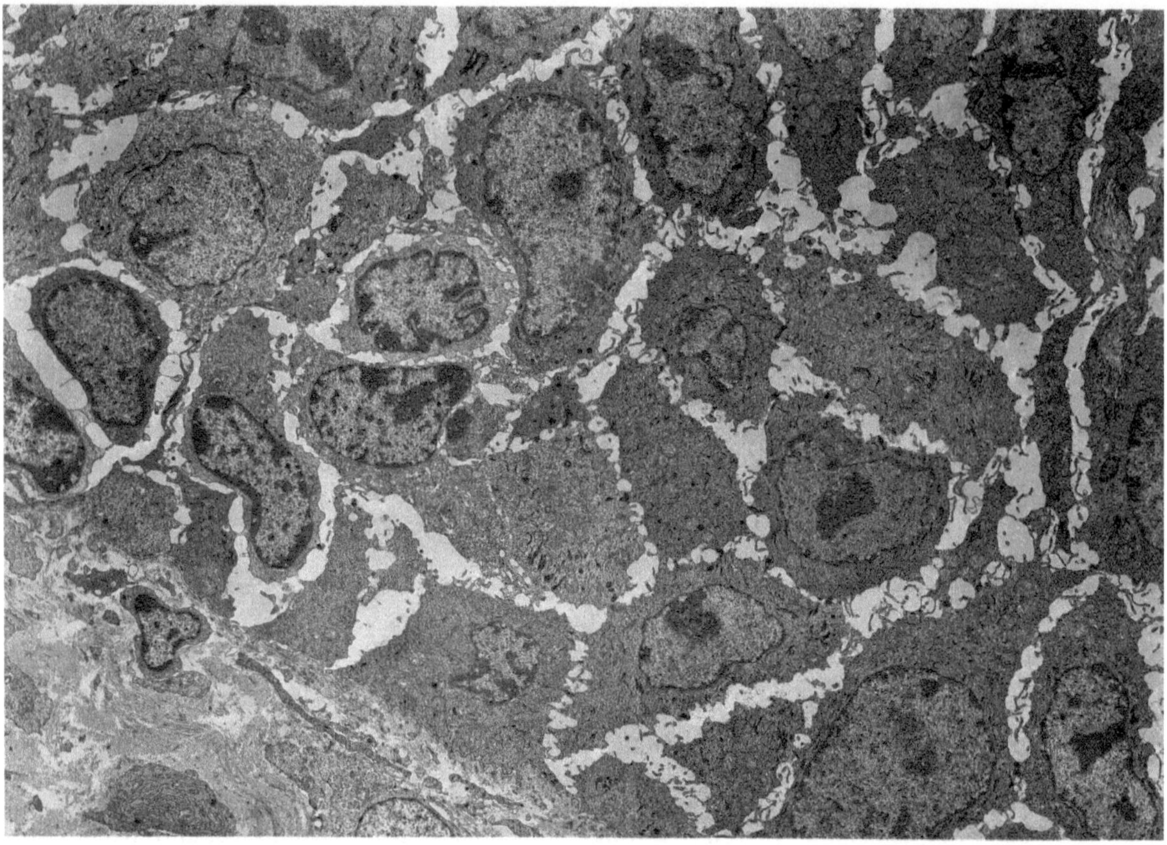

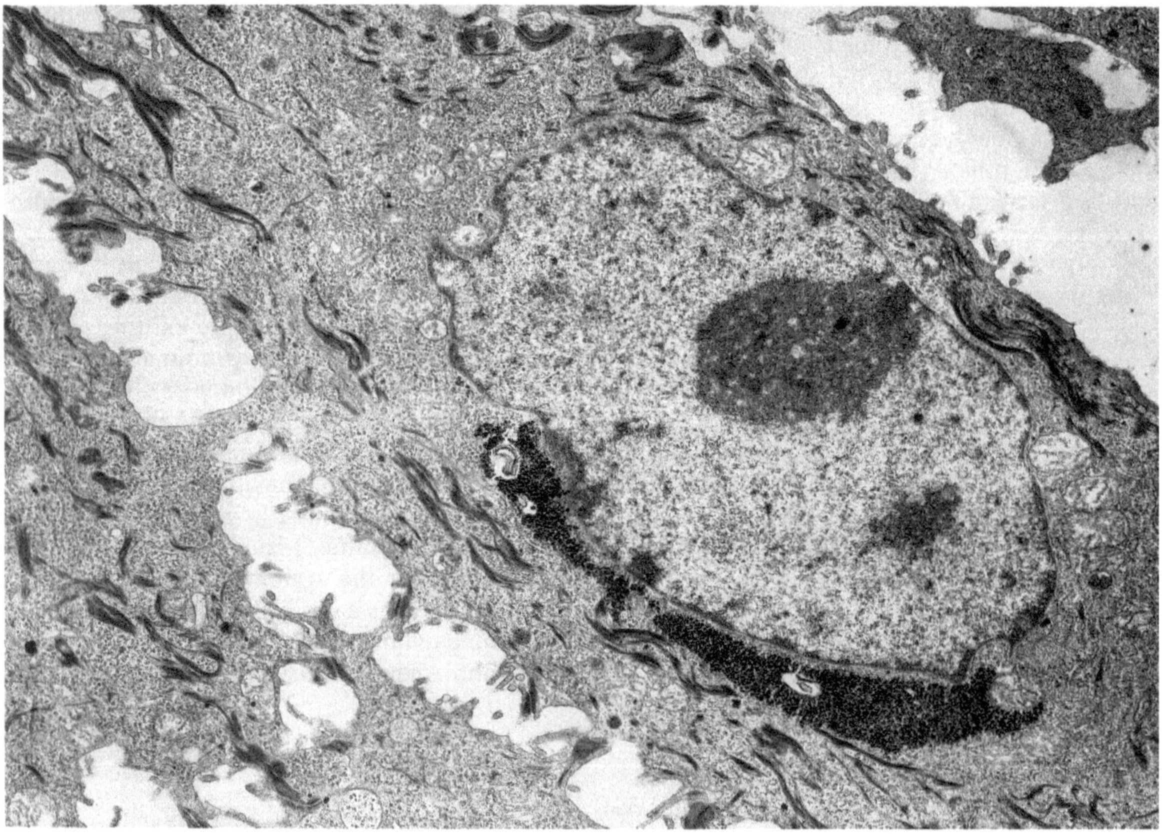

Spontaneous skin tumors in mice are very rare, in general not exceeding 1% of a population of mice (Bogovski 1979). In our studies spontaneous development of squamous cell tumors of the skin were not observed in 800 female mice of the ICR strain. Relatively high incidences of skin tumors reported as appearing spontaneously in earlier publications have been found to be due mostly to the environmental conditions, such as housing in wooden cages with carcinogenic compounds in disinfectants for the cages (Boutwell and Bosch 1958). In the skin-painting carcinogenic bioassays, however, a significantly greater incidence of epidermal neoplasms was reported recently in groups of mice housed in polycarbonate cages with bedding of hard wood chips than in those maintained in stainless-steel wire mesh cages (DePass et al. 1986).

The incidence of spontaneous squamous cell tumors is variable in many genetically distinct strains (Andervont and Edgcomb 1956; Squire et al. 1978). Numerous pure polycyclic aromatic hydrocarbons, such as 7,12-dimethylbenz[a]anthracene, benzo(a)pyrene, and 3-methylcholanthrene, when applied repeatedly, usually induce skin tumors in up to 100% of mice. Single application of high doses of these carcinogens can also induce skin tumors (Turusov et al. 1971). The hair-cycle phase is important in these experiments: The highest incidence was obtained when the single application was made during the resting period of the hair cycle.

Natural History. After the application of carcinogenic substances to the skin, the first tumor, papilloma appears in 1–3 months, as small warts. The smaller tumors may be pink and soft at first. Such tumors harden in a few days and assume a white to yellowish-brown color. Some warts continue to grow and become pedunculated papillomas: Others have a broader base and become less protruding, flat papillomas. Numerous papillomas 1–3 mm in diameter undergo spontaneous involution. Weisburger and Weisburger (1967) considered that if the tumor disappeared within 4 weeks such lesions were not papillomas. Other authors have taken as a criterion 3 weeks (Frei and Kingsley 1968), 2 weeks (Turusov et al. 1971), or 1 week (Slaga and Nesnow 1985). Malignant change in the tumor can occur, usually starting at the base of the tumor.

Pathogenesis. It has been generally considered that squamous cell papillomas originate in the epidermis, while keratoacanthoma arises from hair follicles (Bogovski 1979). However, concerning their origin, there is a different hypothesis which suggests that most squamous cell papillomas arise from the superficial part of the hair follicle. This theory is based on observations in chemical carcinogenesis (Ghadially 1961).

The two-stage hypothesis for chemical carcinogenesis was first established in the mouse skin model: repeated applications of croton oil, phorbol esters, or other "promoting" agents following a single application of a weak or noncarcinogenic dose of a strong carcinogen has been found to result in development of benign and malignant tumors of the skin (Yuspa 1984; Slaga 1983). An implication of this concept is that the appearance of overtly malignant cells is preceded by multiple cellular changes. Chronic physical stimuli such as abrasion (Argyris 1982), wounding (Parkinson 1985), and freezing (Berenblum 1930) of the skin have been demonstrated to be promoting or cocarcinogenic agents in mouse skin carcinogenesis; this suggests that repeated regenerative or proliferative reactions of the skin are strongly related to tumor development (Raick 1974; Yuspa 1984).

Oncogene expression in chemically induced murine skin tumors has been discussed by Balmain et al. (1984) and Roop et al. (1986). Similar phenomena in rats are described by Harper et al. (1987).

Comparison with Other Species

Tumors of epithelial origin are virtually of the same morphologic appearance in all animals (Ghadially 1961). A viral etiology of spontaneous skin tumors has been established in some species.

Most of the oncogenic viruses belong to the classes of papova- and poxviruses, a few are herpesviruses or oncornaviruses (Olson 1963) (although rarely reported in mice). Expression of

◀ **Fig. 31** *(above).* Basal layer of the epithelium of a squamous cell papilloma, skin, ICR mouse. The intercellular spaces are wide. The epithelium is well-demarcated from the dermis by basement membrane. DMBA; TEM, × 3000

Fig. 32 *(below).* Higher magnification of Fig. 31. The epithelial cells contain numerous, electron-dense tonofibrils, some of which make up desmosome-tonofilament complexes. Glycogen granules in the cytoplasm and many intercellular bridges are present. DMBA; TEM, × 8000

oncogenes during the development of skin papilloma has been reported (Pelling et al. 1986).

In general, mice are more sensitive to skin carcinogenesis than rats or hamsters either by the complete carcinogenesis protocol or by the two-stage protocol (Stenbäck 1980). The tumors induced in mice are mostly squamous cell papillomas, whereas similar experimental protocols give rise mainly to basal cell tumors in rats and melanomas in hamsters.

References

Andervont HB, Edgcomb JH (1956) Responses of seven inbred strains of mice to percutaneous applications of 3-methyl cholanthrene. JNCI 17: 481–495

Argyris TS (1982) Tumor promotion by regenerative epidermal hyperplasia in mouse skin. J Cutan Pathol 9: 1–18

Balmain AR, Ramsden M, Bowden GT, Smith J (1984) Activation of the mouse cellular Harvey-ras gene in chemically induced benign skin papillomas. Nature 307: 658–660

Berenblum I (1930) Further investigations on the induction of tumours with carbon dioxide snow. Br J Exp Pathol 11: 208–211

Bogovski P (1979) Tumours of the skin. In: Turusov VS (ed) Pathology of tumours in laboratory animals, vol II. Tumours of the mouse. IARC, Lyon, pp 1–39 (IARC Sci Publ no 23)

Boutwell RK, Bosch DK (1958) The carcinogenicity of creosote oil: its role in the induction of skin tumors in mice. Cancer Res 18: 1171–1175

DePass LR, Weil CS, Ballantyne B, Lewis SC, Losco PE, Reid JB, Simon GS (1986) Influence of housing conditions for mice on the results of a dermal oncogenicity bioassay. Fundam Appl Toxicol 7: 601–608

Frei JV, Kingsley WF (1986) Observations on chemically induced regressing tumors of mouse epidermis. JNCI 41: 1307–1313

Ghadially FN (1961) The role of the hair follicle in the origin and evolution of some cutaneous neoplasms of man and experimental animals. Cancer 14: 801–816

Harper JR, Reynolds SH, Greenkalph DA, Strickland JE, Local JC, Wyspa SH (1987) Analysis of the ras oncogene and its p21 product in chemically induced skin tumors and tumor-derived cell lines. Carcinogenesis 8: 1821–1825

Olson C (1963) Cutaneous papillomatosis in cattle and other animals. Ann NY Acad Sci 108: 1042–1056

Parkinson EK (1985) Defective responses of transformed keratinocytes to terminal differentiation stimuli. Their role in epidermal tumour promotion by phorbol esters and by deep skin wounding. Br J Cancer 52: 479–493

Pelling JC, Ernst SM, Strawhecker JM, Johnson JA, Nairn RS, Slaga TJ (1986) Elevated expression of Ha-ras is an early event in two-stage skin carcinogenesis in SENCAR mice. Carcinogenesis 7: 1599–1602

Raick AN (1974) Cell proliferation and promoting action in skin carcinogenesis. Cancer Res 34: 920–926

Rice JM, Anderson LM (1986) Sebaceous adenomas with associated epidermal hyperplasia and papilloma formation as a major type of tumor induced in mouse skin by high doses of carcinogens. Cancer Lett 33: 295–306

Roop DR, Lowy DR, Tambourin PE, Strickland J, Harper JR, Balaschak M, Spangler EF, Yuspa SH (1986) An activated Harvey ras oncogene produces benign tumours on mouse epidermal tissue. Nature 323: 822–824

Shubik P, Baserga R, Ritchie AC (1953) The life and progression of induced skin tumours in mice. Br J Cancer 7: 342–351

Slaga TJ (1983) Overview of tumor promotion in animals. Environ Health Perspect 50: 3–14

Slaga TJ, Nesnow S (1985) SENCAR mouse skin tumorigenesis. In: Milman HA, Weisburger EK (eds) Handbook of carcinogen testing. Noyes, Park Ridge NJ, pp 230–250

Squire RA, Goodman DG, Valerio MG, Fredrickson T, Strandberg JD, Levitt MH, Lingeman CH, Harshbarger JC, Dawe CJ (1978) Tumors. In: Benirschke K, Garner FM, Jones TC (eds) Pathology of laboratory animals, vol 2. Springer, Berlin Heidelberg New York, pp 1051–1283

Stenbäck F (1980) Skin carcinogenesis as a model system: observations on species, strain and tissue sensitivity to 7,12-dimethylbenz(a)anthracene with and without promotion from croton oil. Acta Pharmacol Toxicol (Copenh) 46: 89–97

Turusov VS, Day N, Andrianov L, Jain D (1971) Influence of dose on skin tumors induced in mice by single application of 7,12-dimethylbenz(a)anthracene. JNCI 47: 105–111

Weisburger JH, Weisburger EK (1967) Tests for chemical carcinogenesis. In: Busch H (ed) Methods in cancer research, vol 1. Academic, New York, pp 307–398

Yuspa SH (1984) Mechanisms of initiation and promotion in mouse epidermis. In: Borzsonyi M, Lapis K, Day NE, Yamasaki Y (eds) Models, mechanisms and etiology of tumor promotion. Oxford University Press, pp 191–204 (IARC Sci Publ no 56)

Squamous Cell Carcinoma, Skin, Rat

Masao Hirose

Synonyms. Epidermoid carcinoma; prickle cell epithelioma; prickle cell carcinoma; spinous cell carcinoma; spindle cell squamous cell carcinoma; spindle cell carcinoma.

Gross Appearance

Small carcinomas that develop within papillomas may be difficult to distinguish from papillomas, but fully developed carcinomas are not difficult to diagnose. These advanced carcinomas are firm nodules of more than 1 cm in diameter attached to the overlying skin which is often ulcerated over the center of the mass. They often infiltrate the underlying supporting structures, but distant metastases to the regional lymph nodes and lungs are not common. Occasionally these carcinomas consist of flat, solid masses with ulceration and crust formation in the overlying skin; this type infiltrates the underlying tissues.

Microscopic Features

The microscopic features of squamous cell carcinoma of the skin are usually more keratinized but otherwise similar to those that occur in other organs. These neoplasms may be classified into well, moderately and poorly differentiated types according to their degree of anaplasia. In well-differentiated squamous cell carcinomas (Figs. 33–35); cords or nests of tumor cells infiltrate the stroma, with maturation from basal to granular cells and with formation of keratin. Intercellular bridges are clearly evident. Keratin pearls may be found in the tumor tissue. Mitoses are frequently seen, mostly in the basal cell layer.

The transition type between the well and the poorly differentiated types is called moderately differentiated squamous cell carcinoma (Figs. 36–38). Frequently, the cancer tissue that has infiltrated the underlying stroma appears less differentiated than the overlying cancer tissue. Focal malignant change may be found in papillomas or keratoacanthomas, and less frequently, atypical cells may be found within the hyperplastic of nonhyperplastic epithelium. Such lesions may be called carcinoma in situ, when present within the epidermis, but are no longer in situ af-

ter they proliferate into the dermis (Fig. 38). In poorly differentiated squamous cell carcinomas (Figs. 39–42), maturation from basal to granular cells and keratinization are not clear. The cells are spindle-shaped or irregular, are basophilic, and contain numerous mitotic figures. The laminar structure and cellular polarity, characteristic of epithelium of squamous origin, are not preserved. Intercellular bridges may not be recognizable in the poorly differentiated lesions. Some poorly differentiated squamous cell carcinomas undergo scirrhous (Fig. 40) growth.

Ultrastructure

Ultrastructural findings are important for discernment between poorly differentiated squamous cell carcinomas and sarcomas, but in the rat no ultrastructural findings have been reported. There are, however, a few reports of such studies on squamous cell carcinomas in mice and on lesions in other organs.

Differential Diagnosis

Squamous cell carcinomas contain connective tissue stroma and epithelium. The epithelium is composed entirely of squamous elements. Although some malignant skin tumors originating from basal cells or sebaceous glands have both malignant squamous elements and basal cells or sebaceous gland elements (Zackheim 1973), these malignant tumors should be called basosquamous cell carcinoma and sebaceous squamous cell carcinoma, respectively.

Fibrosarcomas and rhabdomyosarcomas should be distinguished from poorly differentiated squamous cell carcinomas. In the latter, continuity from more differentiated carcinoma in the epidermis or dermis to deeply invading "pseudosarcomatous" lesions, and dark-staining cords of epithelial cells in the connective tissue stroma may be observed on careful examination.

Differentiation of benign squamous cell papillomas from squamous carcinomas is important. Papillomas may grow downward toward the dermis, but the basement membrane of the tumor tissue is well preserved. In contrast, squamous

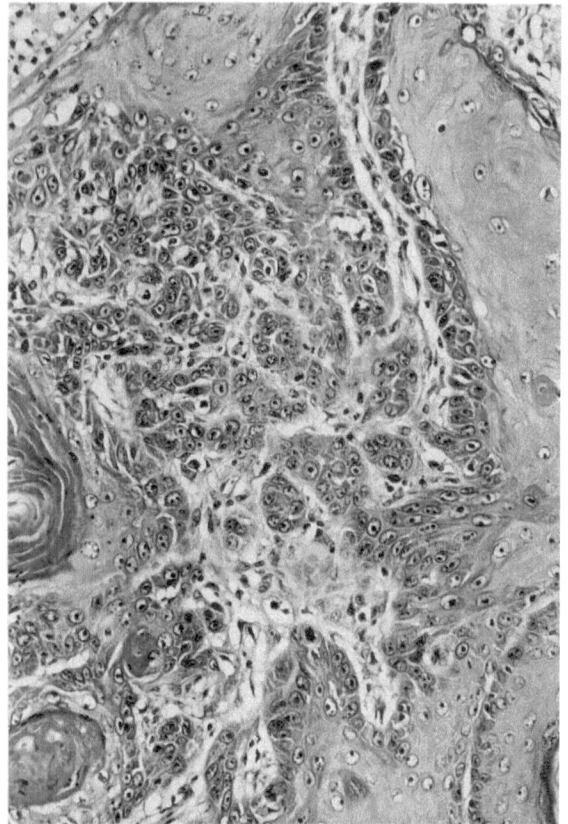

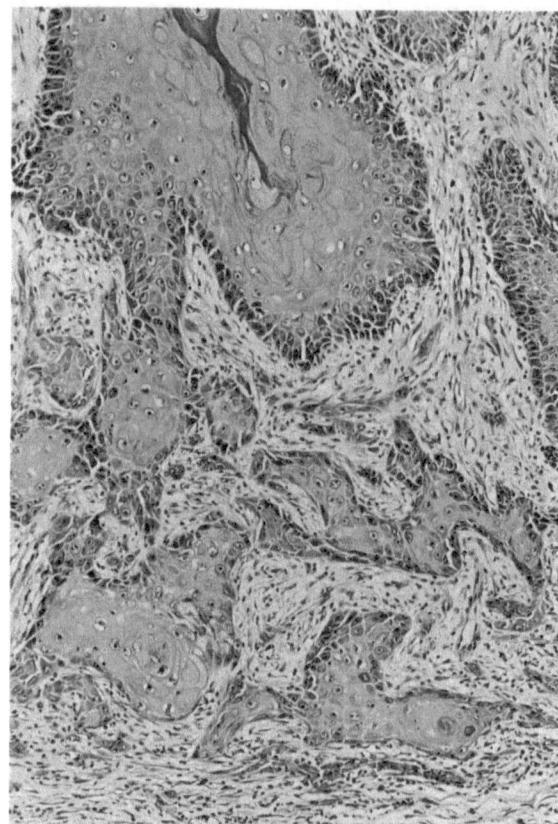

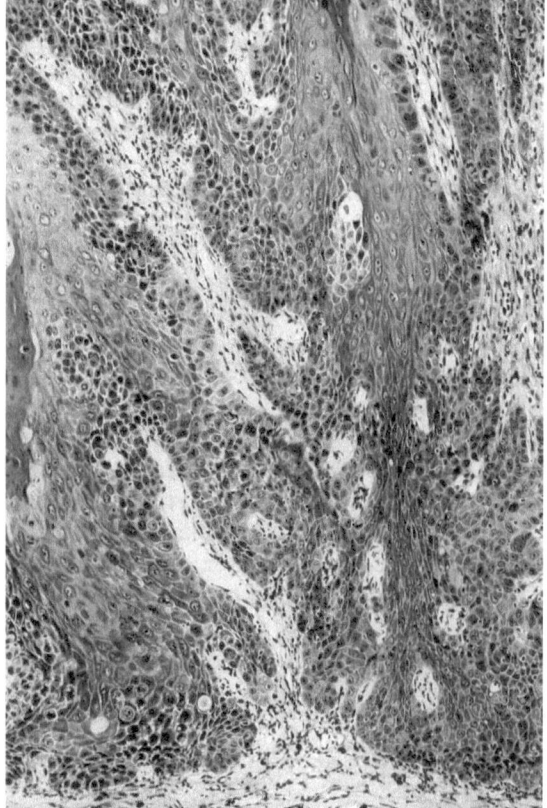

Fig. 33 *(upper left)*. Skin, rat. Well-differentiated squamous cell carcinoma (early stage). Note papillary growth of mature squamous epithelium. Polarity is poorly preserved, and focal invasion is observed in the *left center*. H and E, ×280

Fig. 34 *(lower left)*. Skin, rat. Well-differentiated squamous cell carcinoma with invasive growth into the stromal connective tissue. The border between cancer cells and stromal connective tissue is ill-defined. H and E, ×180

Fig. 35 *(upper right)*. Skin, rat. Well-differentiated squamous cell carcinoma. Islands of atypical cell nests within the stromal connective tissue are a clear indication of invasion. H and E, ×280

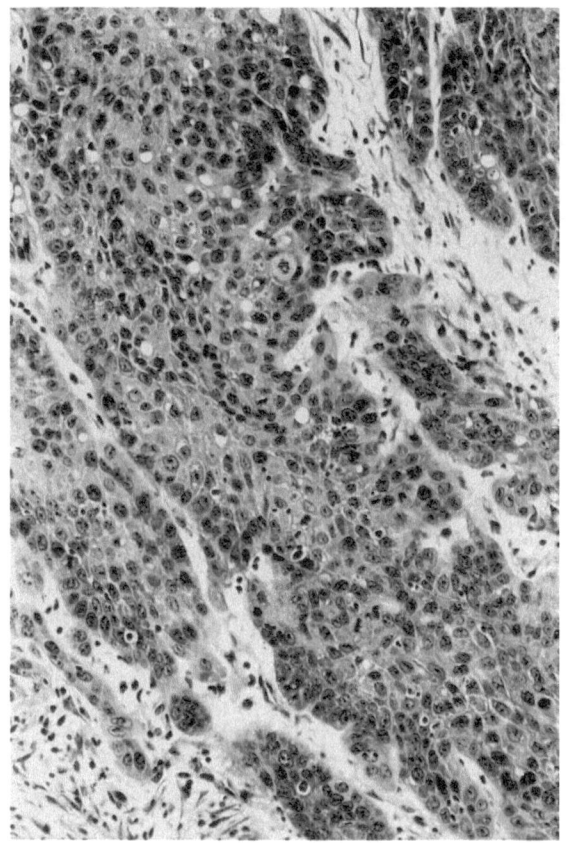

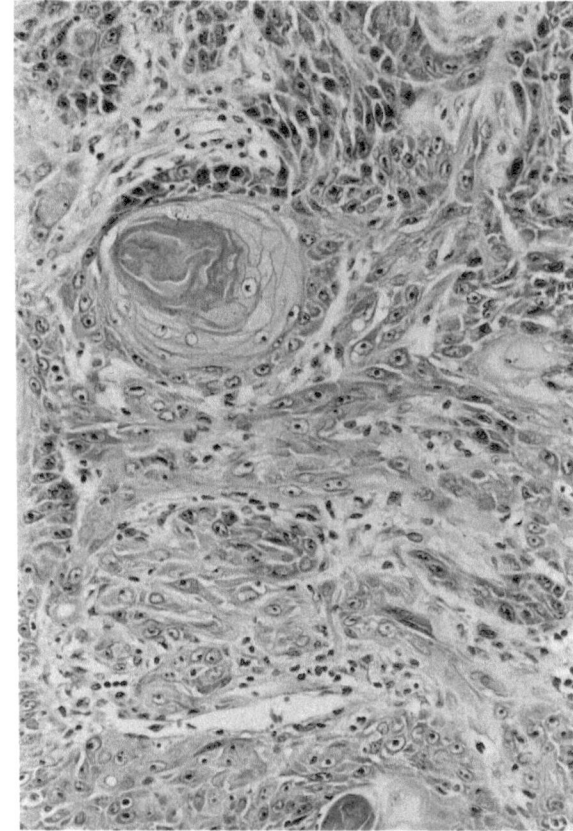

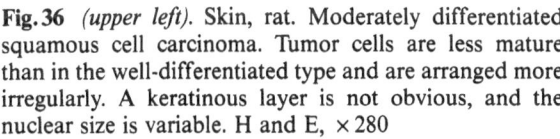

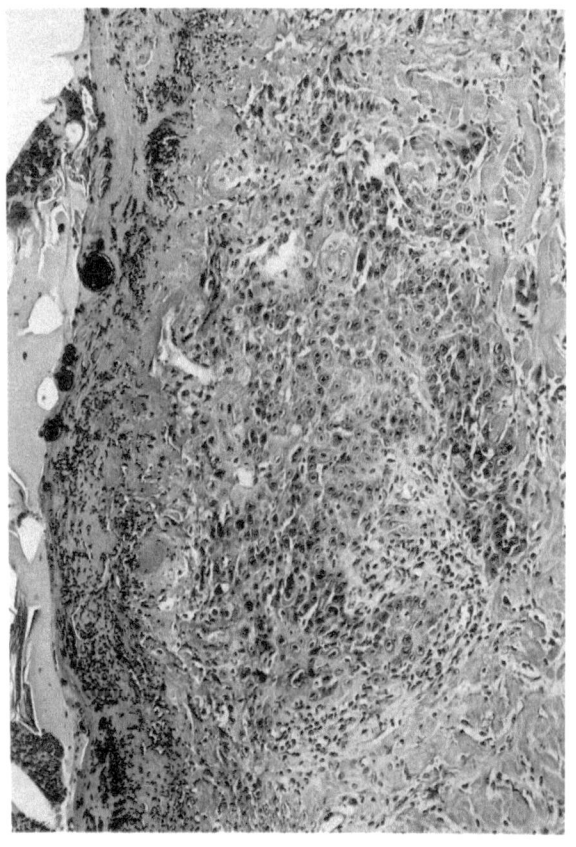

Fig. 36 *(upper left)*. Skin, rat. Moderately differentiated squamous cell carcinoma. Tumor cells are less mature than in the well-differentiated type and are arranged more irregularly. A keratinous layer is not obvious, and the nuclear size is variable. H and E, × 280

Fig. 37 *(upper right)*. Skin, rat. Moderately differentiated squamous cell carcinoma. Less mature squamous cells are more invasive. Note a keratin pearl in the *upper left*. H and E, × 340

Fig. 38 *(lower right)*. Skin rat. Moderately differentiated squamous cell carcinoma. This tumor surface is flat with an eroded surface. The spinous cancer cells have invaded the dermis. This tumor may have originated directly from hyperplastic or nonhyperplastic epithelium. H and E, × 170

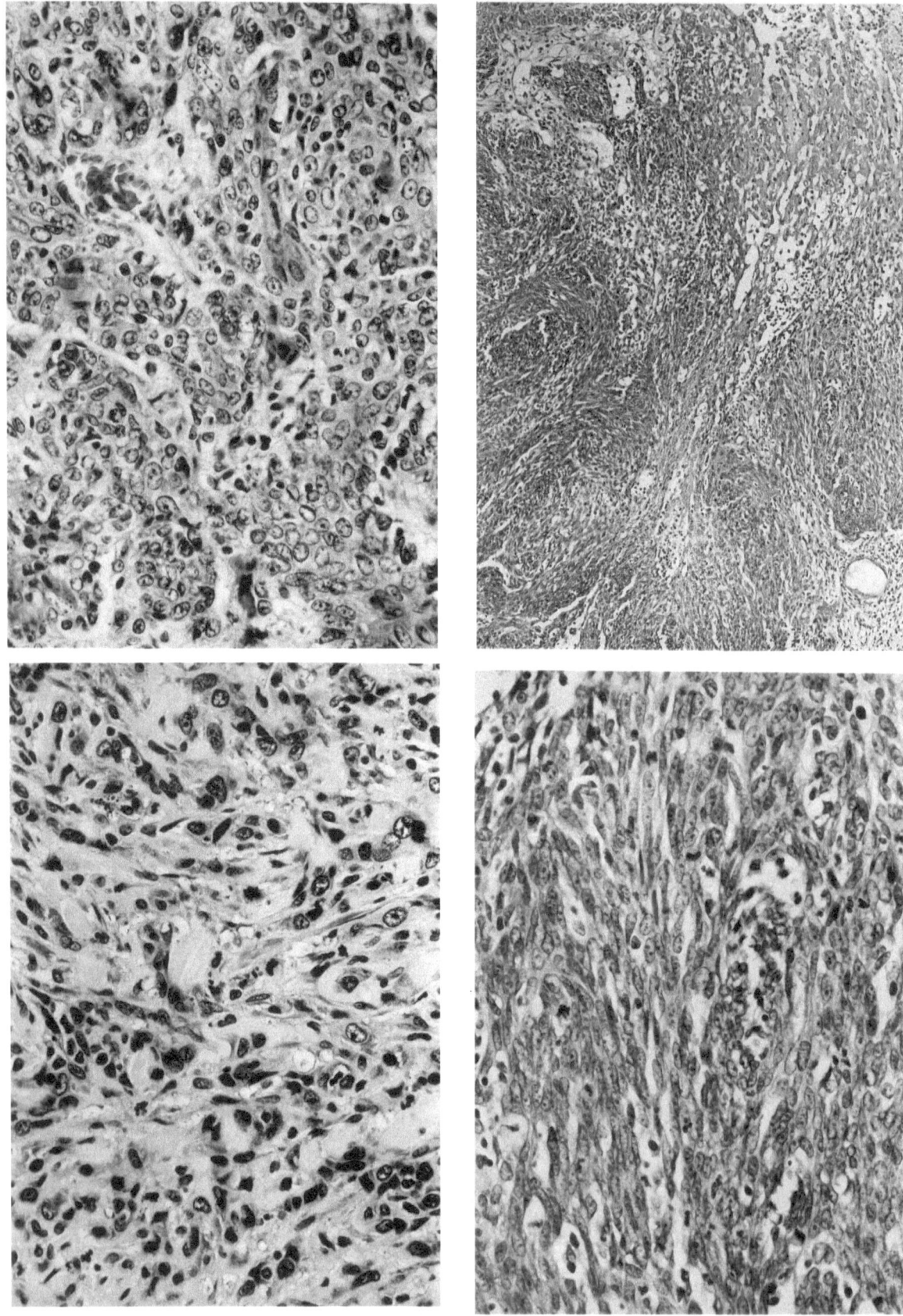

cell carcinomas penetrate the basement membrane and infiltrate the stromal connective tissue or the muscle layer, and the basement membrane is not well preserved. In situ lesion or carcinoma arising in papilloma may be distinguished by the presence of cellular and structural atypia.

Biologic Features

The lesions preceding squamous cell carcinoma may be observed in epidermal hyperplasia, squamous cell papilloma, and keratoacanthoma (Zackheim 1964a, Zackheim 1973). Cells in these antecedent lesions undergo intracellular edema, nuclear hyperchromatism and enlargement; mitotic figures may be found in the basal and suprabasal layers of epidermal hyperplasia. Similar premalignant changes may be found in papillomas. Dyskeratotic cells may be found in the prickle cell layer. These premalignant changes occur diffusely throughout the lesions and simultaneously involve the superficial papilliferous processes as well as the deeper tissue growth.
Early invasion occurs within the basal layer. Less frequently, anaplastic cells may arise directly from nonhyperplastic epidermis (Cherry and Glucksmann 1971; Zackheim 1964a). In such cases, anaplastic cells grow into the underlying stroma, and the epidermis is ulcerated. Growth above the surface of the skin is not seen. Metas-

tases are not common but sometimes occur to local lymph nodes and the lungs.
Squamous call carcinomas can be induced by irradiation (Albert et al. 1969) or chemical carcinogens. However, various histologic types of tumor appear following topical applications of carcinogens. A single topical application of 7,12-dimethylbenz[a]anthracene (DMBA) to rat skin induced a broad spectrum of benign and malignant cutaneous tumors in balanced proportions (Schweizer et al. 1982); repeated applications of DMBA induces predominantly squamous cell carcinomas (Zackheim 1964a; Zackheim 1964b; Rasmussen et al. 1983) or keratoacanthomas (Howell 1962). Repeated treatment with 3-methylcholanthrene (3-MC) induces predominantly trichoepitheliomas and basal cell carcinomas (Howell 1962; Zackheim 1964b). Continuous topical applications of 2-anthramine (2-aminoanthracene) to Fischer rats induces predominantly basal cell epitheliomas with a few tumors of various other types (Zackheim 1964b; Zackheim et al. 1959) or predominantly squamous cell and sebaceous tumors (Lennox 1955).
Rat skin is less susceptible than mouse skin to the carcinogenic effect of benzo(a)pyrene (Arffmann and Hjøorne 1979). Topical applications of some azo dyes (Fare 1966) and nitrosamines (Hirose et al. 1979; Zabezhinski et al. 1985) induced squamous cell carcinomas. Repeated intraperitoneal injections of lasiocarpin induced transplantable squamous cell carcinomas in F344 rats (Svoboda and Reddy 1974).
Intragastric administration of DMBA (Meranze et al. 1969) or 3-MC (Gruenstein et al. 1966) also induced squamous cell carcinoma, although at a low incidence. Topical treatment with 3-MC plus administration of a diet containing 4-dimethylaminostilbene induced about five times as many squamous cell carcinomas as treatment with 3-MC alone (Takayama 1970). Therefore, the histological type of skin tumor may be affected by the type and dose of carcinogen, the duration and route of treatment, and the strain and sex of the rats.
Spontaneous squamous cell carcinomas have been found in several strains of rats, but they usually represent less than 2.5% the total spontaneous tumors as shown in Table 1 (see squamous cell papilloma, p. 17).

◀ **Fig. 39** *(upper left)*. Skin, rat. Poorly differentiated squamous cell carcinoma. The demarcated nests of squamous cells indicate that the tumor is of squamous origin. H and E, × 340

Fig. 40 *(lower left)*. Skin, rat. Poorly differentiated squamous cell carcinoma. Cords of atypical cells proliferate with dense connective tissue. The close-adhering characteristics of squamous epithelium are lost, but small groups of cells adhering to one another indicate their epithelial origin. Mitotic figures are numerous. H and E, × 340

Fig. 41 *(upper right)*. Skin, rat. Poorly differentiated squamous cell carcinoma. Proliferation of spindle-shaped cells may obscure the fact that the tumor is of epithelial origin. However, there is continuity from more differentiated carcinoma. H and E, × 68

Fig. 42 *(lower right)*. Skin rat. Higher magnification of Fig. 41. The tumor cells have lost the adhesive characteristics of epithelial cells. Some are spindle-shaped and suggest the appearance of cells of a fibrosarcoma. H and E, × 340

Comparison with Other Species

Mice and hamsters are more susceptible than rats to induction of squamous cell carcinomas, and they are also more susceptible to the skin tumor promoter 12-0-tetradecanoylphorbol-13-acetate. Therefore, a two-stage skin carcinogenesis model in rats has not yet been fully established (Schweizer et al. 1982), and consequently there have been fewer experiments on skin carcinogenesis in rats.

Squamous cell carcinomas can be induced in the skin of the rabbit (Stenback 1980), hedgehog (Ghadially 1960), and duck, which does not have hair follicles (Rigdon 1952), by the topical applications of a carcinogen, but the same treatment of rat skin induces fewer squamous cell carcinomas. In humans, squamous cell carcinomas mostly arise in sun-damaged skin, either as such or from a senile keratosis (solar keratosis or actinic dermatosis) in irradiated skin from irradiation keratosis or in Bowen's disease. These lesions consist of hyperplastic epithelium with cellular and structural atypia. Thus, they differ histologically from papillomas induced in animals.

Human squamous cell carcinomas have a low potency to metastasize, the incidence of metastases being 2%-3% in all patients with squamous cell carcinomas of the skin. Carcinomas arising from sun-damaged skin have an incidence of 0.5%, and those induced by radiation have an incidence of 20%. About three-quarters of the patients die with metastases (Lever and Schaumberg-Lever 1983).

References

Albert RE, Phillips ME, Bennett P, Burns F, Heimbach R (1969) The morphology and growth characteristics of radiation-induced epithelial skin tumors in the rat. Cancer Res 29: 658-668

Arffmann E, Hjøorne N (1979) Influence of surface lipids on skin carcinogenesis in rats. Acta Pathol Microbiol Immunol Scand [A] 87: 143-149

Cherry CP, Glucksmann A (1971) The influence of carcinogenic dosage and of sex on the induction of epitheliomas and sarcomas in the dorsal skin of rats. Br J Cancer 25: 544-564

Fare G (1966) Rat skin carcinogenesis by topical applications of some azo dyes. Cancer Res 26: 2406-2408

Ghadially FN (1960) Carcinogenesis in the skin of the hedgehog. Br J Cancer 14: 212-215

Gruenstein M, Meranze DR, Shimkin MB (1966) Mammary, sebaceous and cutaneous neoplasms and leukemia in male Wistar rats receiving repeated gastric instillations of 3-methylcholanthrene. Cancer Res 26: 2202-2205

Hirose M, Maekawa A, Kamiya S, Odashima S (1979) Carcinogenic effect of N-ethyl- and N-amyl-N- nitrosourethanes on female Donryu rats. Gann 70: 653-662

Howell JS (1962) Skin tumors in the rat produced by 9,10-dimethyl-1,2-benzanthracene and methylcholanthrene. Br J Cancer 16: 101-109

Lennox B (1955) The production of a variety of skin tumours in rats with 2-anthramine and a comparison with the effects in mice. Br J Cancer 9: 631-639

Lever WF, Schaumberg-Lever G (1983) Histopathology of the skin, 6th edn. Lippincott, Philadelphia PA, pp 499-503

Meranze DR, Gruenstein M, Shimkin MB (1969) Effect of age and sex on the development of neoplasms in Wistar rats receiving a single intragastric instillation of 7,12-dimethylbenz(a)anthracene. Int J Cancer 4: 480-486

Rasmussen KS, Glenthøj A, Arffmann E (1983) Skin carcinogenesis in rats by 3-methylcholanthrene and 7,12-dimethylbenz(a)anthracene. Influence of dose and frequency on tumour response and its histological type. Acta Pathol Microbiol Immunol Scand [A] 91: 445-455

Rigdon RH (1952) Tumors induced by methylcholanthrene in the duck. Papilloma, squamous-cell carcinoma, and hemangioma. Arch Pathol 54: 368-377

Schweizer J, Loehrke H, Hesse B, Goerttler K (1982) 7,12-dimethylbenz(a)anthracene/12-0-tetradecanoylphorbol- 13-acetate-mediated skin tumor initiation and promotion in male Sprague-Dawley rats. Carcinogenesis 3: 785-789

Stenbäck F (1980) Skin carcinogenesis as a model system: observations on species, strain and tissue sensitivity to 7,12-dimethylbenz(a)anthracene with or without promotion from croton oil. Acta Pharmacol Toxicol (Copenh) 46: 89-97

Svoboda DJ, Reddy JK (1974) Lasiocarpine-induced, transplantable squamous cell carcinoma of rat skin. JNCI 53: 1415-1418

Takayama S (1970) Skin tumors in ACI/N rats induced by 3-methylcholanthrene and 4-dimethylaminostilbene. Gann 61: 367-371

Zabezhinski MA, Pliss GB, Okulov VB, Petrov AS (1985) Skin tumours induced by local and systemic action of N-nitroso-compounds in rats. Arch Geschwulstforsch 55: 117-122

Zackheim HS (1964a) Evolution of squamous cell carcinoma in the rat. Arch Pathol Lab Med 77: 434-444

Zackheim HS (1964b) Comparative cutaneous carcinogenesis in the rat. Differential response to the application of anthramine, methylcholanthrene, and dimethylbenzanthracene. Oncology 17: 236-246

Zackheim HS (1973) Tumours of the skin. In: Turusov VS (ed) Pathology of tumours in laboratory animals, vol 1. Tumours of the rat (pt 1). IARC, Lyon, pp 1-21 (IARC Sci Publ no 5)

Zackheim HS, Simpson WL, Langs L (1959) Basal cell epitheliomas and other skin tumors produced in rats and mice by anthramine and methylcholanthrene. J Invest Dermatol 33: 385-402

Squamous Cell Carcinoma, Skin, Mouse

Ryohei Hasegawa, Yoshifumi Miyakawa, and Hidetaka Sato

Synonyms. Cutaneous squamous cell carcinoma; epidermoid carcinoma; prickle cell carcinoma; anaplastic carcinoma; squamous carcinoma.

Gross Appearance

Most squamous cell carcinomas are seen grossly as solid masses of subepidermal induration. Sometimes, small sessile papillary tumors are histologically recognized as carcinomas. The tumor surface is usually irregular, necrotic, and hemorrhagic with erosions and defects that, in advanced carcinomas, give rise to wide annular ulcerations (Fig. 43). The cut surface is whitish to whitish-red, with conspicuous thickening of the skin and prominent subcutaneous growth (Fig. 44). The presence of metastases in regional lymph nodes or in other organs is sometimes observed.

Microscopic Features

Histologically, squamous cell carcinomas may present a wide variety of appearances. Since differentiation in squamous cell epithelium is in the direction of keratinization, squamous cell carcinoma may be classified by morphological type or degree of differentiation. Keratinization is often present in the form of keratin, epithelial or "cancer" pearls, characteristic structures composed of concentric layers of squamous cells with concentrically laminated keratin in the center. Various degrees of differentiation are encountered, and two main types of squamous cell carcinoma may be distinguished, keratinizing and anaplastic. The keratinizing type accounts for approximately 90% of all squamous cell carcinomas in our observations. Both types occasionally include various degrees of differentiation seen in different fields of the same tumor.

Keratinizing Squamous Cell Carcinoma. There is considerable morphological variation in keratinizing squamous cell carcinoma. Infiltration into the subcutis takes place with fingerlike projections extending like the roots of a tree or budding plant (Fig. 45). The cells usually vary greatly in size and staining properties, and the dyskera-

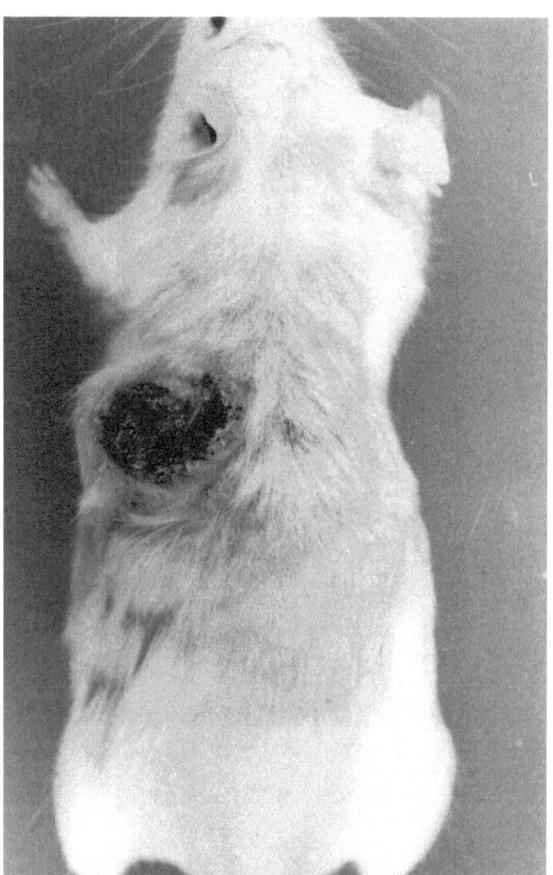

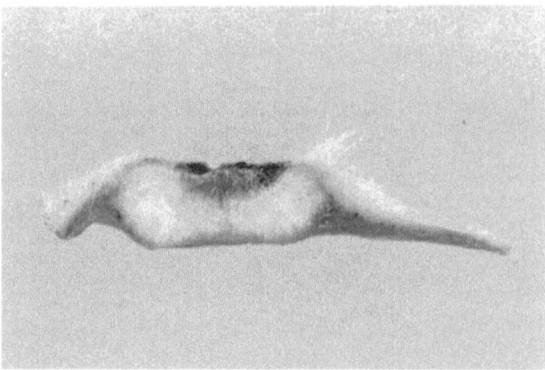

Fig. 43 *(above).* Squamous cell carcinoma, skin, ICR mouse. Following repeated painting with 3-methylcholanthrene

Fig. 44 *(below).* Cut surface of the tumor shown in Fig. 43. It is whitish and compact and has grown into the dermis and subcutis. × 4

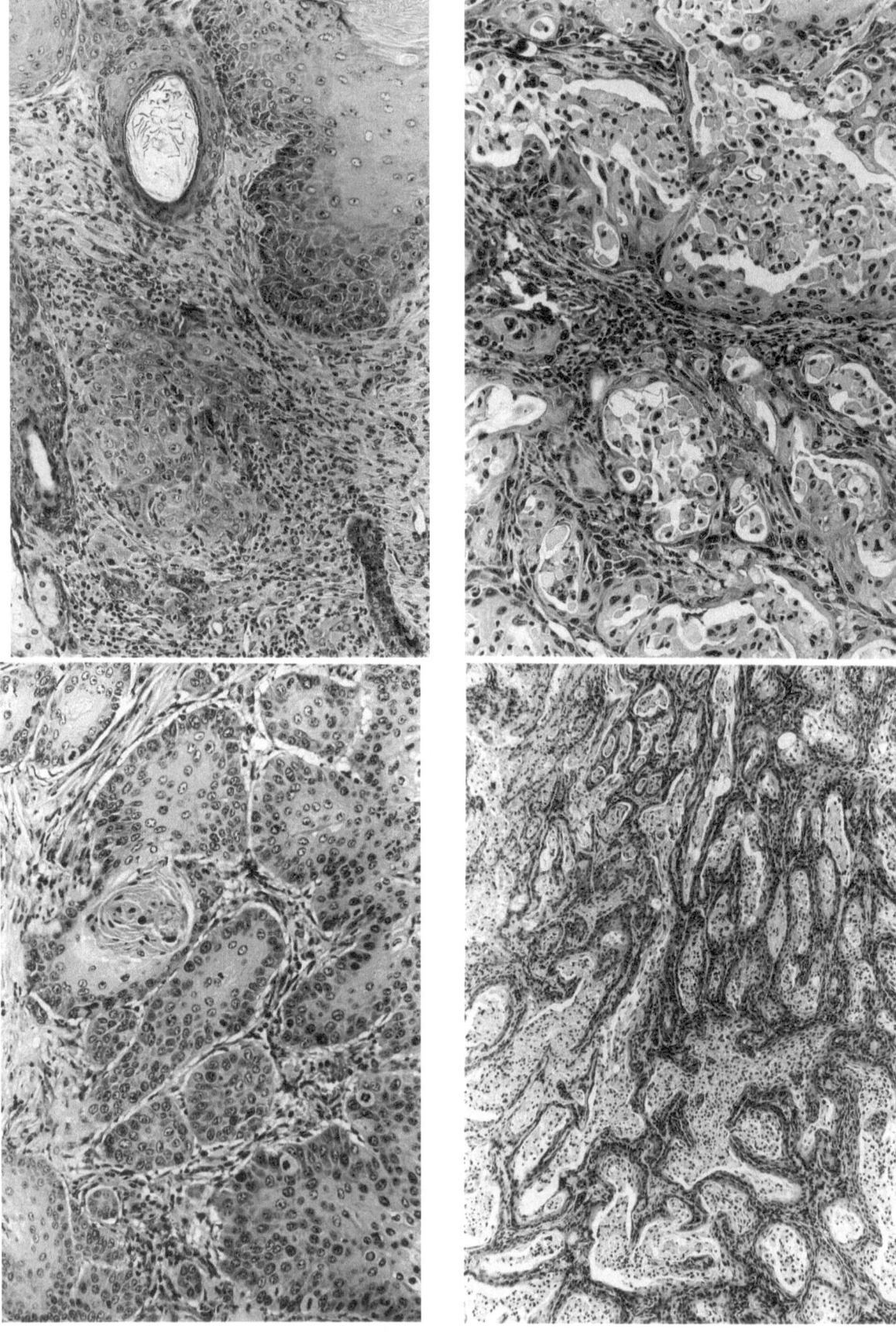

totic and parakeratotic cells, sometimes arranged in a whorled fashion, are characteristic (Fig. 46). Infiltration of inflammatory cells is usually observed.

Well-differentiated tumors imitate the normal structure of stratified, keratinized squamous epithelium. Tumor cells have prominent intercellular bridges and a tendency to differentiate into squamous cells. „Cancer" pearls are usually formed. Keratohyaline granules and keratin are seen in the surface lining areas and in the pearls within the tumor epithelium. The cytoplasm is homogeneous, abundant, and eosinophilic in superficial and intermediate cells, whereas it is basophilic and scanty in basal cell layers. Buds and nests of neoplastic epithelial cells sometimes resemble basal cells with no sign of keratinization. Cellular atypism is less, and cell boundaries are distinct. Mitotic figures are usually common within the basal layer.

As a result of dyskeratosis and subsequent acantholysis, squamous cell carcinomas occasionally undergo tubular or alveolar formation (so-called pseudo-glandular squamous cell carcinoma) (Fig. 47) (Squire et al. 1978). In these cases tubular or alveolar lumina are lined with one or several layers of epithelium. In areas in which the lumina are lined with a single layer of epithelium, the epithelial cells may be simple columnar and resemble glandular cells, but in areas with several layers of epithelium, squamous and partially keratinized cells usually form the inner layers (Figs. 48 und 49). The lumina are filled with desquamated acantholytic cells, many of which are partially or fully keratinized.

Less differentiated tumor cells are markedly irregular in size and shape, and increased numbers of mitotic figures are present. Tumor cells are polymorphic and have hyperchromatic or large, vacuolar nuclei with prominent nucleoli, and vacuolated cytoplasm. Cell boundaries are distinct. Abnormal mitotic figures and absence of intercellular bridges are frequently observed. Keratin pearls are less numerous and not fully keratinized. Small clusters of cells and single, partly keratinized cells are seen invasively proliferating into the subcutis.

Anaplastic Squamous Cell Carcinoma (Spindle Cell Carcinoma; Anaplastic Epidermoid Carcinoma). Cells of most anaplastic tumors or tumor areas are spindle-shaped with elongated nuclei (Fig. 50). Keratinization is almost completely absent. Nearly all tumor cells are atypical and devoid of intercellular bridges. The tumor is difficult to distinguish from sarcomas of connective tissue origin. Normal and abnormal mitotic figures may be seen frequently. Giant, fragmented, multiple nuclei can often be found, as well as bizarre mitotic figures. Neither inflammatory infiltration nor any other connective tissue reaction is observed in the tumor mass or border between tumor and dermal or epidermal tissues. Tumors may be seen in transitional stages streaming away from the basement membrane. The origin and classification of these tumors has remained a matter of dispute. They often show transitions between spindle cells and cells that are undoubtedly epithelium. Immunohistochemical examination with keratin-specific serum and electron microscopy may demonstrate the presence of keratin in the tumor cells, confirming their origin from squamous cells.

Some of the nonkeratinizing squamous cell carcinomas are composed of cells growing in confluent, often large clusters and clumps instead of as spindle cells. The cells are prominently pleomorphic (Fig. 51). Nuclei have various shapes and differing staining properties. Many mitotic figures are seen. Multinucleated giant cells are usually numerous. This histological pattern often forms a part of keratinized tumors. Mast cells are rarely seen.

◀ **Fig. 45** *(upper left)*. Keratinizing squamous cell carcinoma, skin, ICR mouse. A small tumor focus underneath benign squamous cell tumor is associated with inflammatory cell infiltration. DMBA followed by TPA; H and E, × 150

Fig. 46 *(lower left)*. Well-differentiated squamous cell carcinoma, skin, SENCAR mouse. The tumor is composed predominantly of mature squamous cells with relatively slight atypism and few mitoses. Several epithelial pearls are formed. Benzo(a)pyrene followed by TPA; H and E, × 150

Fig. 47 *(upper right)*. Well-differentiated keratinizing squamous cell carcinoma, skin, SENCAR mouse. Note marked acantholysis which may be followed by tubular or alveolar formation by the tumor. DMBA followed by TPA; H and E, × 150

Fig. 48 *(lower right)*. Well-differentiated squamous cell carcinoma, skin, SENCAR mouse. Note severe acantholysis with keratin debris surrounded by a single layer of epithelium. DMBA followed by TPA; H and E, × 80

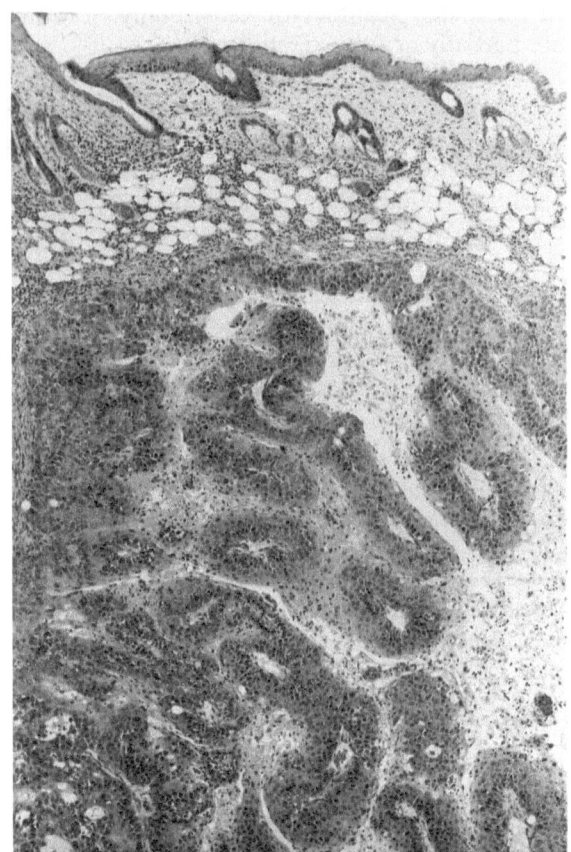
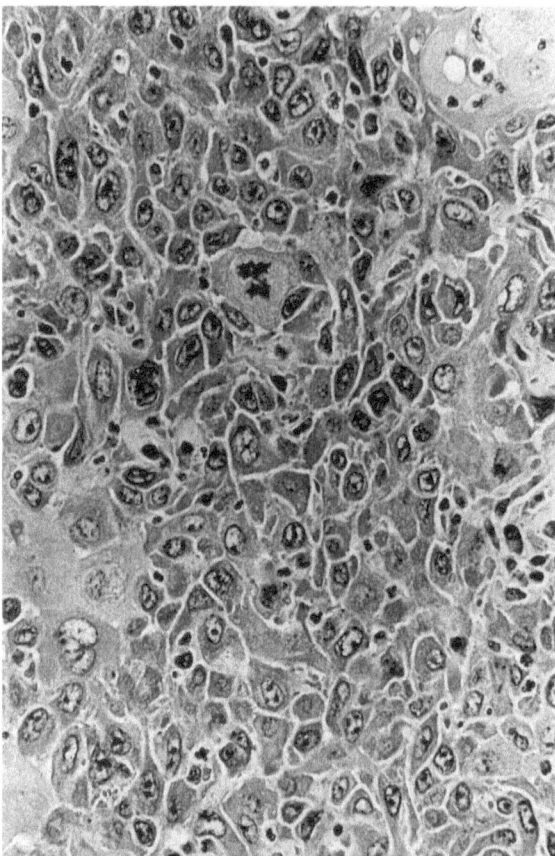

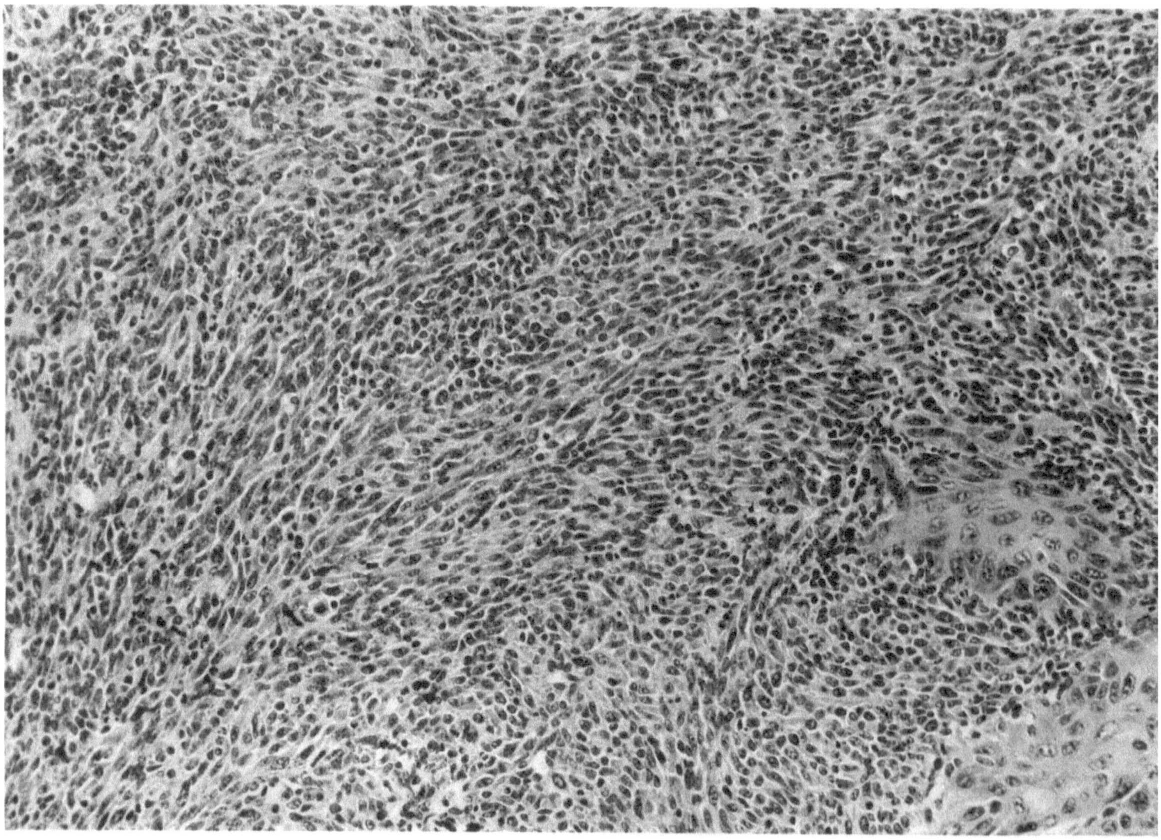

Ultrastructure

Ultrastructural studies are useful to diagnose poorly differentiated squamous cell carcinomas. In comparison with normal epidermal squamous cells, the number of desmosomes is reduced in these tumor cells. The most characteristic feature is the presence of intercellular desmosomes. Bundles of electron-dense tonofilaments are characteristic of squamous cell carcinomas (Figs. 52 and 53). Keratohyaline granules are occasionally seen.

The nuclei have an oval or irregulary shaped nuclear membrane, and aggregated chromatin may be seen in the nucleoplasm. Cytoplasmic membranes are characterized by elaborate intercellular interdigitations. Less keratinizing or poorly differentiated tumors contain fewer desmosomes and tonofilaments (Fig. 54).

Differential Diagnose

Invasive growth breaking through the basement membrane, cellular polymorphism, structural atypism, frequent mitotic figures, and the presence of distant metastasis are obvious signs of malignancy. However, in the case of the keratinizing type, distinction from squamous cell papilloma and keratoacanthoma is sometimes difficult.

In the case of spindle cell carcinoma, the most important differential diagnostic problem is to distinguish this tumor from sarcomas of connective tissue origin. Also distinguishing nonkeratinizing squamous cell carcinoma from anaplastic

tumors of other tissue origin is sometimes difficult. In those cases, transitions between spindle and epithelial cells or the presence of single, partly keratinized cells are indicative of epidermal origin. The tumors sometime include a part of the pre-existing, differentated epithelium. Electron microscopic examination may be helpful in distinguishing between them. Existence of desmosomes, keratohyalin, or tonofilaments strongly supports the tumor being of squamous origin, although desmosomes are sometimes not detectable in the anaplastic type. New histochemical techniques are also available for detection of keratin or other marker materials in tumor tissue (Gown and Vogel 1984).

Biologic Features

Spontaneous squamous cell tumors in mice are rare. In general the prevalence of skin tumors does not exceed 1% (Bogovski 1979), although interstrain differences in tumor incidence is well-known. However, skin tumors can be easily induced by topical application of chemical carcinogens such as polycyclic aromatic hydrocarbons, N-nitroso compounds, and others. Up to this time, carcinogenic hydrocarbons, e. g., 7,12-dimethylbenz[a]anthracene (DMBA), benzo(a)-pyrene (BP), and 3-methylcholanthrene (3-MC), have been the substances most used for induction of skin tumors in mice (Zackheim 1973). It is also reported that tumor incidence is affected by the period of the hair cycle, type of carcinogens employed, dose levels, and vehicles used as well as species and strains of animals.

Most chemical carcinogens applied topically induce squamous cell tumors predominantly. Several authors report that all varieties of skin tumors can be induced by chemical carcinogens through application routes other than topical, and they can also be induced by irradiation with ultraviolet light or beta particles (Morison et al. 1986; Zackheim 1973). It is reported that malignant conversion of mouse skin tumors is increased by strong mutagenic agents, such as N-methyl-N'-nitro-N-nitrosoguanidine (MNNG), topically applied after DMBA initiation and short-term promotion with 12-0-tetradecanoyl-phorbol-13-acetate (TPA) (Hennings et al. 1983).

In mice, both squamous cell papilloma and keratoacanthoma may undergo malignant transformation into squamous cell carcinoma (Zackheim 1973). Occasionally, squamous cell carcinomas

◄ **Fig. 49** *(upper left)*. Keratinizing squamous cell carcinoma, skin, SENCAR mouse. The vascular stroma is covered by several layers of epithelial cells with acantholytic cells and debris, forming a pseudo-adenomatous structure. BP followed by TPA; H and E, × 80

Fig. 50 *(below)*. Anaplastic squamous cell carcinoma of spindle cell type (spindle cell carcinoma), skin, SENCAR mouse. The tumor is composed of bundles of spindle cells without distinct cell borders, and nuclei are elongated but highly variable in shape and size. Small areas of epidermal differentiation with continuous transition to spindle cells are evident. BP followed by TPA; H and E, × 300

Fig. 51 *(upper right)*. Anaplastic squamous cell carcinoma, skin, SENCAR mouse. The tumor is composed of markedly irregular, mostly large cells. The nuclei vary in size and shape. A focus of squamous differentiation is observed. DMBA followed by TPA; H and E, × 300

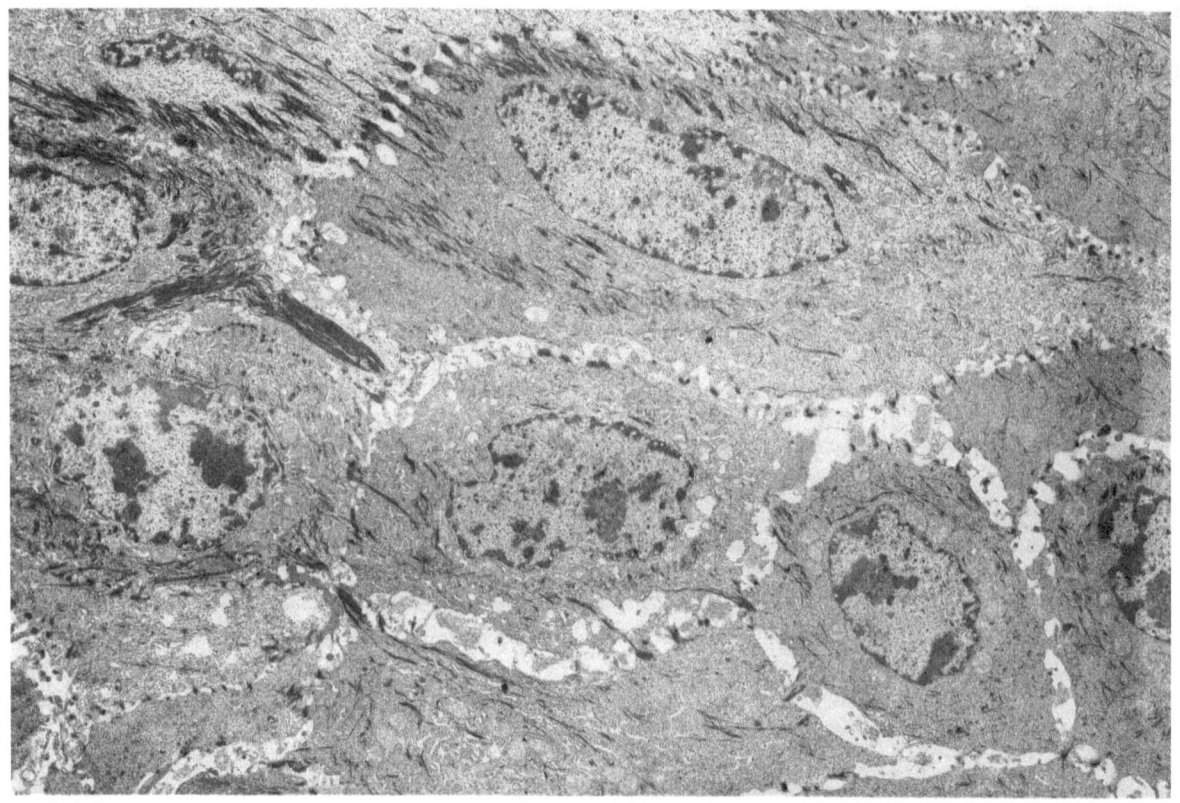

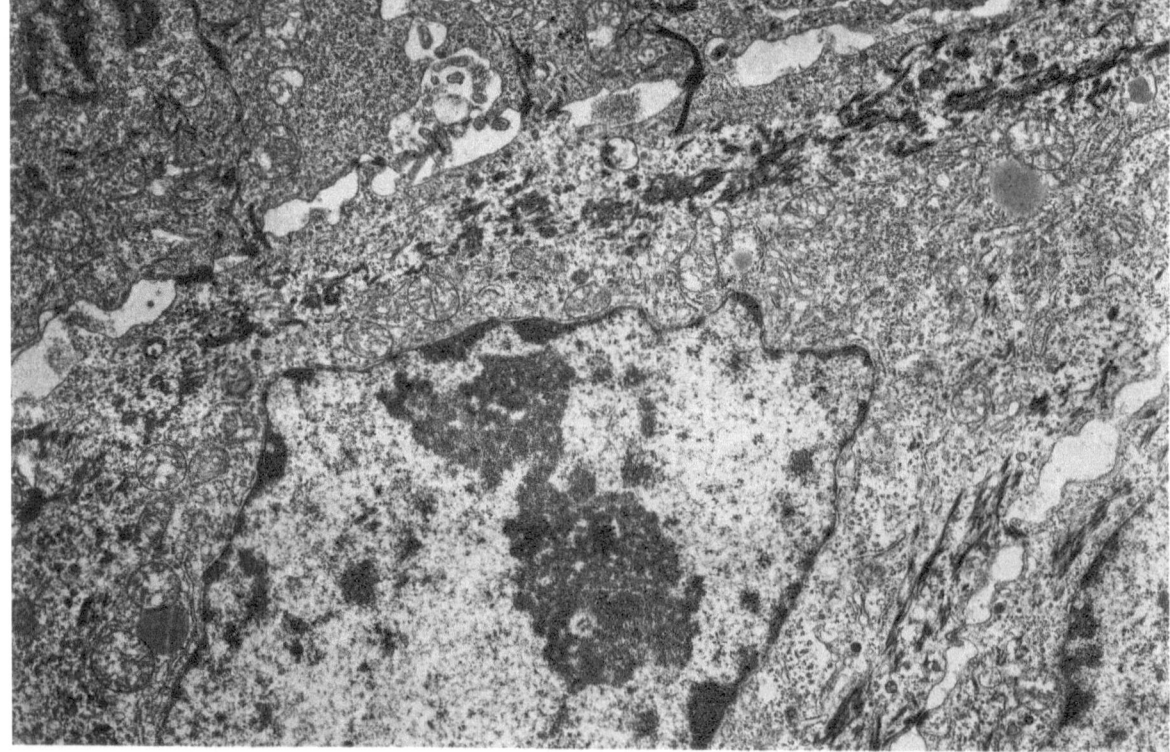

Fig. 52 *(above).* Well-differentiated keratinizing squamous cell carcinoma, skin, ICR mouse. Numerous electron-dense tonofibrils are apparent, many of which are converging perpendicularly onto desmosomes at the apices of cell processes. 3-Methylcholanthrene; TEM, ×8000

Fig. 53 *(below).* Keratinizing squamous cell carcinoma, skin, ICR mouse. Cells are attached by desmosomes. Some lines of tonofibrils converge on desmosomes. The cell contains lipid droplets and numerous glycogen granules. 3-MC; TEM, ×8000

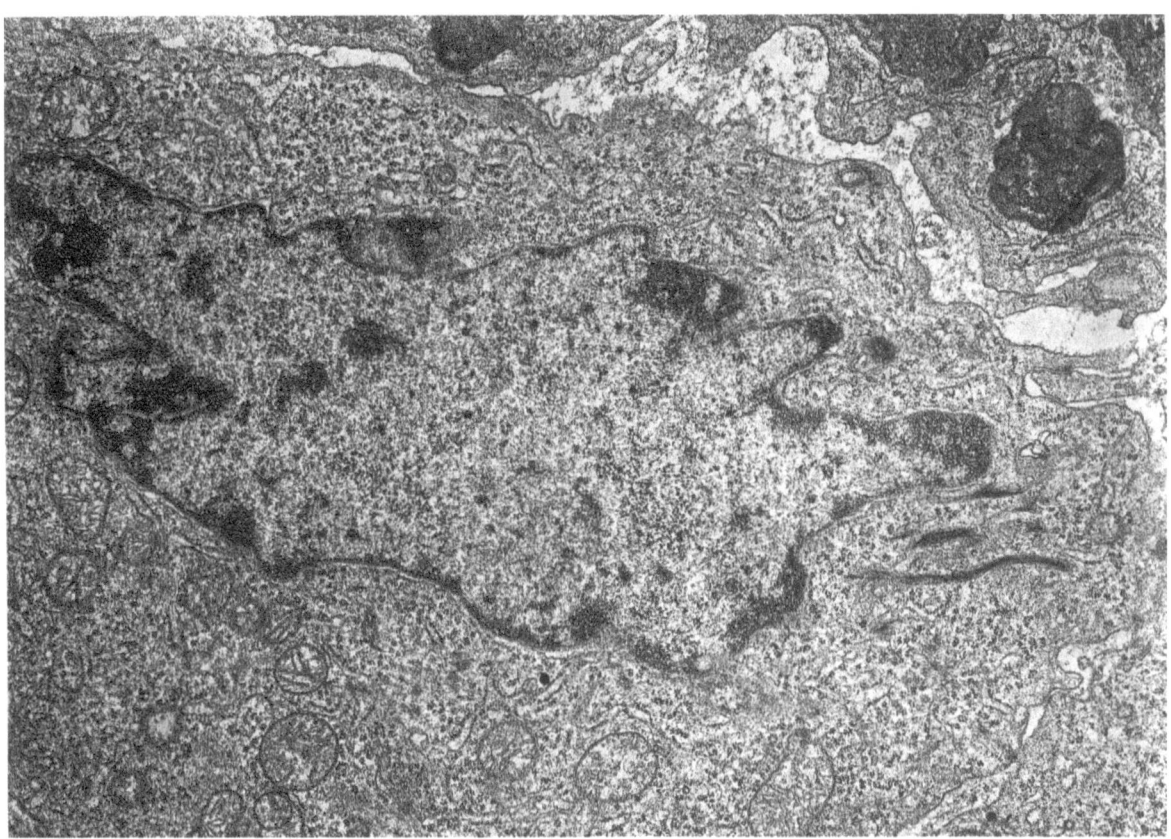

Fig.54. A cell of an anaplastic squamous cell carcinoma, skin, ICR mouse. Note a small number of tonofibrils in the cytoplasm, desmosomes are incompletely developed. 3-MC; TEM, × 12000

will arise from the edge of ulcers and normal or slightly hyperplastic areas without the prior formation of papillomas. The earliest alterations are characterized by focal proliferation at the basal part of benign tumors of hyperplastic squamous epithelium at the edge of the ulcer, which may undergo atypia. These altered foci invade into the subcutis as nests of squamous cells forming whorls of keratin, and as cords or small groups of dark-staining, anaplastic epithelial cells.

The central portion of enlarged tumors becomes depressed and the margins elevated. Fusion with adjacent papules in common. Continued growth results in a firm, centrally ulcerated tumor with elevated borders characteristic of squamous cell carcinoma.

Comparison with Other Species

In general, spontaneous occurrence of skin tumors in rodents is uncommon. However, chemical carcinogens can easily induce all varieties of skin tumors (Bogovski 1979). Histologically, most of the skin tumors observed in mice treated with chemical carcinogens are squamous cell tumors, whereas rats mainly develop basal cell tumors (Squire et al. 1978). Mouse skin is more sensitive to carcinogenic hydrocarbons than rat skin, but less sensitive to N-nitroso compounds (Bock 1983). The reason for this difference in sensitivity is unknown but may be due to interspecies differences in metabolism. In other species of animals such as hamsters, guinea pigs, rabbits, cats, dogs, and primates, spontaneous occurrence of skin tumors is also uncommon (Squire et al. 1978).

References

Bock FG (1983) Comparative anatomy and function of skin as related to experimental chemical carcinogenesis. Prog Exp Tumor Res 26: 5–17

Bogovski P (1979) Tumours of the skin. In: Turusov VS (ed) Pathology of tumours in laboratory animals, vol II. Tumours of the mouse. IARC Lyon, pp 1–41 (IARC Sci Publ no 23)

Gown AM, Vogel AM (1984) Anti-intermediate filament monoclonal antibodies: tissue-specific tools in tumor diagnosis. Surv Synth Pathol Res 3: 369-385

Hennings H, Shores R, Wenk ML, Spangler EF, Tarone R, Yuspa SH (1983) Malignant conversion of mouse skin tumours is increased by tumour initiators and unaffected by tumour promoters. Nature 304: 67-69

Morison WL, Jerdan MS, Hoover TL, Farmer ER (1986) UV radiation-induced tumors in haired mice: identification as squamous cell carcinomas. JNCI 77: 1155-1162

Squire RA, Goodman DG, Valerio MG, Fredrickson T, Strandberg JD, Levitt MH, Lingeman CH, Harshbarger JC, Dawe CJ (1978) Tumors. In: Benirschke K, Garner FM, Jones TC (eds) Pathology of laboratory animals, vol 2. Springer, Berlin, Heidelberg, New York, pp 1051-1283

Zackheim HS (1983) Tumours of the skin. In: Turusov VS (ed) Pathology of tumours in laboratory animals, vol 1. Tumours of the rat (pt 1). IARC, Lyon, pp 1-21 (IARC Sci Publ no 5)

Squamous Cell Carcinoma Arising in Induced Papilloma, Skin, Mouse

Sabine Rehm, Jerrold M. Ward, and Deborah E. Devor

Synonyms. Squamous cell carcinoma; malignant transformation of papilloma.

Gross Appearance

Most frequently, squamous cell carcinomas are studied in skin-painting studies (complete carcinogenesis or initiation-promotion regimens) and are identified as arising from induced papillomas, keratoacanthomas, or epidermal inclusion cysts (Shubik et al. 1953; Foulds 1954). Squamous cell carcinomas are also seen developing within the epidermis without preceding neoplastic lesions or in association with ulcers (Bogovski 1979; Klein-Szanto 1984; Knutsen et al. 1986). Characteristic clinical features of squamous cell carcinomas developing from papillomas are loss of the papillomatous stalk and wartlike appearance, followed by ulceration of the papillomas and crater formation. The borders are elevated and poorly demarcated (Bogovski 1979; Knutsen et al. 1986). The neoplasms grow rapidly and may bleed severely.

Microscopic Features

Induced squamous cell carcinomas may develop deep at the base of benign skin tumors and are initially not observable on gross examination until they appear as large papillomas. Histologically, areas of atypia and dysplasia can be found in the benign tumor (Fig. 55) indicating malignant transformation into a squamous cell carcinoma (Aldaz et al. 1987). Later, squamous cell carcinomas may display a growth pattern with or without keratinization or anaplastic features (Bogovski 1979). Most frequently, keratinizing squamous cell carcinomas are observed arising from papillomas (Figs. 56-58), whereas anaplastic types seem to arise from areas of epidermal hyperplasia or ulcers (Klein-Szanto 1984; Knutsen et al. 1986). Kruszewski et al. (1987) graded dedifferentiation of squamous cell carcinomas according to the extent of keratinization, mitotic index, and degree of cellular atypia as grade I-III. The majority of the squamous cell carcinomas studied were well-differentiated and classified as grade I. Induced squamous cell carcinomas, especially those resulting from fewer doses of TPA following DMBA initiation (Diwan et al. 1985), readily invade the underlying layers (Fig. 57) and

Fig. 55 *(upper left)*. Papilloma with dysplasia arising in ▶ skin of SENCAR mouse initiated with DMBA and promoted with TPA. Loss of regular stratification of cells, disturbed cornification, and increased cellular atypia. H and E, × 100

Fig. 56 *(lower left)*. Squamous cell carcinoma developing at base of papilloma (gross diagnosis) in skin of SENCAR mouse initiatad with DMBA and promoted by TPA. H and E, × 25

Fig. 57 *(upper right)*. Keratinizing squamous cell carcinoma progressing from papilloma as shown in Fig. 56. Poorly differentiated cell clusters invade muscular layer *(arrow)*. H and E, × 250

Fig. 58 *(lower right)*. Squamous cell carcinoma, skin, SENCAR mouse. Anaplastic cells growing in sheets. Squamous cell *(arrow)*. H and E, × 250

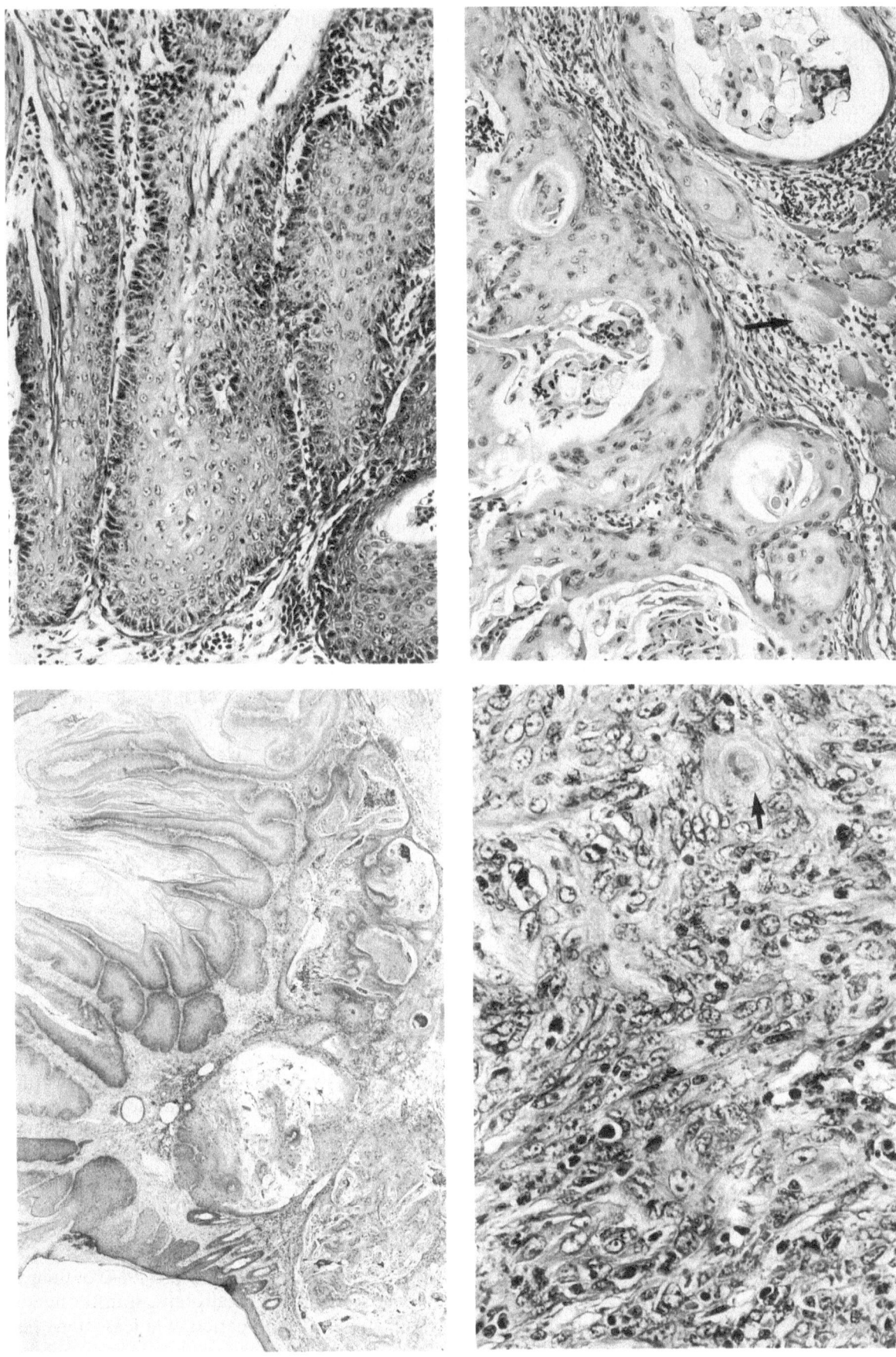

frequently metastasize to regional lymph nodes and the lung (Bogovski 1979).

The gross and histologic features of squamous cell carcinomas arising from induced benign tumors in other experimental systems (such as ultraviolet radiation carcinogenesis with or without the application of carcinogens, promotors, or photosensitizing substances) may be very similar to the neoplastic progression observed in mouse skin-painting studies (Kligman and Kligman 1981; Kripke et al. 1981; Fry and Ley 1984).

Differential Diagnosis

Trichoepitheliomas may sometimes have less well-developed hair follicle formations with extensive central keratinous cores that could be mistaken for a squamous cell carcinoma. Basal cell carcinomas occasionally possess foci of keratinization; however, mitotic figures are usually rare, and the cells are closely packed in uniform sheets (Bogovski 1979). Sarcomas, and in particular fibrosarcomas, have to be differentiated from the rare forms of anaplastic carcinoma. Both neoplasms may be morphologically indistinguishable, but sarcomas are more frequently induced by subcutaneous carcinogen application (Bogovski 1979).

Biologic Features

Natural History. Skin-painting experiments in mice are considered a valubale model with which to study the basic mechanisms of carcinogenesis and to test tumor initiating and/or tumor promoting properties of chemical compounds (Boutwell et al. 1981; Fürstenberger and Marks 1983; Slaga 1984; Bull et al. 1986; Nowell 1986). Based on the tumor initiator 7,12-dimethylbenz[*a*]anthracene (DMBA) and the tumor promoter 12-0-tetradecanoylphorbol-13-acetate (TPA), special mouse strains or stocks were selectively developed that are particularly susceptible to the development of proliferative skin lesions (Slaga 1986; Fischer et al. 1987). These include the SENCAR (sensitive to carcinogenesis) outbred stock and SSIN/UTSP (sensitive SENCAR inbred/University of Texas Science Park) inbred strain. The enhanced response of these mice in the two-stage carcinogenesis model is probably related to the sensitive reaction to TPA (Reiners et al. 1984; Lewis and Adams 1987). SENCAR and other strains and stocks of mice may also develop benign and malignant skin tumors when treated with TPA only (Ward et al. 1986b). If other initiators or promoters are used, papilloma and carcinoma formation in the skin of SENCAR mice can be comparable to those seen in other mouse strains (Slaga 1986; Van Duuren et al. 1986).

Etiology and Pathogenesis. A single application of a complete carcinogen by various routes may cause a genetic alteration of epidermal cells, providing the basis for neoplastic changes of the skin by repetitive local applications of promoters (Loehrke et al. 1983; Burns et al. 1984; Fürstenberger and Marks 1983; Quintanilla et al. 1986). Aldaz et al. (1987) reported a positive correlation between the histologic and cytogenetic features of papillomas at different times during tumor progression. Early hyperplastic lesions were diploid whereas dysplastic changes were associated with hyperdiploid or aneuploid cells. These findings indicate that chromosomal abnormalities are probably of major importance in the sequence of tumor progession (Conti et al. 1986; Nowell 1986). Balmain et al. (1984) demonstrated that induced mouse papillomas possess an activated Harvey-*ras* gene.

In various modifications of the experimental procedure, progression can be demonstrated from hyperplastic and benign neoplastic lesions, to malignant processes with tissue invasion, and, finally, to the formation of distant metastases (Foulds 1954; Klein-Szanto 1984; Hennings et al. 1986; Diwan et al. 1985).

Frequency. In many experiments, results rely on gross clinical observations of skin lesions, with histological evaluations only on occasional, random biopsies and endstage carcinomas. Only in the last few years have more systematic histologic studies been carried out, indicating that early malignant changes are not observable by gross inspection (Knutsen et al. 1986; Ward et al. 1986a). Up to 50% of the grossly identified papillomas, as well as some nonneoplastic lesions (diagnosed clinically) had to be considered carcinomas following histologic evaluation, especially in SENCAR mice (Knutsen et al. 1986). Such a finding is of fundamental importance since carcinomas are an important endpoint in skin-painting studies (Kruszewski et al. 1987), and it was thought that only 5%–10% (O'Connell et al. 1986) or 10%–30% (Klein-Szanto 1984) of the papillomas underwent malignant transformation within an observation period of at least 50 weeks.

There is also evidence, however, that not all papillomas might represent true neoplasms (Shubik 1984) but could be regarded as papillomatous hyperplasias.

Many papillomas regress upon removal of the promoter in those experiments in which the promoter was applied continuously over many weeks (Burns et al. 1976; Hennings et al. 1985), and the papillomas do not recur when promotion is resumed (Reddy et al. 1987). When the promotor is applied for a shorter time period, fewer papillomas develop but do not regress (Diwan et al. 1985), indicating a fundamental difference in papilloma types. Indeed, histopathologic and cytogenetic evaluations show qualitative differences between papillomas (Reddy and Fialkow 1983; Aldaz et al. 1987).

Comparison with Other Species

Among the first studies from which skin painting experiments developed were repeated applications of coal tar on the skin of rabbits (Rous et al. 1941). Shubik (1950) studied skin tumor promotion in mice, rats, rabbits, and guinea pigs, finding that mice are more susceptible to tumor promotion using TPA. Resistance of other species, including hamsters and mini pigs, to two-stage skin carcinogenesis are probably related to the use of TPA as the promoting agent (Reiners et al. 1984).

Squamous cell carcinomas in other species often arise de novo, and there is a general tendency for these neoplasms to develop in areas of unpigmented skin, especially if exposed to sunlight (Witkop 1981; Stannard and Pulley 1978). In humans, several different types of precancerous epidermal lesions have been recognized that may become malignant and others that always become malignant (Laerum 1981).

In goats, squamous cell carcinomas may be associated with papillomas of the udder (Stannard and Pulley 1978) and the "cancer eye" of cattle includes all stages of tumor progression of hyperplasias, papillomas, and squamous cell carcinomas (Stannard and Pulley 1978). The majority of these ocular carcinomas of cattle arise from the conjunctiva and cornea and are related to ultraviolet radiation. Similar proliferative lesions of the eye have been observed in horses and cats (Wilcock 1985).

Squamous cell carcinomas progressing from some viral-induced papillomas are seen in animals (Shope papillomavirus systems) and in humans (zur Hausen 1981). However, virally induced skin papillomas in cattle, warts in humans, and oral papillomatosis in dogs almost never progress to carcinomas (Laerum 1981; Stannard and Pulley 1978; Moulton 1978; Yager and Scott 1985).

References

Aldaz CM, Conti CJ, Klein-Szanto AJP, Slaga TJ (1987) Progressive dysplasia and aneuploidy are hallmarks of mouse skin papillomas: relevance to malignancy. Proc Natl Acad Sci USA 84: 2029–2032

Balmain A, Ramsden M, Bowden GT, Smith J (1984) Activation of the mouse cellular Harvey-*ras* gene in chemically induced benign skin papillomas. Nature 307: 658–660

Bogovski P (1979) Tumours of the skin. In: Turusov VS (ed) Pathology of tumours in laboratory animals, vol 11. Tumours of the mouse. IARC, Lyon, pp 1–41 (IARC Sci Publ no 23)

Boutwell RK, Urbach F, Carpenter G (1981) Experimental models. In: Laerum OD, Iversen OH (eds) Biology of skin cancer (excluding melanomas). UICC, Geneva, pp 109–123 (UICC technical report series, vol 63)

Bull RJ, Robinson M, Laurie RD (1986) Association of carcinoma yield with early papilloma development in SENCAR mice. Environ Health Perspect 68: 11–17

Burns FJ, Vanderlaan M, Sivak A, Albert RE (1976) Regression kinetics of mouse skin papillomas. Cancer Res 36: 1422–1427

Burns FJ, Albert RE, Altshuler B (1984) Cancer progression in mouse skin. In: Slaga TJ (ed) Mechanisms of tumor promotion, vol II. Tumor promotion and skin carcinogenesis. CRC, Boca Raton, pp 17–39

Conti CJ, Aldaz CM, O'Connell J, Klein-Szanto AJP, Slaga TJ (1986) Aneuploidy, an early event in mouse skin tumor development. Carcinogenesis 7: 1845–1848

Diwan BA, Ward JM, Henneman J, Wenk ML (1985) Effects of shortterm exposure to the tumor promoter, 12-0-tetradecanoylphorbol-13-acetate on skin carcinogenesis in SENCAR mice. Cancer Lett 26: 177–184

Fischer SM, O'Connell JF, Conti CJ, Tacker KC, Fries JW, Patrick KE, Adams LM, Slaga TJ (1987) Characterization of an inbred strain of the SENCAR mouse that is highly sensitive to phorbol esters. Carcinogenesis 8: 421–424

Foulds L (1954) The experimental study of tumor progression: a review. Cancer Res 14: 327–339

Fry RJM, Ley RD (1984) Ultraviolet radiation carcinogenesis. In: Slaga TJ (ed) Mechanisms of tumor promotion, vol II. Tumor promotion and skin carcinogenesis. CRC, Boca Raton, pp 73–96

Fürstenberger G, Marks F (1983) Growth stimulation and tumor promotion in skin. J Invest Dermatol 81 [Suppl]: 157s–161s

Hennings H, Shores R, Mitchell P, Spangler EF, Yuspa SH (1985) Induction of papillomas with a high probability of conversion to malignancy. Carcinogenesis 6: 1607–1610

Hennings H, Spangler EF, Shores R, Mitchell P, Devor D, Shamsuddin AKM, Elgjo KM, Yuspa SH (1986) Malignant conversion and metastasis of mouse skin tumors: a comparison of SENCAR and CD-1 mice. Environ Health Perspect 68: 69–74

Klein-Szanto AJP (1984) Morphological evaluation of tumor promoter effects on mammalian skin. In: Slaga TJ (ed) Mechanisms of tumor promotion, vol II. Tumor promotion and skin carcinogenesis. CRC, Boca Raton, pp 41–72

Kligman LH, Kligman AM (1981) Histogenesis and progression of ultraviolet light-induced tumors in hairless mice. JNCI 67: 1289–1297

Knutsen GL, Kovatch RM, Robinson M (1986) Gross and microscopic lesions in the female SENCAR mouse skin and lung in tumor initiation and promotion studies. Environ Health Perspect 68: 91–104

Kripke M, Urbach F, Witkop C (1981) Ultraviolet radiation carcinogenesis. In: Laerum OD, Iversen OH (eds) Biology of skin cancer. UICC, Geneva, pp 195–222 (UICC technical report series, vol 63)

Kruszewski FH, Conti CJ, DiGiovanni J (1987) Characterization of skin tumor promotion and progression by chrysarobin in SENCAR mice. Cancer Res 47: 3783–3790

Laerum OD (1981) Skin cancer in man. Classification. In: Laerum OD, Iversen OH (eds) Biology of skin cancer. UICC, Geneva, pp 73–75 (UICC technical report series, vol 63)

Lewis JG, Adams DO (1987) Early inflammatory changes in the skin of SENCAR and C57BL/6 mice following exposure to 12-0-tetradecanoylphorbol-13-acetate. Carcinogenesis 8: 889–898

Loehrke H, Schweizer J, Dederer E, Hesse B, Rosenkranz G, Goerttler K (1983) On the persistence of tumor initiation in two-stage carcinogenesis on mouse skin. Carcinogenesis 4: 771–775

Moulton JE (1978) Tumors of the alimentary tract. In: Moulton JE (ed) Tumors in domestic animals. University of California Press, Berkeley, pp 240–272

Nowell PC (1986) Mechanisms of tumor progression. Cancer Res 46: 2203–2207

O'Connell JF, Klein-Szanto AJP, DiGiovanni DM, Fries JW, Slaga TJ (1986) Enhanced malignant progression of mouse skin tumors by the free-radical generator benzoyl peroxide. Cancer Res 46: 2863–2865

Quintanilla M, Brown K, Ramsden M, Balmain A (1986) Carcinogen-specific mutation and amplification of Ha-ras during mouse skin carcinogenesis. Nature 322: 78–80

Reddy AL, Fialkow PJ (1983) Papillomas induced by initiation-promotion differ from those induced by carcinogen alone. Nature 304: 69–71

Reddy AL, Caldwell M, Fialkow PJ (1987) Sequential studies of skin tumorigenesis in phosphoglycerate kinase mosaic mice: effect of resumption of promotion on regressed papillomas. Cancer Res 47: 1947–1951

Reiners JJ, Nesnow S, Slaga TJ (1984) Murine susceptibility to two-stage skin carcinogenesis is influenced by the agent used for promotion. Carcinogenesis 5: 301–307

Rous P, Kidd JG (1941) Conditional neoplasms and sub-threshold neoplastic states. A study of the tar tumors of rabbits. J Exp Med 73: 365–389

Shubik P (1950) Studies on the promoting phase in the stages of carcinogenesis in mice, rats, rabbits and guinea pigs. Cancer Res 10: 113–117

Shubik P (1984) Progression and promotion. JNCI 73: 1005–1011 (editorial)

Shubik P, Baserga R, Ritchie AC (1953) The life and progression of induced skin tumors in mice. Br J Cancer 7: 342–351

Slaga TJ (1984) Mechanisms involved in two-stage carcinogenesis in mouse skin. In: Slaga TJ (ed) Mechanisms of tumor promotion, vol II. Tumor promotion and skin carcinogenesis. CRC, Boca Raton, pp 1–16

Slaga TJ (1986) SENCAR mouse skin tumorigenesis model versus other strains and stocks of mice. Environ Health Perspect 68: 27–32

Stannard AA, Pulley LT (1978) Tumors of the skin and soft tissues. In: Moulton JE (ed) Tumors in domestic animals. University of California Press, Berkeley, pp 16–70

Van Duuren BL, Melchionne S, Seidmann I (1986) Phorbol myristate acetate and catechol as skin cocarcinogens in SENCAR mice. Environ Health Perspect 68: 33–38

Ward JM, Rehm S, Devor D, Hennings H, Wenk ML (1986a) Differential carcinogenic effects of intraperitoneal initiation with 7,12-dimethylbenz[a]anthracene or urethane and topical promotion with 12-0-tetradecanoylphorbol-13-acetate in skin and internal tissues of female SENCAR and BALB/c mice. Environ Health Perspect 68: 61–68

Ward JM, Quander R, Devor D, Wenk ML, Spangler EF (1986b) Pathology of aging female SENCAR mice used as controls in skin two-stage carcinogenesis studies. Environ Health Perspect 68: 81–89

Wilcock BP (1985) The eye and ear. In: Jubb KVF, Kennedy PC, Palmer N (eds) Pathology of domestic animals, vol 1, 3rd edn. Academic, Orlando FLA, p 387

Witkop CJ (1981) Skin cancer in man. Genetic factors. In: Laerum OD, Iversen OH (eds) Biology of skin cancer (excluding melanomas). UICC, Geneva, pp 67–72 (UICC technical report series, report 15, vol 63)

Yager JA, Scott DW (1985) The skin and appendages. In: Jubb KVF, Kennedy PC, Palmer N (eds) Pathology of domestic animals, vol 1, 3rd edn. Academic, Orlando FLA, p 506

Zur Hausen H (1981) Viral carcinogenesis. In: Laerum OD, Iversen OH (eds) Biology of skin cancer (excluding melanomas). UICC, Geneva, pp 228–237 (UICC technical report series, report 15, vol 63)

Basal Cell Carcinoma, Skin, Rat

Eva Szabo and Janos Sugar

Synonyms: Basal cell epithelioma; basalioma; Krompecher's carcinoma basocellulare; rodent carcinoma; basal cell tumor.

Gross Appearance

Basal cell carcinomas are first visible as dome-shaped, transparent, and soft papules of pale gray or scarlet to pink color. In the early stage of tumor induction, when about 2–3 cm in diameter, they have a smooth and shining surface. During further stages of development the surface becomes verrucous and covered with keratin. The marginal parts spread laterally, and the central part extends deeper but remains connected with the overlying skin which is mobile over the connective and muscular tissues.

In the final stage of tumor development the tumor center becomes necrotic and ulcerated and is covered by bleeding, necrotic and purulent crust. The base of the ulcer is dense, brownish-red, and finely nodular. At the tumor margins are chains of soft nodules. Basal cell carcinomas usually range from 6 to 10 cm in diameter and from 1 to 2 cm in thickness (Fig. 59).

Microscopic Features

Basal cell carcinoma is characterized by a peculiar and complex histologic picture. The histologic pattern changes and undergoes organoid differentiation during tumor growth. In the early stage, i.e., in the so-called incipient basalioma stage, foci of indistinctive cuboidal and cylindrical cells appear in the basal layer of the epithelium. From these foci narrow, basal-type epithelial bundles grow into the dermis (Fig. 60). These tumor cells resemble embryonal-type epithelial cells. They have large, darkly staining, ovoid nuclei and scant, basophilic cytoplasm. *Solid basalioma* develops from these transformed epithelial bundles. It may appear as a dense tumor nodule with cylindrical tumor cell chains arranged in the so-called palisade pattern at the margins, and in the center, irregularly arranged, indistinctive tumor cells with littel basophilic cytoplasm and a large nucleus (Figs. 61–63). These neoplastic nodules are not well vascularized, the centrally located cells may become necrotic resulting in the development of a pseudocyst (Fig. 64). The solid basalioma foci may assume an adenoid structure. In this case, between the small tumor foci ar-

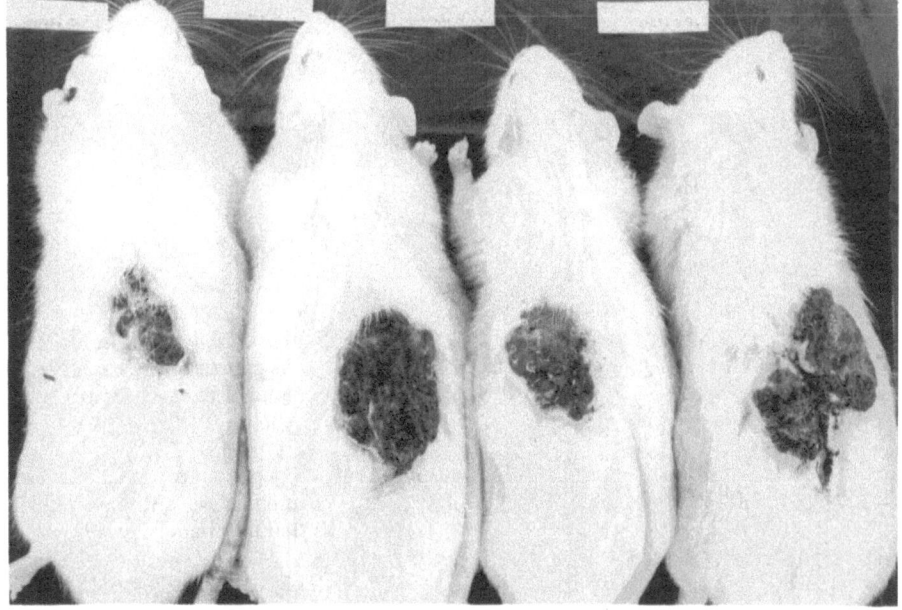

Fig. 59. Basal cell carcinoma induced on the dorsal skin of Wistar H-Riop male rats. The ulcerated, confluent tumor nodules are covered with a bleeding, necrotic crust

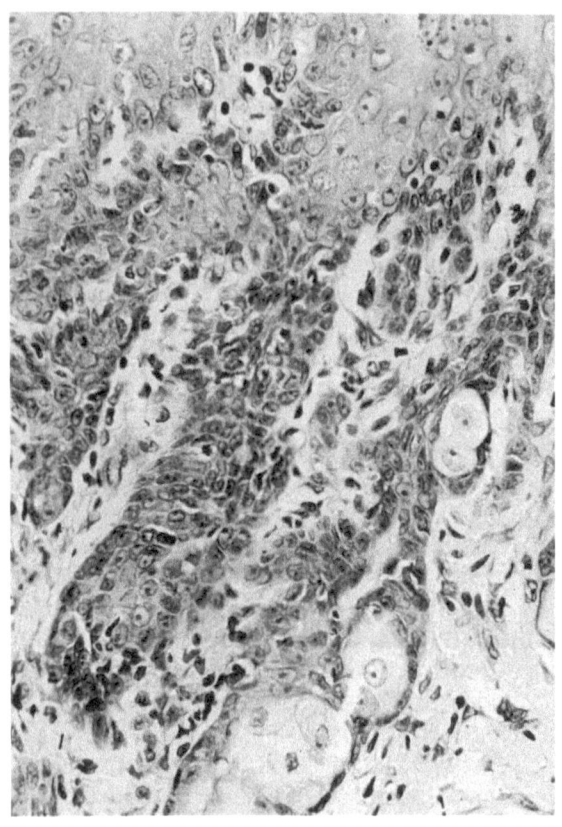

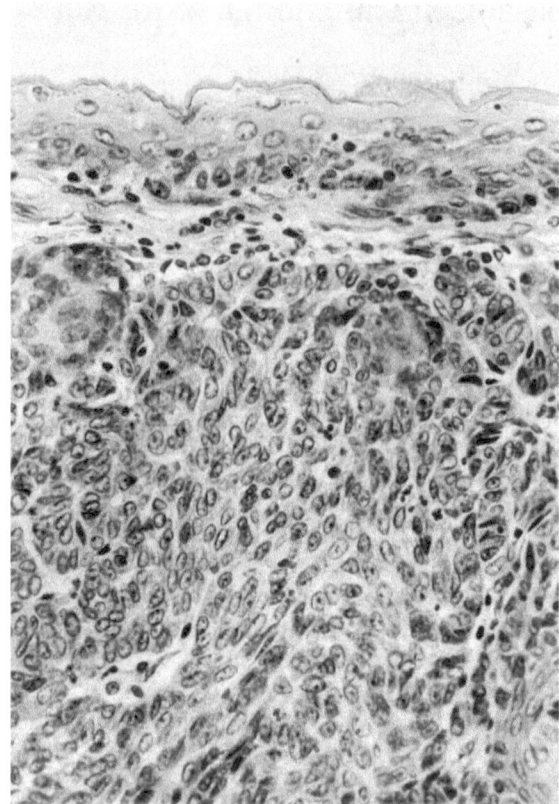

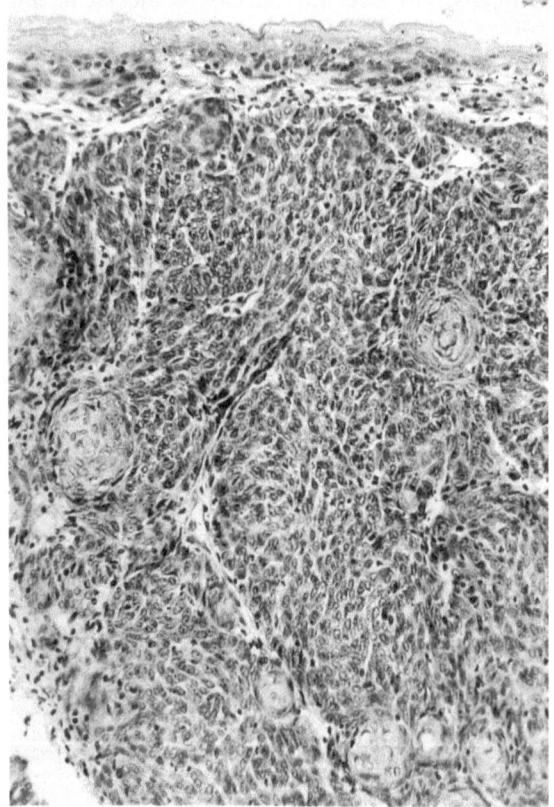

Fig. 60 *(upper left)*. Induced basal cell tumor, skin, rat. Initial growth of the basal type cells of the epidermis. Remnants of the sebaceous glands are still present. H and E, ×350

Fig. 61 *(lower left)*. Solid basalioma, skin, rat. Extensive tumor mass with basocellular character is present in the dermis. H and E, ×175

Fig. 62 *(upper right)*. Detail of the same tumor cells as in Fig. 61. H and E, ×350

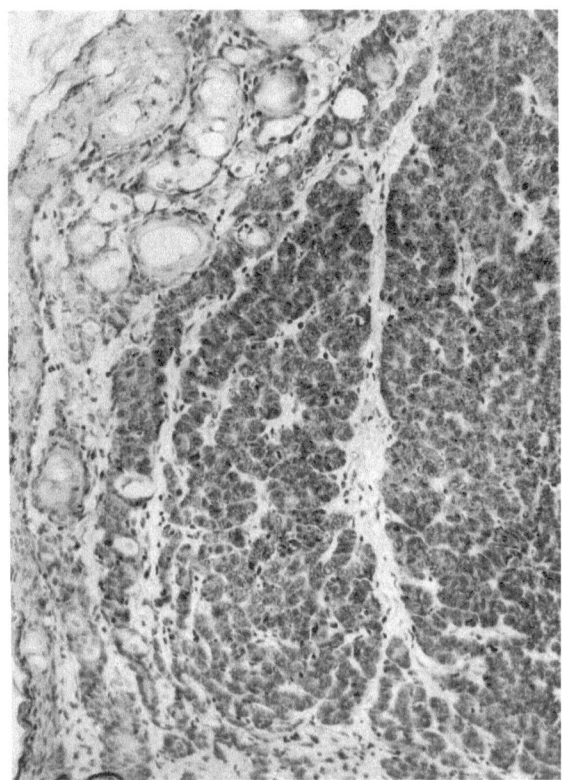

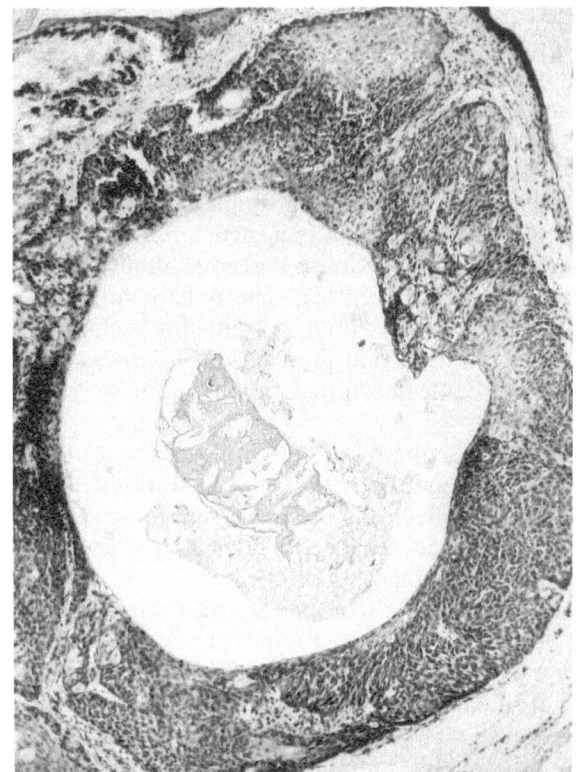

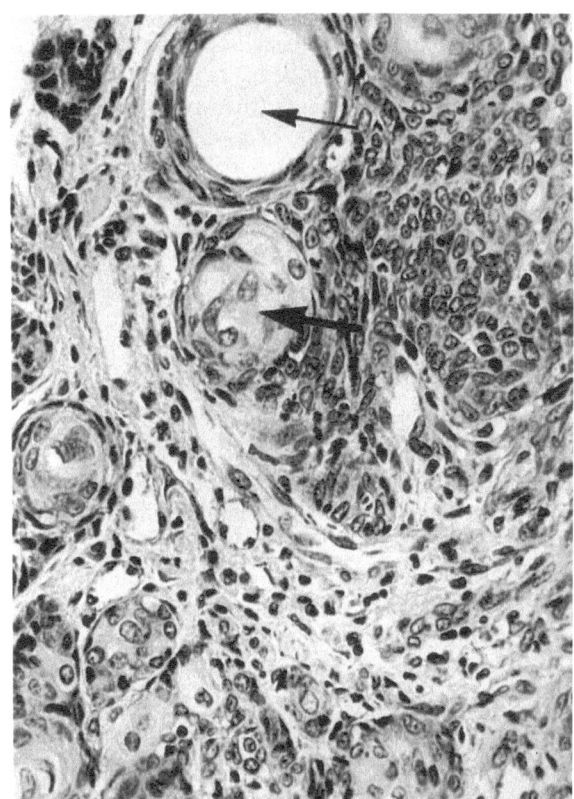

Fig. 63 *(upper left).* Basal cell carcinoma, skin, rat. The tumor cells are arrayed in rows. Note accumulation of sebaceous glands adjacent to the tumor. H and E, × 170

Fig. 64 *(upper right).* Basal cell carcinoma, skin, rat. Note pseudocyst. H and E, × 80

Fig. 65 *(lower right).* Pilosebaceous mixed basalioma, skin, rat. Solid basal cell focus adjacent to structure resembling hair follicle *(thin arrow)* and sebaceous cells *(thick arrow).* H and E, × 350

ranged in glandular pattern and the network of tumor bundles, stroma develops, consisting of fine connective tissue fibers and metachromatic mucoid ground substance.

In the rat, the most frequently observed tumor type is the *solid pilosebaceous mixed basalioma*. In these cases scattered in singles or in small groups in the basalioma foci, structures containing both hair follicle and sebaceous gland components develop (Fig. 65). These hair follicles contain keratin detectable by stains for trichohyalin and citrullin. Cell groups with foamy cytoplasm can be demonstrated to contain fat by specific stains.

In later stages of growth of the pilosebaceous tumor, either keratin cysts lined with stratified epithelium and filled with keratin or sebaceous cysts or hypertrophic sebaceous glands appear between the hair follicles.

Tumors originating from the outset from groups of hair follicles or hypertrophic sebaceous glands may not produce the basalioma component (e.g., trichofolliculoma or sebaceous adenoma), and squamous cell tumors may likewise be induced (e.g., trichoepithelioma). These tumors may also appear in true malignant forms (e.g., sebaceous gland carcinoma, squamous cell carcinoma).

Carcinomas containing both basal cell and squamous epithelial components (the so-called spino basocellular carcinomas) are extremely rare among the induced skin tumors of the rat. Induced rat basaliomas contain numerous mitotic cells; most of the mitoses are, however, not atypical.

Ultrastructure

Tumor cells resemble the basal cells of the embryonal epidermis (Fig. 66). Cell nuclei vary in size, and within one nucleus there are one or more irregular nucleoli. The cytoplasm is poor in organelles and contains fewer tonofilaments than the keratinocytes of the stratum spinosum (Fig. 67). A larger number of desmosomes are found where the cell membrane is undulated (Fig. 68). In areas of invasive growth the basal lamina may completely disappear (Fig. 69), but evidence of microinvasion can also be detected at the sites of gaps in the basal lamina through which cytoplasmic processes protrude into the connective tissue.

Using freeze fracture replicas, different intercellular junctions were found. In basocellular carcinomas, for instance, desmosomes and gap junctions appear, whereas in squamous cell carcinoma tight junctions could be seen (Horak et al. 1984).

Differential Diagnosis

Induced epithelial skin tumors of the rat have differing histologic structure; most of them, however, contain a basal cell component. Zackheim (1973) classified them as follows:

Basal cell tumors: basal cell carcinoma; trichoepithelioma; tricholemmoma; cylindroma; basosquamous carcinoma; pigmented basal cell neoplasm.

Squamous cell tumors: squamous cell papilloma; keratoacanthoma; squamous cell carcinoma.

Sebaceous gland tumors: sebaceous adenoma; sebaceous squamous cell carcinoma; sebaceous carcinoma.

The pure form of basalioma induced in the rat is extremely rare (Slaga et al. 1977; Sugar 1981; Zackheim et al. 1959; Zackheim 1962). As a rule, different forms showing pilosebaceous or squamous epithelial cell differentiation are present simultaneously (Rasmussen et al. 1983; Sugar 1981). Such mixed type basocellular tumors are rather difficult to distinguish, based on their histological structures, from other basal cell tumors.

Trichoepithelioma is characterized by a mosaic picture of tumor foci. The tumor cells have broad, eosinophilic cytoplasm and centrally seated, dark-stained nuclei. Structures suggesting the formation of hair follicles are usually present (see p. 56).

Tricholemmoma exhibits a diversity of lobular tumor foci. The large, clear, and basal tumor cells are characterized by glycogen filling the cytoplasm. Note that true basal cells contain little or no glycogen.

Cylindroma may be mimicked by basalioma if it undergoes hyaline degeneration.

Fig. 66 *(above).* Cells of basal cell tumor, skin, rat. The ▶ cytoplasm contains scanty tonofilaments and many ribosomes. Cell nuclei have irregular shape and contain a few nucleoli. TEM, × 5500

Fig. 67 *(below).* The cells of basal cell tumor, skin, rat, arrayed in palisade pattern. Note cylindrical cell forms, elongated nuclei, few tonofilaments, numerous ribosomes and mitochondria in the cytoplasm. Desmosomes are relatively few in number. TEM, × 4900

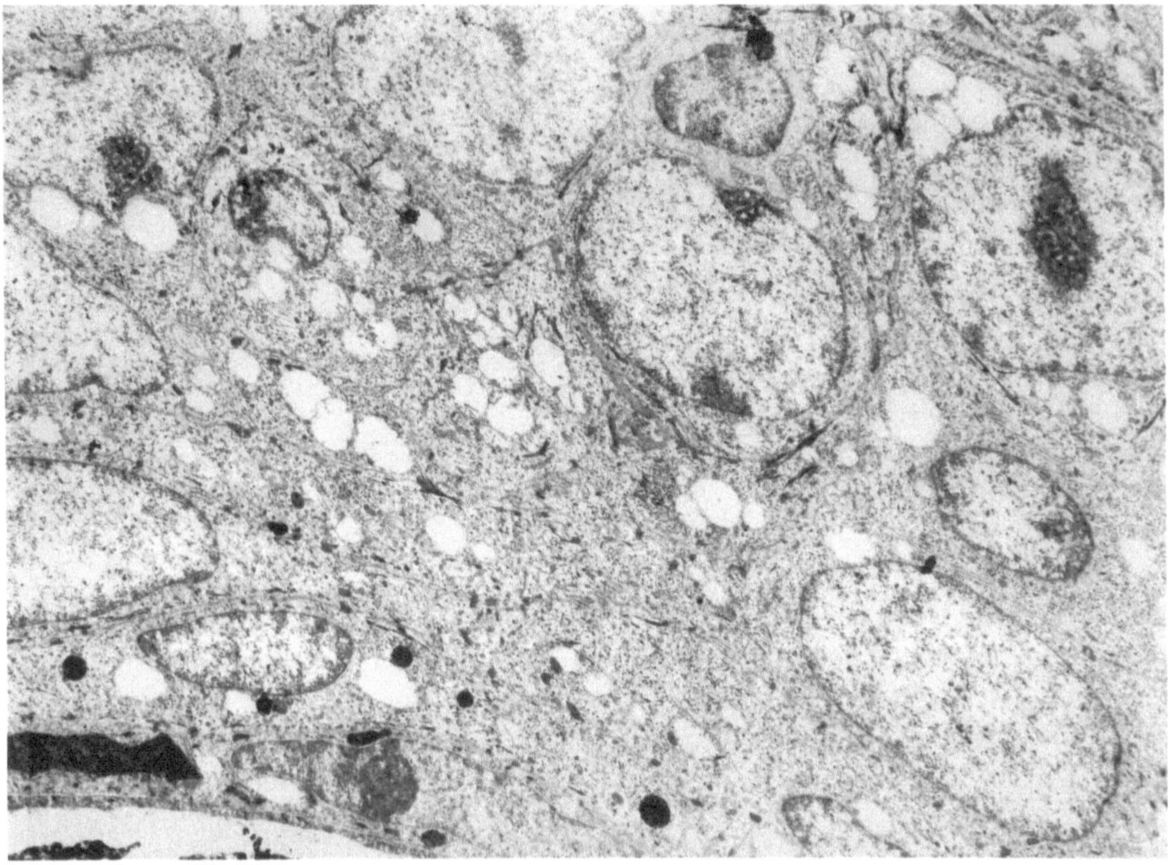

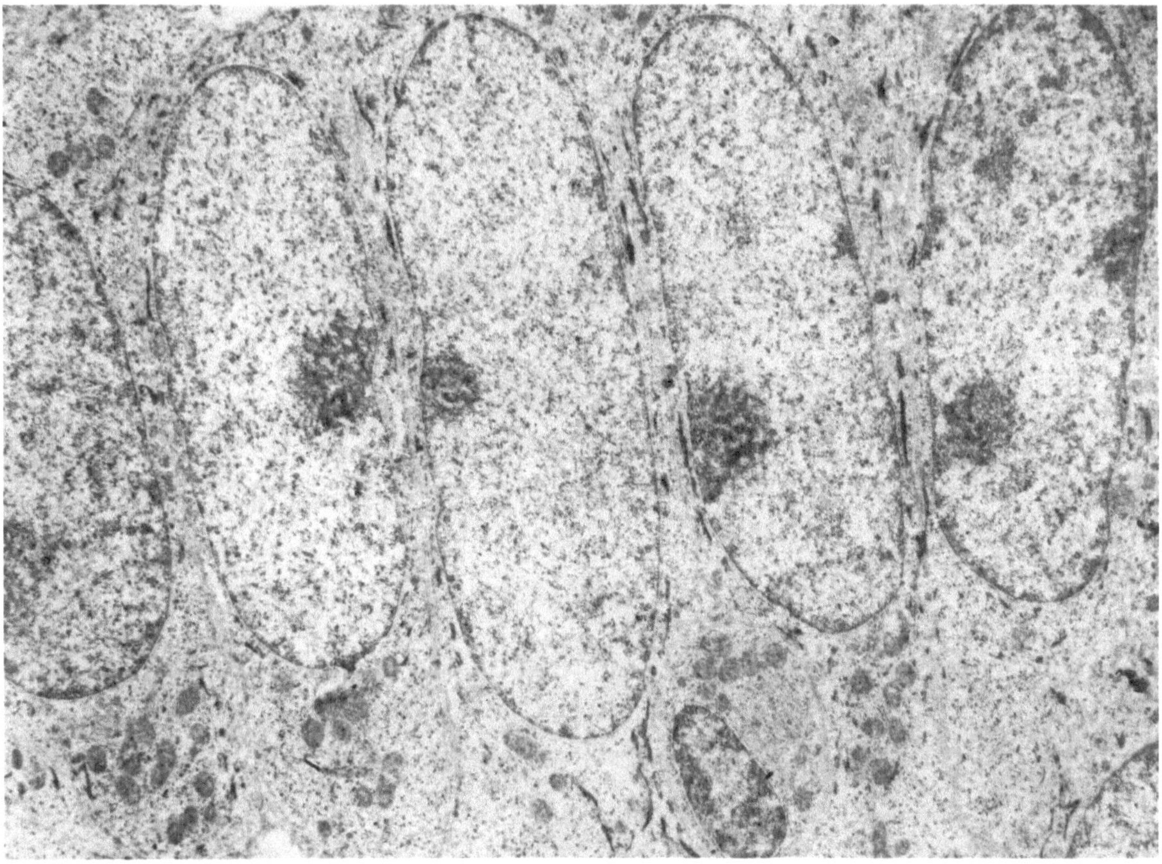

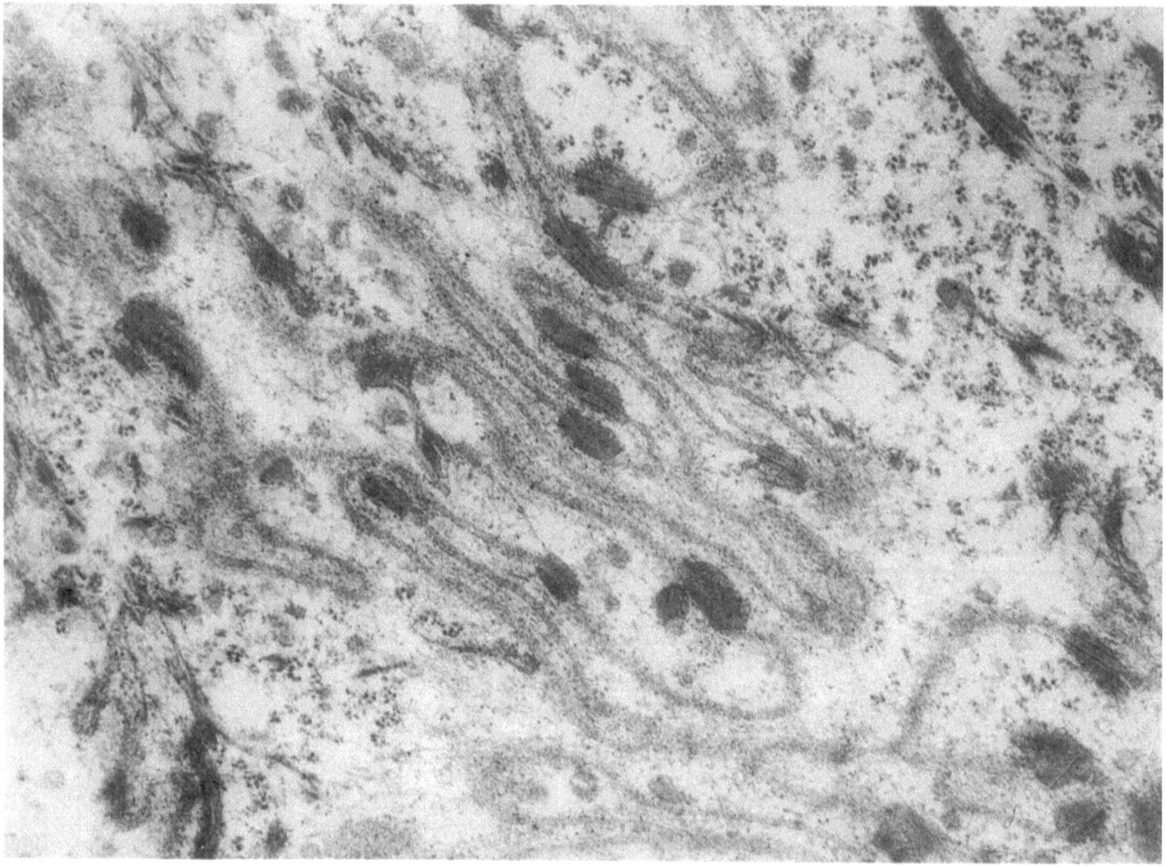

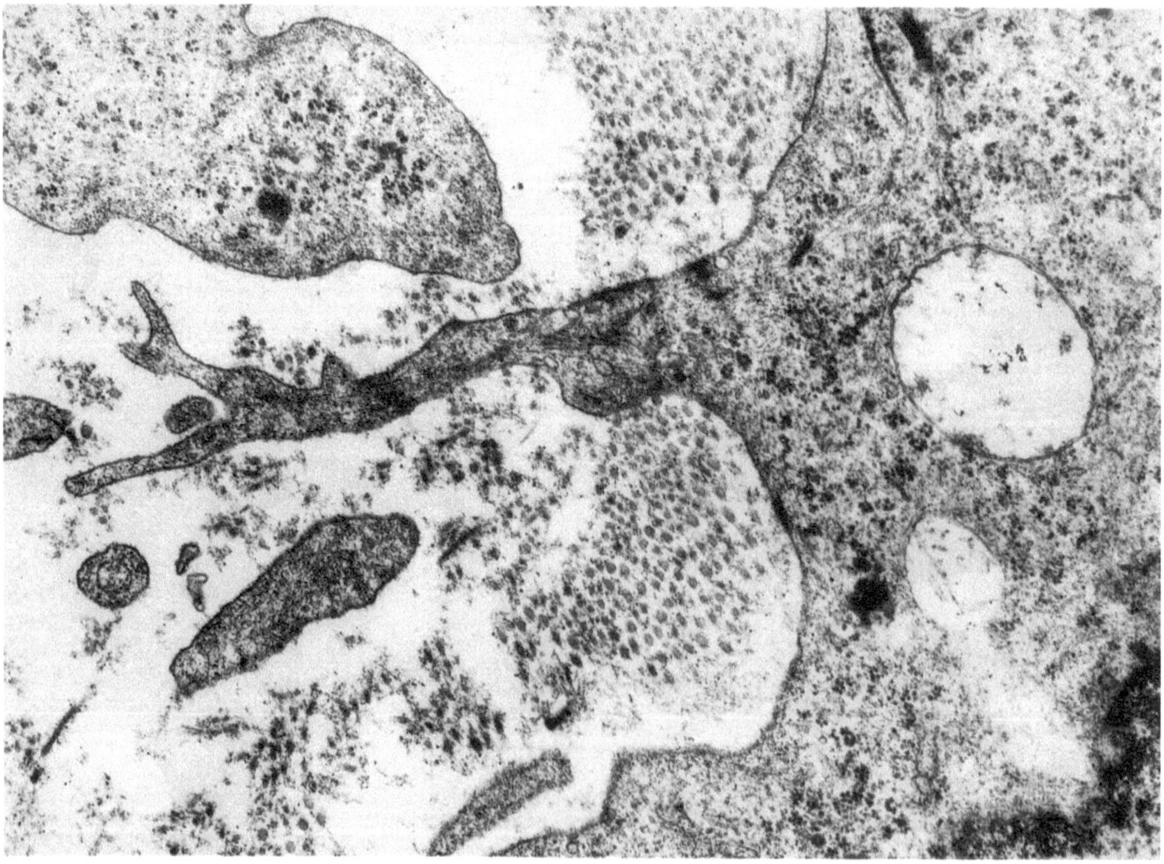

In *basalioma,* if present, hyaline degeneration involves the entire stroma in contrast to cylindroma in which the basal lamina surrounding the tumor foci undergoes hyaline degeneration.

The immature cell components of *anaplastic squamous cell carcinoma* may be similar to the basalioma cells. In the squamous cell tumors, however, differences in nuclear atypia, cell size and shape, and staining intensity are always more pronounced than those observed in the cells of basal cell carcinoma.

In the less developed forms of *sebaceous adenoma,* groups of immature basal cells may accumulate in the lobules of a few sebaceous glands. The majority of mature, vacuolized sebaceous cells, however, form hypertrophic sebaceous glands. Conversely, in pilosebaceous basalioma only small islands of mature sebaceous cells appear in the immature basal cell tumor.

Anaplastic sebaceous carcinoma structures reveal similarities to basalioma; the immature elements remind one of the epithelial cells of glandular ductules. In the apical cytoplasm of cylindrical cells glycogen or lipid vacuoles can be seen.

Biologic Features

Natural History. Basal cell tumor can be induced under strict experimental conditions (Cherry and Glucksmann 1971; Dobson 1963; Rasmussen et al. 1983; Zackheim et al. 1959) only in a few animal species, e.g., in the rat (Bachmann et al. 1937; Zackheim et al. 1959), mouse (Bielschowsky 1946; Lau et al. 1972; Lennox 1955; Rice et al. 1986), and guinea pig (Rasanen 1979). A limited number of chemical agents are effective, such as 3-methylcholanthrene (3-MC) (Thiers et al. 1954; Zackheim et al. 1959; Sugar 1981; Horak et al. 1984); 2-anthramine (Lennox 1955; Zackheim et al. 1959; Dobson 1963; Bielschowsky 1946); 9,10-dimethyl-1,2-benz(α)anthracene (DMBA) (Brown et al. 1977; Zackheim et al. 1959); polycyclic hydrocarbons (Bachmann et al. 1937; Daniel et al. 1967; Slaga et al. 1977); 7,12-diethylbenz[a]anthracene (Bennington et al. 1976); 7,12-dimethylbenz[a]anthracene (Benning-

ton et al. 1976); and nitroso-2,6-dimethylmorpholine (Lijinsky et al. 1980).

Among the different rat strains the males of the Wistar and Lister strains are the most suitable for induction of this tumor (Zackheim 1973). Tumor induction requires a relatively long latency period (200–280 days). It is performed with frequently administered (3–5 paintings a week), low percutaneous doses of 3-MC (Sugar 1981). Tumor incidence is five times higher in males compared with females (Zackheim et al. 1959). Differences are noted also in the sensitivity of various skin regions (Bennington et al. 1976; Cherry and Glucksmann 1971; Ghadially 1961; Zackheim et al. 1959). The induced tumor grows slowly; tumor doubling time is 3–5 weeks (Ghadially 1961; Rasmussen et al. 1983; Zackheim et al. 1959). After 6–9 months of tumor growth, the deeper connective tissues also become infiltrated. Animals bearing basal cell tumors have long survival times, 300–500 days (1–1.5 years), and their vitality is not decreased by the presence of extended tumors (8–10 cm in diameter).

In those basaliomas in which pilosebaceous differentiation takes place and sebaceous or keratinous cysts develop, the tumor doubling time slows down (8–10 weeks), and the diameter of the tumor does not exceed 2–3 cm. From the sebaceous cell or squamous epithelial cell components of some basaliomas, sebaceous gland tumor or squamous cell carcinoma may develop; the latter can give rise to metastases.

In rats only autologous transplantation results in successful take of basalioma (Rasanen 1979; Sugar 1981). It cannot be transplanted by means of homologous transplantation, but the autologous transplant develops (Fig. 70).

Pathogenesis. Bachmann et al. (1973) were the first to induce basal cell tumors successfully in the rat. The histogenesis was studied by Zackheim (1962) during the growth of induced basal cell tumors. He stated that most of the primary tumor foci developed in the hair follicles, rarely from the interfollicular "epidermis proper." They arose first as a simple basocellular hyperplasia (near the 180th day of MCA painting of the skin). On day 194 he detected characteristic basocellular proliferation with adenoid, tubuloalveolar pattern. Based on these studies, Zackheim considered basalioma to be a tumor of hair follicle origin.

Lupulescu and Pinkus (1976) followed the development of induced basal cell tumor at the electronmicroscopic level. They considered this neo-

◀ **Fig. 68** *(above).* Tumor cell membranes with undulated course and numerous desmosomes. TEM, × 18 000

Fig. 69 *(below).* Basal cell tumor, skin, rat. The basement membrane has almost disappeared at the interface of the epithelium and connective tissue. TEM, × 18 000

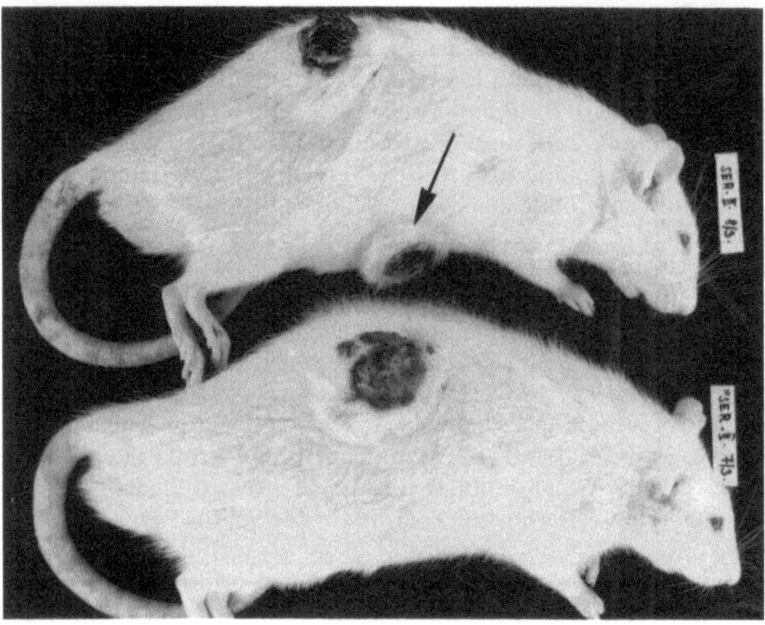

Fig. 70. Basal cell carcinoma of the rat is successfully transplanted from the back skin into the abdominal wall of the same host (autologous transplantation) *(arrow)*. Following homologous transplantation to another rat, however, it is rejected

plastic transformation to be a stepwise process from the normal basal cells into tumorous ones. This transformation is characterized by the gradual disorganization not only of epithelial cells but also of the cellular junctions and basal lamina, and by the structural disintegration of the subepidermal connective tissues.

Our studies (Sugar 1981) have revealed that basalioma may stem either from the epidermis, hair follicle, or sebaceous gland. By means of serial excision the tumors' transformation can be monitored.

Etiology and Frequency. Although a great many chemical carcinogens are known, only a few coal derivates [7,12-dimethylbenz[a]anthracene (9,10-dimethyl-1,2-benz(α)anthracene; DMBA) and 3-methylcholanthrene (MCA)] are suitable to induce basalioma by topical application to the rat (Rasmussen et al. 1983). The application of DMBA mainly results in squamous cell carcinomas, but MCA can produce basocellular carcinomas. Other chemical agents have been only occasionally used for the induction of basalioma (Lijinsky and Reuber 1980; Slaga et al. 1977; Tucker 1975).

In the course of experimental tumor induction, particularly when tumor induction is to be modelled and studied, these carcinogens are usually applied in combination with other agents with various promoting or inhibitory effects (Slaga et al. 1977; Tucker 1975). For instance, retinyl palmitate (Brown et al. 1977) and vitamin A acid (Lupulescu 1986) have inhibitory action on the development of basal cell tumor. The so-called skin surface lipid extraction (Arffmann and Hjøorne 1979), a chemical agent similar to sebum, or exposure to ultraviolet light are known to act as promoting factors (Lijinsky et al. 1980; Schweizer et al. 1982; Zabeshinski et al. 1985).

Spontaneously occurring basal cell tumor has been observed infrequently in rats (Zackheim 1973). In dogs and cats, however, spontaneous basal cell tumors occur much more frequently (Drommer 1968; Seldmeier et al. 1967).

Comparison with Other Species

Induced basal cell carcinoma of the rat is most frequently of follicular origin. The developing tumor, however, often gets mixed with tumors of pilosebaceous origin. In the tumor composition the epidermal basal cell character prevails.

In different forms of rat basal cell tumor the stroma is insignificant. In humans, however, the given form and integrity of basalioma are determined mainly by the variety of stroma near the tumor parenchyma (Zackheim 1963). Since in animals both spontaneous and induced basaliomas are uncommon, comparison is somewhat difficult. The induced basal cell tumors of monkeys (Palotay et al. 1976) and the spontaneous basal cell tumors of dogs and cats (Seldmeier et al. 1967), due to their predominantly basal cell character, sharply differ from the induced basal cell tumor of rats with pilosebaceous character. In mice, basaliomas in very low numbers can be induced by chemical carcinogens (Lau et al. 1972; Lennox 1955).

References

Arffmann E, Hjøorne N (1979) Influence of surface lipids on skin carcinogenesis in rats. Acta Pathol Microbiol Immunol Scand [A] 87: 143-149

Bachmann WE, Cook JW, Dansi A, de Worms CGM, Haslewood GAD, Hewett CL, Robinson AM (1937) The production of cancer by pure hydrocarbons IV. Proc R Soc Lond [Biol] B 123: 343-368

Bennington JL, Holmes EJ, Combs JW (1976) Tumors of the pilosebaceus unit induced in the rat by the intravenous administration of 7,12-dimethylbenz(A)anthracene. J Invest Dermatol 66: 183-187

Bielschowsky F (1946) Tumors produced by 2-anthramine. Br J Exp Pathol 27: 54-61

Brown IV, Lane BP, Pearson J (1977) Effects of depot injections of retinyl palmitate on 7,12-dimethylbenz[a]-anthracene-induced preneoplastic changes in rat skin. JNCI 58: 1347-1355

Cherry CP, Glucksmann A (1971) The influence of carcinogenic dosage and of sex on the induction of epitheliomas and sarcomas in the dorsal skin of rats. Br J Cancer 25: 544-564

Daniel PM, Pratt OE, Prichard MML (1967) Metabolism of labeled carcinogenic hydrocarbons in rats. Nature 215: 1142-1146

Dobson RL (1963) Anthramine carcinogenesis in the skin of rats. I. The epidermis. JNCI 31: 841-859

Drommer W (1968) Submikroskopische Untersuchungen am Basaliom des Hundes. Pathol Vet 5: 174-185

Ghadially FN (1961) The role of the hair follicle in the origin and evolution of some cutaneous neoplasms of man and experimental animals. Cancer 14: 801-816

Horak E, Lelkes G, Sugar J (1984) Intercellular junction: of methylcholanthrene-induced rat skin basocellular and squamous carcinomas. Br J Cancer 49: 637-644

Lau M, Rohrbach R, Thomas C (1972) Zur Morphologie der experimentell induzierten Hauttumoren bei der Ratte und der haarlosen Maus. Beitr Pathol Anat 146 (1): 33-54

Lennox B (1955) The production of a variety of skin tumors in rats with 2-anthramine, and a comparison with the effects in mice. Br J Cancer 9: 631-639

Lijinski W, Reuber MD (1980) Comparison of carcinogenesis by two isomers of nitroso-2,6-dimethylmorpholine. Carcinogenesis 1: 501-503

Lijinski W, Saavedra JE, Reuber MD, Blackwell BN (1980) The effect of deuterium labeling on the carcinogenicity of nitroso-2,6-dimethylmorpholine in rats. Cancer Lett 10: 325-331

Lupulescu A (1986) Inhibition of DNA synthesis and neoplasmic cell growth by vitamin A (retinol). JNCI 77: 149-156

Lupulescu A, Pinkus H (1976) Electron microscopic observations on rat epidermis during experimental carcinogenesis. Oncology 33: 24-28

Palotay JL, Adachi K, Dobson RL, Pinto JS (1976) Carcinogen-induced cutaneous neoplasms in nonhuman primates. JNCI 57: 1269-1274

Rasanen O (1979) Transplantability of chemically induced skin tumors in synergeneic strains of mice, rats and guinea pigs. Exp Pathol 17: 121-127

Rasmussen KS, Glenthøj A, Arffmann E (1983) Skin carcinogenesis in rats by 3-methylcholanthrene and 7,12-DMBA. Influence of dose and frequency on tumour response and its histological type. Acta Pathol Microbiol Immunol Scand [A] 91: 445-451

Rice JE, Hosted TJ Jr, DeFloria MC, LaVoie EJ, Fischer DL, Wiley JC Jr (1986) Tumor-initiating activity of major in vivo metabolites of indeno/1,2,3-cd/pyrene on mouse skin. Carcinogenesis 7: 1761-1764

Schweizer J, Loehrke H, Hesse B, Goerttler K (1982) 7,12-dimethylbenz[a]anthracene, 12-0-tetradecanoyl-phorbol-12-acetate mediated skin tumor initiation and promotion in male Sprague-Dawley rats. Carcinogenesis 3: 785-789

Seldmeier H, Weiss E, Schäffer E (1967) Die histologische Klassifizierung der Basalzellenkarzinome der Haut des Hundes und der Katze. DTW 74: 176-179

Slaga TJ, Thompson S, Berry DL, Digiovanni J, Juchauss MR, Viaje A (1977) The effects of benzoflavones on polycyclic hydrocarbon metabolism and skin tumor initiation. Chem Biol Interact 17: 297-312

Sugar J (1981) Experimentally induced basalioma. Magy Onkol 25: 145-156

Thiers H, Vontilainen A, Kiljunen A (1954) Effects on white rats of MCA painting of the skin and simultaneous intraperitoneal injections of skin suspensions. I. Tumor induction in the painted skin. Acta Pathol Microbiol Immunol [A] 34: 218-225

Tucker MJ (1975) Carcinogenic action of quinoxaline 1,4-dioxide in rats. JNCI 55: 137-146

Zabezhinski MA, Pliss GB, Okulov VB, Perov AS (1985) Skin tumours induced by local and systemic action of N-nitroso-compounds in rats. Arch Geschwulstforsch 55: 117-122

Zackheim HS (1962) The origin of experimental basal cell epitheliomas in the rat. J Invest Dermatol 38: 57-68

Zackheim HS (1963) Origin of the human basal cell epithelioma. J Invest Dermatol 40: 283-297

Zackheim HS (1973) Tumours of the skin. In Turusov VS (ed) Pathology of tumours in laboratory animals, vol 1. Tumours of the rat, pt 1. IARC, Lyon, pp 1-22

Zackheim HS, Simpson WL, Langs L (1959) Basal cell epitheliomas and other skin tumors produced in rats and mice by anthramine and methylcholanthrene. J Invest Dermatol 33: 385-402

Basal Cell Tumor, Skin, Mouse

Ryohei Hasegawa, Yoshifumi Miyakawa, and Hidetaka Sato

Synonyms. Basalioma; basaloma; basal cell epithelioma; basal cell carcinoma; basaloid tumor.

Gross Appearance

The gross appearance of basal cell tumors may vary considerably. Some are superficial with a granular surface, and others are protuberant nodules. The tumors are usually solitary but are occasionally multiple. Sometimes, the tumor is palpable under the intact skin as a hard nodule. The cut surface is solid and grayish-white.

Microscopic Features

Tumors are composed of cells resembling basal cells of the epidermis and its appendages (Fig. 71). The tumors consist of demarcated, comparatively uniform sheets or strands of closely packed cells with round or oval nuclei and a scanty amount of basophilic cytoplasm (Figs. 72 and 73). Mitotic figures are commonly observed. The tumors are sometimes multicentric underneath hyperplastic epidermis. A continuous transition from the tumor tissue into the basal layer of the epidermis can often be observed. Various morphological forms of the basal cell neoplasm can be distinguished by their differentiation toward keratinization, sebaceous glands, or hair follicles. Small whorls and foci of keratinization often appear (Fig. 74). It is not uncommon to observe several different patterns within the same tumor (Fig. 75). The tumors differentiating into hair follicles are usually solid and sometimes have a palisading pattern of nuclei in the basal layer, whereas other nuclei are arranged in a haphazard fashion. Cystic spaces in the centers of the sheets of tumor cells and intertwining strands which consist of one, two, or three rows of palisading cells are sometimes included. Nests of tumor basal cells are circumscribed by thin connective tissue sheaths (Fig. 73). Malignant conversion of the tumor can be identified by the irregularity of cells, variations in staining properties, or invasion into deeper parts of subepidermal tissues (Fig. 76). Della Porta et al. (1960) termed malignant basal cell tumor as basal cell carcinoma.

Excessive proliferation of basal cells is sometimes associated with papillomas and keratoacanthomas. Possible early foci of basal cell tumors can be seen arising from the follicular epithelium of the carcinogen-treated skin (Fig. 77).

Ultrastructure

The tumor cells in basal cell neoplasms have a squamoid appearance in the form of short cytoplasmic projections extending into relatively wide intercellular spaces, cytoplasmic tonofibrils, and desmosome-tonofilament complexes. The cytoplasm contains numerous free ribosomes. The nuclei are large in proportion to the cytoplasm and contain prominent nucleoli and abundant euchromatin. The nests of tumor cells are invested by a basal lamina (Johnson et al. 1978). The basal cells of this tumor usually lack intercellular bridges.

Differential Diagnosis

Various morphological forms of basal cell neoplasm can be observed, and it is sometimes difficult to distinguish squamous cell tumor and sebaceous cell tumor. In mice, the pure type of trichoepithelioma is rarely observed. Basal cell tumors are uniformly composed of cells resembling normal epidermal basal cells. Some benign tumors have the appearance of human seborrheic keratosis. Malignant basal cell tumors or basal cell carcinomas are distinguishable from being one by the morphological presence of irregular epithelial cells varying in shape, size, and staining properties. They invade deeper parts of the subepidermal tissues, often penetrating the cutaneous muscle. The term basalioma has been used to describe malignant basal cell tumors (Lau et al. 1972). Extensive downward proliferation of basal cells is sometimes seen in papillomas and especially in keratoacanthomas.

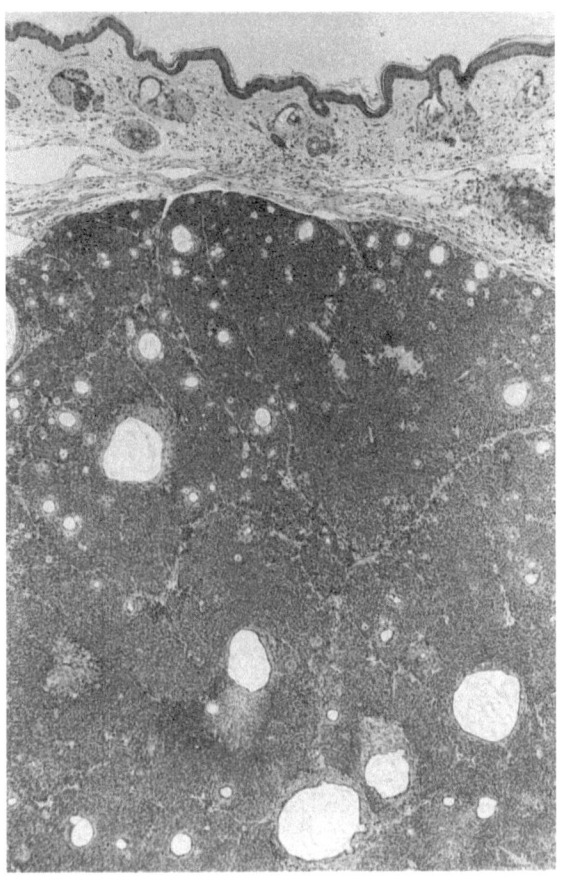

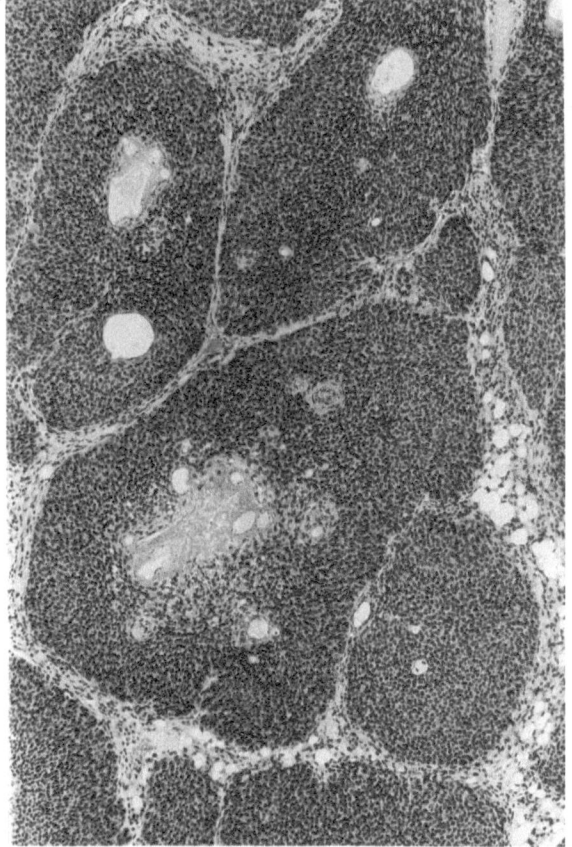

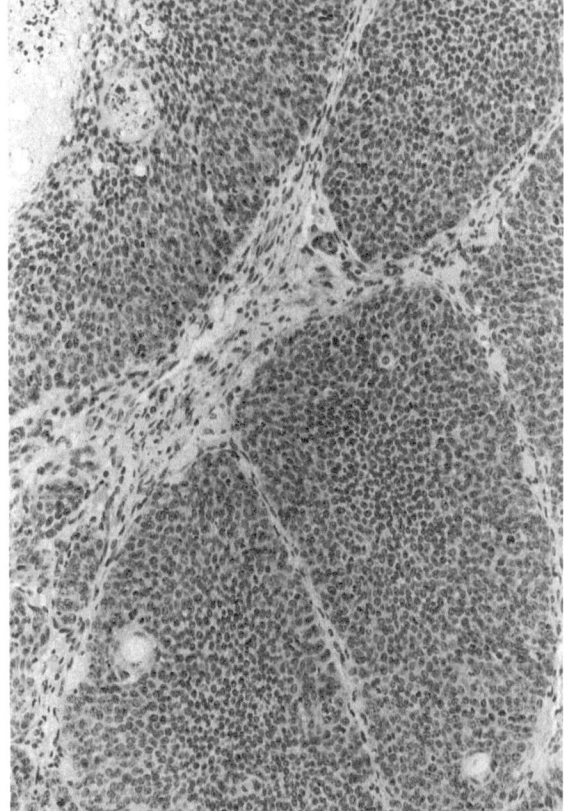

Fig. 71 *(upper left).* Basal cell tumor, subcutis, BDF mouse. Note sharp demarcation from the surrounding connective tissue. Many cysts resembling dilated hair follicles lined by a flat single layer of squamous cells are observed. Single DMBA, 100 weeks; H and E, × 15

Fig. 72 *(upper right).* Basal cell tumor, subcutis, BALB/c mouse. Note circumscribed nests of dark-staining tumor cells resembling basal cells. DMBA followed by TPA; H and E, × 75

Fig. 73 *(lower right).* Basal cell tumor, subcutis, BALB/c mouse. Nests of cells of the tumor are circumscribed by thin connective tissue sheaths. DMBA followed by TPA; H and E, × 150

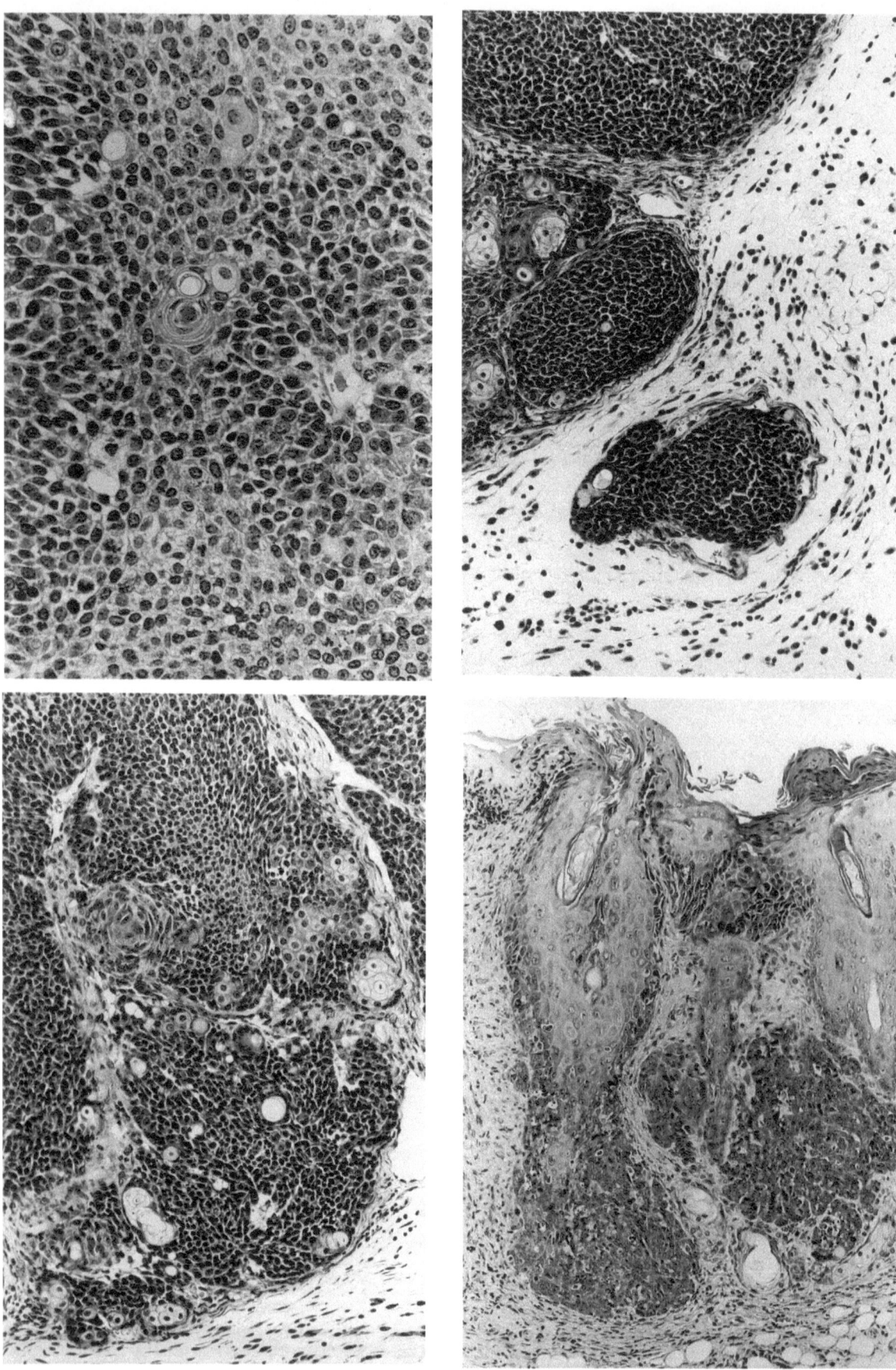

Biologic Features

Unlike in rats, basal cell tumors are rare and mostly benign in mice (Bogovski 1979). Basal cell tumors are first visible as small, smooth, dome-shaped papules, 1–2 mm in size. They are usually slow growing and tend to remain encapsulated. The nodules are usually soft and tend to ulcerate. Early foci of basal cell tumors are most commonly seen arising from the broad layer of follicular epithelium, and less often from the interfollicular epidermis. The tumor cells from the follicular wall often migrate into the sebaceous gland. The tumor may also undergo differentiation toward keratinization or formation of hair follicle. As a result, the tumor includes various morphological forms. Tumors having features of both the basal cell tumor and the squamous cell carcinoma are sometimes termed baso-squamous carcinoma. It has been suggested that the solid type of the tumor is more aggressive than the other histologic types (Nielsen and Cole 1960). A high incidence of tumors of hair follicle origin in female Swiss albino mice is obtained by a single subcutaneous injection of 3-methylcholanthrene followed by repeated topical applications of 12-0-tetradecanoylphorbol-13-acetate (Bhisey et al. 1982). It is noteworthy that in mice treated with a single dose of 7,12-dimethylbenz[*a*]anthracene (DMBA) followed by painting with Tween-60 (Della Porta et al. 1960), the proportion of basal cell tumors was higher than in experiments in which stronger carcinogenic substances, such as tars and oil, were applied for long periods. Also

Johnson et al. (1978) reported the induction of basal cell tumors in mice by six subcutaneous injections of dehydroretronecine, a metabolite of the pyrrolizidine alkaloid monocrotaline.

Comparison with Other Species

Basal cell tumors are common in dogs and cats (Squire et al. 1978). The rat is unique among laboratory animals with regard to the high incidence of basal cell tumors that can be induced with various carcinogenic agents. Basal cell tumors in laboratory animals are most often of folicular origin, while in humans the epidermis appears to be the most common site of origin, although the upper protion of the hair follicle is also a frequent source (Zackheim 1963). The etiology of basal cell neoplasms in humans in firmly associated with solar irradiation.

References

Bhisey RA, Iyengar B, Sirsat SM (1982) Effect of the active tumor promoter, 12-0-tetradecanoylphorbol-13-acetate on hair follicular growth and development of hair anlage tumors in the mouse skin: a comparison with human adnexal lesions. J Cancer Res Clin Oncol 102: 245–252

Bogovski P (1979) Tumours of the skin. In: Turusov VS (ed) Pathology of tumours in laboratory animals, vol II. Tumours of the mouse. IARC, Lyon, pp 1–41 (IARC Sci Publ no 23)

Della Porta G, Terracini B, Dammert K, Shubik P (1960) Histopathology of tumors induced in mice trated with polyoxyethylene sorbitan monostearate. JNCI 25: 573–605

Johnson WD, Robertson KA, Pounds JG, Allen JR (1978) Dehydroretronecine-induced skin tumors in mice. JNCI 61: 85–89

Lau M, Rohrbach R, Thomas C (1972) Zur Morphologie der experimentell induzierten Hauttumoren bei der Ratte und der haarlosen Maus. Beitr Pathol Anat 146 (1): 33–54

Nielsen SW, Cole CR (1960) Cutaneous epithelial neoplasms of the dog. A report of 153 cases. Am J Vet Res 21: 931–948

Squire RA, Goodman DG, Valerio MG, Fredrickson TN, Strandberg JD, Levitt MH, Lingeman CH, Harshbarger JC, Dawe CJ (1978) Tumors. In: Benirschke K, Garner FM, Jones TC (eds) Pathology of laboratory animals, vol 2. Springer, Berlin, Heidelberg, New York, pp 1051–1283

Zackheim HS (1963) Origin of the human basal cell epithelioma. J Invest Dermatol 40: 283–297

◀ **Fig. 74** *(upper left)*. Basal cell tumor, subcutis, BALB/c mouse. Note small whorls and foci of keratinization, and several individual cells with foamy cytoplasm resembling sebaceous cells. Single DMBA, 100 weeks; H and E, ×300

Fig. 75 *(lower left)*. Basal cell tumor, subcutis, BALB/c mouse. Note differentiation into hair follicles and sebaceous glands. Single DMBA, 100 weeks; H and E, ×75

Fig. 76 *(upper right)*. Malignant basal cell tumor, subcutis, BALB/c mouse. Tumor cells invade a blood vessel adjacent to a tumor mass. These cells are morphologically indistinguishable from benign ones. Metastasis to the lung was detected in this case. Single DMBA, 100 weeks; H and E, ×75

Fig. 77 *(lower right)*. Proliferation of basal cells of a C57BL mouse skin painted with a carcinogen. These may be early lesions of basal cell tumor. Single *N*-methyl-*N'*-nitro-*N*-nitrosoguanidine, 100 weeks; H and E, ×120

Trichoepithelioma, Skin, Rat

Akihiko Maekawa

Synonyms. Keratotic basal cell epithelioma; keratotic basalioma.

Gross Appearance

Skin tumors are found on all parts of the rat skin. Basal cell tumors including trichoepithelioma are first detected as small papules beneath the intact epidermis and are easily distinguishable from squamous cell papillomas. The lesions slowly enlarge to form red or brown, occasionally pale, smooth, soft to moderately firm nodules which sometimes ulcerate when larger. Many tumors, however, remain large nodules without any ulceration; this is in contrast to squamous cell carcinomas which often ulcerate and are secondarily infected.

Microscopic Features

In general, trichoepithelioma is considered to be the tumor originating from pluripotential cells present either in the epidermis or in the follicular wall. Histologically, horn (keratin) cysts represent the most characteristic feature of this tumor (Figs. 78–85), although they may be absent in some lesions. Horn cysts have a keratinized center surrounded by basophilic cells with the same appearance as the cells in basal cell tumors. When cut transversely, the basophilic cells are seen to be arranged in concentric rings (whorls) surrounding a keratinous center (Fig. 78–81).
Tumor islands composed a basaliomatous cells, arranged in a ribbon or tendril pattern radiating from the center of the islands to the periphery (Fig. 82), or solid aggregates (Figs. 83–85) are also detectable. A few epithelial nests or whorls are also intermingled in these cells (Figs. 82–85). Peripheral palisading of cells is sometimes seen in these tumor islands. Neoplastic basal cells are relatively small, with scanty, basophilic cytoplasm and large, oval or elongated nuclei. Mitotic figures are not common. Immunohistochemical studies have been used for histological diagnosis of skin tumors. Keratin proteins are one class of intermediate-sized filamentous proteins which are specifically distributed in epithelial cells and epidermis-derived tissues. Immunohis-tochemical staining of keratin proteins in epithelial tumors has shown that basal layer cells of the human epidermis do not contain keratins. Hyun et al. (1984) reported that the most prominent lecitin-binding sites in basal cell tumor of human beings were those adjacent to the keratinizing regions or those surrounding the horny cyst. There is, however, no available report concerning immunohistochemical study of basal cell tumors or trichoepithelioma in the rat.

Ultrastructure

There is little reliable information of the ultrastructural features of trichoepithelioma or trichilemmoma in rats (Inazu and Mishima 1984, 1985). In human beings, however, some information is available, and studies have confirmed that the horn cysts of trichoepithelioma represent immature hair structures, with abrupt development of the horn cells from the hair matrix cells.

Differential Diagnosis

In well-differentiated typical cases, a diagnosis of trichoepithelioma is not difficult. In poorly differentiated forms, however, the most important differential diagnostic problem lies in distinguishing this tumor from a basal cell tumor. In rats, most basal cell tumors are thought to rise from the follicular epithelium and less often from the interfollicular epidermis. Many basal cell tumors have small whorls and foci of keratinization which resemble hair structures (Fig. 86), although some basal cell tumors undergo either differentiation toward sebaceous glands or no differentiation. Therefore, there is often no clear-cut separation in the histologic diagnosis

Fig. 78 *(above).* Trichoepithelioma in a rat treated with ▶ topical application of 3-methylcholanthrene (3-MC). Horn cysts are surrounded by characteristic basophilic (basal) cells. H and E, × 115

Fig. 79 *(below).* Higher magnification of Fig. 78. Besides horn cysts, a few epithelial nests (whorls) are also evident. H and E, × 180

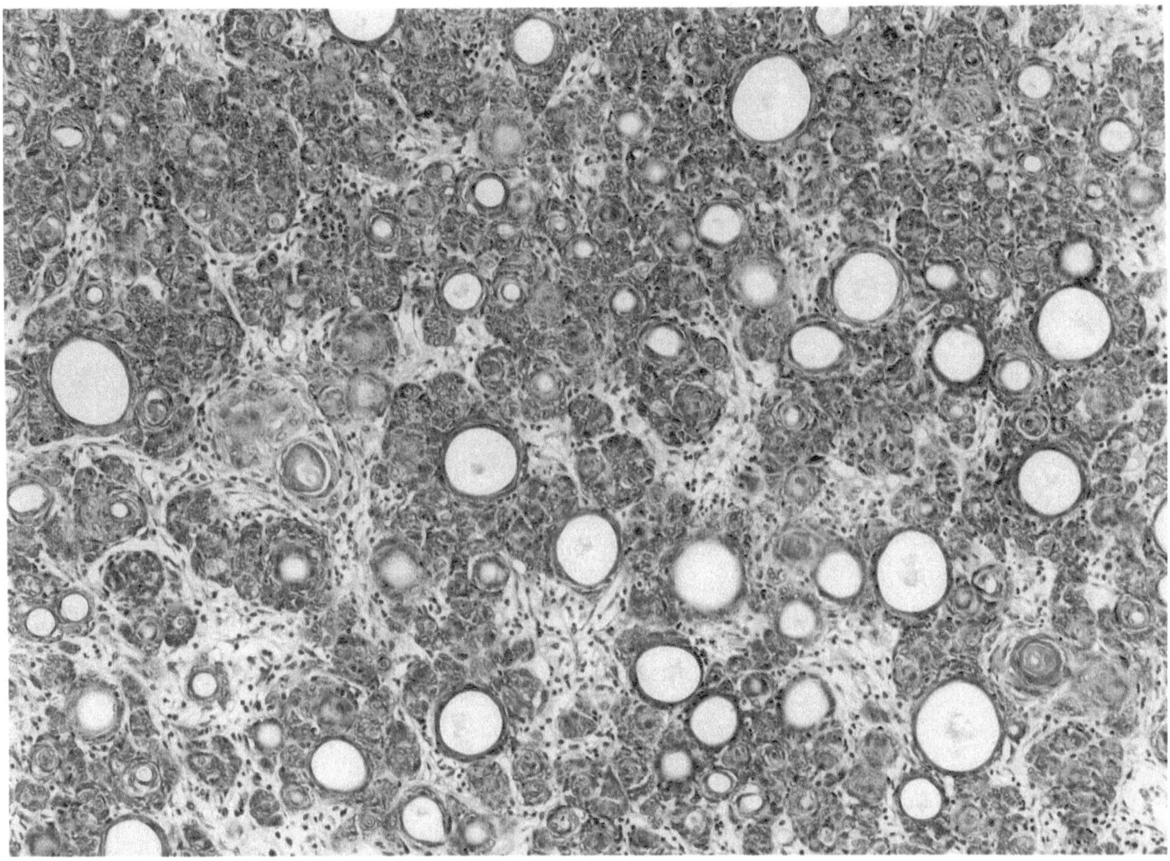

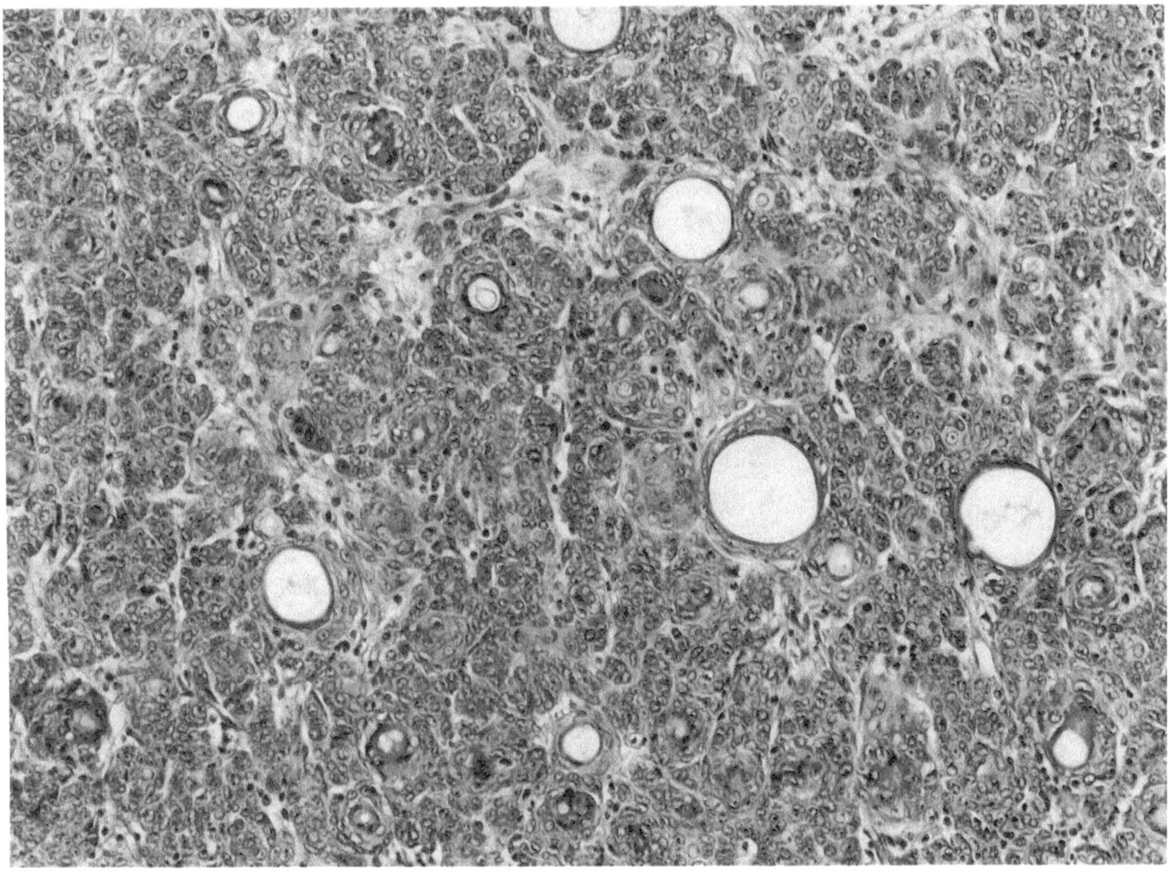

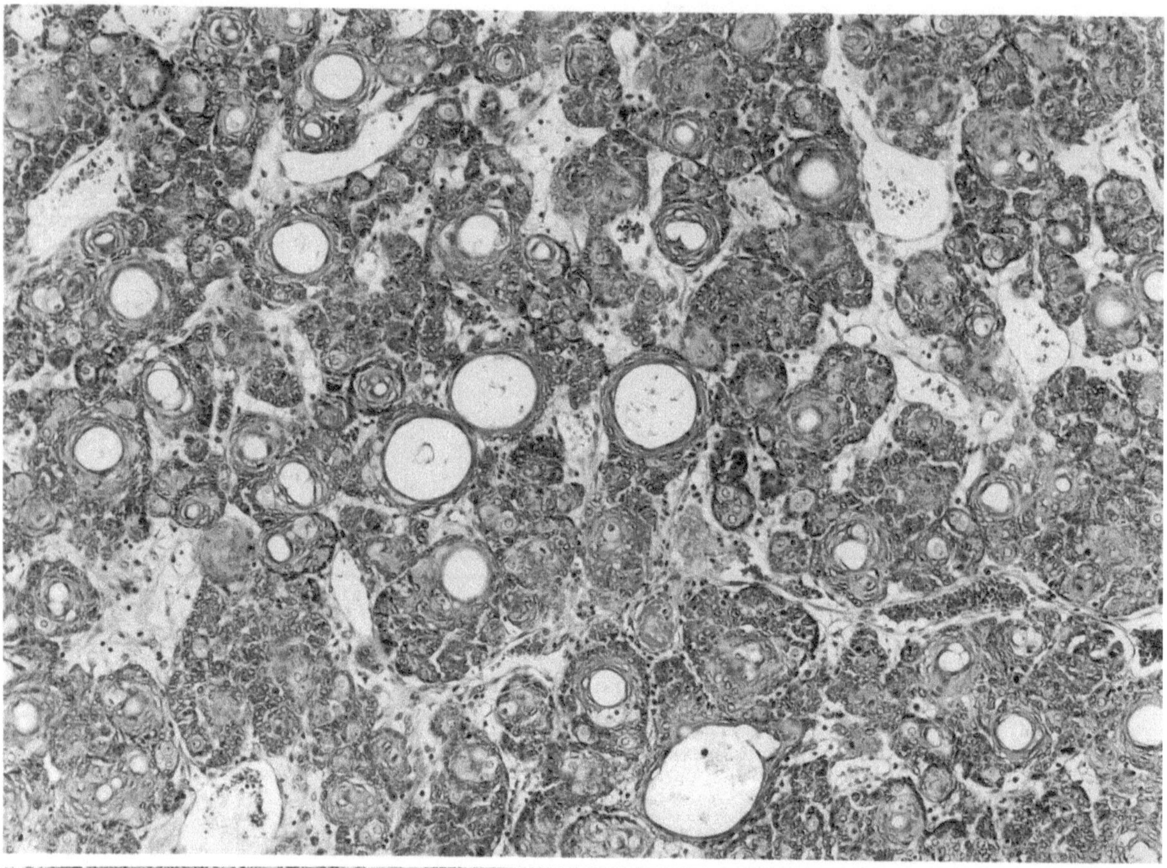

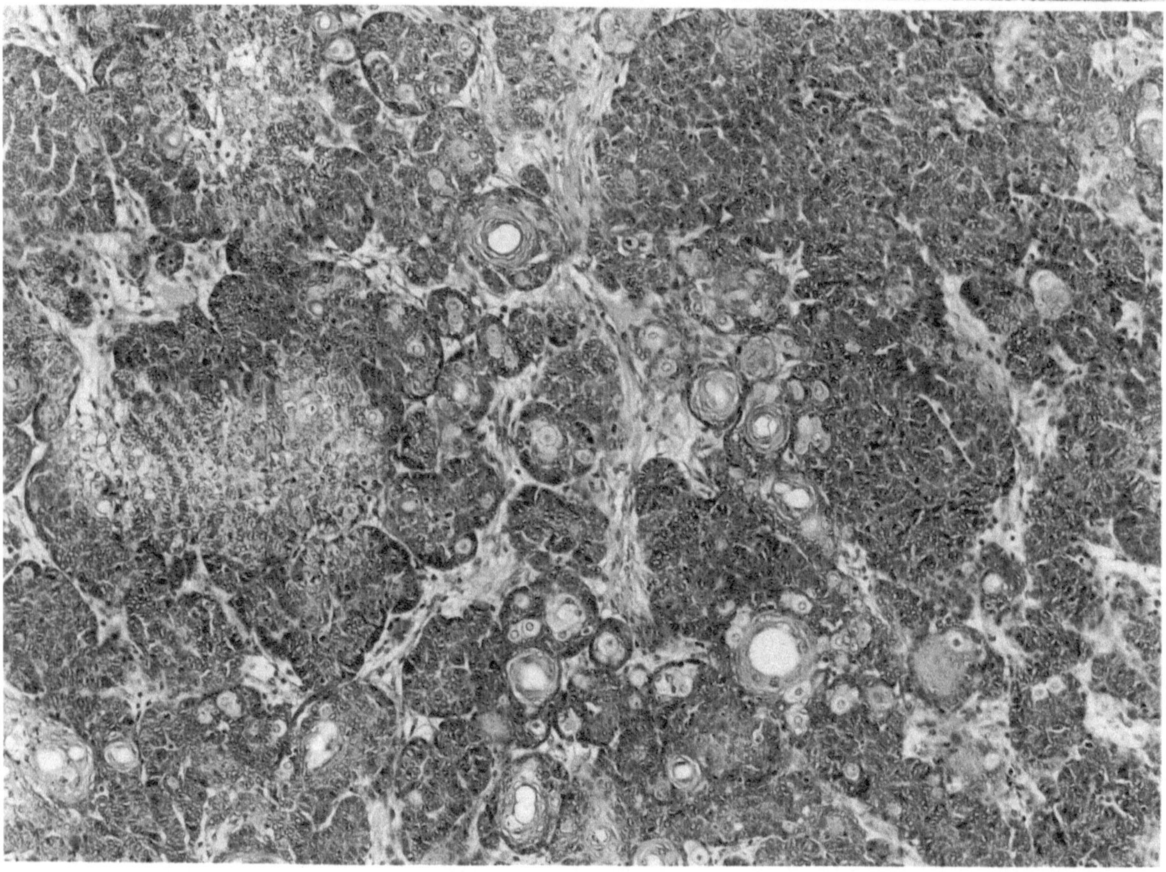

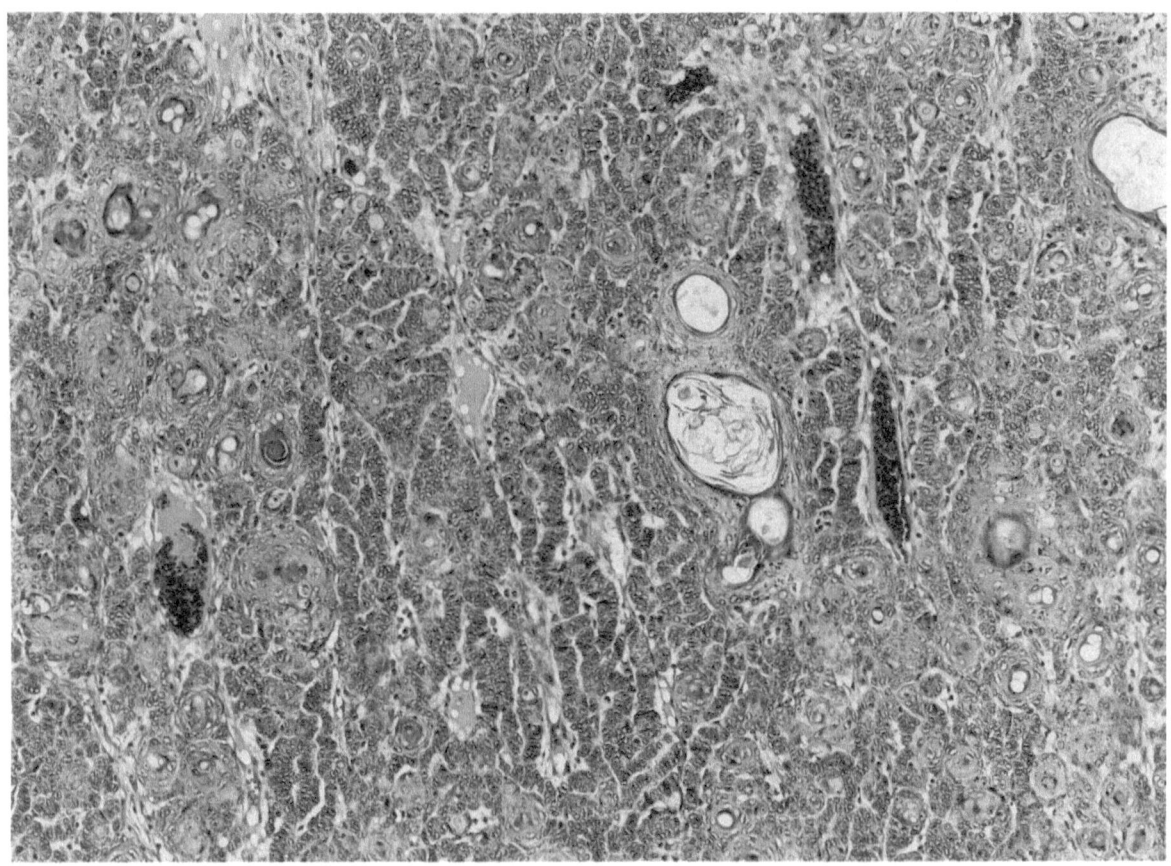

Fig. 82. Trichoepithelioma induced by 3-MC, skin, rat. Note characteristic horn cysts or whorls and arrangement of basal cells in a ribbon pattern. In this case, differentiation from basal cell tumor is difficult. H and E, × 115

between trichoepithelioma and basal cell tumor. A diagnosis of basal cell tumor seems more appropriate than that of trichoepithelioma if differentiation is detected not only toward hair follicles but also sebaceous glands. Keratoacanthoma, which also arises from the hair follicles, has the architecture of a crater surrounded by buttresses. Histologic features of keratoacanthoma have a resemblance to squamous cell carcinoma, but with more keratinization than is usually seen in the latter. Differentiation between trichoepithelioma and keratoacanthoma, with its large keratin-filled cysts, is generally not difficult.

◀ **Fig. 80** *(above)*. Trichoepithelioma, skin, rat, induced by 3-MC. Numerous horn cysts are surrounded by basal cells. H and E, × 115

Fig. 81 *(below)*. Another area of the same tumor as in Fig. 80. Basal cells are arranged in nests or a ribbon pattern. H and E, × 115

Inazu et al. (1984) reported that skin tumors were spontaneously observed with relatively high incidence in the hairless mutant rat ("bald" rat). These skin tumors were histologically diagnosed as infundibular (trichilemmal) epitheliomas. A diagnosis of trichilemmoma may be more appropriate when a variable number of cells have the appearance of clear cells owing to their content of glycogen. Trichilemmoma is a primary neoplasm of the outer root sheath of the hair follicles. They are lobular and extend into the dermis. The tumor cells are similar to clear cells of the outer root sheath of growing hair follicles. In the center of the tumor lobules, thin cores of keratin are usually present, reminiscent of the core of hair shafts. In the periphery of the lobules palisading of columnar cells can usually be seen. The trichilemmoma, however, seems to be very rare in rats.

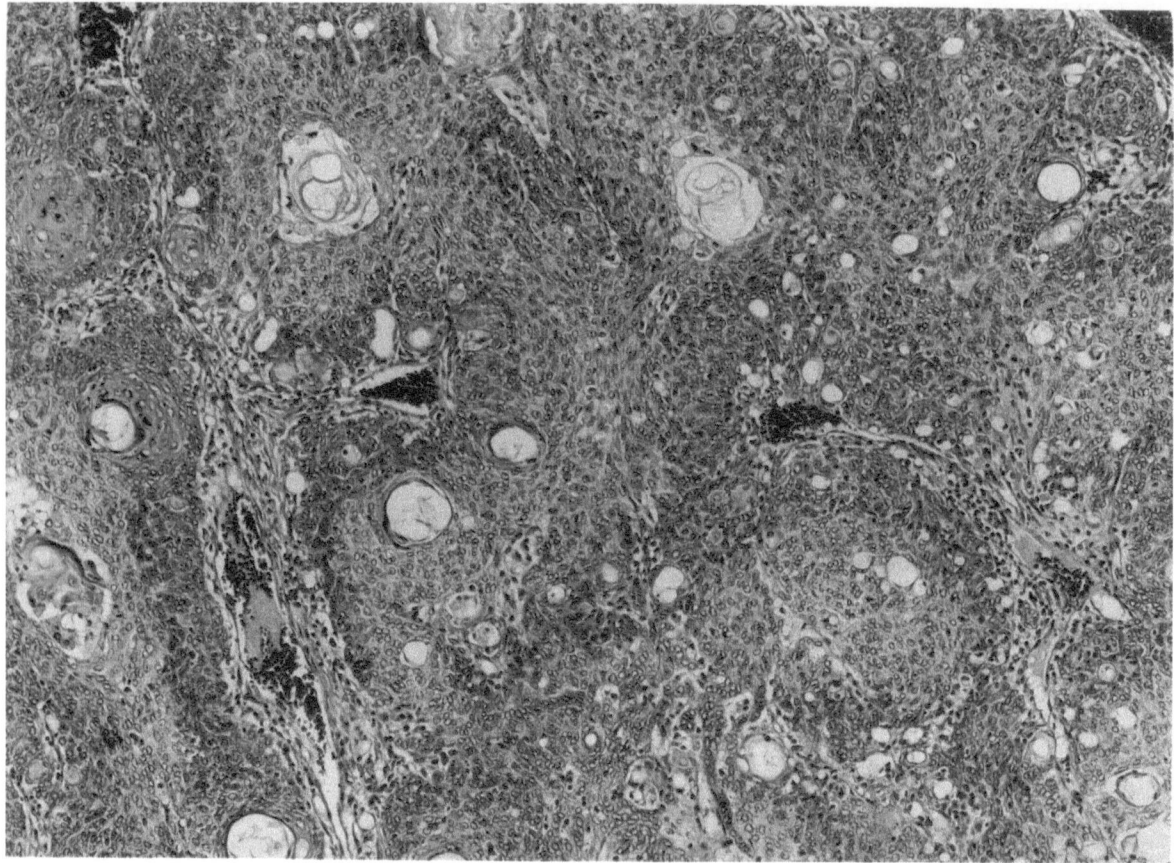

Fig. 83. Trichoepithelioma induced by 3-MC, skin, rat. Tumor islands are composed of basal cells arranged in a solid pattern. Horn cysts and whorls are intermingled among these cells. H and E, × 115

Biologic Features

Spontaneous skin tumors, including trichoepithelioma, are uncommon in all strains of rats (Zackheim 1973). Of the few spontaneous skin tumors arising in F344 rats, trichoepitheliomas were not the most frequent; they were observed in 5 out of 2320 males and 1 out of 2370 females (Solleveld et al. 1984). In 2000 Wistar rats (1000 males and 1000 females), only 1 trichoepithelioma was found in a male (Bomhard et al. 1986).

On the other hand, it is well-known that the rat is quite susceptible to the carcinogenic effect of topically applied carcinogens such as polycyclic aromatic hydrocarbons. In particular 7,12-dimethylbenz[a]anthracene (DBMA) and 3-methylcholanthrene (3-MC) have been used for the induction of skin tumors including trichoepithelioma; Zackheim (1973) further reported that the rat exhibits a different response to the topical application of various carcinogens. For example, basal cell tumors including trichoepithelioma are induced most frequently by anthramine (2-aminoanthracene) or 3-MC. On the contrary, DMBA induces predominantly squamous cell carcinomas. Rasmussen et al. (1983) also investigated skin carcinogenesis in rats by 3-MC and DMBA and confirmed Zackheim's reported results.

Several reports indicate that skin tumors may be induced by application methods other than topical. In one, ethyldiazoacetate (EDA), a substance which has been shown to induce skin tumors when administered intravenously to rats, was tested with regard to its initiative activity on two-stage skin carcinogenesis; the combination EDA-

Fig. 84 *(above).* Trichoepithelioma induced by 3-MC, ▶ skin, rat. Tumor islands are composed of basal cells in a solid pattern surrounding a few horn cysts. H and E, × 180

Fig. 85 *(below).* Trichoepithelioma induced by 3-MC, skin, rat. Horn cysts and whorls are intermingled with basal cells in a solid pattern. H and E, × 180

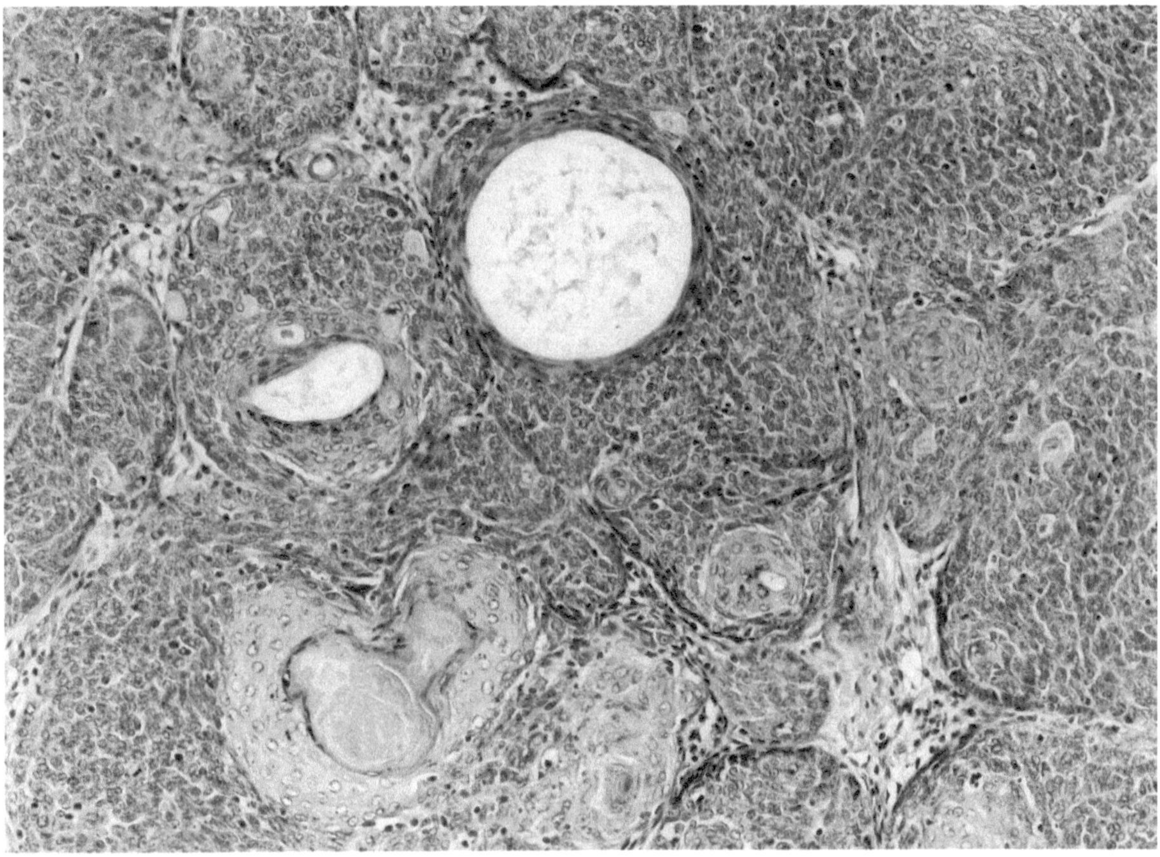

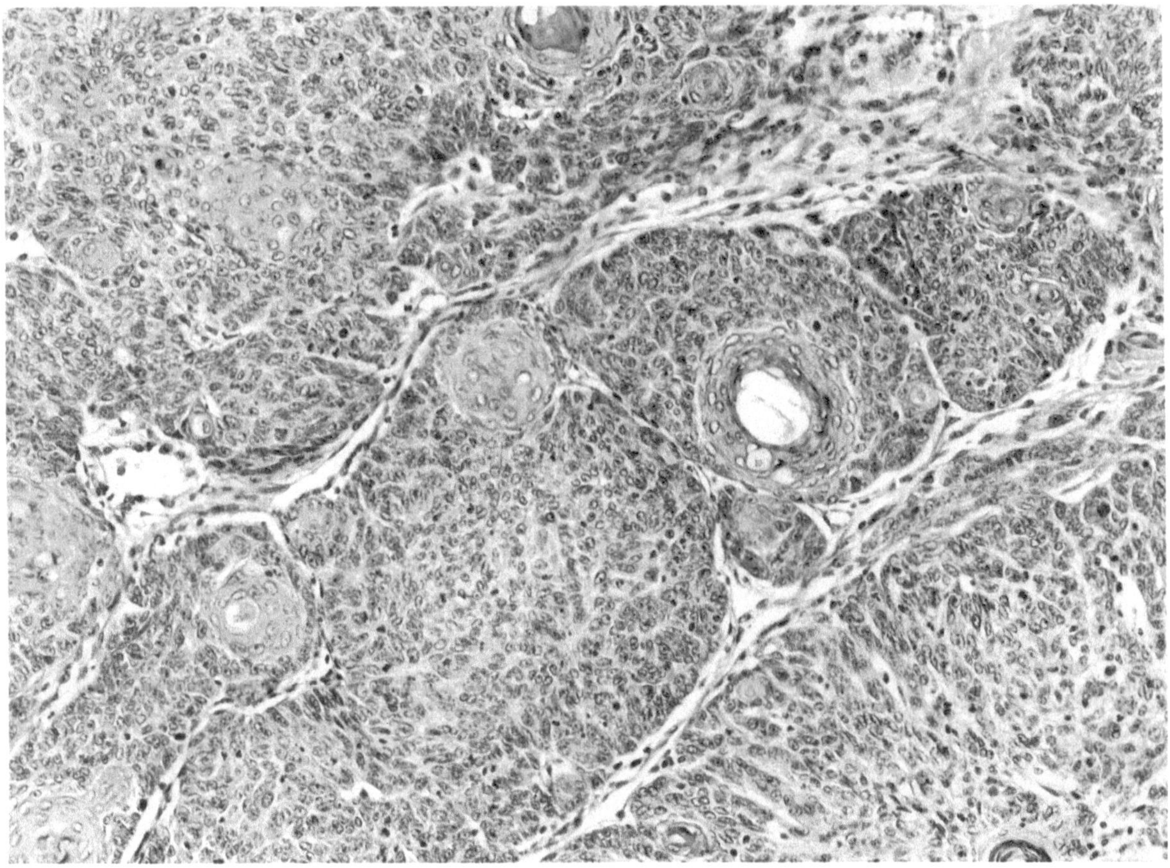

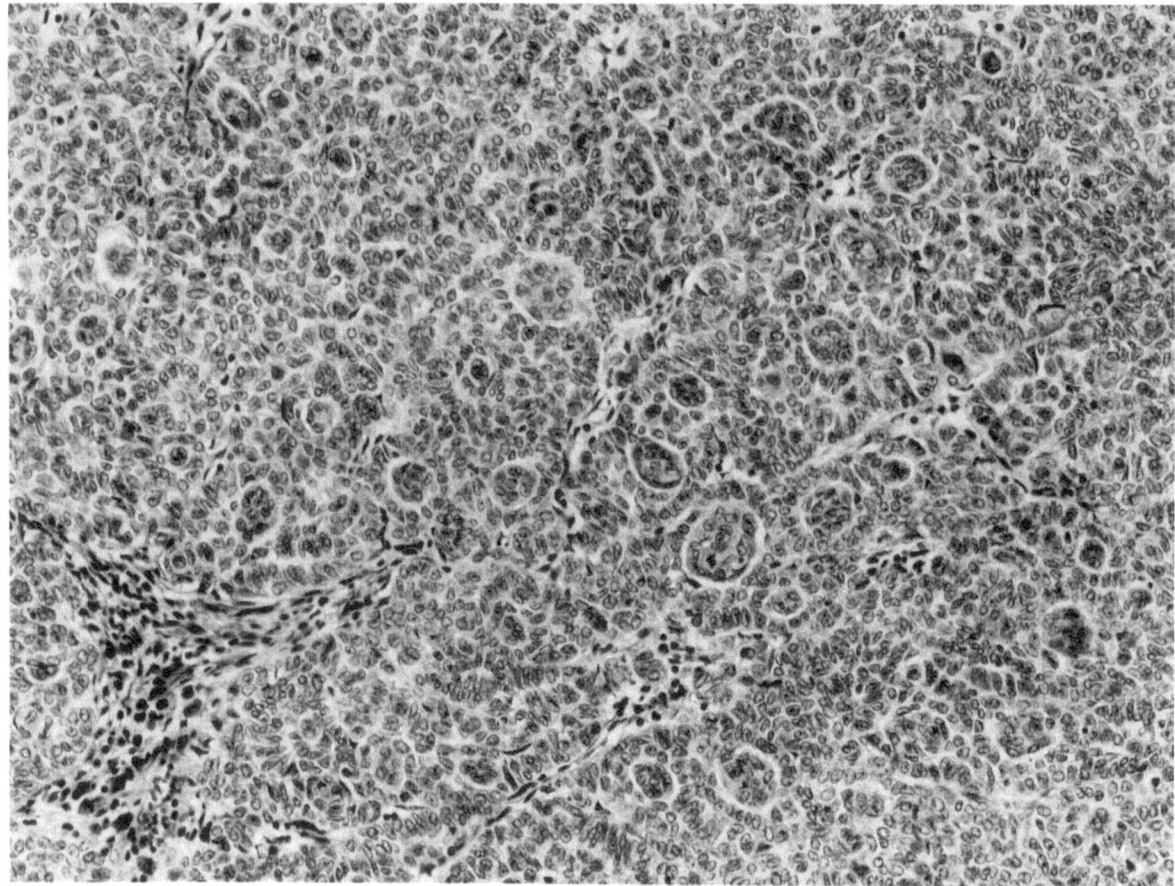

Fig. 86. Basal cell tumor (basalioma), induced by 3-MC, skin, rat. The tumor is composed of small basophilic cells (basalioma cells) arranged in a ribbon pattern or in whorls. These structures suggest differentiation toward hair follicles, but no horn cysts are observed. H and E, ×230

TPA (12-0-tetradecanoylphorbol-13-acetate) produced a skin tumor spectrum comparable to that of DMBA-TPA (Schweizer et al. 1982). All varieties of skin tumors including trichoepithelioma can be induced by irradiation, as well as by chemical carcinogens (Zackheim 1973).

Comparison with Other Species

Although histologic features of basal cell tumors, including trichoepithelioma, in the rat are quite similar to those in human beings, there are certain differences. As mentioned above, basal cell tumors in the rat more often originate from hair follicles, and many of them have features of trichoepithelioma, even though the epidermis appears to be the most common site of origin in human beings.

In mice, spontaneous occurrence of skin tumors is uncommon, but tumor can be easily induced by topical application of chemical carcinogens (Bogovski 1979). Histologically, however, most of the skin tumors observed in mice treated with chemical carcinogens were squamous cell carcinomas, whereas rats developed basal cell tumors, including trichoepithelioma. Rat skin was less sensitive than mouse skin when treated with carcinogenic hydrocarbons, but much more sensitive to anthramine. The reason for this difference in sensitivity is unknown but may be due to differential activation of the respective carcinogens (Bock 1983).

Tumors of the skin and subcutaneous tissues are the most common neoplasms in dogs, while trichoepitheliomas and/or basal cell tumors do not predominate. In cats, however, tumors of the skin and adnexa are more frequent. Basal cell tumors and their differentiated forms toward the sweat gland, sebaceous gland, or hair matrix are most commonly found on the external ear and trunk in cats. In other species such as hamsters, guinea pigs, rabbits and primates, spontaneous occurrence of skin tumors, including trichoepithelioma, is less frequent (Squire et al. 1978).

References

Bock FG (1983) Comparative anatomy and function of skin as related to experimental chemical carcinogenesis. Prog Exp Tumor Res 26: 5–17

Bogovski P (1979) Tumours of the skin. In: Turusov VS (ed) Pathology of tumours in laboratory animals, vol II. Tumours of the mouse. IARC, Lyon, pp 1–41 (IARC Sci Publ no 23)

Bomhard E, Karbe E, Loeser E (1986) Spontaneous tumors of 2000 Wistar TNO/W.70 rats in two-year carcinogenicity studies. J Environ Pathol Toxicol Oncol 7: 35–52

Hyun K-H, Hosaka M, Fukui S, Sugimoto A, Mori M (1984) Lectin-binding sites in basal cell epitheliomas and carcinomas. Acta Histochem Cytochem 17: 507–523

Inazu M, Mishima Y (1984) Electron microscopic study of infundibulo-trichilemmal epithelioma which occurred in a bald rat. J Clin Electron Micoscopy 17: 5–6

Inazu M, Mishima Y (1985) Cytopathologic study of trichilemmal epithelioma which occurred in a bald rat. Proc Jpn Soc Invest Dermatol 9: 122–123

Inazu M, Kasai K, Sakaguchi T (1984) Characteristics of a new hairless mutation (bald) in rats. Lab Anim Sci 34: 577–583

Rasmussen KS, Glenthøj A, Arffmann E (1983) Skin carcinogenesis in rats by 3-methylcholanthrene and 7,12-dimethylbenz(a)anthracene. Influence of dose and frequency on tumour response and its histological type. Acta Pathol Microbiol Immunol Scand [A] 91: 445–455

Schweizer J, Loehrke H, Hesse B, Goerttler K (1982) 7,12-Dimethylbenz[a]anthracene/12-0-tetradecanoyl-phorbol-13-acetate-mediated skin tumor initiation and promotion in male Sprague-Dawley rats. Carcinogenesis 3: 785–789

Solleveld HA, Haseman JK, McConnel EE (1984) Natural history of body weight gain, survival, and neoplasia in the F344 rat. JNCI 72: 929–940

Squire RA, Goodman DG, Valerio MG, Fredrickson T, Strandberg JD, Levitt MH, Lingeman CH, Harsbarger JC, Dawe GJ (1978) Tumors. In: Benirschke K, Garner FM, Jones TC (eds) Pathology of laboratory animals, vol II. Springer, Berlin Heidelberg New York, pp 1051–1283

Zackheim HS (1973) Tumours of the skin. In: Turusov VS (ed) Pathology of tumours in laboratory animals, vol 1. Tumours of the rat (p 1). IARC, Lyon, pp 1–21 (IARC Sci Publ no 5)

Melanocytic Tumors, Skin, Mouse

Jun Kanno

Synonyms. Malignant melanoma; melanotic tumor; melanoma.

Gross Appearance

Melanocytic tumors are recognized as black or blue-black pigmented spots or soft elevated nodules usually measuring up to 5 mm in diameter and, in a small number of case, reaching 1 cm in size. On cut section, the tumors are well demarcated and usually heavily pigmented.

Miscroscopic Features

Chemically induced melanocytic tumors are seen as small pigmented spots in an early stage of their induction. Histologically they resemble human cellular blue nevi (Fig. 87). The pigmented dendritic tumor cells are located in the reticular dermis. In a later stage of induction, melanocytic tumors grow expansively in the dermal adipose layer (Fig. 88). The tumor consists mainly of oval cells which are heavily pigmented and closely packed and manifest slight cellular atypism. The tumors are accompanied by melanophages in varying numbers. The melanophages contain coarse cytoplasmic melanin granules, i.e., compound melanosomes (Fig. 89) which can be distinguished from the fine granular melanosomes of the tumor cells.

Ultrastructure

The tumor cells are filled with single membrane-bound melanosomes and some single membrane-bound premelanosomes (Fig. 90). Golgi apparatus, mitochondria, and smooth endoplasmic re-

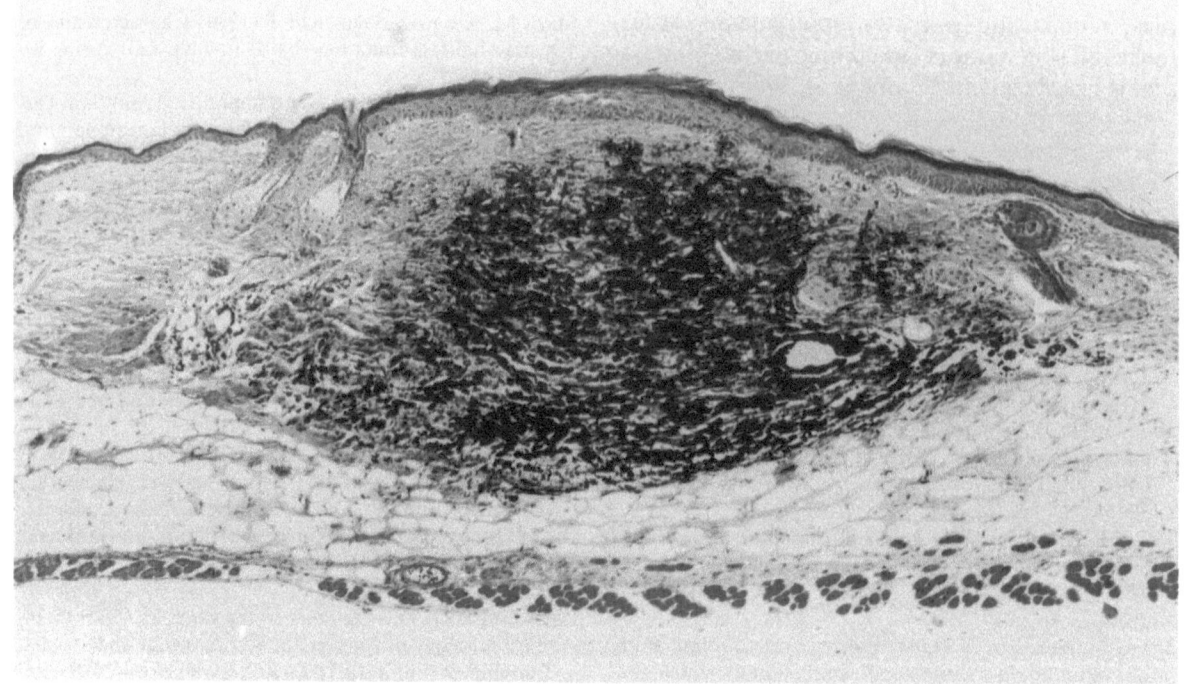

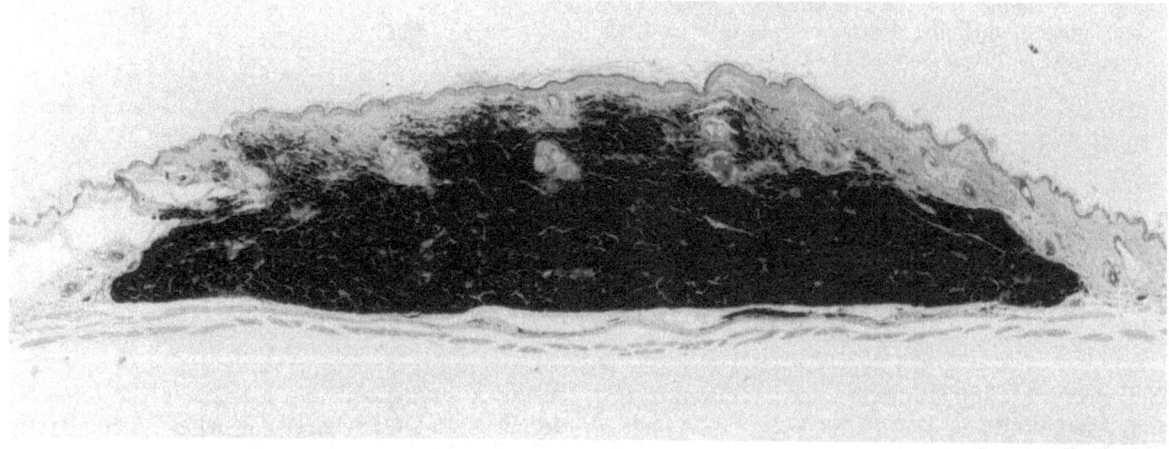

Fig.87 *(above).* Chemically induced melanocytic tumor, skin, BDF₁ mouse. Blue nevus-like lesion is confined to the reticular dermis; five weeks after DMBA and TPA treatment. H and E, ×80

Fig.88 *(below).* Melanocytic tumor with expansive growth into dermal adipose layer, skin, BDF₁ mouse; 1.5 years after DMBA treatment. H and E, ×40

ticulum are found among the melanosomes. One can also see short pseudopodia (Fig.91) and poorly formed basement membranes (Fig.92). It is possible to find a few fusiform or dendritic tumor cells, which have many single membrane-bound premelanosomes and well-developed basement membranes. Phagocytic cells (melanophages) containing compound melanosomes are also found among the tumor cells (Fig.93). Schwann cells and perineural cells of the nerve bundles involved in the tumors often contain sin-

gle membrane-bound melanosomes and, occasionally, single membrane-bound premelanosomes, indicating that these cells can produce melanin under certain circumstances (Kanno et al. 1987).

Differential Diagnosis

The diagnosis of melanotic tumor of the skin is usually easy since other pigmented tumors are very rare.

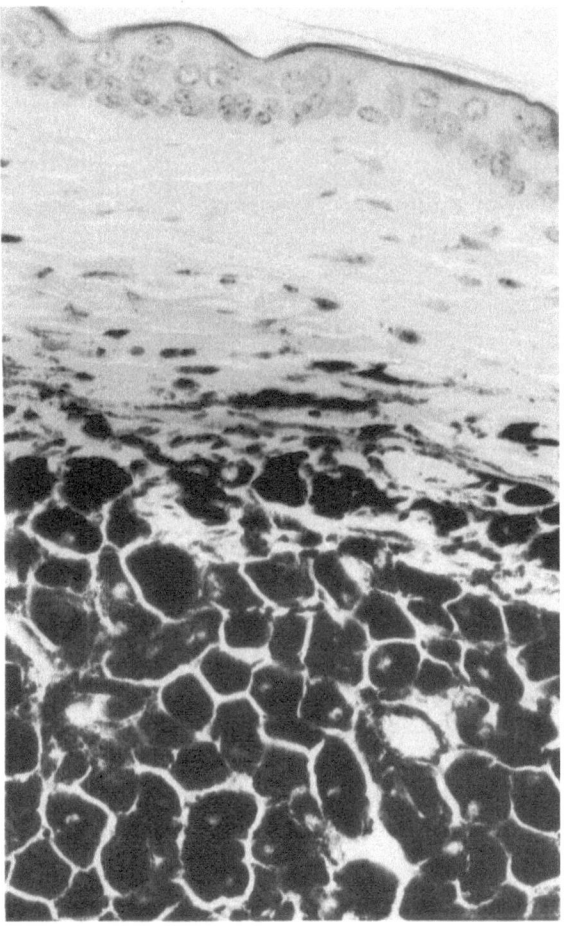

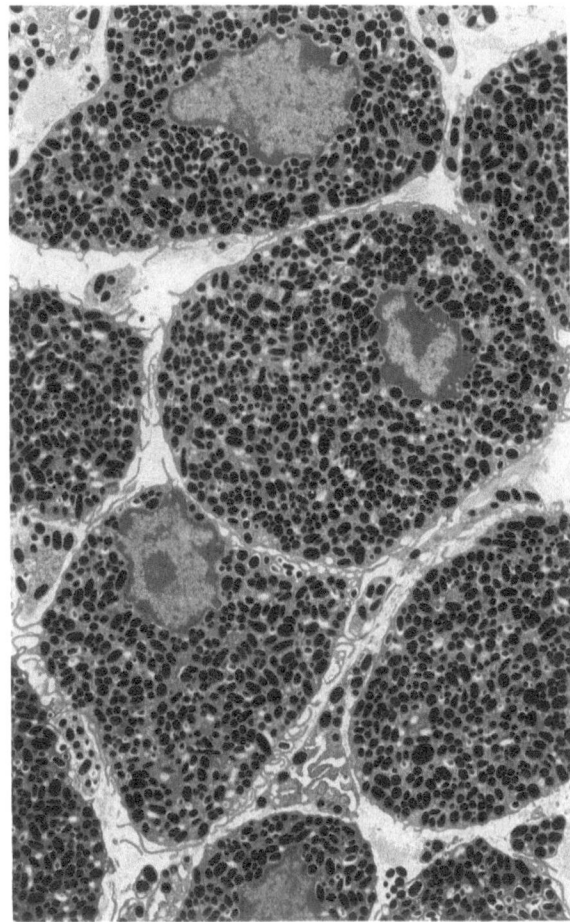

Fig. 89. Higher magnification of the melanocytic tumor in Fig. 88. The tumor consists of oval or polygonal cells heavily pigmented with slight atypism; 1.5 years after DMBA treatment. H and E, × 400

Fig. 90. Higher magnification of the melanocytic tumor in Fig. 88 induced by DMBA. TEM, × 3000

Demonstration of melanogenesis by electron microscopic detection of single membrane-bound melanosomes and premelanosomes or cytochemical confirmation by positive dopa reaction is essential for diagnosis.

The induced melanocytic tumors usually have slight cellar atypia, but no obvious invasion and metastasis. However, they and some of their draining lymph nodes contain tumor cells transplantable to syngeneic or nude mice (Berkelhammer and Oxenhandler 1987; Takizawa et al. 1985; Kanno et al., unpublished data) and usually grow in vitro to produce cell lines (Kanno, unpublished data). Taking these facts into consideration, these induced tumors could be described as malignant melanomas or their precursors.

Biologic Features

Spontaneous Melanocytic Tumors. Found very rarely in mice, only a few reports of spontaneous melanomas are available (Bogovski 1979). The famous murine melanoma cell lines, Harding-Passey melanoma (Harding and Passey 1930), S91 melanoma (Algire 1944; Cloudman 1941), and B16 melanoma (Roscoe B Jackson Memorial Laboratory 1962), are melanoma of spontaneous origin. However, the incidence and histogenesis of the melanoma are not described in the literature.

Ward et al. (1979) reported two cutaneous malignant melanomas (incidence = 0.03%) and one ocular melanoma in 5065 untreated B6C3F1 mice. Haseman et al. (1985) reported that no malignant melanoma was observed in 1791 untreated B6C3F1 mice, indicating that the incidence of

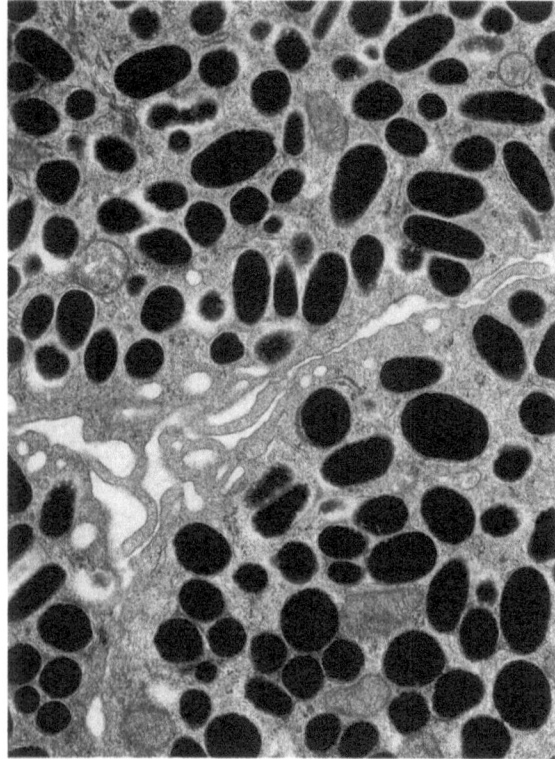

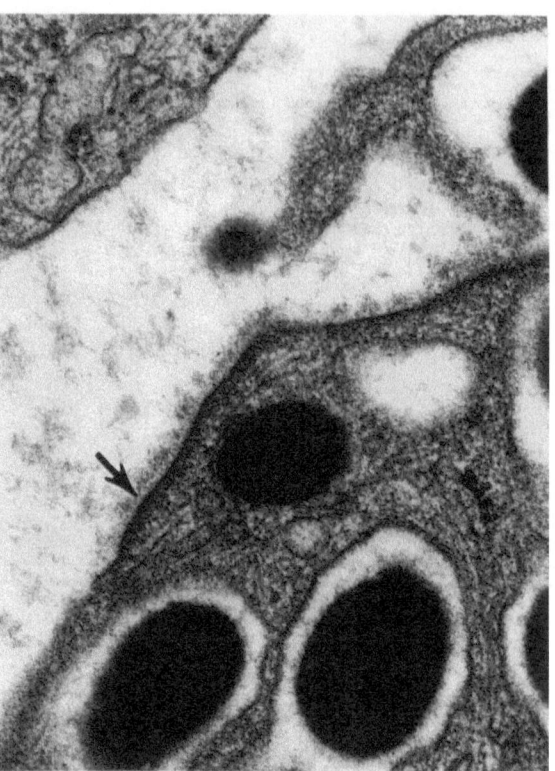

Fig. 91. Higher magnification of the melanocyitc tumor cells in Fig. 90 with single membrane-bound melanosomes, organelles, and pseudopodia. There are no obvious intercellular junctions. TEM, × 15 000

Fig. 92. Poorly formed basement membrane *(arrow)* of a tumor cell. TEM, × 52 000

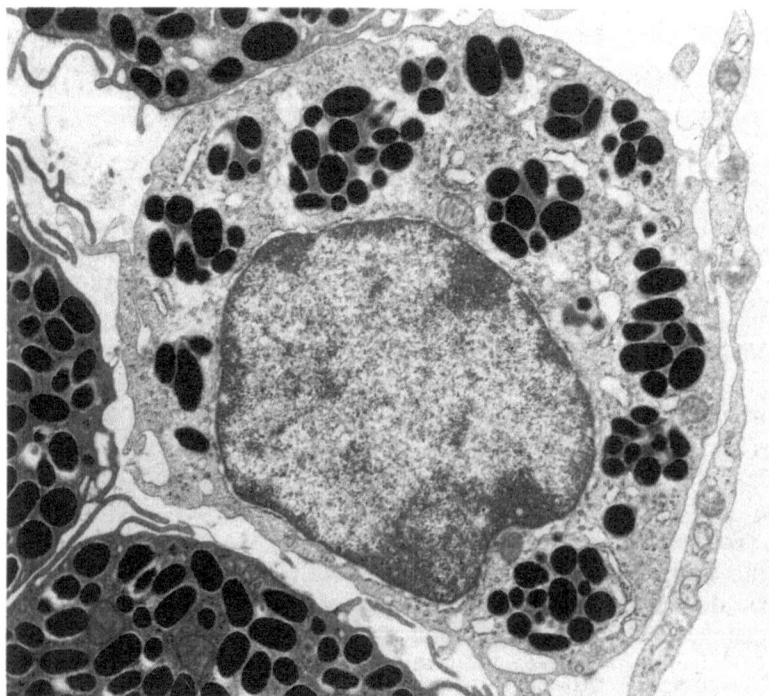

Fig. 93. Skin, mouse, melanophage containing compound melanosomes. TEM, × 9000

Table 2. Chemically induced melanocytic tumors in mice

Author	Year	Mouse	Age	Treatment[a] Initiation	Promotion	Tumor incidence	Latent period	Histology of the primary site	Metastasis
Burgoyne et al.	1949	DBA	6–8 w	TMBA	–	46/73	7 m	1 invasive/ localized	no
		C57BL	6–8 w	TMBA	–	36/58	7 m	localized	no
		(DBA × C57BL)F1	6–8 w	TMBA	–	51/67	7 m	localized	no
		(C57BL × DBA)F1	6–8 w	TMBA	–	59/77	7 m	localized	no
Rocha and Winkelmann	1962	hairless (C57 brown)	adult	gas-oil	UV	2/2	6 m	blue nevus-like	no
Forbes	1965	C57BL-hr+ (haired)	adult	DMBA	–	6/6	4 w	blue nevus-like	no
		C57BL-hr+ (hairless)	adult	DMBA	–	6/6	4 w	blue nevus-like	no
		rhino mice	adult	DMBA	–	6/6	4 w	blue nevus-like	no
		C57BL-hr+ (haired)	adult	MC	–	6/6	4 w	blue nevus-like	no
Epstein et al.	1967	hairless (pigmented)	8–11 w	DMBA	UV	5/11	5 m	invasive	no
		hairless (pigmented)	8–11 w	DMBA	–	0/25	5 m	–	
		hairless (pigmented)	8–11 w	–	UV	0/34	5 m	–	
		hairless (pigmented)	8–11 w	–	–	0/19	5 m	–	
Berkelhammer et al.	1982	C57BL/6	4 day	DMBA	croton oil	2/20	39 w	invasive	yes[b]
Takizawa et al.	1985	BDF$_1$	4 w	DMBA	croton oil	24/30	25 w	localized and invasive	no yes[c]
		CDF1	4 w	DMBA	croton oil	21/30	25 w	localized	no
		C57BL/6	4 w	DMBA	croton oil	9/30	25 w	localized	no
		DBA/2	4 w	DMBA	croton oil	0/30	25 w	localized	no
Kanno et al.	1986	BDF$_1$	6 w	DMBA	TPA	21/21	20 w	nevus-like	no
Berkelhammer and Oxenhandler	1987	C57BL/6	2–6 day	DMBA	croton oil	11/70	11 m	invasive	yes[b]

[a] Topical application.
[b] Lymph node metastases.
[c] Lung metastases.
w, weeks; m, months.

spontaneous malignant melanoma in B6C3F1 mice is much lower than 0.1%.

Spontaneous melanomas are reported to metastasize to the lung and other organs (Harding and Passey 1930; Algire 1944; Cloudman 1941; Roscoe B Jackson Memorial Laboratory 1962). Although the histogenesis of the reported spontaneous melanotic tumors are equivocal (Algire 1944), some are thought to be of dermal melanocyte origin (Harding and Passey 1930).

Induced Melanocytic Tumors. Various strains of mice produce melanocytic tumors after topical application of carcinogens (Takizawa et al. 1985). These induced melanocytic tumors are of dermal origin and confined to the primary site with a few exceptions (Table 2).

Four types of dendritic melanocytes occur in the skin of colored mice, i.e., in the epidermis, hair bulbs, perifollicular melanocytic networks (PFM), and deep dermis (Kanno et al. 1986). The PFM surround some hair follicles recognized as tylotrich (sensory) hair follicles (Straile 1960) (Fig. 94) and are closely associated with the tactile nerve endings of the follicles (Fig. 95). The deep dermal melanocytes are large dendritic pig-

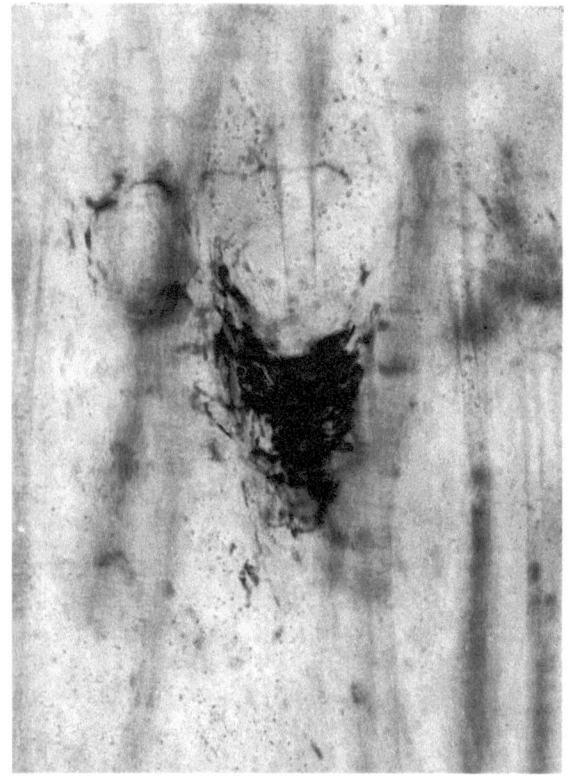

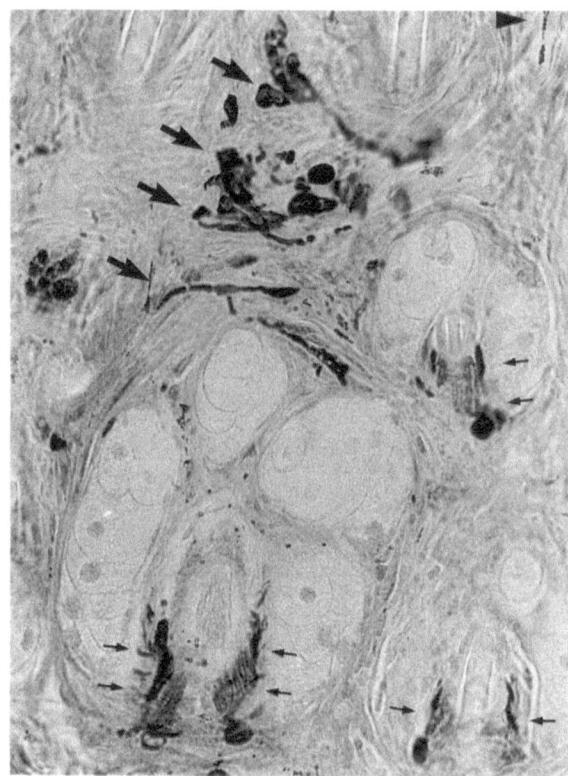

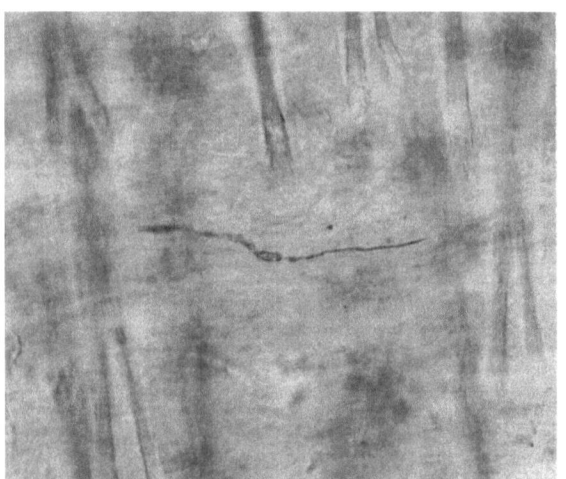

Fig. 94 *(upper left).* Perifollicular melanocytic network (PFM) before treatment, skin, BDF$_1$ mouse. Cleared skin preparation after dopa-tyrosine reaction, × 200

Fig. 95 *(upper right).* Tangential section of a PFM of an untreated mouse skin. The dendritic cells of the PFM are positive for S100 protein and contain fine melanin pigments *(large arrows).* Sheaths of nerve bundles and nerve endings of the hair follicles are positive for S100 protein *(small arrows).* Note the coarse compound melanosomes in melanophages *(arrowhead).* ABC method against S100 protein (Dako) without counter staining, × 320

Fig. 96 *(lower left).* Cleared skin preparation of an untreated mouse focused on a deep dermal melanocyte at the bottom of the reticular dermis, × 160

mented cells, located at the bottom of the reticular dermis, and distributed without obvious relation to the hair follicles and nerves (Fig. 96).

Melanocytes of the PFM are considered to be the origin of induced melanocytic tumors. An initial skin reaction to topically applied carcinogens is transient hyperpigmentation of the epidermis (Figs. 97 and 98) (Klaus and Winkelmann 1965; Kanno et al. 1986). This change is very sensitive and occurs in a dose-time-dependent manner (Iwata et al. 1981). If carcinogen is applied to the skin in telogen, the hair follicles in telogen move into anagen. Some 3 or 4 weeks later, the dendritic melanocytes in some of the PFMs begin proliferating (Fig. 99) to form small, pigmented spots resembling blue nevi (Fig. 87). In 20–30 weeks, the lesions grow expansively in the dermal adipose layer to form slightly elevated nodules measuring about 2–5 mm in diameter (Figs. 88 and 89). In 1 or 1.5 years, some of the nodules reach the approximate size of 10 × 10 × 5 mm. Distant metastasis rarely occurs, even though local invasion may be seen with advanced lesions.

Fig. 97 *(above).* Melanosis of the epidermal melanocytes, ▶ skin, BDF₁ mouse; one week after DMBA application. Cleared skin preparation after dopa-tyrosine reaction, × 130

Fig. 98 *(middle).* Melanosis of epidermal melanocytes, skin, BDF₁ mouse; one week after DMBA application. H and E, × 200

Fig. 99 *(below).* Perifollicular melanocytic network, skin, BDF₁ mouse. Note proliferation and melanosis of melanocytes around hair follicles; five weeks after DMBA and TPA treatment. H and E, × 200

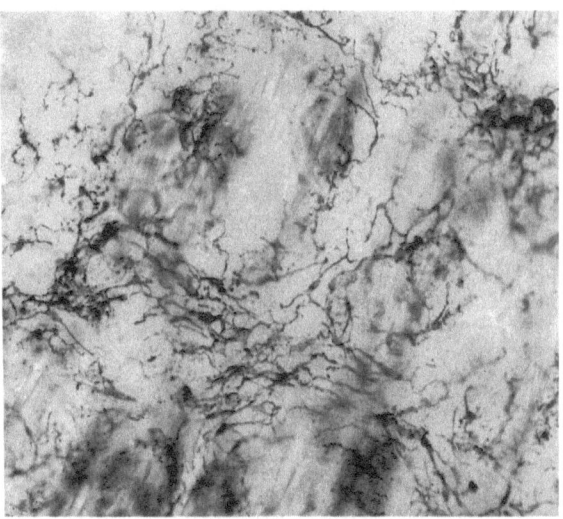

Comparison with Other Species

Melanocytic tumors are found or induced more frequently in hamsters than in mice. Hamsters possess special structures called the costovertebral spot with small pigmented spots around it, and the latter structures are believed to be much more susceptible to melanocarcinogenesis (Ghadially and Barker 1960) (see p. 70).

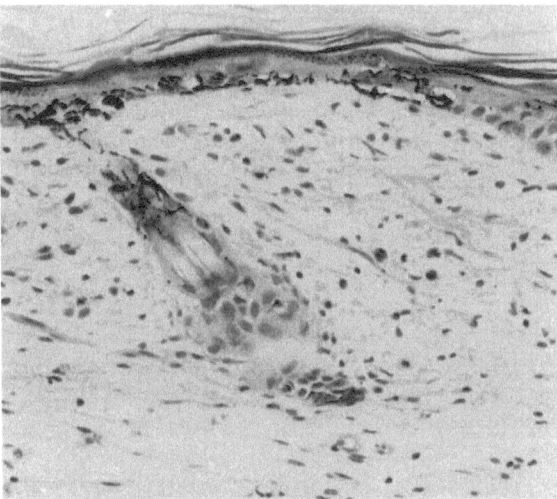

Guinea pigs also produce melanomas following DMBA treatment, and some of them are reported to be of junctional origin (Clark et al. 1976; Pawlowski et al. 1976, 1980).

References

Algire GH (1944) Growth and pathology of melanoma S91 in mice of strains dba, A and C. JNCI 5: 151–160

Berkelhammer J, Oxenhandler RW (1987) Evaluation of premalignant and malignant lesions during the induction of mouse melanomas. Cancer Res 47: 1251–1254

Berkelhammer J, Oxenhandler RW, Hook RR Jr, Hennessy JM (1982) Development of a new melanoma model in C57BL/6 mice. Cancer Res 42: 3157–3163

Bogovski P (1979) Tumours of the skin. In: Turusov VS (ed) Pathology of tumours in laboratory animals, vol II. Tumours of the mouse. IARC, Lyon, pp 1–42 (IARC Sci Publ no 23)

Burgoyne FH, Heston WE, Hartwell JL, Stewart HL (1949) Cutaneous melanin production in mice following application of the carcinogen 5,9,10-trimethyl-1,2-benzanthracene. JNCI 10: 665–672

Clark WH Jr, Min BH, Kligman LHL (1976) The developmental biology of induced malignant melanoma in guinea pigs and a comparison with other neoplastic systems. Cancer Res 36: 4079–4091

Cloudman AM (1941) The effect of an extra-chromosomal influence upon translated spontaneous tumors in mice. Science 93: 380–381

Epstein JH, Epstein WL, Nakai T (1967) Production of melanomas from DMBA-induced blue nevus in hairless mice with ultraviolet light. JNCI 38: 19–30

Forbes PD (1965) Experimentally-induced neoplasms in the skin of mice. I. Single-dose effects of DMBA in

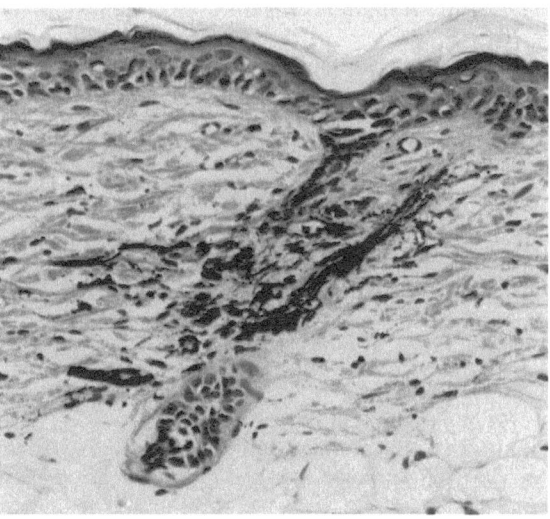

haired, hairless, and rhino mice. J Invest Dermatol 44: 388-398

Ghadially FN, Barker JF (1960) The histogenesis of experimentally induced melanotic tumours in the Syrian hamster *(Cricetus auratus).* J Pathol Bacteriol 79: 263-271

Harding HE, Passey RD (1930) A transplantable melanoma of the mouse. J Pathol Bacteriol 33: 417-427

Haseman JK, Huff JE, Rao GN, Arnold JE, Boorman GA, McConnell EE (1985) Neoplasms observed in untreated and corn oil gavage control groups of F344/N rats and (C57BL/6N × C3H/HeN)F$_1$ (B6C3F$_1$) mice. JNCI 75: 975-984

Iwata K, Inui N, Takeuchi T (1981) Induction of active melanocytes in mouse skin by carcinogens: a new method for detection of skin carcinogens. Carcinogenesis 2: 589-593

Kanno J, Matsubara O, Kasuga T (1986) Histogenesis of the intradermal melanocytic tumor in BDF1 mice induced by topical application of 9,10-dimethyl-1,2-benzanthracene (DMBA) and 12-0-tetradecanoylphorbol-13-acetate (TPA). Acta Pathol Jpn 36: 1-14

Kanno J, Matsubara O, Kasuga T (1987) Induction of melanogenesis in Schwann cell and perineural epithelium by 9,10-dimethyl-1,2-benzanthracene (DMBA) and 12-0-tetradecanoylphorbol-13-acetate (TPA) in BDF1 mice. Acta Pathol Jpn 37: 1297-1304

Klaus SN, Winkelmann RK (1965) Pigment changes induced in hairless mice by dimethylbenzanthracene. J Invest Dermatol 45: 160-167

Pawlowski A, Haberman HF, Menon IA (1976) Junctional and compound pigmented nevi induced by 9,10-dimethyl-1,2-benzanthracene in skin of albino guinea pigs. Cancer Res 36: 2813-2821

Pawlowski A, Haberman HF, Menon IA (1980) Skin melanoma induced by 7,12-dimethylbenzanthracene in albino guinea pigs and its similarities to skin melanoma of humans. Cancer Res 40: 3652-3660

Rocha G, Winkelmann RK (1962) Induced dermal melanocytosis in hairless mice. Arch Dermatol 86: 229-231

Roscoe B, Jackson Memorial Laboratory (1962) Handbook on genetically standardized JAX mice. Bar Harbor Times, Bar Harbor

Straile WE (1960) Sensory hair follicles in mammalian skin: the tylotrich follicle. Am J Anat 106: 133-147

Takizawa H, Sato S, Kitajima H, Konishi S, Iwata K, Hayashi Y (1985) Mouse skin melanoma induced in two stage chemical carcinogenesis with 7,12-dimethylbenz[a]anthracene and croton oil. Carcinogenesis 6: 921-923

Ward JM, Goodman DG, Squire RA, Chu KC, Linhart MS (1979) Neoplastic and nonneoplastic lesions in aging (C57BL/6N × C3H/HeN)F$_1$ (B6C3F$_1$) mice. JNCI 63: 849-854

Melanocytic Tumors, Skin, Hamster

Jun Kanno

Synonyms. Malignant melanoma; melanotic tumor; melanoma.

Gross Appearance

Melanocytic tumors are black or blue-black, elevated nodules usually measuring up to 1 cm in diameter. On cut sections, the tumors are well demarcated and pigmented to a variable degree.

Microscopic Features

Melanocytic tumors undergo nodular growth in the dermal adipose layer (Fig. 100). The tumor cells are fusiform, oval or polygonal in shape, heavily pigmented, closely packed together, and with slight atypism (Fig. 101). The tumors are accompanied by melanophages to differing extent.

Ultrastructure

The oval tumor cells are usually filled with fully melanized melanosomes. Phagocytic cells containing compound melanosomes are also found among the tumor cells (Rappaport et al. 1963). Schwann cells and perineural cells of the nerve bundles involved in the tumors often contain melanosomes (Nakai and Rappaport 1963).

Differential Diagnosis

The diagnosis of melanotic tumor of the skin is usually easy since other pigmented tumors are very rare in hamsters (Ghadially 1982). Diagnosis may be confirmed by demonstration of melanogenesis by electron microscopic detection of single membrane-bound melanosomes and premelanosomes or cytochemical confirmation of positive dopa reaction.

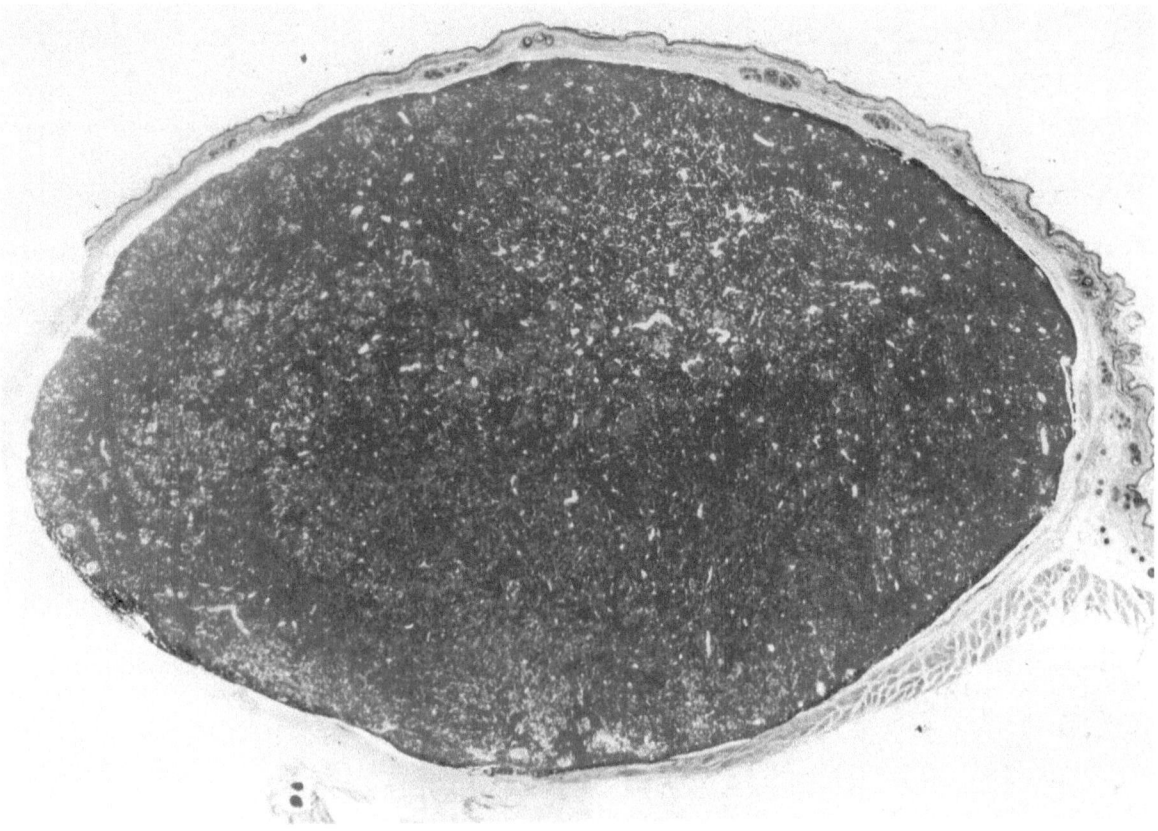

Fig. 100. Melanocytic tumor induced in skin of a Syrian golden hamster. H and E, × 20

Biologic Features

Spontaneous Melanocytic Tumors. The appearance of spontaneous malignant melanoma is more common in hamsters than in mice. Fortner and Allen (1959) reported 10 malignant melanomas in 523 Syrian golden hamsters (1.9%). However, the incidence of the melanoma was different among hamster strains: five melanomas (3.8%) and no blue nevus in 132 cream hamsters, no melanomas and two blue nevi (1.4%) in 141 white hamsters (Pour et al. 1979). Ghadially (1982) also commented that only in certain colonies of Syrian golden hamsters do spontaneous melanotic tumors occur.

Spontaneous melanotic tumors are reported to develop sporadically in the skin at any place over the body without any relation to the costovertebral spot or small pigmented spots around it (Fortner and Allen 1959).

Spontaneous melanomas may be invasive and occasionally metastasize (Fortner and Allen 1959).

Histologically, in spontaneous melanomas one can see junctional activity, indicating that they were derived from epidermal melanocytes (Fortner and Allen 1959).

Chemically Induced Melanocytic Tumors. Many reports are available of chemically induced melanocytic tumor of hamsters (Table 3). Melanocytic tumors are induced by single topical application of 7,12-dimethylbenz[*a*]anthracene (DMBA) (Nakai and Rappaport 1963; Della Porta et al. 1956; Rappaport et al. 1961; Shubik et al. 1960), single subcutaneous injection (Walters et al. 1967), or repeated topical application (Ghadially and Barker 1960; Ghadially and Illman 1963; Mishima and Oboler 1965; Shubik et al. 1960). Experiments based on two-stage carcinogenesis induced more melanocytic tumors without an increase in the incidence of other neoplasms (Goerttler et al. 1980, 1982; Della Porta et al. 1956; Quevedo et al. 1961). Urethan (Pietra and Shubik 1960; Vesselinovitch et al. 1970) and ethylnitrosourea (Pelfrene and Love 1977) also induce melanocytic tumors in hamsters. Chemically induced melanocytic tumors are believed to originate from PFM (Ghadially and Barker 1960; Ghadially and Illman 1963)

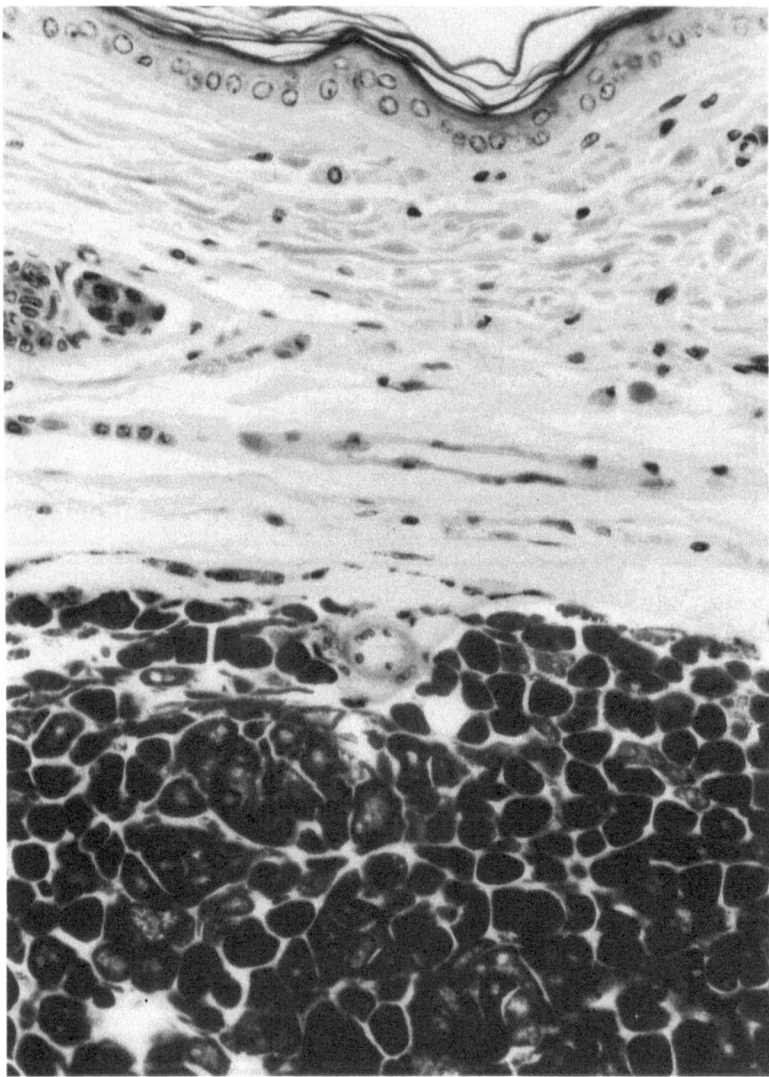

Fig. 101. Melanocytic tumor, skin, hamster, same case as in Fig. 100. H and E, ×320

and are usually localized and seldom metastasize (see Table 3).

The dendritic melanocytes of the nonalbino hamster skin can be divided into four types. There seems to be no fundamental differences between the cutaneous melanocytic system in hamsters and mice (see p. 63).

The costovertebral spots [flank organs or organs of Kupperman (1944)] are paired spots in the skin of the flank measuring about 5 mm in diameter. Histologically, they are made up of about 40 clusters of hair follicles with large sebaceous glands and dense perifollicular melanocytic networks (PFM) (Figs. 102 and 103). The PFM are seen in the costovertebral spots and in the so-called small pigmented spots around it. The small pigmented spots (Fig. 104) are identical

structures to PFMs in mice skin irrespective of their difference in size. Melanocytic tumors are not induced in the costovertebral spots but rather in the small pigment spots possibly because, in costovertebral spots, continual secretion from large sebaceous glands washes out the carcinomas (Ghadially and Barker 1960).

The pigmented spots are under the control of the sex hormones. Estrogens reduce the size of the costovertebral spots and increase the size of the small pigmented spot (Illman and Ghadially 1966). However, the relation between the sex hormones and melanocarcinogenesis is obscure.

Transplantable Melanoma. Greene (1958) and Fortner et al. (1961) reported transplantable spontaneous melanomas; most of them had a

Table 3. Chemically induced melanocytic tumors in hamsters

Author	Year	Hamster	Age or wgt	Treatment[a] Initiation	Promotion	Melanoma incidence	Latent period	Primary site histology	Metastasis
Della Porta et al.	1956	Syrian (golden)	adult	DMBA	–	4/14	41 w	blue nevus-like	no
		Syrian (golden)	adult	DMBA	croton oil	5/14	41 w	blue nevus-like	no
Ghadially and Barker	1960	Syrian	35 g	DMBA	–	3/40	9 w	blue nevus-like	–
		Syrian	50 g	DMBA	–	24/30	27 w	blue nevus-like	–
Illman and Ghadially	1966	Syrian (brown coat)	4–6 m	DMBA	–	19/19	17 w	blue nevus-like	no
		Syrian (white coat)	4–6 m	DMBA	–	18/23	17 w	blue nevus-like	no
		Syrian (cream coat)	4–6 m	DMBA	–	0/24	31 w	–	–
Pietra and Shubik	1960	Syrian (golden)	8–10 w	urethan (dw)	–	8/20	55–76 w	localized	no
		Syrian (golden)	8–10 w	urethan	–	0/20	95 w	–	–
Shubik et al.	1960	Syrian (golden)	10–12 w	DMBA	–	49/60	90 w	blue nevus-like plus 1 invasive	no yes[c]
		Syrian (golden)	10–12 w	BP	–	1/30	89 w	pigmented spot	no
Quevedo et al.	1961	Syrian (white coat)	4 m	DMBA	–	18/19	15 w	blue nevus-like	no
Rappaport et al.	1961	Syrian (white)	10–12 w	DMBA	–	41/47	79 w	blue nevus-like	no
Mishima and Oboler	1965	Syrian (golden)	30–50 g	DMBA	–	30/30	55 w	blue nevus-like	no
Walters et al.	1967	Syrian (golden)	1 day	DMBA (sc)	–	17/40	60 w	blue nevus-like plus invasive	no yes[d]
		Syrian (golden)	1 day	urethan (sc)	–	0/12	60 w	–	–
Vesselinovitch et al.	1970	Syrian (white)	in utero	urethan (ip)	–	19/54	45–48 w	localized plus invasive	no yes[e]
Pelfrene and Love	1977	Syrian (golden)	in utero	ENU (transp)	ENU	9/59[b]	17–43 w	localized	no
		Syrian (golden)	in utero	ENU (transp)	–	5/64[b]	23–50 w	localized	no
		Syrian (golden)	in utero	–	ENU	2/62	60 w	localized	no
Goerttler et al.	1980	Syrian (golden)	6 m	DMBA	–	4/20	22 w	blue nevus-like	
		Syrian (golden)	6 m	DMBA	TPA	20/40	16 w	blue nevus-like	
Goerttler et al.	1982	Syrian (golden)	8 w	DMBA	–	80%[f]	22 w	blue nevus-like	no
		Syrian (golden)	8 w	DMBA	TPA	100%[f]	18 w	blue nevus-like	no

[a] Topical application if not specified in the table as follows: dw, drinking water; sc, subcutaneous injection; ip, intraperitoneal injection; transp, transplacental application.
[b] Other neurogenic tumors such as schwannomas are also induced in high incidence.
[c] Lung and lymph node metastases.
[d] Lung metastases.
[e] Lung, lymph node, kidney, and liver metastases.
[f] 20 animals each at the beginning.
m, month; w, week.

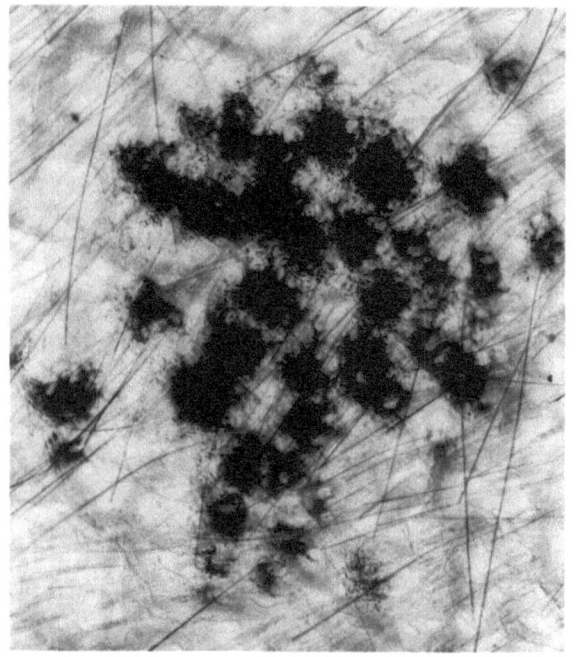

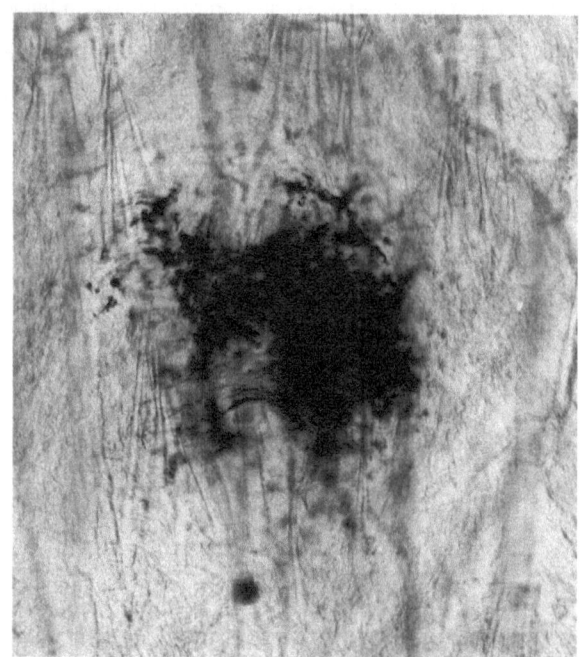

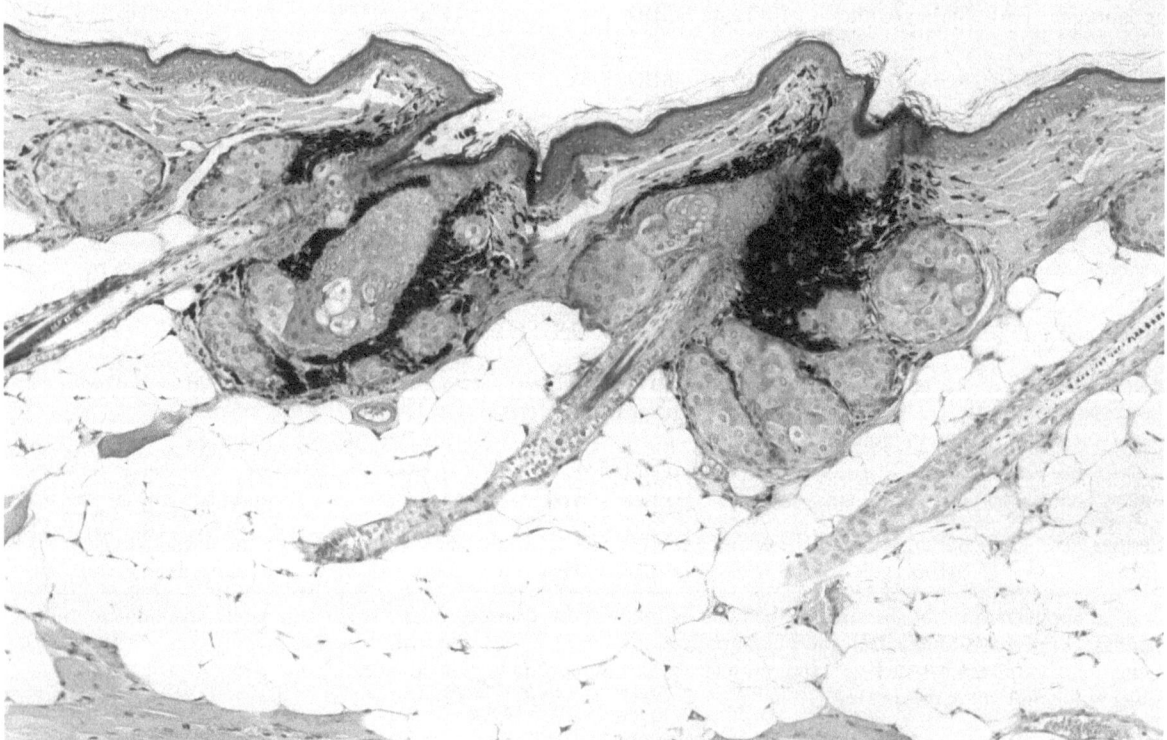

Fig. 102 *(upper left)*. A costovertebral spot in the skin of a Syrian golden hamster. It consists of about 40 clusters of highly pigmented, perifollicular melanocytic networks. Cleared skin preparation, × 20

Fig. 103 *(below)*. Costovertebral spot, skin of flank, Syrian hamster. Many dendritic melanocytes surround the necks of hair follicles and sebaceous glands. H and E, × 100

Fig. 104 *(upper right)*. Skin, Syrian hamster. A small pigmented spot near the costovertebral spot. Cleared skin preparation, × 80

tendency to become amelanotic and/or sarcomatous upon transplantation. Shubik et al. (1956) reported a transplantable, induced, melanotic tumor which originated from a blue nevus-like lesion.

Comparison with Other Species

Induced melanocytic tumors in mice are of intradermal origin, i.e., PFM origin without junctional activity. Guinea pigs, on the other hand, produce melanomas of junctional origin, which are similar to human skin melanomas (Clark et al. 1976; Pawlowski et al. 1976, 1980). Spontaneous malignant melanomas in the skin of the extremities were reported in 2% of females (5 of 236) and 4% of males (3 of 74) in an aging population of BN/Bi rats (Burek 1978).

References

Burek JD (1978) Pathology of aging rats. CRC, Boca Raton, pp 162-163

Clark WH Jr, Min BH, Kligman LHL (1976) The developmental biology of induced malignant melanoma in guinea pigs and a comparison with other neoplastic systems. Cancer Res 36: 4079-4091

Della Porta G, Rappaport H, Saffiotti U, Shubik P (1956) Induction of melanotic lesions during skin carcinogenesis in hamster. Arch Pathol 61: 305-313

Fortner JG, Allen AC (1959) Comparative oncology of melanomas in hamsters and man. In: Gordon M (ed) Pigment cell biology. Academic, New York, pp 85-98

Fortner JG, Mahy AG, Schrodt GR (1961) Transplantable tumors of the Syrian (golden) hamster, pt I. Tumors of the alimentary tract, endocrine glands and melanomas. Cancer Res 21 [Suppl]: 161-198

Ghadially FN (1982) Tumours of the skin. In: Turusov VS (ed) Pathology of tumours in laboratory animals, vol 3. Tumours of the hamster. IARC, Lyon, pp 1-32 (IARC Sci Publ no 34)

Ghadially FN, Barker JF (1960) The histogenesis of experimentally induced melanotic tumours in the Syrian hamster *(Cricetus auratus).* J Pathol Bacteriol 79: 263-271

Ghadially FN, Illman O (1963) The histogenesis of experimentally produced melanotic tumours in the Chinese hamster *(Cricetulus criseus).* Br J Cancer 17: 727-730

Goerttler K, Loehrke H, Schweizer J, Hesse B (1980) Two-stage tumorigenesis of dermal melanocytes in the back skin of the Syrian golden hamster using systemic initiation with 7,12-dimethylbenz(a)anthracene and topical promotion with 12-0-tetradecanoylphorbol-13-acetate. Cancer Res 40: 155-161

Goerttler K, Loehrke H, Hesse B, Pyerin WG (1982) Tumor initiation by 7,12-dimethylbenz[a]anthracene in dermal melanocytes of hamster: inhibition through 7,8-benzoflavone. Carcinogenesis 3: 791-795

Greene HSN (1958) A spontaneous melanoma in the hamster with a propensity for amelanotic alteration and sarcomatous transformation during transplantation. Cancer Res 18: 422-425

Illman O, Ghadially FN (1966) Effect of oestrogen on the small pigmented spots in hamsters. Nature 211: 1303-1304

Kupperman HS (1944) Hormonal control of a dimorphic pigmentation area in the golden hamster *(Cricetus auratus).* Anat Rec 88: 442

Mishima Y, Oboler AA (1965) Differential chemical carcinogenesis in three distinct melanocyte systems of Syrian (golden) hamsters. J Invest Dermatol 44: 157-169

Nakai T, Rappaport H (1963) A study of the histogenesis of experimental melanotic tumors resembling cellular blue nevi: the evidence in support of their neurogenic origin. Am J Pathol 43: 175-199

Pawlowski A, Haberman HF, Menon IA (1976) Junctional and compound pigmented nevi induced by 9,10-dimethyl-1,2-benzanthracene in skin of albino guinea pigs. Cancer Res 36: 2813-2821

Pawlowski A, Haberman HF, Menon IA (1980) Skin melanoma induced by 7,12-dimethylbenzanthracene in albino guinea pigs and its similarities to skin melanoma of humans. Cancer Res 40: 3652-3660

Pelfrene AF, Love LA (1977) Experimental induction of melanotic tumors in Syrian golden hamsters by transplacental and topical application of ethylnitrosourea. Z Krebsforsch 90: 233-239

Pietra G, Shubik P (1960) Induction of melanotic tumors in the Syrian golden hamster after administration of ethyl carbamate. JNCI 25: 627-630

Pour P, Althoff J, Salmasi SZ, Stepan K (1979) Spontaneous tumors and common diseases in three types of hamsters. JNCI 63: 797-811

Quevedo WC Jr, Cairns JM, Smith JA, Bock FG, Burns RJ (1961) Induction of melanotic tumours in the white ('partial albino') Syrian hamster. Nature 189: 936-937

Rappaport H, Pietra G, Shubik P (1961) The induction of melanotic tumors resembling cellular blue nevi in the Syrian white hamster by cutaneous application of 7,12-dimethylbenz[a]anthracene. Cancer Res 21: 661-666

Rappaport H, Nakai T, Swift H (1963) The fine structure of normal and neoplastic melanocytes in the Syrian hamster, with particular reference to carcinogen-induced melanotic tumors. J Cell Biol 16: 171-186

Shubik P, Della Porta G, Rappaport H, Spencer K (1956) A transplantable induced melanotic tumor of the Syrian golden hamster. Cancer Res 16: 1031-1032

Shubik P, Pietra G, Della Porta G (1960) Studies of skin carcinogenesis in the Syrian golden hamster. Cancer Res 20: 100-105

Vesselinovitch SD, Mihailovich N, Richter WR (1970) The induction of malignant melanomas in Syrian white hamster by neonatal exposure to urethan. Cancer Res 30: 2543-2547

Walters MA, Roe FJC, Levene A (1967) The induction of tumours and other lesions in hamsters by a single subcutaneous injection of 9,10-dimethyl-7-1,2-benzanthracene or urethane on the first day of life. Br J Cancer 21: 184-190

Melanocytic Tumors, Rat

Chris Zurcher and P.J.M.Roholl

Synonyms. Melanoma.

Gross Appearance

Most spontaneous melanocytic tumors reported in rats are located in the skin. They appear as tiny black spots or raised firm black nodules generally less than 1 cm in diameter or as local, dark-stained, diffuse, irregularly delineated, thickened areas of the skin. Ulceration and crust formation are common. When located in the uveal tract, protrusion of the eye bulb, conjunctival discharge, and corneal opacities may occur (see p.78).

Predilection sites are: skin of the external ear (Fig.105), genitalia, tail, and eye. In 15%–30% of cases metastases can be observed as evidenced by enlarged, black, regional lymph nodes or black spots in the lungs (Hollander et al. 1974; Burek 1978).

Microscopic Features

The earliest signs of melanocyte proliferation are seen at the predilection sites of melanocytic tumor formation. They can be considered as premalignant. In the skin, focal hyperplasia of scattered dermal melanocytes without any epidermal junctional involvement is observed (Fig.106). Such lesions are grossly visible as a flat, dark spot.

Small melanocytic tumors are characterized by expansive growth in the loose connective tissue of dermis and subcutis (Fig.107) and consist of dense aggregates of dermal melanocytes with many melanin-containing macrophages (melanophages) interspersed between the melanocytes. Cellular and nuclear pleomorphism are moderate. Mitoses are infrequent.

Larger tumors may invade and destroy pre-existent adjacent structures (Fig.108). Most of the cells are filled with dark-brown pigment granules, staining positively by the Fontana or Schmorl's reaction for melanin; bleaching is often necessary to allow microscopic examination

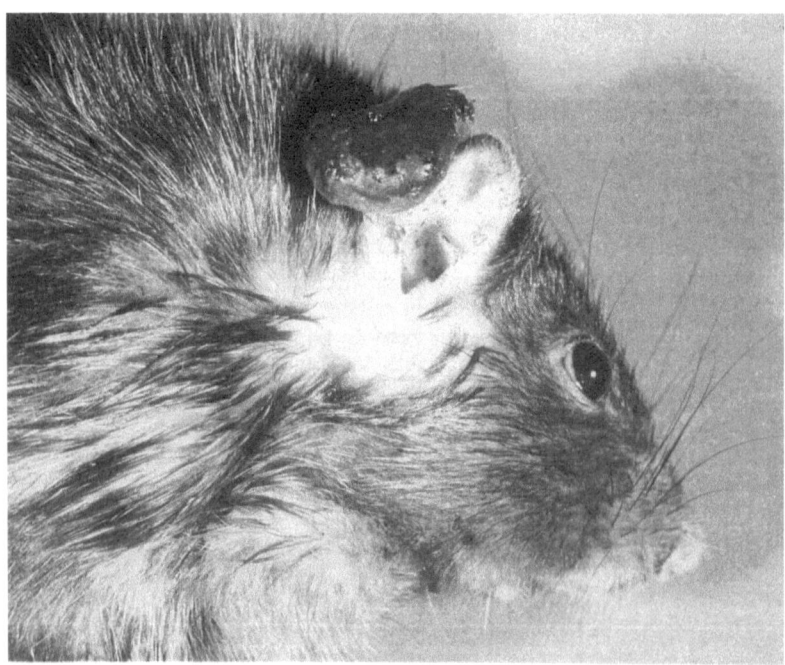

Fig. 105. Ulcerated, partly melanized, malignant melanocytic tumor in the pinna of an untreated male (WAG × BN)F$_1$ rat, 23 months of age

for cytological details (Fig. 109). Generally, the more densely pigmented cells are macrophages characterized by a large amount of cytoplasm filled with fine, dustlike or coarse melanin granules and a small round or oval, eccentric nucleus. The nonadherent tumor cells have a moderate amount of cytoplasm containing scattered, fine melanin granules and an irregular, large nucleus with coarse or finely granular chromatin and one or two small nucleoli. Mitoses are frequent.

In later stages of tumor development diversification of growth pattern, cellular characteristics, and melanin production occurs. Epithelial, spindle cell, schwannoma-type, and anaplastic areas may be recognized even within the same tumor. In the histologically more malignant areas, often characterized by an epitheloid or anaplastic growth pattern, the tumor cells generally contain less melanin.

While melanin within the tumor cells may be inapparent under light microscopy, its production by these cells is suggested by many heavily melanized macrophages in the intervening stromal

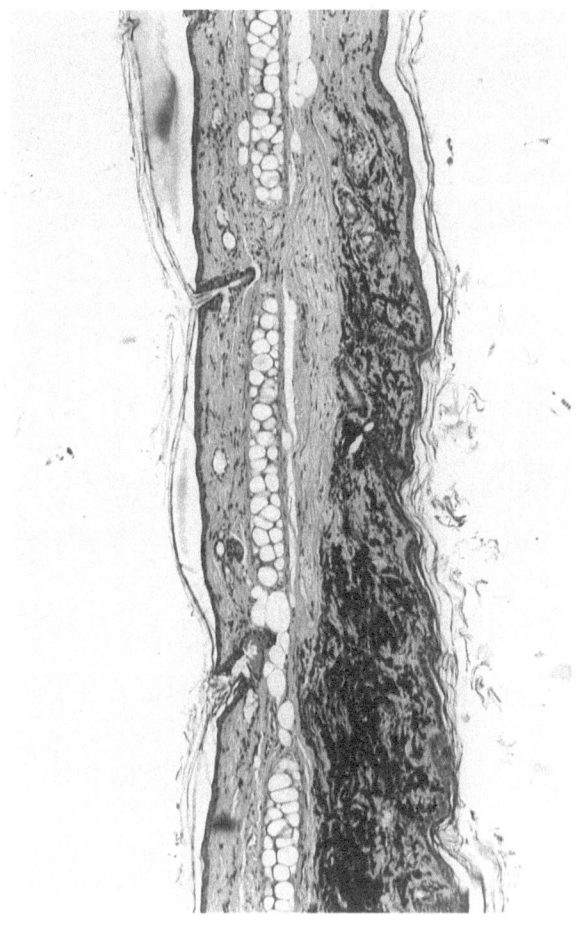

Fig. 106. Hyperplasia of dermal melanocytes in the pinna ▶ of a 10-month-old male BN rat treated with cyclophosphamide 100 mg kg⁻¹ i.p. and total body irradiation. Hematoxylin phloxine saffron, × 75

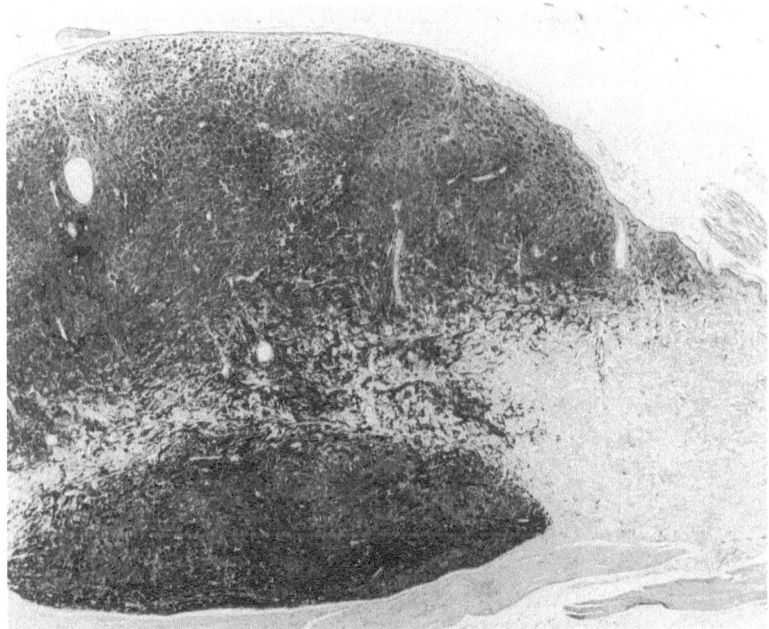

Fig. 107. Melanocytic tumor at the base of the tail of a 16-month-old BN rat treated with cyclophosphamide and total body irradiation. Hematoxylin phloxine saffron, × 35

78   Chris Zurcher and P. J. M. Roholl

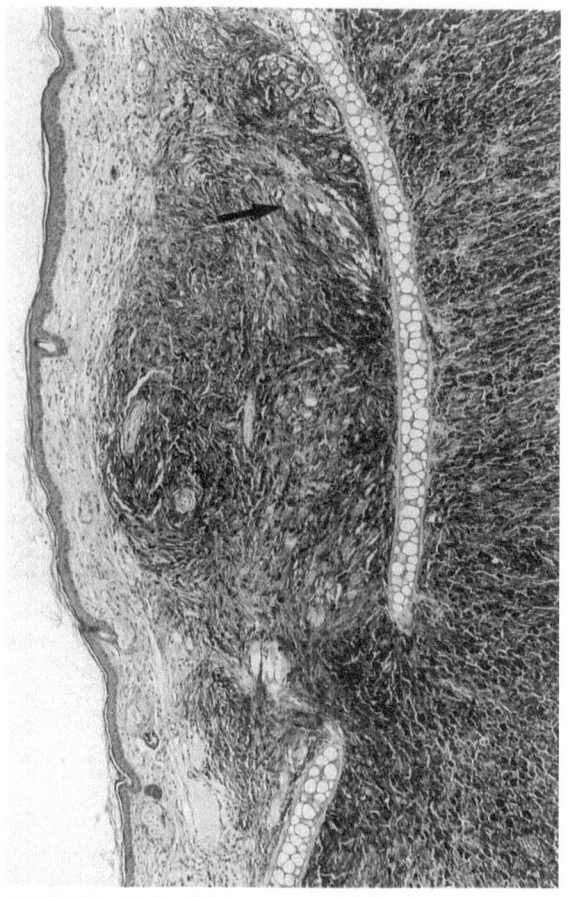

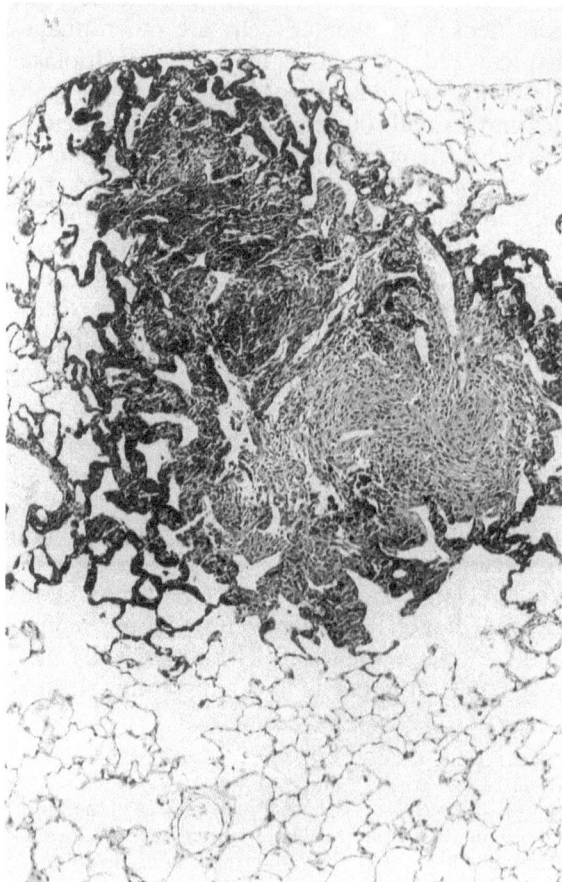

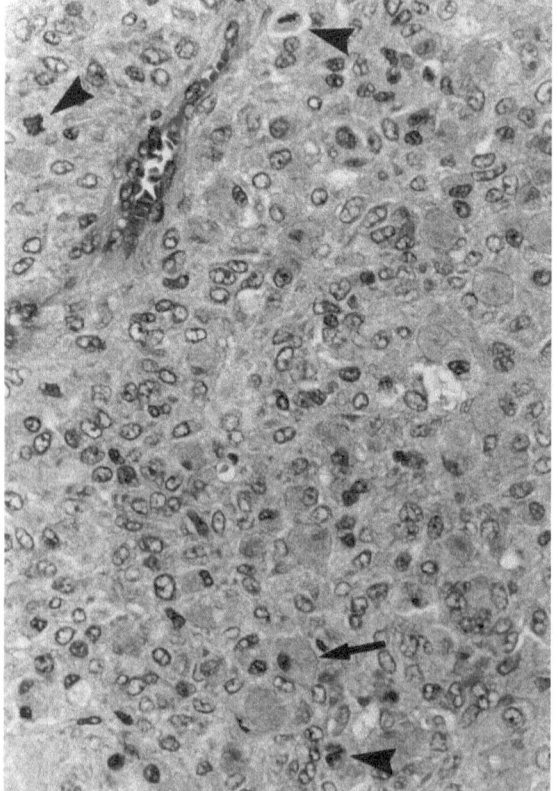

Fig. 108 *(upper left).* Part of a large malignant melanocytic tumor in the pinna of a 25-month-old male BN rat treated with cyclophosphamide and total body irradiation. Note destruction of cartilage and invasion into striated muscle *(arrow).* Hematoxylin phloxine saffron, × 55

Fig. 109 *(lower left).* Malignant melanocytic tumor in the ear of an untreated 16-month-old male (WAG × BN)F₁ rat. Note melanocytes with moderately pleomorphic nuclei and many interspersed macrophages *(arrow).* Mitotic figures are frequent *(arrowheads).* Biopsy specimen, bleached preparation, hematoxylin phloxine saffron, × 340

Fig. 110 *(upper right).* Metastasis to lung from a melanocytic tumor of the chorioid of the eye in an untreated 10-month-old male hooded U rat. Hematoxylin phloxine saffron, × 85

compartment or at the edge of apparently amela-notic metastases (Fig. 110). Smaller and larger areas of necrosis can be found in epitheloid and anaplastic areas and ulceration of the overlying skin may be severe.

Spindle cell areas may differ considerably from each other. In the histologically less malignant form, tumor cells are fusiform, nuclear pleomorphism is moderate, and mitoses are infrequent. The intervening stroma may be substantial and contains many melanophages. In the more malignant-appearing variant the slender fusiform cells generally contain less melanin and are arranged in loose bundles with a minimal amount of connective tissue (Fig. 111). Nuclei are oval with stippled or coarse chromatin, and mitoses are frequent. Transition into anaplastic areas is common (Fig. 112).

In *epitheloid cell* areas (Figs. 113 and 114) the tumor grows in irregularly sized fields or nests, separated by thin strands of connective tissue, and consists of loosely adherent large cells with pale-staining, sometimes vacuolated, cytoplasm with scant or no melanin granules and pleomorphic nuclei. Mitoses may be frequent.

Anaplastic melanocytic tumor areas (Fig. 115) consist of loosely adherent small cells with a small amount of eosinophilic cytoplasm and moderately pleomorphic, round to oval, hyperchromatic nuclei. Mitoses are frequent.

In exceptional cases a pattern resembling a Schwann's cell may occur with fusiform cells, focal nuclear palisading, and a finely wavy, fibrillar, acellular stromal component. In one case of an amelanotic melanoma of the ear of a WAG/Rij rat, this latter pattern was predominant, with focal epitheloid junctional activity (Fig. 116 and 117).

In all growth patterns, nuclei and to a lesser degree cytoplasm generally stain positively with polyclonal antibodies to S-100 protein. This characteristic is suggestive, although not proof, of a neural crest origin.

Inflammatory cells other than macrophages are generally absent. Notably, lymphoid cell infiltration suggestive of an immunological reaction to this tumor type, as may be seen in some other species, is not conspicuous.

Ultrastructure

In order to allow a proper interpretation of the few data available on the ultrastructural aspects of melanocytic tumors in rats, it is necessary to

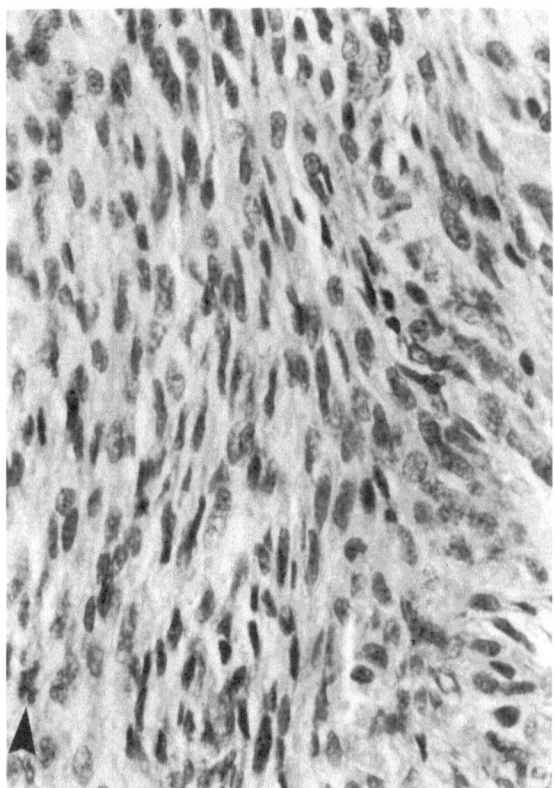

Fig. 111. Biopsy of the same tumor as in Fig. 109 but 4 months later, with spindle cell areas not present in the first biopsy. Plump cells with pleomorphic, elongated nuclei with fine or coarse granular chromatin. Sporadic mitoses are present *(arrowhead)*. Bleached preparation, hematoxylin phloxine saffron, × 525

provide some basic information derived from studies on melanogenesis in other species.

Melanocytes of mammalian species are characterized by melanin production and deposition within specialized cytoplasmic organelles, so-called melanosomes. Four stages of melanosomes development can be recognized: stages I and II, unmelanized; stage III, partly melanized; stage IV, completely melanized (Szpak et al. 1988).

Two types of melanin may be formed through oxidation of tyrosine and DOPA in the presence of tyrosinase: brown-black eumelanin and reddish-brown pheomelanin. Under normal conditions, as revealed by studies on melanogenesis in mice, eumelanogenesis is associated with ellipsoid mature melanosomes and pheomelanogenesis with spherical mature melanosomes. In mice, stage I melanosomes (derived from dilatation of agranular portions of the rough endoplasmic reticulum) are spherical, single membrane-limited,

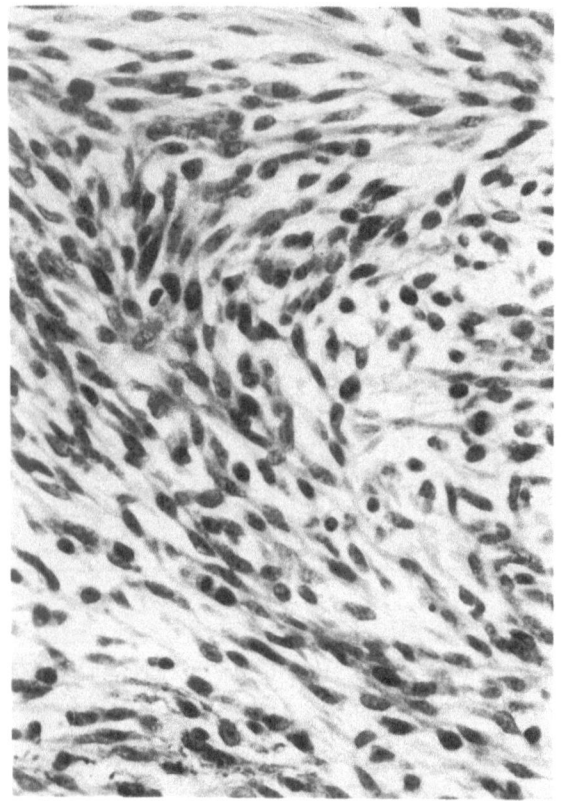

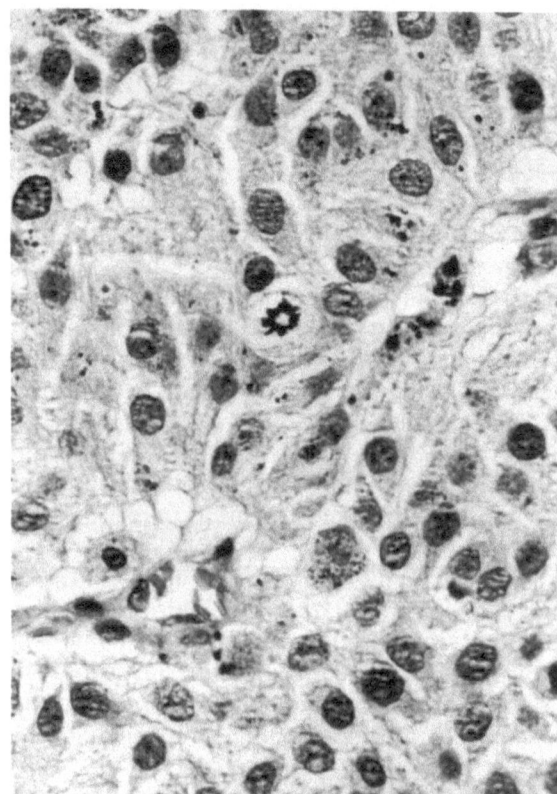

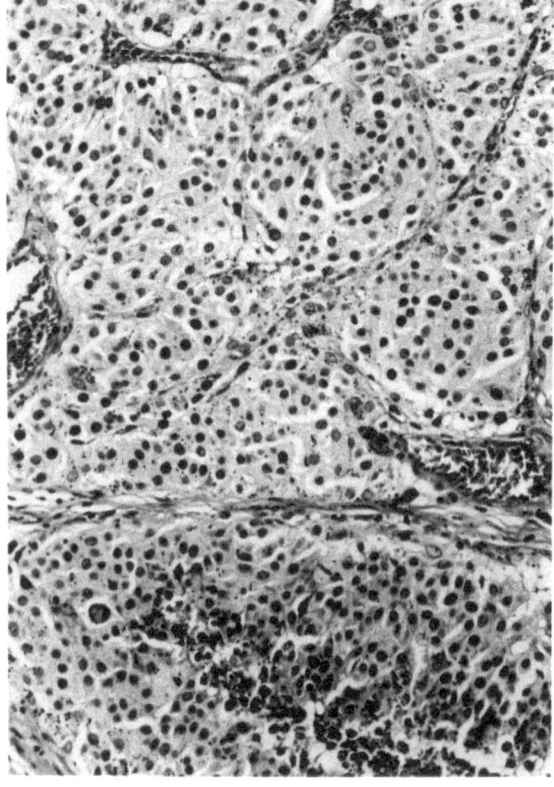

Fig. 112 *(upper left)*. Spindle cell area of the same malignant melanocytic tumor as in Fig. 109 and 111 at time of death, 3 months after the last biopsy. The gross appearance is seen in Fig. 105. The loosely arranged slender spindle cells have scant eosinophilic cytoplasm with sporadic melanin granules and pleomorphic oval nuclei. Scattered pleomorphic anaplastic tumor cells are present. Melanophages are infrequent. Hematoxylin phloxine saffron, × 420

Fig. 113 *(lower left)*. Melanocytic tumor, male, 24 month-old BN rat. Fields of loosely arranged epithelioid cells with focal central necrosis separated by thin strands of connective tissue. Hematoxylin phloxine saffron, × 170

Fig. 114 *(upper right)*. Higher magnification view of Fig. 113. Epithelioid cells with pale stained or vacuolated cytoplasms containing scattered melanin granules. Mitotic figures are common. Hematoxylin phloxine saffron, × 525

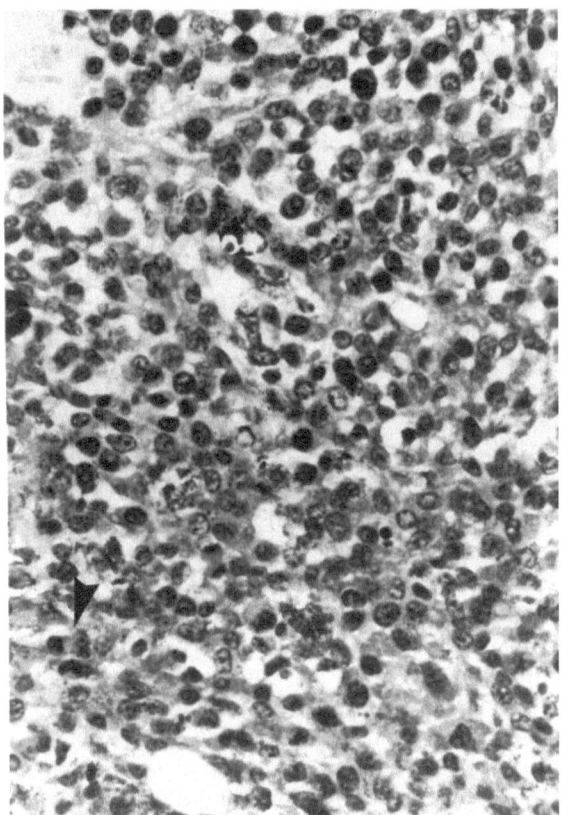

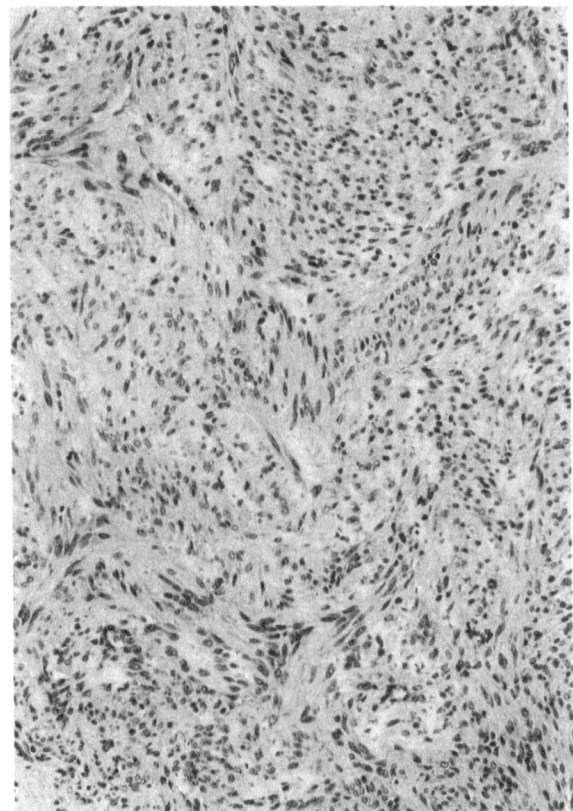

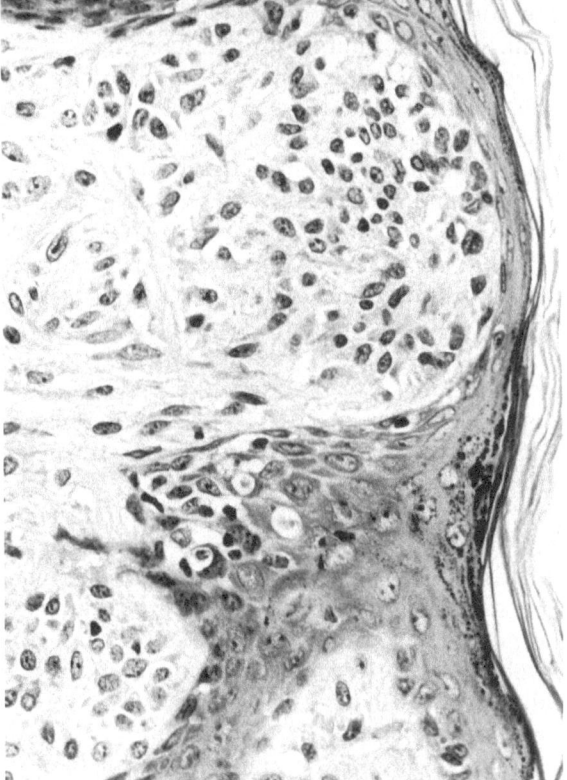

Fig. 115 *(upper left)*. Anaplastic cell area of same tumor as presented in Fig. 112 showing loosely adherent small cells with scant eosinophilic cytoplasm without melanin granules and with small round or oval hyperchromatic pleomorphic nuclei. Some mitotic figures are present *(arrowhead)*. Hematoxylin phloxine saffron, × 420

Fig. 116 *(upper right)*. Amelanotic malignant melanocytic tumor in the pinna of a 37-month-old untreated female WAG/Rij rat. Note predominant Schwann cell growth pattern. Spindle cells with faintly eosinophilic cytoplasm are arranged in small bundles. Focal nuclear palisading is present, bordering acellular areas in a fine fibrillar appearance. Hematoxylin phloxine saffron, × 140

Fig. 117 *(lower right)*. Same case as in Fig. 116. Tumor cells in dermis form cell nests in direct contact and invade the epidermis. Hematoxylin phloxine saffron, × 440

cytoplasmic organelles, containing a few so-called vesiculo-globular bodies (Jimbow et al. 1979). They are identical in eumelanogenesis and pheomelanogenesis. Starting with stage II melanosomes (premelanosomes) development is different for both types of melanin production. Stage II eumelanosomes are ellipsoid with an internal oblong fibrillar or lamellar matrix organization with cross-striations and parallel arrangement of the vesiculo-globular bodies (Jimbow et al. 1979). Stage II pheomelanosomes are spherical with many vesiculo-globular bodies and no lamellar organization of the internal matrix. In stage III eumelanin is deposited along the lamellae, and pheomelanin is deposited on the surface and inner core of the vesiculo-globular bodies with subsequent fusion into larger aggregates. Finally in stage IV completely melanized ellipsoid eumelanosomes and spherical granular pheomelanosomes result. These are difficult to distinguish from melanin granules taken up by macrophages and other cells.

While the presence of ellipsoid stage II melanosomes with a lamellar internal organization and cross-striations is generally considered to be the hallmark of human malignant melanoma (Ackerman 1981; Ghadially 1985), this may not be the case for melanocytic tumors of other species. Form, size, and internal organization may differ between species and between genotypes of the same species (Jimbow et al. 1979; Lever and Schaumburg-Lever 1983). Moreover, in tumors, melanosome morphogenesis does not directly reflect the amount or the type of melanin produced (Jimbow et al. 1984). They generally contain eumelanin and pheomelanin in varying quantities and proportions, and the ultrastructural organization of their melanosomes may differ completely even when they are predominantly eumelanogenic, e.g., the spherical granular melanosomes of the Harding-Passey (HP) and ellipsoid laminated melanosomes of the B 16 mouse melanoma cell lines (Jimbow et al. 1984).

Other ultrastructural characteristics of melanocytic tumors as described in various species (Ghadially 1985; Kanno et al. 1986; Junker and Chemnitz 1981; Demopoulos et al. 1965) include the presence of cytoplasmic protrusions, a well-developed endoplasmic reticulum, and Golgi apparatus. Intercellular junctions are infrequent, as are external lamina.

Ultrastructural studies on rat melanocytic tumors are few and incomplete and therefore have to be interpreted based on the data derived from studies in other species as detailed above. Ultra-structural examination of melanin-containing malignant melanomas of the uveal tract (iris, ciliary body, chorioid), induced in Fischer 344 rats by intraocular injection of nickel subsulfide (Ni_3S_2) (Albert et al. 1982) and in Wistar rats by intraocular injection of N-methyl-N-nitrosourea (Albert et al. 1986), revealed the presence of completely melanized melanosomes and partly melanized premelanosomes. No data were provided on the internal structure of the premelanomes. The depicted premelanosomes, however, had a spherical, granular appearance (Albert et al. 1982).

Electron microscopic studies performed on a melanocytic tumor in the skin of one of our (WAG × BN)F_1 rats disclosed the presence of melanocytes and many macrophages. Cells of the latter type contain a variable number of melanin granules of different sizes engulfed within secondary lysosomes. Peripherally in the cytoplasms of the melanocytes many more or less regular sized, round or oval, single membrane-delineated, and partly or completely melanized melanosomes were observed (Fig. 118). Sporadic, round, stage III melanosomes had various sized granules without any internal laminated structures. The latter aspect was similar to that presented by Albert et al. (1982). Depending on the stage of melanogenesis, melanin accumulates within the melanosomes, dispersed as fine granules or in needle shapes (Figs. 119 and 120). Vesiculo-globular bodies as described in normal melanogenesis in mice (Jimbow et al. 1979) were not seen. Other ultrastructural cytoplasmic characteristics of the melanocytic tumor cells were: many small, round, agranular, single membrane-bound vesicles, most probably derived from the smooth endoplasmic reticulum; a well-developed rough endoplasmic reticulum (RER) and Golgi apparatus; and sparse mitochondria. The nuclei were irregular with much euchromatin. Nucleoli were sometimes seen (Fig. 118). External laminae and cellular protrusions were not observed in this case.

Differential Diagnosis

Melanocytic tumors have to be distinguished from other heavily pigmented tumors. Pigmented squamous cell, basal cell, and adnexal skin tumors can easily be recognized as such by routine light microscopy. Ultrastructurally they can contain melanosomes and premelanosomes which may have been transferred from neighbouring melanocytes.

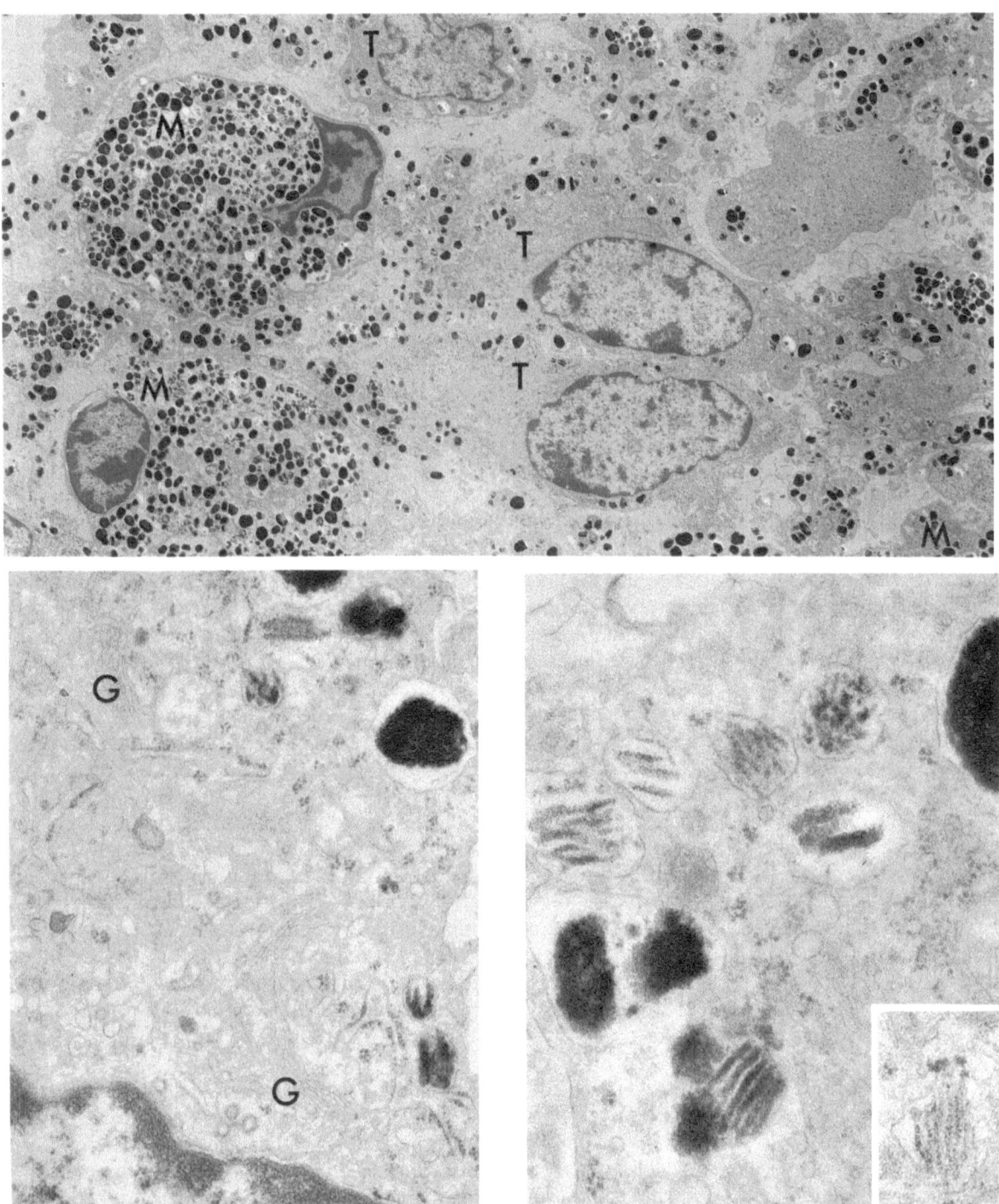

Fig. 118 *(above)*. Malignant melanocytic tumor in the pinna of a 24-month-old, female, UV-irradiated BN rat. Tumor cells *(T)* and macrophages *(M)*. The pigmented tumor cells are elongated; the nuclei are large, slightly irregular, and contain much euchromatin. Melanosomes in the periphery of the cytoplasm are partly or completely melanized. The macrophages possess an abundance of ingested melanosomes within lysosomes. TEM, × 4500

Fig. 119 *(lower left)*. Cytoplasm of a malignant melanocyte. Same case as in Fig. 118. Melanosomes in varying

degrees of melanization are present. The Golgi apparatus *(G)* is prominent with many adjacent formative vesicles. TEM, × 27 500

Fig. 120 *(lower right)*. Enlargement of melanosomes. Several irregular round melanosomes are in various stages of development, with laminar or granular melanin deposition. The banded material present within one of the melanosomes *(inset)* is suggestive of the characteristic transverse striation pattern seen in other species. TEM, × 47 500

Problems arise with tumors of neural crest origin, as some of them can produce melanin, e.g., nerve sheath tumors, and outside the skin, meningiomas and others such as medullary thyroid carcinoma. These tumors, too, can consist of epithelioid cells as well as spindle-shaped cells. Melanin and S100 positivity are often not discriminatory in such cases. Ultrastructural characteristics and extensive immunohistochemical investigations for specific differentiation products may be necessary to reach a diagnosis. Such methods are regularly applied in human diagnostic pathology (Ruiter et al. 1987; Van Duinen et al. 1984). By using a panel of monoclonal and polyclonal antibodies to intermediate filaments and other antigenic differentiation markers, a melanoma-specific pattern may result. For instance, positive reactions for vimentin, S100, and NKI/C-3 and negative ones for cytokeratin, desmin, neurofilament, and epithelial membrane antigen are highly suggestive of a diagnosis of malignant melanoma in man (Ruiter et al. 1987). In a comparable way antibodies to polypeptide hormones may be used to determine whether a specific hormone is produced (Nieuwenhuyzen Kruseman 1987).

However, experience with immunohistochemistry applied the studies in rodents is rare. With the increasing availability of monoclonal antibodies for use in formalin-fixed material, this may change in the future. In most instances, however, location and light microscopic features such as the presence of focal nuclear palisading and Verocay bodies and cyst formation (in case of a nerve sheath tumor in the skin) will be sufficient to reach a diagnosis.

Biologic features

No systematic studies on the histogenesis and biological behavior of rat melanocytic tumors have been reported.

Reports of spontaneous melanocytic tumors in rats are few and are mostly part of a survey of neoplastic and nonneoplastic changes occurring with age in a particular strain of rats (Hollander et al. 1974; Burek 1978; Ward et al. 1983). Only Burek provides data on gross appearance, location, and size of the tumors and age of the rats affected. All eight tumors from his series measured less than 0.8 cm and were observed in rats aged between 26 and 35 months. Three of them had black, enlarged regional lymph nodes due to metastases. In the remaining rats regional lymph nodes were not remarkable at gross necropsy and not included for routine histology. In the course of a series of lifelong experiments at the REP TNO Institutes an additional 18 melanocytic tumors were observed in BN/BiRij ($n=14$), (WAG × BN)F$_1$ ($n=2$), U ($n=1$), and WAG/Rij ($n=1$) rats. Of these, 9 occurred in the ear, 5 in the anogenital region or tail and 3 in the uveal tract. Three of them had metastasized to lungs and lymph nodes. One case described by Deerberg et al. (1986) was located in the scrotal skin and had metastasized to the regional lymph node.

This high frequency of metastasis and the histological signs of malignancy, such as invasion and destruction of surrounding tissues in those tumors which did not metastize, confirm the malignant potential of the rat melanocytic tumors. Some of the BN/Bi melanocytic tumors of the skin proved to be transplantable in syngeneic rats (Maat, personal communication, 1974).

Spontaneous incidence in rats is low. Apart from incidental findings, a small series of malignant melanocytic tumors has been described in male (3 out of 73) and female (5 out of 218) BN/BiRij rats (Burek 1978) and in male (7 out of 216) ACI rats (Ward et al. 1983). The majority of spontaneous melanocytic tumors in rats are melanin producing and occur in pigment-forming rat strains (such as ACI, BN/Bi, (WAG × BN)F$_1$, and U). Strangely, also those induced in albino rats by intraocular injection of carcinogenic substances were reported to be melanin positive (Albert et al. 1982, 1986). Spontaneously occurring amelanotic melanocytic tumors may occur in albino rats (Magnusson et al. 1978), but diagnosis without additional ultrastructural or immunohistochemical studies is difficult in most cases due to the protean nature of these tumors.

Histogenesis. The tumors arise from melanocytes, one of the cell types originating from the neural crest. They are specialized cells characterized by the presence of tyrosinase within premelanosomes, catalyzing the oxidation of tyrosine to melanin. They are predominant in the skin and eye but may occur in various other tissues such as the meninges and perivascular tissue in the brain. Under certain conditions other cells of neural crest origin such as various neuroendocrine tissues may develop melanin-producing activity.

Whether the predilection of melanocytic tumors to occur in certain areas is related to the presence of a greater number of melanocytes in these regions such as in the anogenital area, or to a greater exposure to high energy photons such as on the ears, or to both as in the eye is unknown.

Melanocytes in the skin may occur in close association with or within the epidermis and adnexal structures but also within the dermis. The smallest melanocytic tumors in the rat skin are found in the dermis and have no contact with the epidermis or skin adnexa. The majority, therefore, seem to arise from dermal melanocytes. Their human counterpart would then be the so-called malignant cellular blue nevus and not the more common malignant melanoma. The dermal origin of rat melanocytic tumors is comparable to those induced in hamsters (Goerttler et al. 1980; Nakai and Rappaport 1963) and mice (Berkelhammer et al. 1982; Kanno et al. 1986). Sequential light microscopic and ultrastructural studies in mice treated with topical 9,10-dimethyl-1,2-benzanthracene (DMBA) and 12-0-tetradeca-noylphorbol-13-acetate (TPA) revealed that melanocytic tumors did arise from melanocytes of the perifollicular melanocytic network (Kanno et al. 1986).

Induced tumors. Melanocytic tumors apparently are more difficult to induce in rats (Zackheim 1973) than in other rodent species (Nakai et al. 1963; Goerttler et al. 1980; Berkelhammer et al. 1982; Kanno et al. 1986). Documented reports on high yield melanocytic tumor induction in rats are limited to those induced in the uveal tract by subcutaneous injections of urethan or N-hydroxyurethan in neonatal rats (Kendrey and Roe 1969). Spontaneous intraocular melanomas in rats are reportedly infrequent (Magnusson et al. 1978). Some of the tumor originating in the eye were histologically malignant with invasion into surrounding tissues, and in a single case distant metastasis was observed.

No significantly increased incidence of malignant melanocytic tumors was observed in BN rats treated supralethal total body irradiation with or without cyclophosphamide followed by bone narrow transplantation (Zurcher et al. 1987).

Comparison with Other Species

Spontaneous melanocytic tumors occur in various species ranging from fish (Sobel et al. 1976) to humans. Among animals they are frequent in grey horses, dogs, some breeds of miniature pigs

(Jubb et al. 1985; Hook et al. 1982), and humans. They are rare in cats and sheep (Weiss and Frese 1974; Jubb et al. 1985).

They may be benign or malignant and originate from clusters of epidermal or dermal melanocytes of the skin and mucous membranes, from uveal tract melanocytes, but also from dispersed melanocytes elsewhere in the body. Histogenetically, skin melanomas of dogs and pigs with a pronounced intraepidermal component are most comparable to the predominant types of malignant melanoma in man.

Transplantation of rat skin melanocytic tumors is feasible (Maat 1974) but has been limited, in contrast to the experience in mice.

The rat (and mouse) melanocytic tumors are in most instances of dermal melanocytic origin and therefore more comparable with the human malignant cellular nevus tumors than with the more common malignant melanomas of epidermal melanocytic origin in that species. However, the availability of rodent models for human malignant melanocytic tumors in the skin and eye is advantageous to study problems common to all malignant melanocytic tumors such as: etiology, pathogenesis, melanogenesis, host immunological resistance, metastatic capacity, and treatment (see p.63).

Acknowledgements. We are grateful to Mrs. E.Blauw, Mr. A.A.Glaudmans, and Mr. E.H. Offerman for their expert technical assistance.

References

Ackerman AB (1981) Pathology of malignant melanoma. Masson, New York

Albert DM, Gonder JR, Papale J, Craft JL, Dohlman HG, Reid MC, Sunderman FW Jr (1982) Induction of ocular neoplasms in Fischer rats by intraocular injection of nickel subsulfide. Invest Ophthalmol Vis Sci 22: 768–782

Albert DM, Puliafito CA, Haluska FG, Kimball GP, Robinson NL (1986) Induction of ocular neoplasms in Wistar rats by N-methyl-N-nitrosurea. Exp Eye Res 42: 83–86

Berkelhammer J, Oxenhandler RW, Hook RR Jr, Hennessy JM (1982) Development of a new melanoma model in C57BL/6 mice. Cancer Res 42: 3157–3163

Burek JD (1978) Pathology of aging rats. A morphological and experimental study of the age-associated lesions in aging BN/Bi, WAG/Rij and (WAG × BN)F$_1$ rats. CRC, Boca Raton

Deerberg F, Knupp F, Rehm S (1986) Spontaneous epithelial tumors of the skin of HAN:WIST and DA/Han rats. Z Versuchstierkd 28: 45–57

Demopoulos HB, Kasuga T, Channing AA, Bagdoyan H (1965) Comparison of ultrastructure of B-16 and S91 mouse melanomas and correlation with growth patterns. Lab Invest 14: 108-121

Ghadially FN (1985) Diagnostic electron microscopy of tumours, 2nd edn., Butterworths, London

Goerttler K, Loehrke H, Schweizer J, Hesse B (1980) Two-stage tumorigenesis of dermal melanocytes in the back skin of the Syrian golden hamster using systemic initiation with 7,12-dimethylbenz(a)anthracene and topical promotion with 12-0-tetradecanoylphorbol-13-acetate. Cancer Res 40: 155-161

Hollander CF, Boorman GA, Zurcher C (1974) Classification of malignant tumours in rodents. In: Severi L (ed) Multiple primary malignant tumors. Proceedings of the 5th Perugia Quadrennial International Conference on Cancer. Division of Cancer Research, Perugia

Hook RR Jr, Berkelhammer J, Oxenhandler RW (1982) Animal model of human disease: Sinclair swine melanoma. Am J Pathol 108: 130-133

Jimbow K, Oikawa O, Sugiyama S, Takeuchi T (1979) Comparison of eumelanogenesis and pheomelanogenesis in retinal and follicular melanocytes; role of vesiculo-globular bodies in melanosome differentiation. J Invest Dermatol 73: 278-284

Jimbow K, Miyake Y, Homma K, Yasuda K, Izumi Y, Tsutsumi A, Ito S (1984) Characterization of melanogenesis and morphogenesis of melanosomes by physiochemical properties of melanin and melanosomes in malignant melanoma. Cancer Res 44: 1128-1134

Jubb KVD, Kennedy PC, Palmer N (1985) Pathology of domestic animals, 3rd edn. Academic, Orlando

Junker S, Chemnitz J (1981) Ultrastructural characterization of a mouse melanoma cell line, a mouse fibroblastic cell line, and hybrids between them. Eur J Cell Biol 24: 16-19

Kanno J, Matsubara O, Kasuga T (1986) Histogenesis of the intradermal melanocytic tumor in BDF1 mice induced by topical application of 9,10-dimethyl-1,2-benzanthracene (DMBA) and 12-0-tetradecanoylphorbol-13-acetate (TPA). Acta Pathol Jpn 36: 1-14

Kendrey G, Roe FJC (1969) Melanotic lesions of the eye in August hooded rats induced by urethan or N-hydroxyurethan given during the neonatal period: a histopathological study. JNCI 43: 749-762

Lever WF, Schaumburg-Lever G (1983) Histopathology of the skin. Lippincott Medical, Philadelphia

Maat B (1974) New animal model for melanoma: identification of factors modifying tumour growth. In: Annual report REPGO-TNO, Rijswijk, pp 59-60

Magnusson G, Majeed S, Offer JM (1978) Intraocular melanoma in the rat. Lab Anim 12: 249-252

Nakai T, Rappaport H (1963) Carcinogen-induced melanotic tumors in animals. NCI Monogr 10: 297-322

Nieuwenhuyzen Kruseman AC (1987) Endocrine tumors. In: Ruiter DJ, Fleuren GJ, Warnaar SO (eds) Applications of monoclonal antibodies in tumor pathology. Development in oncology series. Kluwer Academic/Nijhoff, The Hague, pp 255-263

Ruiter DJ, Broecker EB, Vennegoor C, Ferrone S (1987) Monoclonal antibodies recognizing melanoma associated antigens. In: Ruiter DJ, Fleuren GJ, Warnaar SO (eds) Applications of monoclonal antibodies in tumor pathology. Nijhoff, The Hague, pp 131-166

Sobel HJ, Marquet E, Kallman KD, Corly GJ (1976) Animal model of human disease malignant melanoma. Hereditary malignant melanomas in Platy/Swordtail hybrids. Am J Pathol 82: 441-444

Szpak CA, Shelburne J, Linder J, Klintworth GK (1988) The presence of stage II melanosomes (premelanosomes) in neoplasms other than melanomas. Modern Pathol 1: 35-43

Van Duinen SG, Ruiter DJ, Hageman PH, Vennegor C, Dickersin GR, Scheffer E, Rumke PH (1984) Immunohistochemical and histochemical tools in the diagnosis of amelanotic melanoma. Cancer 53: 1566-1573

Ward JM, Hamlin MH II, Ackerman LJ, Lattuada CP, Longfellow DG, Cameron TP (1983) Age-related neoplastic and degenerative lesions in aging male virgin and ex-breeder ACI/segHapBR rats. J Gerontol 38: 538-548

Weiss E, Frese K (1974) Tumours of the skin. International histological classification of tumours of domestic animals. Bull WHO 50: 79-100

Zackheim HS (1973) Tumours of the skin. In: Turusov VS (ed) Pathology of tumours in laboratory animals, vol I. Tumors of the rat, pt 1. (IARC Sci Publ no 5) IARC, Lyon, pp 1-22

Zurcher C, Varekamp AE, Solleveld HA, Durham SK, De Vries AJ, Hagenbeek A (1987) Late effects of cyclophosphamide and total body irradiation as a conditioning regimen of the bone marrow transplantation in rats (a preliminary report). Int J Radiat Biol 51: 1059-1068

Fibroma, Dermis and Subcutis, Rat

Laura Hart-Elcock, Stephen G. Lake, Robert E. Mueller, and Barry P. Stuart

Gross Appearance

Fibromas are described as well-circumscribed, firm, grayish-white, dermal or subcutaneous masses with a whorled appearance on cut section. They are usually focal, flat or raised masses and can vary from less than 1 cm to several centimeters in size. Some of the fibromas may become ulcerated and/or infected. They are usually mobile in relation to the epidermis and underlying tissue. Fibromas and fibrosarcomas can occur within the same animal (Bogovski 1979; Greaves and Faccini 1984; Stannard and Pulley 1978; Zackheim 1973).

Microscopic Features

Fibromas consist of varying amounts of mature collagen arranged into bundles, interwoven with well-differentiated fibroblasts (Figs. 121 and 122). The tumors are sparsely cellular, with collagen the primary component. There is also an extensive reticulin framework that tends to course parallel to the collagen and envelops individual cells. Mitotic figures are rare. Ground substance is usually minimal, but occasional myxomatous areas may be seen. Fibromas are well-vascularized, show no evidence of invasion, and are commonly encapsulated (Bogovski 1979; Greaves and Faccini 1984; Squire et al. 1978; Zackheim 1973).

Ultrastructure

There is little information in the literature concerning the ultrastructural characteristics of fibromas. Ultrastructural features of fibromas examined at our laboratory include abundant collagen fibrils (64-nm periodicity) interspersed with

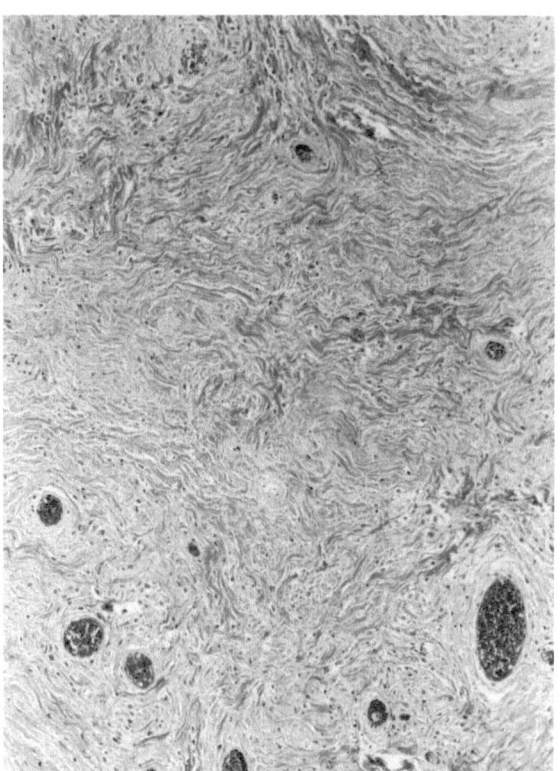

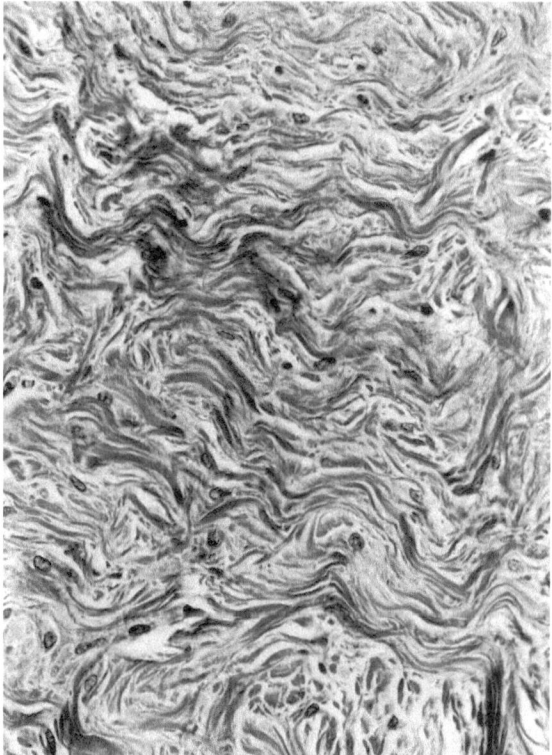

Fig. 121 *(above).* Fibroma, skin, F344 rat. The primary ▶ component is collagen. Occasional fibroblasts are interspersed between fibers. H and E, × 80

Fig. 122 *(below).* Fibroma, skin, F344 rat. Note the densely packed collagen fibers with sparse numbers of fibroblasts. H and E, × 600

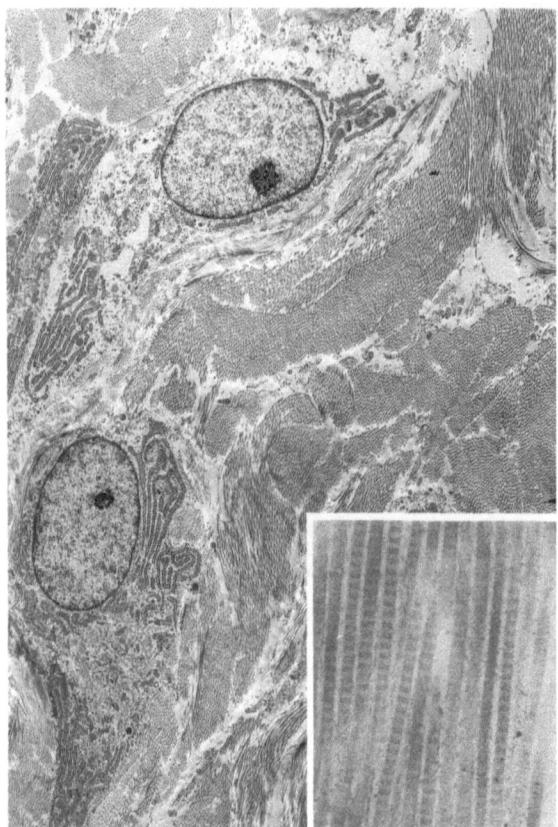

Fig. 123. Fibroma, skin, F344 rat. Note that two fibroblasts with abundant rough endoplasmic reticulum are surrounded by bundles of collagen fibrils. TEM, ×7500. *Inset:* Collagen fibrils with 64-nm periodicity. TEM, ×60000

fibroblasts which, according to Ham and Cormack (1979) are typified by prominent rough endoplasmic reticulum (Fig. 123). Intercellular ground substance is minimal. Their ultrastructural characteristics may be difficult to distinguish from those of mature scar tissue.

Differential Diagnosis

Fibromas adjacent to or encroaching on mammary gland tissue need to be differentiated from mammary gland fibroadenomas, which contain both epithelial and connective tissue elements. Distinction may be difficult when remnants of normal glandular tissue are trapped in the midst of a fibroma (Greaves and Faccini 1984; Zackheim 1973). Fibromas must also be differentiated from leiomyomas and neurofibromas, but light microscopic criteria are poorly defined and often contradictory. Special stains such as Masson

trichrome stain (collagen stains light green, muscle fibers stain red), Mallory's phosphotungstic acid-hematoxylin (PTAH) technique (collagen stains reddish-orange, muscle fibers stain blue), or van Gieson's stain (the cytoplasm of neurofibroma cells stains yellow, collagen stains reddish-orange, muscle fibers stain blue) and ultrastructural analysis may provide sufficient evidence to allow differentiation (Sheehan and Hrapchak 1980). Immunocytochemistry methods may also be particularly helpful. Markers such as desmin (muscle specific), vimentin (mesenchymal cells such as fibroblasts and myofibroblasts), and S100 protein (neuroectodermal tissue) can be used to distinguish these tumors (Gough et al. 1986; Hayden et al. 1986; Meuten et al. 1985; Sandusky et al. 1985).

Biologic Features

Fibromas are benign in behavior and appearance (Zackheim 1973).

Etiology and Frequency. Fibromas can occur spontaneously in a variety of rodent strains (Table 4). They are usually age related and in most instances occur in less than 5% of rats and mice. The literature also contains reports of rodent fibromas following exposure to ionizing radiation (Greaves and Faccini 1984; Zackheim 1973) and at the site of repeated injections of iron-dextran (Zackheim 1973).

Comparison with Other Species

Fibromas in other animal species resemble those in rodents. They occur in all domestic animal species, and have no known breed or sex prevalence (Stannard and Pulley 1978). No fibromas were seen in 100 male and 100 female CD1 mice from our laboratory's historical control data. Viral-induced fibromas are known to occur in rabbits (the Shope fibroma virus). These eventually undergo necrosis and slough after 1–5 months (Squire t al. 1978; Weisbroth 1974).

References

Bogovski P (1979) Tumours of the skin. In: Turusov VS (ed) Pathology of tumours in laboratory animals, vol II. Tumours of the mouse. IARC, Lyon, p 11
Burek JD (1978) Pathology of aging rats. CRC, West Palm Beach, pp 161–162 (Age-associated pathology)

Table 4. Occurrence of fibromas in the skin and subcutaneous tissues of aging rodents

Species	Strain	Age (months)	Sex	No. with fibroma/ no. examined	Percentage	References
Rat	CD	24	Male	27/806	3.3	Charles River Laboratories 1985
Rat	CD	24	Female	11/795	1.4	Charles River Laboratories 1985
Rat	BN/Bi	26	Male	1/74	1.0	Burek 1978
Rat	WAG/Rij	21	Male	1/124	< 1.0	Burek 1978
Rat	(WAG X BN) F$_1$	36	Male	1/67	1.0	Burek 1978
Rat	F344	24	Male	48/1794	2.6	Goodman et al. 1979
Rat	F344	24	Female	17/1754	< 1.0	Goodman et al. 1979
Rat	F344	18–24	–	6/37	16.2	Coleman et al. 1977
Rat	F344	24–30	–	1/46	2.2	Coleman et al. 1977
Rat	F344	30–33	–	2/15	13.3	Coleman et al. 1977
Rat	F344	24	Male	107/2320	4.6	Haseman et al. 1984; NTP 1983
Rat	F344	24	Female	34/2370	1.4	Haseman et al. 1984; NTP 1983
Rat	F344	24	Male	5/200	2.5	Mobay Corporation, unpublished
Rat	F344	24	Female	2/200	1.0	Mobay Corporation, unpublished
Mouse	CD-1	24	Male	0/100	0.0	Mobay Corporation, unpublished
Mouse	CD-1	24	Female	0/100	0.0	Mobay Corporation, unpublished
Mouse	B6C3F1	24	Male	34/2343	1.5	Haseman et al. 1984; NTP 1983
Mouse	B6C3F1	24	Female	39/2486	1.6	Haseman et al. 1984; NTP 1983

Charles River Laboratories (1985) Historical data for spontaneous neoplastic lesions in the Crl: CD BR rat. Charles River, Wilmington MA, pp 3–5

Coleman GL, Barthold SW, Osbaldiston GW, Foster SJ, Jonas AM (1977) Pathological changes during aging in barrier-reared Fisher 344 male rats. J Gerontol 32 (3): 258–278

Goodman DG, Ward JM, Squire RA, Chu KC, Linhart MS (1979) Neoplastic and nonneoplastic lesions in aging F344 rats. Toxicol Appl Pharmacol 48: 237–248

Gough AW, Hanna W, Barsoum NJ, Moore J, Sturgess JM (1986) Morphologic and immunohistochemical features of two spontaneous peripheral nerve tumors in Wistar rats. Vet Pathol 23: 68–73

Greaves P, Faccini JM (1984) Rat histopathology. Elsevier, Amsterdam, p 5 (Integumentary system)

Ham AW, Cormack DH (1979) Histology, 8th edn. Lippincott, Philadelphia, pp 229–235 (The origins, morphologies, and functions (including immunological functions) of the cells of loose connective tissue)

Haseman JK, Huff J, Boorman GA (1984) Use of historical control data in carcinogenicity studies in rodents. Toxicol Pathol 12 (2): 126–135

Hayden DW, Ghobrial HK, Johnson KH, Buoen LC (1986) Feline mammary sarcoma composed of cells resembling myofibroblasts. Vet Pathol 23: 118–124

Meuten DJ, Calderwood Mays MB, Dillman RC, Cooper BJ, Valentine BA, Kuhajda FP, Pass DA (1985) Canine laryngeal rhabdomyoma. Vet Pathol 22: 533–539

National Toxicology Program (NTP) (1983) Incidences of primary tumors in untreated control F344 rats and B6C3F1 mice. National Institute of Environmental Health Sciences Research, Triangle Park NC, p 9 (Technical bulletin no 10)

Sandusky GE Jr, Carlton WW, Wightman KA (1985) Immunohistochemical staining for S-100 protein in the diagnosis of canine amelanotic melanoma. Vet Pathol 22: 577–581

Sheehan DC, Hrapchak BB (1980) Theory and practice of histotechnology, 2nd edn. Mosby, St Louis, pp 180–201 (Connective tissue and muscle fiber stains)

Squire RA, Goodman DG, Valerio MG, Fredrickson TN, Strandberg JD, Levitt MH, Lingeman CH, Harshbarger JC, Dawe CJ (1978) Tumors. In: Benirschke K, Garner FM, Jones TC (eds) Pathology of laboratory animals, vol II. Springer, Berlin Heidelberg New York, p 1062

Stannard AA, Pulley LT (1978) Tumors of the skin and soft tissues. In: Moulton JE (ed) Tumors in domestic animals. University of California Press, Berkeley, pp 16–22

Weisbroth SH (1974) Neoplastic diseases shope fibroma. In: Weisbroth SH, Flatt RE, Kraus AL (eds) The biology of the laboratory rabbit. Academic, New York, pp 361–363

Zackheim HS (1973) Tumours of the skin. In: Turusov VS (ed) Pathology of tumours in laboratory animals, vol I. Tumours of the rat, p 1. IARC, Lyon, pp 5–6

Fibrosarcoma, Dermis and Subcutis, Rat

Laura Hart-Elcock, Stephen G. Lake, Robert E. Mueller, and Barry P. Stuart

Gross Appearance

Fibrosarcomas can appear grossly as elevated dermal or subcutaneous masses that are often ulcerated and attached firmly to surrounding tissues. They frequently reach several centimeters in size and vary from grayish-white to red or purple depending on the amount of hemorrhage and necrosis. They have a firm or fleshy consistency and can appear lobulated on cut section (Carter 1973; Stannard and Pulley 1978; Yager and Scott 1985).

Microscopic Features

Fibrosarcomas are less well-differentiated than fibromas, characterized by a high degree of cellularity and by variable, often scant amounts of collagen formation. There may be little cellular orientation, but interwoven bundles forming a herringbone pattern are characteristic (Carter 1973; Greaves and Faccini 1984) Fig. 124). Reticulin fibers may be abundant and tend to envelop fibroblasts. Ground substance is usually minimal, but myxomatous changes can occur. Tumor cells are spindle-shaped with a variable chromatin pattern and prominent nucleoli. Mitotic figures are frequent (Fig. 125) (Carter 1973; Squire et al. 1978; Stewart 1979). Areas of hemorrhage and necrosis with accompanying inflammation are common. Blood vessels are numerous and thin-walled, sometimes with an incomplete endothelial lining so that tumor cells may border and/or infiltrate them (Stewart 1979). Fibrosarcomas are usually locally invasive and nonencapsulated (Carter 1973).

Ultrastructure

Fibrosarcomas contain variable amounts of collagen fibrils (64-nm periodicity) interspersed between fibroblastic cells (Fig. 126) and usually have a well-developed Golgi complex and lack a basal lamina and cell junctions. Distended rough endoplasmic reticulum cisternae within these cells is characteristic but can also occur with malignant fibrous histiocytomas and liposarcomas. A few intracellular lipid droplets may be found, and myofibroblasts (fibroblasts containing smooth muscle myofilaments in the peripheral cytoplasm) may occur in more well-differentiated fibrosarcomas (Mackay 1981).

Differential Diagnosis

Fibrosarcomas must be differentiated from leiomyosarcomas, rhabdomyosarcomas, neurofibrosarcomas, malignant fibrous histiocytomas, and hemangiosarcomas. Light microscopic differentiation may be exceedingly difficult in anaplastic tumors; however, special stains such as Masson trichrome stain (collagen stains light green, muscle fibers stain red), Mallory's phosphotungstic acid-hematoxylin (PTAH) technique (collagen stains reddish-orange, muscle fibers stain blue), van Gieson's stain (the cytoplasm of neurofibrosarcoma tumor cells stains yellow, collagen stains reddish-orange, muscle fibers stain blue) (Sheehan and Hrapchak 1980) and ultrastructural analysis may provide sufficient evidence to allow differentiation. Immunocytochemistry methods may also be particularly helpful. Markers such as desmin (muscle specific), vimentin (mesenchymal cells such as fibroblasts and myofibroblasts), and S100 protein (neuroectodermal tissue) can be used to distinguish between muscle, neuroectodermal, and fibroblastic tumors (Gough et al. 1986; Hayden et al. 1986; Meuten et al. 1985; Sandusky et al. 1985). In addition, myoglobin immunoreactivity is skeletal muscle specific and can be used to differentiate between smooth and skeletal muscle tumors (Meuten et al. 1985), and factor VIII-related antigen is a marker for endothelial cells which can identify hemangiosarcomas (Moore et al. 1986).

Biologic Features

Fibrosarcomas are locally invasive but do not often metastasize. When metastasis does occur, the most frequent sites are the regional lymph nodes and lungs (Carter 1973).

Etiology and Frequency. Fibrosarcomas can occur spontaneously in various strains, their incidence

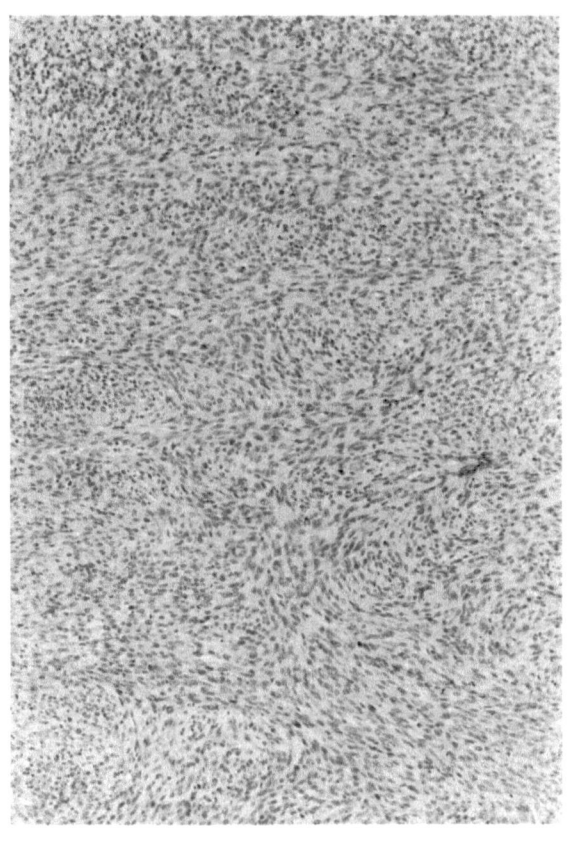

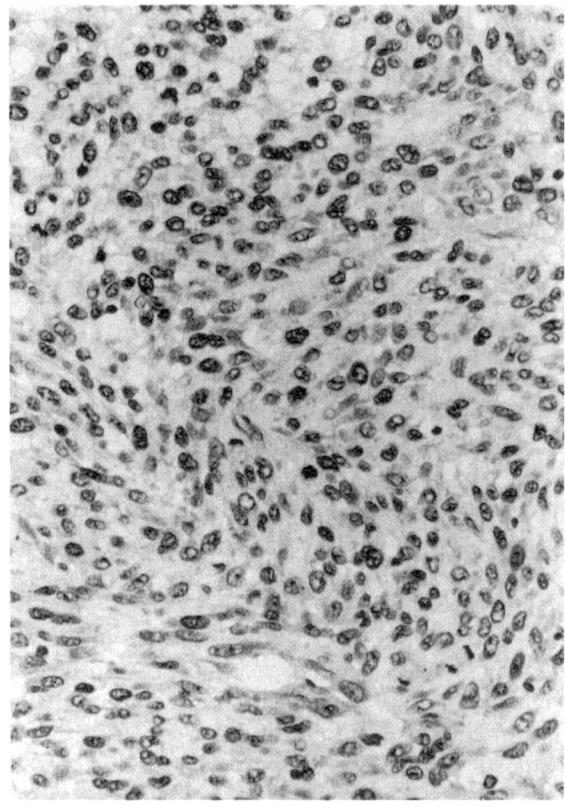

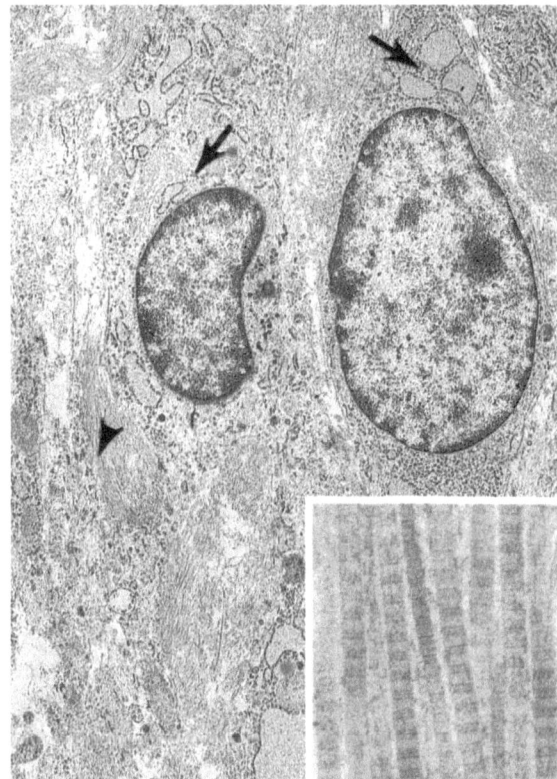

Fig. 124 *(upper left)*. Fibrosarcoma, skin, F344 rat. Cells are densely packed and arranged in a herringbone pattern. H and E, ×75

Fig. 125 *(upper right)*. Fibrosarcoma, skin, F344 rat. Cells are densely packed and have pleomorphic, hyperchromatic nuclei. Mitoses are numerous. H and E, ×330

Fig. 126 *(lower right)*.Fibrosarcoma, skin, F344 rat. Fibroblastic cells with distended rough endoplasmic reticulum cisternae *(arrows)* and intercellular collagen fibrils *(arrowhead)*. TEM, ×6000. *Inset,* collagen fibrils with a 64-nm periodicity. TEM, ×30000

varying from less than 1% to 7% in Fischer 344 rats and less than 1% to 6% in B6C3F1 mice (Burek 1978; Goodman et al. 1979; Haseman et al. 1984; NTP 1983). In our laboratory, fibrosarcomas have been observed in 3 out of 200 (1.5%) male and 0 out of 200 female control Fischer 344 rats. No fibrosarcomas were seen in 100 male and 100 female CD1 mice from our laboratory s historical control data. Fibrosarcomas can also be induced in rodents by exposure to 3-methylcholanthrene and 5,9,10-trimethylbenzanthracene (Stewart 1979).

Comparison with Other Species

Fibrosarcomas occur in most other animal species and are similar to those occurring in rodents. Of the domestic animals, they occur most frequently in the dog and cat. There is no breed or sex predilection. In dogs, they are found most frequently in the subcutis, dermis, oral, and nasal cavities. In cats, they occur most commonly in the subcutis. No predilection sites occur in other domestic animals (Stannard and Pulley 1978). The feline sarcoma virus (FeSV), a C-type virus, can cause fibrosarcomas in cats usually less than 5 years of age. The virus is a recombinant hybrid of the feline leukemia virus (FeLV) and host genome and is found only in FeLV-positive cats. Tumors are usually multiple and anaplastic (Yager and Scott 1985). Cutaneous fibrosarcomas have also been observed in several rhesus monkeys during a recent outbreak of immunodeficiency syndrome at the California Primate Research Center. Two different viruses have been isolated at the center: a type D retrovirus (SRV-1) and a type C retrovirus (STLV-III), which is antigenically related to the human immunodeficiency virus, HIV (HTLV-III/LAV). A condition termed retroperitoneal fibromatosis has occurred in various macaques with an immunodeficiency syndrome at the Washington and Oregon Primate Centers, characterized by retroperitoneal and/or subcutaneous proliferative fibrovascular tissue. The subcutaneous form is identical to the fibrosarcomas described at the California center. A group of type D retroviruses (SRV-2) have been isolated at the Washington and Oregon centers (King 1986).

References

Burek JD (1978) Pathology of aging rats. CRC West Palm Beach, pp 161–162 (Age-associated pathology)

Carter RL (1973) Tumours of the soft tissues. In: Turusov VS (ed) Pathology of tumours in laboratory animals, vol I. Tumours of the rat, pt 1 IARC, Lyon, pp 152–153 (IARC Sci publ no 5)

Goodman DG, Ward JM, Squire RA, Chu KC, Linhart MS (1979) Neoplastic and nonneoplastic lesions in aging F344 rats. Toxicol Appl Pharmacol 48: 237–248

Gough AW, Hanna W, Barsoum NJ, Moore J, Sturgess JM (1986) Morphologic and immunohistochemical features of two spontaneous peripheral nerve tumors in Wistar rats. Vet Pathol 23: 68–73

Greaves P, Faccini JM (1984) Rat histopathology. Elsevier, Amsterdam, p 5 (Integumentary system)

Haseman JK, Huff J, Boorman GA (1984) Use of historical control data in carcinogenicity studies in rodents. Toxicol Pathol 12 (2): 126–135

Hayden DW, Ghobrial HK, Johnson KH, Buoen LC (1986) Feline mammary sarcoma composed of cells resembling myofibroblasts. Vet Pathol 23: 118–124

King NW (1986) Simian models of acquired immunodeficiency syndrome (AIDS): a review. Vet Pathol 23: 345–353

Mackay B (1981) Diagnostic electron microscopy. Appleton-Century-Crofts, New York, pp 239–249 (Tumor diagnosis)

Meuten DJ, Calderwood Mays MB, Dillman RC, Cooper BJ, Valentine BA, Kuhajda FP, Pass DA (1985) Canine laryngeal rhabdomyoma. Vet Pathol 22: 533–539

Moore PF, Hacker DV, Buyukmihci NC (1986) Ocular angiosarcoma in the horse: morphological and immunohistochemical studies. Vet Pathol 23: 240–244

National Toxicology Program (NTP) (1983) Incidences of primary tumors in untreated control F344 rats and B6C3F1 mice. NTP, Research Triangle Park, North Carolina, p 9

Sandusky GE Jr, Carlton WW, Wightman KA (1985) Immunohistochemical staining for S-100 protein in the diagnosis of canine amelanotic melanoma. Vet Pathol 22: 577–581

Sheehan DC, Hrapchak BB (1980) Theory and practice of histotechnology 2nd edn. Mosby, St Louis, pp 180–201 (Connective tissue and muscle fiber stains)

Squire RA, Goodman DG, Valerio MG, Fredrickson TN, Strandberg JD, Levitt MH, Lingeman CH, Harshbarger JC, Dawe CJ (1978) Tumors. In: Benirschke K, Garner FM, Jones TC (eds) Pathology of laboratory animals, vol II. Springer, Berlin Heidelberg New York, p 1062

Stannard AA, Pulley LT (1978) Tumors of the skin and soft tissues. In: Moulton JE (ed) Tumors in domestic animals. University of California Press, Berkeley, pp 17–18

Stewart HL (1979) Tumours of the soft tissues. In: Turusov VS (ed) Pathology of tumours in laboratory animals, vol II. Tumours of the mouse. IARC, Lyon, pp 488–489 (IARC Sci Publ no 23)

Yager JA, Scott DW (1985) The skin and appendages. In: Jubb KVF, Kennedy PC, Palmer N (eds) Pathology of domestic animals, 3rd edn. Academic, Orlando, p 519

Fibroma, Dermis and Subcutis, Mouse (Especially B6C3F1 Mouse)

Gary A. Boorman, Michael R. Elwell, and Scot L. Eustis

Synonyms. Fibromatosis; collagenous nevus.

Gross Appearance

Fibromas are benign neoplasms that occur in the dermis and subcutis of the back, thorax, abdomen, head, and legs of mice. These neoplasms usually appear as firm, rounded, nodular masses; some may be somewhat pedunculated with a broad stalk. Alopecia or ulceration of the skin overlying the mass may occur. The cut surface is usually smooth, grayish-white, and glistening.

Microscopic features

Fibromas are circumscribed masses of collagenous connective tissue located between the epidermis and the panniculus carnosus or other underlying structures; the borders are relatively well-defined as compared with fibrosarcomas (Fig. 127). The overlying epidermis may undergo acanthosis and hyperkeratosis, and narrow ridges of epidermis may extend down into the neoplasms. The neoplasms are comprised of interlacing bundles of moderate to well-differentiated fibroblasts with variable amounts of mature collagen interspersed among the fibroblasts (Fig. 128). The neoplastic cells are usually fusi-

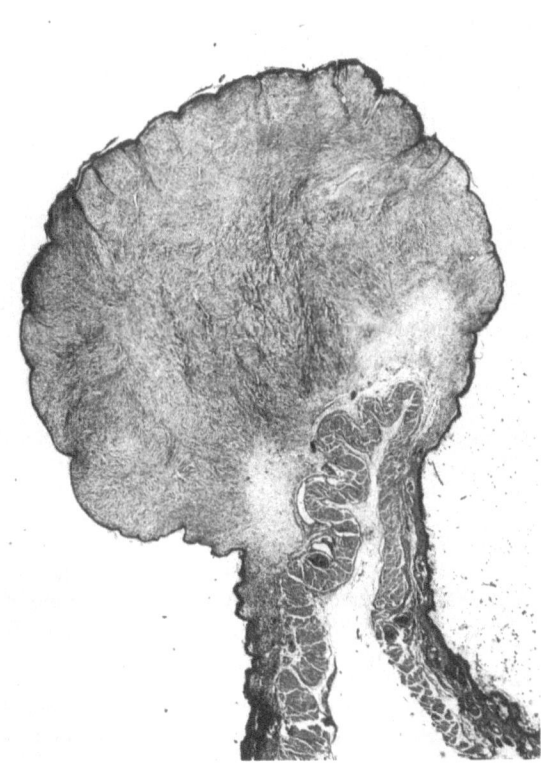

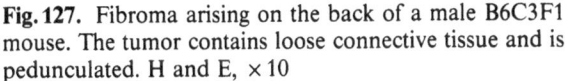

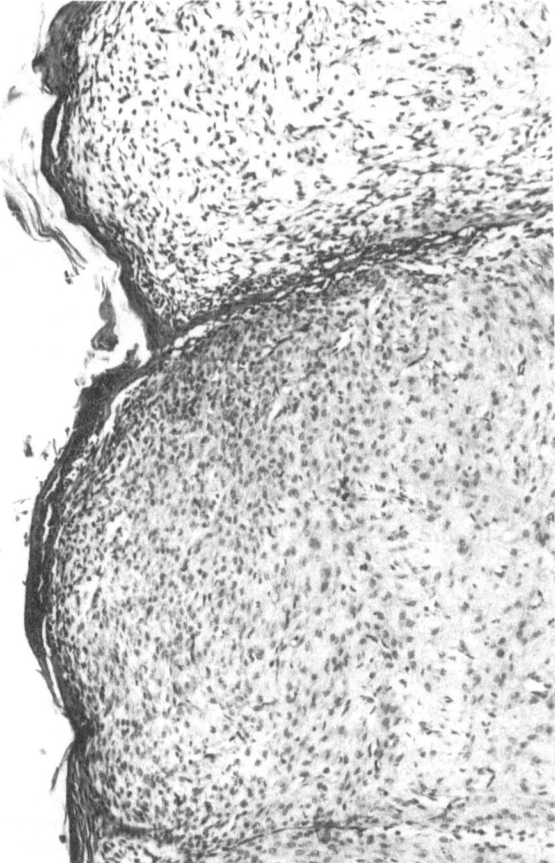

Fig. 127. Fibroma arising on the back of a male B6C3F1 mouse. The tumor contains loose connective tissue and is pedunculated. H and E, × 10

Fig. 128. Higher magnification of the fibroma shown in Fig. 127. The fibroblasts are relatively well-differentiated and there is abundant intercellular collagen. Note that the density of the collagen varies within the tumor. H and E, × 110

form with elongated nuclei that may appear hyperchromatic or vesicular, with one or more nucleoli. In some cases the collagenous stroma is loose and edematous or contains abundant mucinous ground substance, and the neoplastic cells may be stellate in shape.

Ultrastructure

We are unaware of any reports of ultrastructural studies of subcutaneous fibromas in mice.

Differential Diagnosis

Fibroma must be differentiated from fibrosis that results from the healing of wounds (particular in group-housed male mice among whom fighting is not uncommon) and fibrosarcoma, its malignant counterpart. Fibrosis tends to be less extensive with limited elevation of the epidermis; inflammatory cells may be present if the lesion is active. Fibroma must also be differentiated from connective tissue nevus (Fox et al. 1973; Scott 1981), which are nonneoplastic lesions consisting of dense collagen and are relatively acellular. While connective tissue nevus has been described in the dog, we are not aware of any reports of this lesion in mice. Fibrosarcoma generally is less well-circumscribed than fibroma, and there is invasion of the surrounding tissue; the malignant neoplasms are more cellular, show celluluar atypia and pleomorphism, and contain less collagen.

Biologic Features

Lesions diagnosed as fibroma may be relatively early stages of fibrosarcoma. True endstage benign fibromas that are relatively acellular and that contain predominantly hyalinized mature collagen are extremely uncommon in the B6C3F1 mouse.

Etiology and Frequency. The etiology of integumentary fibromas is not known. Fibromas of the subcutis are uncommon in the mouse including the B6C3F1 hybrid. The incidence of fibroma in the untreated B6C3F1 mouse is 41 out of 2040 (2%) for males and 0 out of 2040 for females (NTP Carcinogenesis Bioassay Data System 1987). Sheldon and Greenman (1980) did not report a single fibroma occurring in 2592 female

BALB/c mice. Stewart (1979) does not even list fibromas as one of the tumors that may occur in the soft tissue of the mouse.

Comparison with Other Species

In rats, fibromas occur in subcutaneous tissue in a variety of sites and usually are well-differentiated (Carter 1973). They tend to be relatively acellular and contain dense collagen in contrast to those that occur in mice. In the dog, fibromas of the dermis or subcutis are common, and there is no sex or breed predisposition (Stannard and Pulley 1978). A distinctive type of fibroma (or fibrosarcoma) is common in the horse. It tends to be locally invasive and will recur following excision but rarely metastasizes; it is referred to as equine sarcoid (Ragland et al. 1966) and has a viral etiology (Watson and Larson 1974). Fibromas occur in rabbits and are caused by pox viruses (Marshall and Regnery 1963; Shope 1932; Woodroofe and Fenner 1965; Weisbroth 1974). In guinea pigs, fibrosarcomas are not uncommon, but fibromas were not reported in a review of neoplasms in this species (Manning 1976). Soft tissue tumors in humans are common, of which a vast majority are benign (Stout and Lattes 1967).

References

Carter RL (1973) Tumours of soft tissues. In: Turusov VS (ed) Pathology of tumours in laboratory animals, vol I. Tumours of the rat, pt 1. International Agency for Research on Cancer, Lyon, pp 151–168 (IARC Sci Publ no 5)

Fox JG, Snyder SB, Campbell LH (1973) Connective tissue nevus in a dog. Vet Pathol 10: 65–68

Manning PJ (1976) Neoplastic diseases. In: Wagner JE, Manning PJ (eds) The biology of the guinea pig. Academic, New York, pp 211–227

Marshall ID, Regnery DC (1963) Studies in the epidemiology of myxomatosis in California. III. The response of brush rabbits *(Sylvilagus bachmani)* to infection with exotic and enzootic strains myxoma virus and the relative infectivity of the tumors for mosquitos. Am J Hyg 77: 213–219

National Toxicology Program (NTP) (1987) Carcinogenesis bioassay data system. Tumor incidences for selected control groups. National Institute of Environmental Health Scien us Research, Triangle Park NC

Ragland WL, Keown GH, Spencer GR (1966) An epizootic of equine sarcoid. Nature 210: 139

Scott DW (1981) Examination of the integumentary system. Vet Clin North Am [Small Anim Pract] 11: 499–510

Sheldon WG, Greenman DL (1980) Spontaneous lesions in control BALB/C female mice. J Environ Pathol Toxicol 3: 155–167

Shope RE (1932) A transmissible tumor-like condition in rabbits. J Exp Med 56: 793-802

Stannard AA, Pulley LT (1978) Tumors of the skin and soft tissues. In: Moulton JE (ed) Tumors in domestic animals. University of California Press, Berkeley, p 18

Stewart HL (1979) Tumours of the soft tissues. In: Turusov VS (ed) Pathology of tumours in laboratory animals. II. Tumours of the mouse. International Agency for Research on Cancer, Lyon, pp 487-526 (IARC Sci Publ no 23)

Stout AP, Lattes R (1967) Tumors of the soft tissues. Armed Forced Institute of Pathology, Washington DC (Atlas of tumor pathology, 2nd series, fasc I)

Watson RE Jr, Larson FA (1974) Detection of tumor-specific antigens in an equine sarcoid cell line. Infect Immun 9: 714-718

Weisbroth SH (1974) Neoplastic diseases. In: Weisbroth SH, Flatt RE, Kraus AL (eds) The biology of the laboratory rabbit. Academic, New York, pp 332-376

Woodroofe GM, Fenner F (1965) Viruses of the myxoma-fibroma subgroup of the poxviruses. I. Plaque production in culture cells, plaque reduction tests, and cross-protection tests in rabbits. Aust J Exp Biol Med Sci 43: 123-142

Fibrosarcoma, Dermis and Subcutis, Mouse

Gary A. Boorman, Scot L. Eustis, and Michael R. Elwell

Synonyms. Sarcoma; undifferentiated sarcoma; neurofibrosarcoma.

Gross Appearance

Fibrosarcomas are malignant neoplasms that occur in the dermis and subcutis of the back, thorax, abdomen, head, and legs of mice. These neoplasms may appear as flattened elevations or as nodular masses. Alopecia frequently occurs in the skin overlying the mass, and ulceration of the skin may also be present. The cut surface is grayish-white; areas of hemorrhage are commonly seen within the larger masses.

Microscopic Features

Fibrosarcomas of the integumentary system in the B6C3F1 mouse are characterized by a wide spectrum of histologic features. The boundaries of these neoplasms are poorly defined; neoplastic cells extend into surrounding tissues. The neoplasms often invade the panniculus carnosus (Fig. 129). Larger neoplasms may contain hemorrhage, acute inflammation, and areas of necrosis, particularly those with ulceration of the overlying skin. The neoplastic cells vary from moderately well-differentiated fibroblasts arranged in interweaving bundles or in whorled patterns (Fig. 130) to poorly differentiated pleomorphic cells arranged in sheets (Fig. 131). Some of the large pleomorphic cells have abundant eosinophilic cytoplasm and giant or multiple nuclei and may resemble the "strap cells" of rhabdomyosarcoma. Collagen fibers are interspersed between the cells; the amount of collagen varies with the degree of differentiation of the neoplasm.

Ultrastructure

Fibrosarcomas exhibit a wide range of ultrastructural features according to the degree of differentiation of the neoplastic cells; these ultrastructural features may not be definitively diagnostic but they may be helpful in ruling out other neoplasms. The neoplastic cells are separated by variable amounts of collagen, but they are not invested by a basal lamina (Fig. 132). Nuclei are elongated and irregular with a thin marginal zone of heterochromatin and one or more nucleoli. The cytoplasm contains variable numbers of round or oval mitochondria, rough endoplasmic reticulum, free ribosomes, and a Golgi apparatus (Fig. 133). Thin filaments 5-7 nm in diameter may be present and aggregated near the cell membrane. When filaments are abundant, a careful search for Z bands is necessary to rule out rhabdomyosarcoma. Peripheral filaments and dense bodies are present in neoplastic smooth muscle cells, but the cells are invested by a basal lamina. Neoplastic Schwann cells are invested by basal lamina and lack myofilaments and dense bodies.

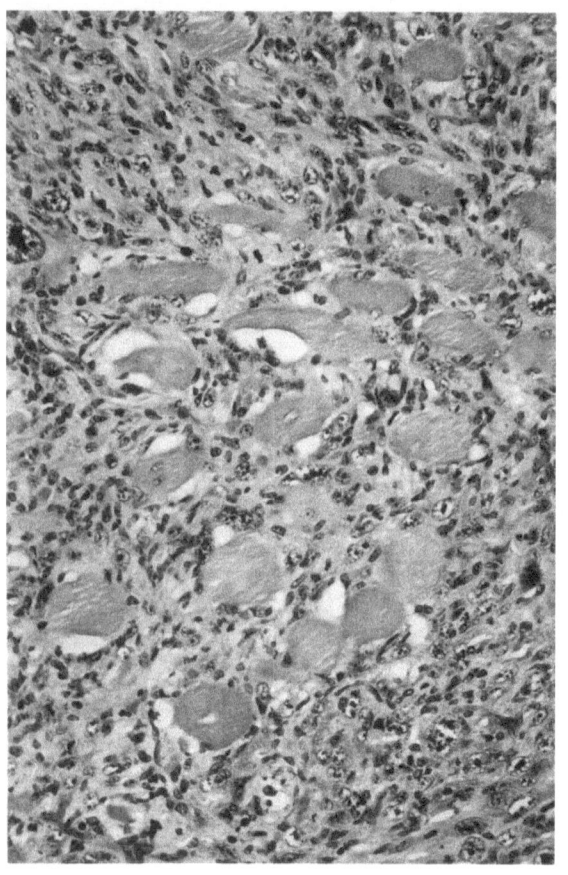

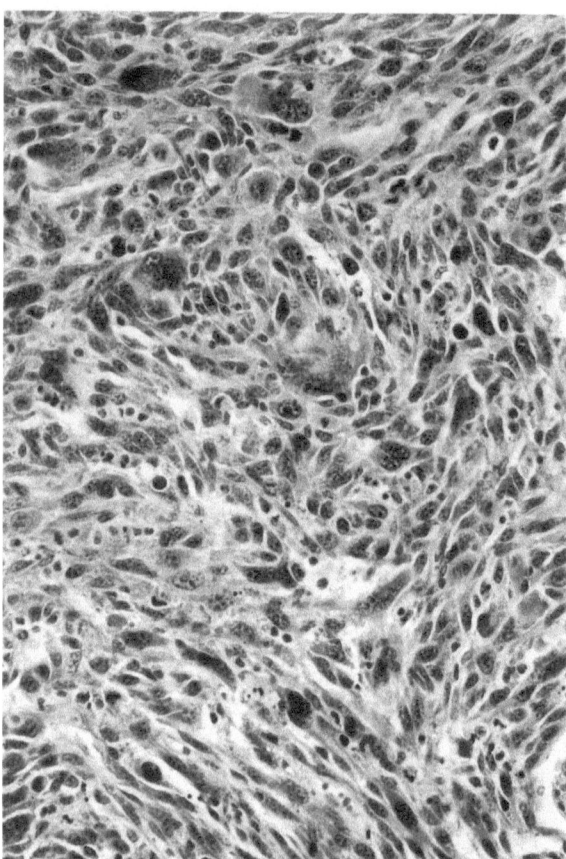

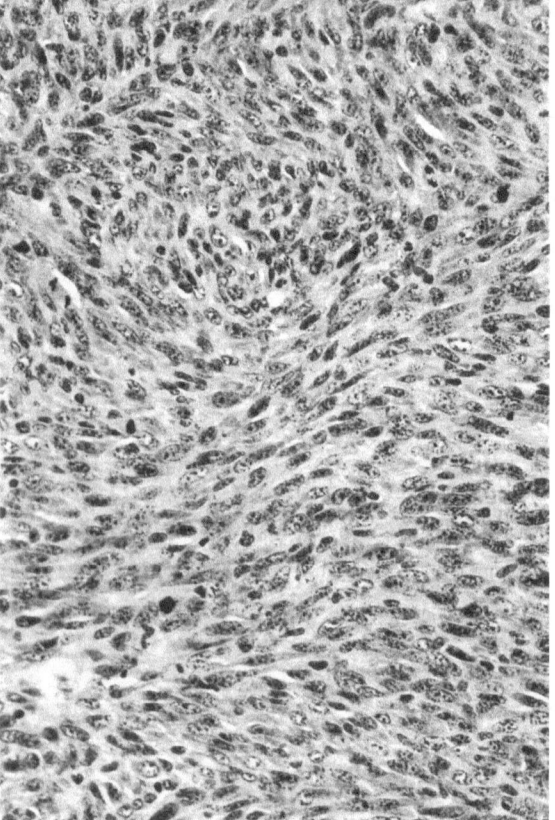

◄ **Fig. 129** *(upper left)*. Fibrosarcoma, male B6C3F1 mouse. Neoplastic cells invading the skeletal muscle of the panniculus carnosus. H and E, × 200

Fig. 130 *(lower left)*. Fibrosarcoma, male B6C3F1 mouse. Interlacing bundles of fusiform-shaped fibroblasts with elongated nuclei and scant fibrillar cytoplasm. H and E, × 325

Fig. 131 *(upper right)*. Fibrosarcoma, male B6C3F1 mouse. Neoplastic cells are highly anaplastic and pleomorphic. H and E, × 400

Fig. 132 *(above)*. Fibrosarcoma, male B6C3F1 mouse. ▶ Neoplastic fibroblasts have elongated nuclei and variable amounts of cytoplasm. TEM, × 2800

Fig. 133 *(below)*. Fibrosarcoma, male B6C3F1 mouse. Note the elongated nucleus with a narrow rim of heterochromatin and prominent nucleoli. The cytoplasm contains round or oval mitochondria and profiles of rough endoplasmic reticulum. Collagen fibers are present in the intercellular space. TEM, × 10000

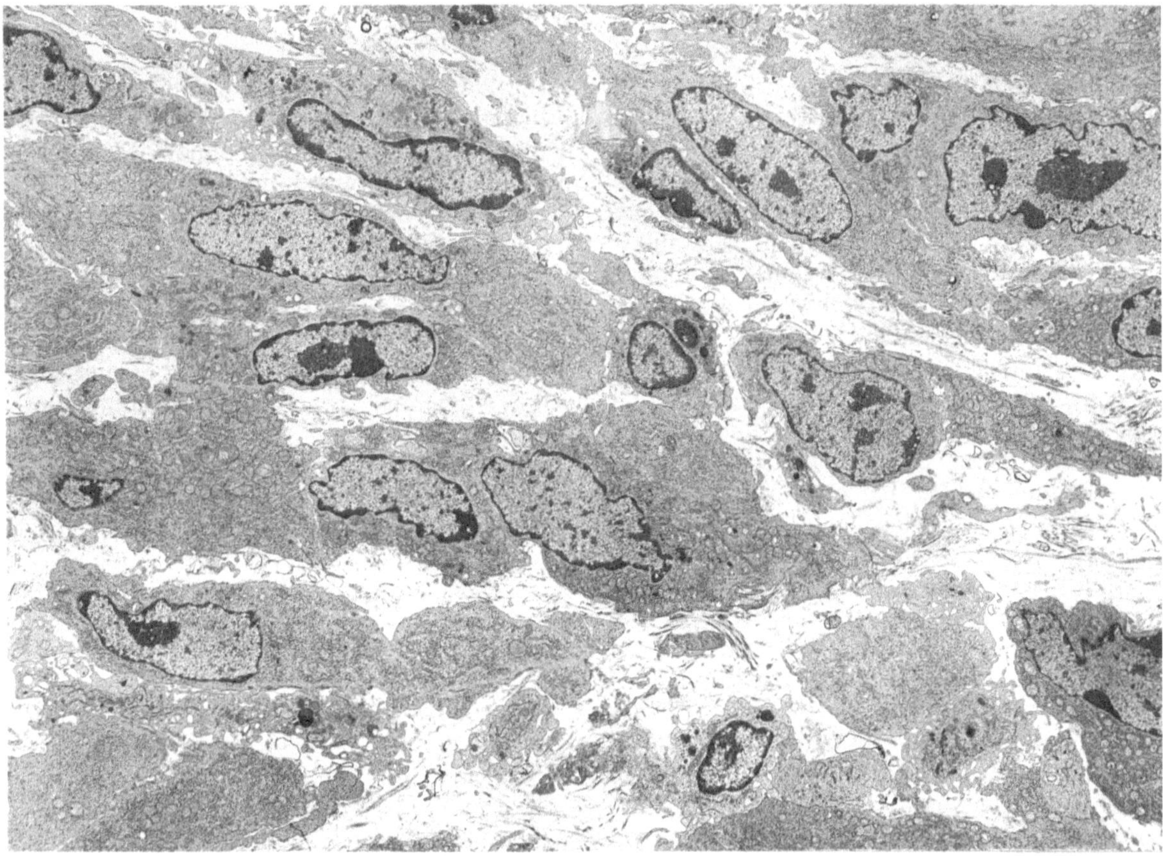

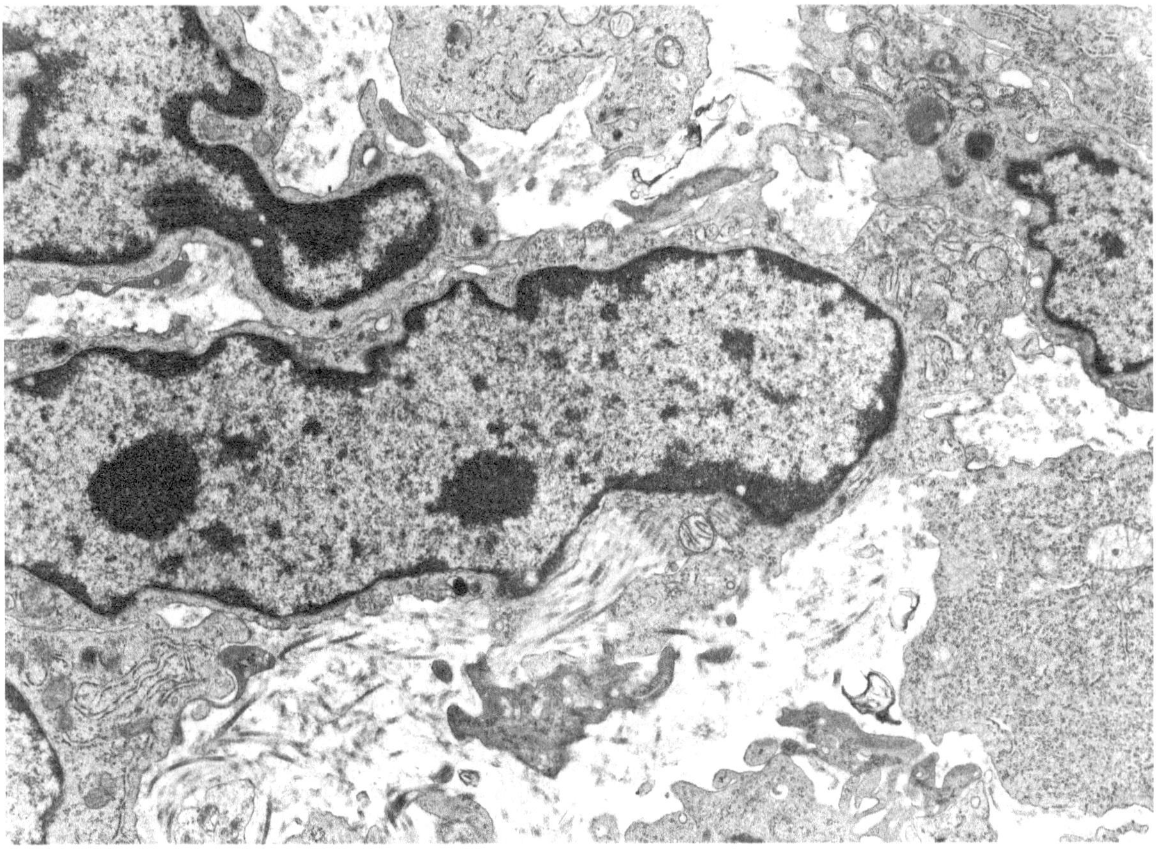

Differential Diagnosis

The variation of histologic patterns and cellular differentiation in dermal and subcutaneous sarcomas has resulted in a number of morphological diagnoses for these neoplasms. Fibrosarcoma must be differentiated from leiomyosarcoma, rhabdomyosarcoma, and malignant schwannoma. Well-differentiated fibrosarcomas with interweaving bundles of spindle cells typical of fibroblasts with interspersed collagen fibers pose no diagnostic problems. Subcutaneous neoplasms that consist of poorly differentiated cells are difficult to classify without special techniques such as electron microscopy, immunocytochemical stains for intermediate filaments, or histochemical stains. A battery of histologic stains was used in one study in an attempt to determine the cell of origin for 156 spindle cell neoplasms of mice (Stewart 1979). No conclusive results were obtained for nearly 20% of the neoplasms. Others were considered to be derived from fibroblasts, smooth muscle, striated muscle, or Schwann cells. Well-differentiated leiomyosarcomas consist of interlacing bundles of spindle cells with relatively abundant eosinophilic cytoplasm and elongated nuclei with blunt ends. Collagen is minimal or absent. Rhabdomyosarcomas are composed of pleomorphic cells arranged in poorly organized bundles and solid sheets. Strap cells with multiple nuclei, longitudinal myofibrils, and cross striations are characteristic for these neoplasms. Stewart (1979) notes that the presence of giant cells or straplike cells does not necessarily warrant a diagnosis of rhabdomyosarcoma. Myofibrils and cross striations must be demonstrated. He appropriately cautions that fibrosarcomas frequently invade skeletal muscle, and regenerating skeletal muscle cells may be trapped within the neoplasm. The trapped muscle cells intermixed with the pleomorphic neoplastic cells has led some to classify these tumors erroneously as rhabdomyosarcomas. Although rhabdomyosarcomas may occur in the skin, they are probably overdiagnosed. Schwannomas usually have the typical Antoni's type A fibrillar pattern and/or Antoni's type B reticular pattern. There is minimal collagen present. Ultrastructural examination and immunocytochemical stains for intermediate filaments (vimentin and desmin), microfilaments (actin), neurofilaments, and S100 antigen are sometimes useful for differentiating subcutaneous mesenchymal neoplasms. Neoplasms that are so anaplastic as to preclude identification are simply diagnosed as sarcomas.

Biologic Features

In the B6C3F1 mouse, fibrosarcomas arise relatively late in life; most are seen after 90 weeks of age. In one study in which 42 tumors were found in 150 male mice, only 3 tumors were found before 91 weeks of age and nearly half (20 out of 42) were found upon killing at 114 weeks of age. These neoplasms appear to develop in the dermis and subcutis, and most are found over the back. They are locally invasive; some metastasize to the lung and less frequently to other organs. Metastatic potential for methylcholanthrene-induced sarcomas in mice have been correlated with specific oncogene expression and major histocompatibility complex antigens (Alon et al. 1987).

Etiology and Frequency. The overall incidence of spontaneously occurring subcutaneous neoplasms in 2-year-old control male and female B6C3F1 mice from current National Toxicology Program studies is about 10% and 2%, respectively (NTP Carcinogenesis Bioassay Data System 1987). Fibrosarcomas and anaplastic sarcomas account for the majority of subcutaneous neoplasms observed. Neurofibrosarcoma, leiomyosarcoma, rhabdomyosarcoma, and malignant schwannoma are rare (incidence less than 1%). Subcutaneous injection (Carter et al. 1968; Zajdela et al. 1980; Toth and Nagel 1981) or topical application of carcinogens to the skin (Searle and Spencer 1966) will induce fibromas and fibrosarcomas. Extracts of mushrooms given orally have been reported to induce subcutaneous tumors in Swiss mice (Toth 1986). Repeated localized freezing of the skin on the back of mice resulted in the development of subcutaneous sarcomas (Berenblum 1929). In a recent study in rats, sarcomas occurred at the site of persistent inflammation associated with metallic ear tags; in a second study in which local inflammation was not present, neoplasms did not occur (Waalkes et al. 1987). There may be an association between chronic wounds and the risk of sarcoma in humans (Abbes and Barety 1978).

In a few NTP studies the control groups of male mice had an unusually high incidence (three times the historical control incidence) of subcutaneous neoplasms. In each of these studies the neoplasms were found throughout all groups with no evidence of a treatment effect. These studies were conducted at different laboratories, and the mice were obtained from different production colonies. The mice were housed five per

Table 5. Cage distribution of mice with subcutaneous neoplasms

Affected mice/cage	Number of cages[a]	
	Expected	Actual
0	5.8	11
1	11.3	7
2	8.8	5
3	3.4	3
4	0.7	4
5	0.0	0

[a] A total of 42 tumors were found in one study of 150 mice. The mice were housed 5 per cage in 30 cages. The expected number of cages is the number of cages with mice having either 0, 1, 2, 3, etc. number of tumors if the distribution of tumors occurred at random. There was a significant cage effect with more than half of the tumors occurring in cages where 3 or 4 mice/cage had subcutaneous tumors.

cage, and the distribution of tumor-bearing mice by cage showed that there were more cages without tumor-bearing mice and more cages with three or four tumor-bearing mice than would be predicted by random distribution (Boorman, unpublished observations, 1987) (Table 5). The cause of the apparent "cage effect" is unknown, but clinical records indicate that a high incidence of skin lacerations due to fighting occurred in the cages of animals with tumors. It needs to be stressed that the association of bite wounds with the occurrence of subcutaneous neoplasms in mice is anecdotal. Clearly the role of wounds and inflammation in rodent studies needs further study before conclusions can be made. The National Toxicology Program has instituted a requirement for individual housing of mice for long-term toxicity and carcinogenicity studies to preclude any potential effects of fighting.

Comparison with Other Species

The incidence of subcutaneous neoplasms in mouse strains is generally low, and most of the neoplasms are malignant (Percy and Jonas 1971; Shelden and Greenman 1979; Stewart 1979). The subcutaneous neoplasms in the B6C3F1 mouse are usually fibrosarcomas or undifferentiated sarcomas. They are generally locally invasive, and some metastasize to the lungs. In the rat subcutaneous fibromas occur more frequently than fibrosarcomas, and the fibrosarcomas of rats tend to be more differentiated that those in the

B6C3F1 mouse (Carter 1973; Ward et al. 1979). For the F344/N rat the incidence of fibroma, neurofibroma, fibrosarcoma, neurofibrosarcoma, and sarcoma combined is 6.5% for males and 2% for females (NTP Carcinogenesis Data System 1987). In humans, the majority of subcutaneous neoplasms are benign and fibrosarcomas that occur tend to be well-differentiated neoplasms which are not highly malignant and rarely metastasize. In the dog, human, and guinea pig, lipomas and liposarcomas are not uncommon, in the mouse they are exceedingly rare (Stewart 1979).

Acknowledgment. We thank Mr. Fred Talley for his expert assistance in the preparation of the electron micrographs.

References

Abbes M, Barety M (1978) Cancers on chronic wounds or the risks of disturbed cicatrization (Study of 33 cases). Ann Chir Plast Esthet 23: 80–85 (in French with Engl abstract)

Alon Y, Hammerling GJ, Segal S, Bar-Eli M (1987) Association in the expression of Kirsten-ras oncogene and the major histocompatibility complex class I antigens in fibrosarcoma tumor cell variants exhibiting different metastatic capabilities. Cancer Res 47: 2553–2557

Berenblum I (1929) Tumour-formation following freezing with carbon dioxide snow. Br J Exp Pathol 10: 179–187

Carter RL (1973) Tumours of soft tissues. In: Turusov VS (ed) Pathology of tumours in laboratory animals, vol I, pt 1. Tumours of the rat. IARC, Lyon, pp 151–168

Carter RL, Mitchely BC, Roe FJ (1968) Induction of tumours in mice and rats with ferric sodium gluconate and iron dextran glycerol glycoside. Br J Cancer 22: 521–526

National Toxicology Program (NTP) (1987) Carcinogenesis bioassay data system. Tumor incidences for selected control groups. National Institute of Environmental Health Sciences Research, Triangle Park NC

Percy DH, Jonas AM (1971) Incidence of spontaneous tumors in CD-1 HaM/ICR mice. JNCI 46: 1045–1065

Searle CE, Spencer AT (1966) Induction of tumours of connection tissue by repeated applications of 4-nitroquinoline N-oxide to mouse skin. Br J Cancer 20: 877–885

Shelden WG, Greenman DL (1979) Spontaneous lesions in control BALB/c female mice. J Environ Pathol Toxicol Oncol 3: 155–167

Stewart HL (1979) Tumours of the soft tissues. In: Turusov VS (ed) Pathology of tumours in laboratory animals. II. Tumours of the mouse. IARC, Lyon, pp 487–525

Toth B (1986) Carcinogenesis by N2-[gamma-L(+)-glutamyl-4-carboxyphenylhydrazine of *Agaricus bisporus* in mice. Anticancer Res 6: 917–920

Toth B, Nagel D (1981) Studies of the tumorigenic potential of 4-substituted phenylhydrazines by the subcutaneous route. J Toxicol Environ Health 8: 1–9

Waalkes MP, Rehm S, Kasprzak KS, Issaq HJ (1987) In-
flamatory, proliferative and neoplastic lesions at the
site of metallic indentification ear tags in Wister
[Crt:(Wi)BR] rats. Cancer Res 47: 2445-2450

Ward JM, Goodman DG, Squire RA, Chu KC, Linhart MS (1979) Neoplastic and nonneoplastic lesions in
aging (C57BL/6N x C3H/HeN)F$_1$ (B6C3F1) mice.
JNCI 63: 849-854

Zajdela F, Croisy A, Barbin A, Malaveille C, Tomatis L,
Bartsch H (1980) Carcinogenicity of chloroethylene ox-
ide, an ultimate reactive matabolite of vinyl chloride,
and bis(chloromethyl)ether after subcutaneous administration and in initiation-promotion experiments in
mice. Cancer Res 40: 352-356

Lipoma, Subcutis, Rat

Miriam R. Anver

Synonym. Benign fatty tumor.

Gross Appearance

Lipomas are smooth, soft, well-demarcated
masses which may be lobulated. The cut surface
is white to yellow and may have a slightly greasy
texture (Altman and Goodman 1979; Carter
1973).

Microscopic Appearance

Lipomas are composed of mature adipocytes
that have no unusual histologic characteristics.
The tumor may compress surrounding tissue
(Altman and Goodman 1979; Carter 1973). The
adipocytes contain a large droplet of lipid that
distends and occupies much of the cytoplasm,
which is reduced to a small rim at the periphery
(Fig. 134 and 135). In frozen section, lipid droplets stain with oil-red-O and other stains for neutral fat; the droplets are extracted by the fat solvents during routine tissue processing. The nucleus of the cell is displaced to one side of the cell
and compressed by the cytoplasmic lipid droplet
(Wheater et al. 1979).

Ultrastructure

Lipoma cells have the same ultrastructural characteristics as normal adipocytes. The lipid droplet
which occupies most of the cell volume is not enclosed by a membrane. The compressed cytoplasm
retains small Golgi complexes, small mitochondria which may be spherical or filamentous, and
a few free ribosomes. The nucleus is compressed
to a crescent shape, is eccentrically located, and
has a single nucleolus. Pinocytotic invaginations
are common at the cell surface (Lentz 1971).

Differential Diagnosis

Lipomas are tumors of "white" adipose tissue.
The primary differential diagnosis is with hibernoma, which is a tumor of "brown" adipose tissue (see p. 126). Hibernomas are rare tumors in
rats. They occur either in the posterior thoracic
cavity or in the subcutis (Stefanski et al. 1987).
When located subcutaneously, hibernomas are
generally found in the interscapular region (Carter 1973). While the gross appearance is similar
to lipoma, the microscopic appearance of hibernomas differs considerably. Hibernomas are
composed of cells with granular eosinophilic cytoplasm which may contain finely granular, gold-
en-brown pigment as well as clear vacuoles of
variable size. In frozen sections the vacuoles
stain positively for fat (Port et al. 1979; Stefanski
et al. 1987). Port et al. (1979) described a subcutaneous neoplasm in a female Sprague-Dawley
rat which had cells with light microscopic characteristics of both types of adipocytes. The origin
from brown fat was determined by ultrastructural features typical of normal and neoplastic
brown fat. Specifically, these features were the
presence of abundant pleomorphic mitochondria
with transverse, closely packed cristae and intra-
matrical granules, poorly developed Golgi apparatus and endoplasmic reticulum, and close apposition of neoplastic adipocytes to the abundant
capillaries in the intercellular space. Lipomas can
be differentiated.

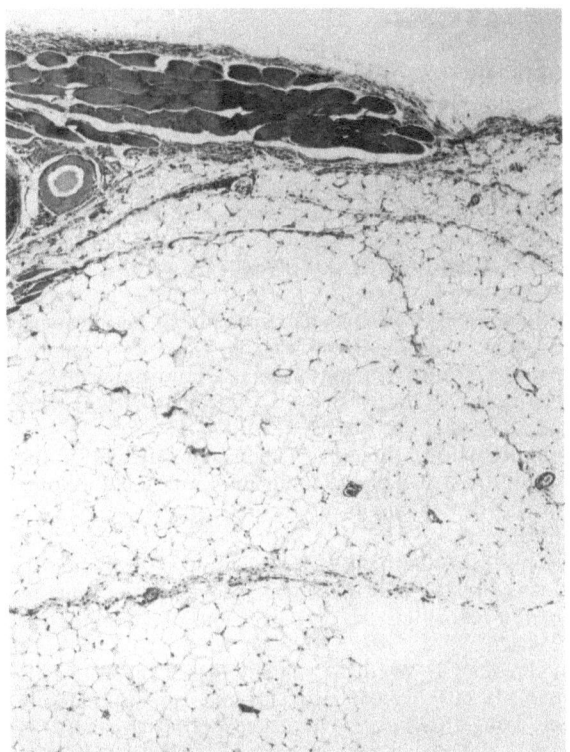

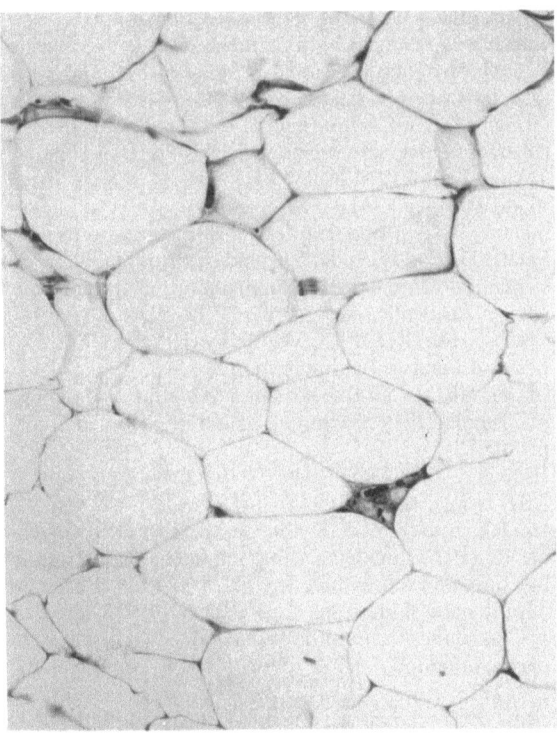

Fig. 134 *(above)*. Lipoma, axillary subcutis, rat. The tumor has a partial connective tissue capsule and is composed of mature adipocytes. H and E, × 20

Fig. 135 *(below)*. Higher magnification of the tumor in Fig. 134. The adipocytes contain a large lipid droplet which compresses the nucleus and cytoplasm to the periphery of the cell. H and E, × 400

Biologic Features

Spontaneous, subcutaneous, mesenchymal tumors are more common in rats than epithelial skin tumors, and lipoma is one of the most common subcutaneous neoplasms (Altman and Goodman 1979). However, the incidence of lipoma in most strains is generally less than 1% as noted in Table 6. This table includes control rats from 2-year bioassays as well as several life-span studies.

Lipomas undergo an exaggerated lipolytic response to hormones such as l-epinephrine, glucagon, corticotropin (ACTH), thyroid-stimulating hormone (TSH), and growth hormone as compared with cells from normal adipose tissue (Schwenzer and Kang 1980).

Hibernomas are very rare tumors. From all the studies listed in Table 6, only one integumentary hibernoma was reported; this occurred in a female Osborne Mendel rat (0.1% incidence). In addition, hibernomas of the subcutis have been reported in only 2 out of 115 000 F344 rats in the National Toxicology Program's data base (Stefanski et al. 1987).

Table 6. Frequency of lipomas in the subcutis in five strains of rats

Strain	Incidence		Reference
	Male	Female	
ACI/N	0/55	1/209 (0.4%)	Maekawa and Odashima 1975
ACI/segHapBR	1/216 (0.4%)	–	Ward et al. 1983
F344	3/144[a] (2.0%)	–	Coleman et al. 1977
	4/1794 (0.22%)	2/1754 (0.11%)	Goodman et al. 1979
	12/2320 (0.5%)	1/2370 (<0.1%)	Haseman et al. 1984
	3/529[a] (0.6%)	6/529[a] (1.0%)	Solleveld et al. 1984
Holtzman	1/3387 (<0.1%)	0/1699	Schardein et al. 1968
Osborne-Mendel	3/975 (0.3%)	4/970 (0.4%)	Goodman et al. 1980
Sprague-Dawley			Anver et al. 1982
HAP	0/62[a]	–	
CD	1/113[a] (0.9%)	–	
CD	0/60	1/105[b] (0.1%)	Prejean et al. 1973

[a] Life span; all other studies, 2 years.
[b] "Myxolipoma".

Comparison with Other Species

Subcutaneous lipomas occur in a wide variety of mammals including nonhuman and human primates and are also reported in avian species. The tumors generally occur in adult and aged animals. The gross and histologic appearance are similar in most species. Lipomas are most common in dogs, occur less frequently in horses and cattle, and are rare in cats, sheep, and swine. These neoplasms may be multiple and are often found in obese animals (Jones and Hunt 1983; Squire et al. 1978; Stannard and Pulley 1978; Yager and Scott 1985).

Hibernomas have been reported in dogs, wild animal species, and humans. Standard and Pulley (1978) note that because dogs do not normally have brown fat or a hibernating gland, the reported hibernomas may represent a variant of lipoma. These tumors are usually located on the dorsal midline of the thorax or in the axilla. They have a similar histologic appearance to the tumor in rats but generally are brown grossly (Jones and Hunt 1983; Stefanski et al. 1987; see p. 126).

Subcutaneous lipoma is an extremely rare, spontaneous tumor in mice. It was not discussed in several reviews of tumors of the integument and subcutis of mice (Holland and Fry 1982; Squire et al. 1978; Stewart 1979). An occasional lipoma, site not specified, was recorded in a tabulation of literature on tumor incidence in control mice (Sher 1974). Subcutaneous lipomas were not present in 2056 breeder and retired breeder BALB/cCr mice (Peters et al. 1972). Integumentary lipomas were reported in 4 out of 2543 (0.15%) male and 3 out of 2522 (0.11%) female B6C3F1 control mice used in bioassays by the National Cancer Institute (Ward et al. 1979). B6C3F1 mice in the National Toxicology Program historical control data had an incidence of lipoma of less than 0.5% in 2343 males and 2486 females (Haseman et al. 1984).

Chemically induced, benign, lipomatous integumentary tumors of mice have not been reported. Skin neoplasms which develop in the initiation/promotion model of carcinogenesis are of epithelial origin (Berenblum 1975).

Acknowledgment. The photographs of lipoma and liposarcoma were kindly provided by Col. John M. Pletcher, Veterinary Pathology Division, Armed Forces Institute of Pathology, Washington D.C.

References

Altman NH, Goodman DG (1979) Neoplastic diseases, Integumentary System. In: Baker HJ, Lindsey JR, Weisbroth SH (eds) The laboratory rat. Biology and diseases, vol I. Academic, London

Anver MR, Cohen BJ, Lattuada CP, Foster SJ (1982) Age-associated lesions in barrier-reared male Sprague-Dawley rats: a comparison between Hap: (SD) and Crl: COBS[R]CD[R](SD) stocks. Exp Aging Res 8: 3–24

Berenblum I (1975) Sequential aspects of chemical carcinogenesis: skin. In: Becker FF (ed) Cancer. A comprehensive treatise. Etiology: chemical and physical carcinogenesis, vol I, chap 10. Plenum, New York, pp 323–344

Carter RL (1973) Tumours of the soft tissues. In: Turusov VS (ed) Pathology of tumours in laboratory animals, vol 1. Tumours of the rat, pt 1. IARC, Lyon, pp 151–156

Coleman GL, Barthold W, Osbaldiston GW, Foster SJ, Jonas AM (1977) Pathological changes during aging in barrier-reared Fischer 344 male rats. J Gerontol 32: 258–278

Goodman DG, Ward JM, Squire RA, Chu KC, Linhart MS (1979) Neoplastic and non-neoplastic lesions in aging F344 rats. Toxicol Appl Pharmacol 48: 237–248

Goodman DG, Ward JM, Squire RA, Paxton MB, Reichardt WD, Chu KC, Linhart MS (1980) Neoplastic and non-neoplastic lesions in aging Osborne-Mendel rats. Toxicol Appl Pharmacol 55: 433–447

Haseman JK, Huff J, Boorman GA (1984) Use of historical control data in carcinogenicity studies in rodents. Toxicol Pathol 12: 126–135

Holland JM, Fry RJM (1982) Neoplasms of the integumentary system and Harderian gland. In: Foster HL, Small JD, Fox JG (eds) The mouse in biomedical research, vol IV, chap 29. Experimental biology and oncology. Academic, New York, pp 513–528

Jones TC, Hunt RD (1983) Veterinary pathology, 5th edn. Lea and Febiger, Baltimore, p 1126

Lentz TL (1971) Cell fine structure. An atlas of drawings of whole-cell structure. Saunders, Philadelphia, pp 70–72

Maekawa A, Odashima S (1975) Spontaneous tumors in ACI/N rats. JNCI 55: 1437–1445

Peters RL, Rabstein LS, Spahn GJ, Madison RM, Huebner RJ (1972) Incidence of spontaneous neoplasms in breeding and retired breeder BALB/cCr mice throughout the natural life span. Int J Cancer 10: 273–282

Port CD, Nunez C, Battifora H (1979) An unusual neoplasm of adipose tissue in a rat. Lab Anim Sci 29: 214–217

Prejean JD, Peckham JC, Casey AE, Griswold DP, Weisburger EK, Weisburger JH (1973) Spontaneus tumors in Sprague-Dawley rats and Swiss mice. Cancer Res 33: 2768–2773

Schardein JL, Fitzgerald JE, Kaump DH (1968) Spontaneous tumors in Holtzman-source rats of various ages. Pathol Vet 5: 238–252

Schwenzer K, Kang ES (1980) Hormone responsiveness of the lipoma: a tumor of adipose tissue. Horm Metab Res 12: 444–449

Sher SP (1974) Tumors in control mice: liberature tabulation. Toxicol Appl Pharmacol 30: 337-359

Solleveld HA, Haseman JK, McConnell EE (1984) Natural history of body weight gain, survival, and neoplasia in the F344 rat. JNCI 72: 929-940

Squire RA, Goodman DG, Valerio MG, Frederickson TN, Strandberg JD, Levitt MH, Lingeman CH, Harshbarger JC, Dawe CJ (1978) Tumors. In: Benirschke K, Garner FM, Jones TC (eds) Pathology of laboratory animals, vol II. Springer, Berlin Heidelberg New York, pp 1068-1070

Stannard AA, Pulley LT (1978) Tumors of the skin and soft tissues. In: Moulton JE (ed) Tumors in domestic animals, 2nd edn, chap 2. University of California Press, Berkeley, pp 22-23

Stefanski SA, Elwell MR, Yoshitomi K (1987) Malignant hibernoma in a Fischer 344 rat. Lab Anim Sci 37: 347-349

Stewart HL (1979) Tumours of the soft tissues. In: Turusov VS (ed) Pathology of tumours in laboratory animals, vol II. Tumours of the mouse. IARC, Lyon, pp 487-501

Ward JM, Goodman DG, Squire RA, Chu KC, Linhart MS (1979) Neoplastic and nonneoplastic lesions in aging (C57BL/6N X C3H/HeN(F₁ (B6C3F1) mice. JNCI 63: 849-854

Ward JM, Hamlin MH II, Ackerman LJ, Lattuada CP, Longfellow DG, Cameron TP (1983) Age-related neoplastic and degenerative lesions in aging male virgin and ex-breeder ACI/segHapBR rats. J Gerontol 38: 538-548

Wheater PR, Burkitt HG, Daniels VG (1979) Functional histology. A text and color atlas. Churchill Livingstone, Edinburgh

Yager JA, Scott DW (1985) The skin and appendages. In: Jubb KVF, Kennedy PC, Palmer N (eds) Pathology of domestic animals, vol I, 3rd end. Academic, Orlando, p 519

Liposarcoma, Subcutis, Rat

Miriam R. Anver

Synonyms. Malignant lipoma; myxoliposarcoma.

Gross Appearance

The gross appearance of this neoplasm in the rat has not been described in the literature other than to note that it is an infiltrating neoplasm (Carter 1973).

Microscopic Features

Liposarcomas are composed primarily of pleomorphic fat cells (Fig. 136). These tumor cells are round or oval and may have single or multiple, clear, cytoplasmic vacuoles that stain positively on frozen section for neutral fat (e.g., oil-red-O and osmium stains). Nuclei may be large and centrally located or eccentric and compressed by the cytoplasmic lipid; a single nucleolus is present (Fig. 137). Some tumor cells are binucleate but multinucleated or giant cells are not usually present. The tumor has a collagenous stroma containing areas with many large fibroblasts. Some liposarcomas also have areas of intercellular myxoid tissue (Carter 1973; Port et al. 1979).

Ultrastructure

While ultrastructural features of subcutaneous liposarcoma of rats have not been detailed, a pleomorphic liposarcoma of the omentum and mesentery of a KBL rat has been described (Minato et al. 1986). On light microscopy, the tumor was composed of two different cell types: round cells with abundant cytoplasm and large clear nuclei, and spindle-shaped cells with oval to spheroidal nuclei. Both types of cells had cytoplasmic lipid vacuoles of various sizes.

Ultrastructurally, the round cells have irregularly outlined nuclei with deeply invaginated nuclear membranes. These round cells have sparsely distributed, small, round mitochondria and dilated, round endoplasmic reticulum. Lipid droplets are present in the dilated cisternae of the rough endoplasmic reticulum or in the cytoplasm with no limiting membrane. Spindle cells have a scanty cytoplasm, few organelles, nuclei with marginated chromatin, and cytoplasmic lipid droplets with no surrounding limiting membrane.

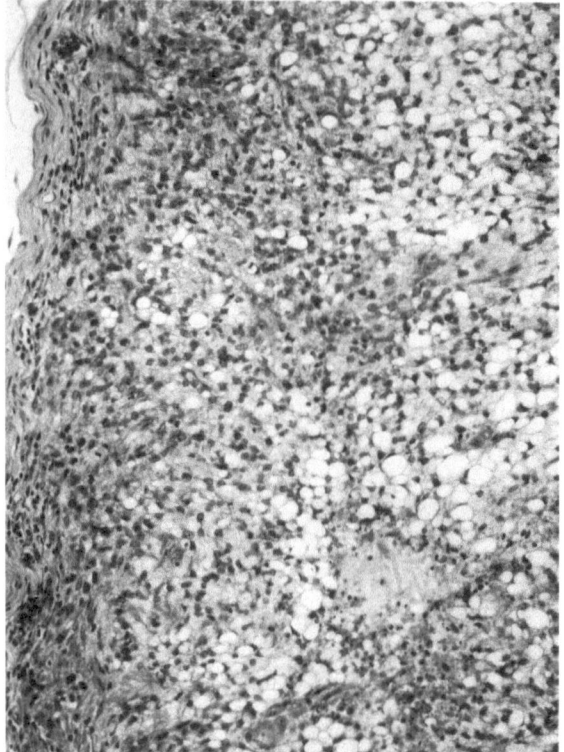

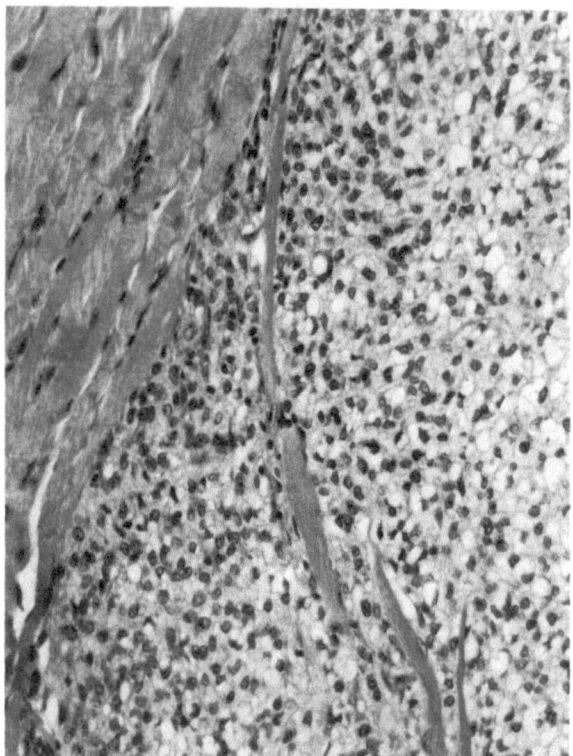

Fig. 136. Liposarcoma, subcutis, thorax, rat. The tumor is composed of a pleomorphic population of cells. Many of the cells have large lipid droplets which compress the nucleus and cytoplasm to the periphery of the cell. H and E, × 160

Fig. 137. Another field from the same tumor as in Fig. 136. Tumor cells have invaded and destroyed the skeletal muscle of the thorax. A number of tumor cells have large central nuclei, which are round or spindle shaped. At the invasive border of the tumor, lipid droplets in tumor cell cytoplasm are small or absent. H and E, × 250

Differential Diagnosis

Anaplastic liposarcomas should be differentiated from other tissue sarcomas. Stains for neutral fat on frozen sections of the tumor should demonstrate cytoplasmic fat. In addition, liposarcoma should be differentiated from malignant hibernoma, a rare tumor of brown fat. A cervical or interscapular location is suggestive at gross necropsy of the latter neoplasm. Microscopically, malignant hibernomas have many of the features of liposarcoma, including cells with vacuolated cytoplasm that stain positively for neutral fat. In contrast to liposarcomas, hibernomas have a highly vascular stroma composed of many capillaries. The most reliable differential diagnostic feature is an ultrastructural one: hibernoma tumor cells contain abundant mitochondria with elongated cristae, as opposed to liposarcoma cells which contain only scattered small mitochondria similar to their normal cell of origin,

the adipocyte (Lentz 1971; Port et al. 1979; Stefanski et al. 1987; see p. 126).

Lipomas may be distinguished from liposarcomas by their uniform pattern of mature cells with cytoplasm distended by a large droplet of fat and peripherally displaced nuclei (Fig. 135).

Biologic Features

Liposarcomas of the subcutis are very uncommon spontaneous findings in rats. Based on review of data, the frequency is generally less than 0.1%. Liposarcomas may occur sporadically in association with subcutaneous implants of plastic films (Altman and Goodman 1979; Carter 1973). Some reports also associate liposarcoma with: vinylidene fluoride administered in olive oil by gavage to Sprague-Dawley rats (Maltoni and Tovoli 1979); neutron irradiation to male Sprague-Dawley rats (Jones et al. 1968); and polyoma virus BB/T2 (Gimmy and Graffi 1963).

Comparison with Other Species

Liposarcomas are rare tumors in domestic animals and other species (Jones and Hunt 1983; Squire et al. 1978; Stannard and Pulley 1978; Yager and Scott 1985). Their histologic appearance is similar to that of rats. However, tumor cell nuclei usually are not compressed, and karyomegaly and multinucleated cells are frequently found (Stannard and Pulley 1978). In dogs, well-defined but invasive lipoid tumors may be considered to be a form of liposarcoma (Yager and Scott 1985). Liposarcoma in domestic animals, although locally invasive, rarely metastasizes (Stannard and Pulley 1978). In humans, liposarcomas are usually located intermuscularly (intramuscularly in the extremities), in contrast to lipoma which is usually located in the subcutis. Human liposarcomas may be well-differentiated, myxoid, round cell, pleomorphic, or mixed. A characteristic ultrastructural feature of these tumors is the presence of uni- or multivacuolated lipoblasts with hyperchromatic nuclei that have been scalloped by the impression of lipid droplets (Walaas and Kindblom 1985). Some human liposarcomas have shared cell surface antigenicity with malignant fibrous histiocytoma, perivascular mesenchymal cells, and fibroblasts (Iwasaki et al. 1987).

Liposarcomas in mice are rare, spontaneous neoplasms. In his review, Stewart (1979) noted a spontaneous liposarcoma that was transplantable in WB/Rd mice at the Jackson Laboratories. He also noted infrequent older reports about induction of liposarcoma. Squire et al. (1978) and Holland and Fry (1982) did not mention liposarcoma in their reviews of mouse skin tumors.

Liposarcoma of the integument was not reported in a tabulation of literature on tumor incidence in control mice (Sher 1974) or in a lifetime study of 2056 breeder and retired breeder BALB/cCr mice (Peters et al. 1972). B6C3F1 mice used in the National Cancer Institute's Carcinogenesis Testing Program had no liposarcomas in 2543 males and 1 out of 2522 (0.03%) liposarcomas in females (Ward et al. 1979). Liposarcomas were not present at 0.5% or greater incidence in the NTP historical control data base of 2343 male and 2486 female B6C3F1 mice (Haseman et al. 1984). Liposarcomas are not described as being induced in the initiation/promotion model of mouse skin carcinogenesis. The tumor discussed under "Ultrastructure" was induced in a female Swiss mouse that received a single subcutaneous injection of 3-methylcholanthrene followed 6 weeks later by skin painting with 12-0-tetradecanoylphorbol-13-acetate (TPA) in acetone (Ramchandani et al. 1985). A fibroliposarcoma was reported in a male C3H mouse which had been injected subcutaneously with a transformed cell line derived from an organ culture of C3H ventral prostate treated with 3-methylcholanthrene (Heidelberger and Iype 1967). Liposarcomas have been induced in guinea pigs which received subcutaneous injections of carcinogenic hydrocarbons (Stewart 1979).

Acknowledgement. The photographs of lipoma and liposarcoma were kindly provided by Col. John M. Pletcher, Veterinary Pathology Division, Armed Forces Institute of Pathology, Washington D.C.

References

Altman NH, Goodman DG (1979) Neoplastic diseases. Integumentary System. In: Baker HJ, Lindsey JR, Weisbroth SH (eds) The laboratory rat. Biology and diseases, vol I. Academic, New York, pp 336–340

Carter RL (1973) Tumours of the soft tissues. In: Turusov VS (ed) Pathology of tumours in laboratory animals, vol 1. Tumours of the rat, pt 1. IARC, Lyon, pp 151–156

Gimmy J, Graffi A (1963) Zur Transplantabilität der durch den BB/T2-Polyoma Virusstamm induzierten Tumoren. Arch Geschwulstforsch 20: 1–21

Haseman JK, Huff J, Boorman GA (1984) Use of historical control data in carcinogenicity studies in rodents. Toxicol Pathol 12: 126–135

Heidelberger C, Iype PT (1967) Malignant transformation in vitro by carcinogenic hydrocarbons. Science 155: 214–217

Holland JM, Fry RJM (1982) Neoplasms of the integumentary system and Harderian gland. In: Foster HL, Small JD, Fox JG (eds) The mouse in biomedical research, vol IV, chap 20. Experimental biology and oncology. Academic, New York, pp 513–528

Iwasaki H, Isayama T, Johzaki H, Kikuchi M (1987) Malignant fibrous histiocytoma. Evidence of perivascular mesenchymal cell origin immunocytochemical studies with monoclonal anti-MFH antibodies. Am J Pathol 128: 528–537

Jones DC, Castanera TJ, Kimeldorf DJ, Rosen VJ (1968) Radiation induction of skin neoplasms in the male rat. J Invest Dermatol 50: 27–35

Jones TC, Hunt RD (1983) Veterinary pathology, 5th edn. Lea and Febiger, Baltimore, p 1126

Lentz TL (1971) Cell fine structure. An atlas of drawings of whole-cell structure. Saunders, Philadelphia, pp 70–72

Maltoni C, Tovoli D (1979) First experimental evidence of the carcinogenic effects of vinylidine fluoride. Long-term bioassays on Sprague-Dawley rats by oral administration. Med Lav 70: 363–368

Minato Y, Takada H, Yamanaka H, Kojima A, Wada I, Takeshita M, Okaniwa A (1986) Pleomorphic liposarcoma in an aged rat. Jpn J Vet Sci 48: 429-432

Peters RL, Rabstein LS, Spahn GJ, Madison RM, Huebner RJ (1972) Incidence of spontaneous neoplasms in breeding and retired breeder BALB/cCr mice throughout the natural life span. Int J Cancer 10: 273-282

Port CD, Nunez C, Battifora H (1979) An unusual neoplasm of adipose tissue in a rat. Lab Anim Sci 29: 214-217

Ramchandani AG, Bhisey RA, Sirsat SM (1985) Ultrastructure of chemicaly induced mouse skin tumours. Indian J Cancer 22: 46-58

Sher SP (1974) Tumors in control mice: literature tabulation. Toxicol Appl Pharmacol 30: 337-359

Squire RA, Goodman DG, Valerio MG, Frederickson TN, Strandberg JD, Levitt MH, Lingeman CH, Harshbarger JC, Dawe CJ (1978) Tumors. In: Benirschke K, Garner FM, Jones TC (eds) Pathology of laboratory animals, vol II. Springer, Berlin Heidelberg New York, pp 1068-1070

Stannard AA, Pulley LT (1978) Tumors of the skin and soft tissues. Lipoma and liposarcoma. In: Moulton JE (ed) Tumors in domestic animals, 2nd edn, chap 2. University of California Press, Berkeley, pp 22-23

Stefanski SA, Elwell MR, Yoshitomi K (1987) Malignant hibernoma in a Fischer 344 rat. Lab Anim Sci 37: 347-349

Stewart HL (1979) Tumours of the soft tissues. In: Turusov VS (ed) Pathology of tumours in laboratory animals, vol II. Tumours of the mouse. IARC, Lyon, pp 487-501

Walaas L, Kindblom LG (1985) Lipomatous tumors: correlative cytologic and histologic study of 27 tumors examined by fine needle aspiratio cytology. Hum Pathol 16: 6-18

Ward JM, Goodman DG, Squire RA, Chu KC, Linhart MS (1979) Neoplastic and non-neoplastic lesions in aging (C57BL/6N X C3H/HeN)F$_1$ (B6C3F1) mice. JNCI 63: 849-854

Yager JA, Scott DW (1985) The skin and appendages. In: Jubb KVF, Kennedy PC, Palmer N (eds) Pathology of domestic animals, vol I, 3rd edn. Academic, Orlando, p 519

Fibrous Histiocytoma, Malignant, Subcutis, Rat

Peter Greaves

Synonyms. Malignant fibrous histiocytoma; fibrosarcoma; pleomorphic fibrosarcoma; pleomorphic sarcoma; dermatofibrosarcoma.

Gross Appearance

Both spontaneous and induced malignant fibrous histiocytoma occur in the rat as firm, pale nodules or masses which are often lobulated and infiltrated into the surrounding soft tissues and adjacent structures.

Size is to some extent dictated by experimental conditions, but these tumors reach on average about 5 cm in diameter in most series studied (Greaves and Faccini 1981; Mii et al. 1982; Greaves et al. 1985). They can, however, grow as large as 15 cm in diameter if they are allowed to progress (Greaves and Faccini 1981). The tumor cut surface is usually white or yellowish in color with zones or foci of necrosis and hemorrhage. A focal gelatinous appearance may also be seen (Konishi et al. 1982). Ulceration of the overlying skin is a frequent finding.

X-ray examination of malignant fibrous histiocytomas arising in or near bones and joints reveals

Fig. 138 *(upper left).* Malignant fibrous histiocytoma, male ▶ Sprague-Dawley rat. Note spindle cells arranged in a storiform of cartwheel pattern. This neoplasm developed 57 weeks after subcutaneous implantation of a Millipore filter, 2.4 cm diameter, pore size 0.125 mm. H and E, × 220

Fig. 139 *(lower left).* Malignant fibrous histiocytoma, aged male Wistar rat. This tumor developed spontaneously as a mass on the left side of the chest wall. Although less cellular, with more abundant connective tissue than the example in Fig. 138, the storiform pattern is evident. This neoplasm infiltrated surrounding tissues and local lymph nodes. H and E, × 100

Fig. 140 *(upper right).* Malignant fibrous histiocytoma, aged Sprague-Dawley rat. A spontaneous tumor in subcutaneous tissues. The storiform pattern of spindle cells is present but considerable cellular pleomorphism and both giant cells and foam cells are visible in this field. H and E, × 140

Fig. 141 *(lower right).* Pleomorphic malignant fibrous histiocytoma, male Sprague-Dawley rat. Note irregular giant cells and smaller, rounded histiocytic cells which developed at the site of an implanted Millipore filter after 72 weeks. H and E, × 220

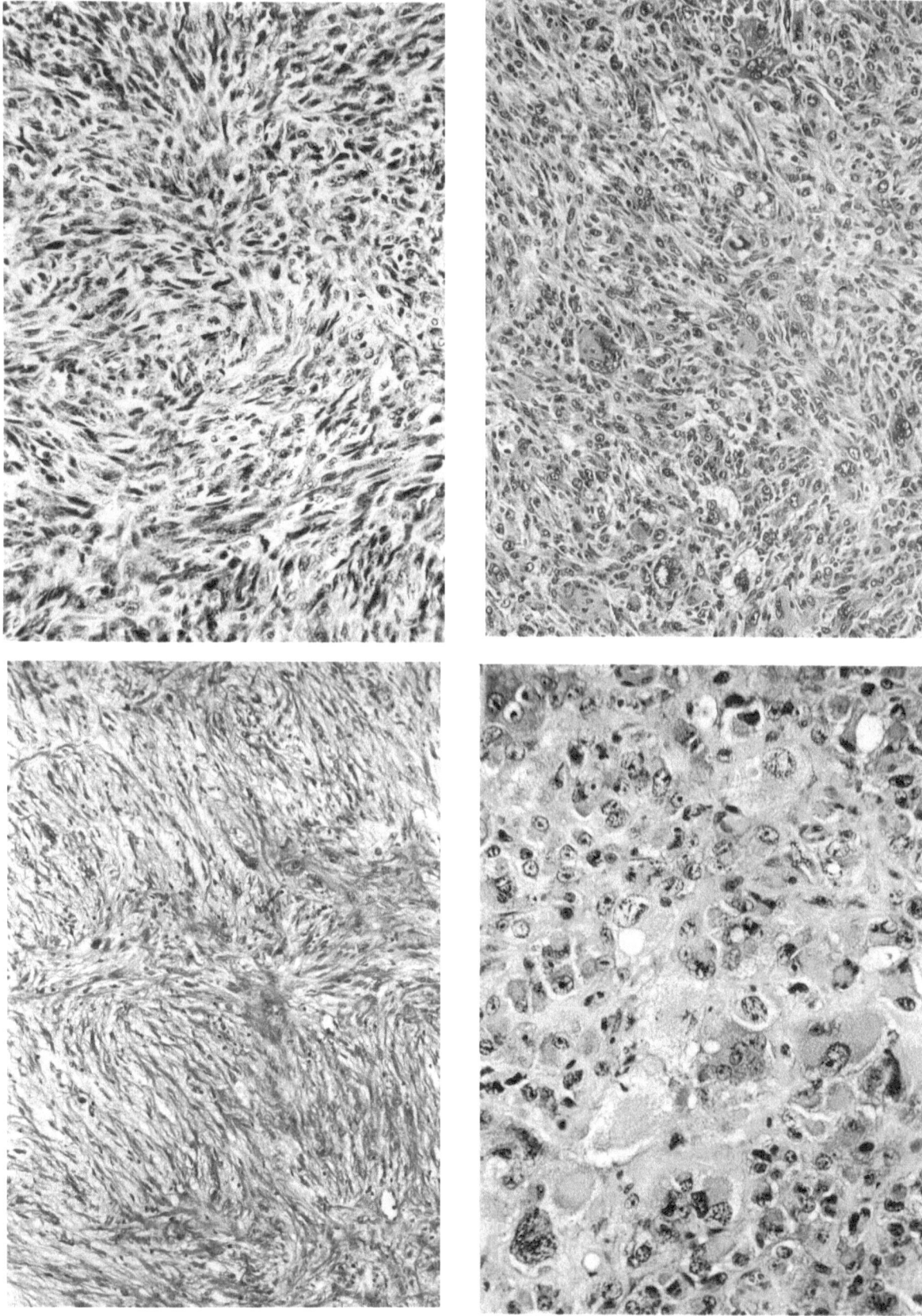

destruction of bone cortex, intramedullar involvement, and invasion of the joint space (Mii et al. 1982).

Microscopic Features

Histologic features vary between different tumors and within the same neoplasm. Appearances range from a well-ordered storiform or cartwheel pattern of plump spindle cells (Figs. 138 and 139) to a highly pleomorphic cellular pattern comprising bizarre giant cells, multinucleated cells, spindle cells, and smaller undifferentiated cells (Figs. 140 and 141) (Greaves and Faccini 1981). Giant cells may phagocytize cells and cell debris. Foam cells in foci are sometimes also evident (Fig. 140).

Giant or spindle cells possessing abundant eosinophilic cytoplasm can suggest myogenic differentiation, but cross striations, even with the aid of special stains, are not seen. Mitotic activity is variable but may be extensive. A mononuclear or lymphoid cellular infiltrate is common and can be quite intense in some tumors. Less frequently a diffuse, polymorphonuclear, cellular infiltration is seen. A myxomatous appearance is frequently observed. A prominent vasculature suggestive of hemangiopericytoma may also be evident in some tumors (Sakamoto 1986), and the presence of foci of nonneoplastic osteoid is also described (Mii et al. 1982). Although pigment is usually not prominent in sections stained by hematoxylin and eosin, Perls' stain may reveal the presence of iron.

Enzyme cytochemical studies of these rat neoplasms demonstrate the presence of lysosomal enzymes in both spindle and pleomorphic cells, as shown by abundant activity of acid phosphatase (EC 3.1.3.2) (Fig. 142), β-glucuronidase (EC 3.2.1.31), and alpha-naphthyl butyrate or alpha-naphthyl acetate esterase (Greaves et al. 1985; Sakamoto 1986). Immunocytochemical studies indicate myoglobin is absent from the tumor cells. As these tumors show considerable individual variation in histologic features, some authors subdivide malignant fibrous histiocytomas in the rat into fibrous, giant cells, myxoid, and imflammatory subgroups as have been defined for human neoplasms (Mii et al. 1982). Such detailed subdivisions may be inappropriate when small numbers of these neoplasms are being studied, particularly as histologic features vary within the same tumor. Nevertheless, these neoplasms fall fairly easily into two distinct types, a

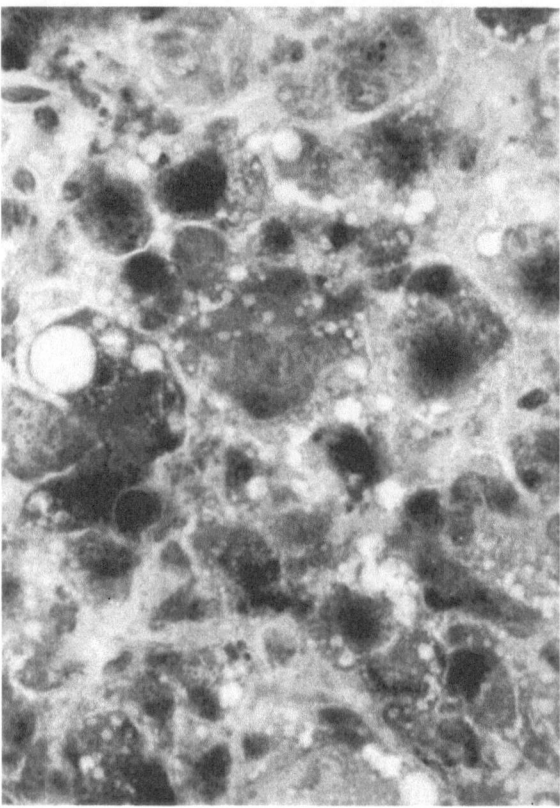

Fig. 142. Similar case to that in Fig. 141 with intense acid phosphatase activity. Frozen section, azo coupling method for acid phosphatase, counterstained with hematoxylin, × 560

fibrous (or spindle cell) group and a pleomorphic group (Greaves et al. 1985).

Malignant fibrous histiocytomas often infiltrate locally into the surrounding muscle and other soft tissues. Metastases are found relatively late in development, principally in local lymph nodes, lungs, and liver (Greaves and Faccini 1981; Mii et al. 1982).

Ultrastructure

Spindle cells contain oval nuclei with infolded nuclear membranes, abundant euchromatin, and prominent nucleoli. The cell cytoplasm contains profiles of granular endoplasmic reticulum of variable size and number, often dilated by moderately electron dense material (Fig. 143). Mitochondria, lysosomal structures, and lipid droplets may be prominent. Cytoplasmic filaments are present in some cells, and very occasionally focal densities suggestive of myofibroblast differentiation may be seen. Structures diagnostic of skele-

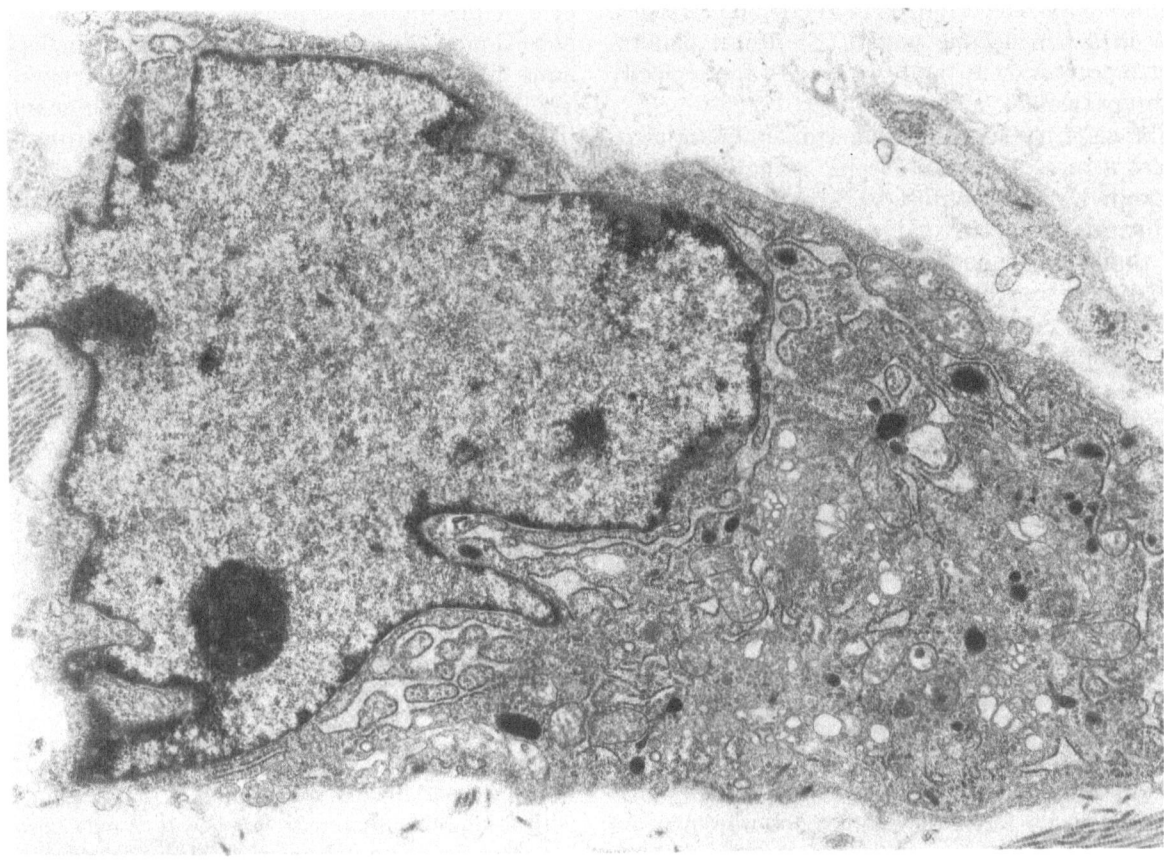

Fig. 143. A cell with both fibroblastic and histiocytic features from the tumor seen in Fig. 139. The cell possesses a large indented nucleus with prominent nucleolus and abundant rough endoplasmic reticulum, mitochondria, and dense lysosomal bodies. Glutaraldehyde fixation, post-osmicated, TEM, × 10700

tal muscle differentiation such as Z bands are absent. Cytoplasmic margins are fairly smooth with a few, elongated, cytoplasmic processes. Cells are separated by electron lucent ground substance and collagen fibers (Fig. 143).

Pleomorphic cells have essentially similar features, although the nuclei appear more irregular, often with cytoplasmic pseudo-inclusions. Cytoplasmic filaments may be focally abundant. Lysosomes and lipid droplets may be especially numerous in some cells. Cell margins may be more ruffled or irregular than in spindle cells. In addition, smaller primitive cells with few or no distinctive features are scattered among these various cell types.

Differential Diagnosis

It is important to make the distinction between malignant fibrous histiocytoma and the so-called histiocytic sarcoma or malignant histiocytoma.

Although malignant fibrous histiocytoma and histiocytic sarcoma have certain overlapping histological characteristics, notably their histiocytic appearance, these tumors appear to be distinct types. Histiocytic sarcomas have well-differentiated histiocytic features with generally little or no spindle cell differentiation. The cells are principally oval or rounded, histiocytic or epithelioid cells mixed with multinucleated giant cells of foreign body type, and there is often characteristic, well-defined, zonal necrosis. These tumors may develop as soft tissue masses but metastatic spread occurs early, or they may arise in a diffuse lymphomatous manner (Greaves and Faccini 1981; Squire et al. 1981).

Malignant fibrous histiocytomas have in the past been understandably classified as pleomorphic fibrosarcomas or rhabdomyosarcomas (see "Pathogenesis"). Fibrosarcomas are distinguished from malignant fibrous histiocytomas by their *monomorphic* pattern of spindle cells with some chromatin-rich, oval nuclei and pale, basophilic cytoplasm arranged in interlacing fascicles, or in a herringbone pattern. Storiform pattern, pleomorphic cells, and giant cells are typically absent (Katenkamp and Neupert 1982).

The giant pleomorphic cells with abundant cytoplasm present in pleomorphic malignant histiocytomas may be confused with rhabdomyoblasts. However, the cells in malignant fibrous histiocytomas have none of the diagnostic features of rhabdomyosarcomas such as the presence of cross striations, immunocytochemical evidence of cytoplasmic myoglobin, or ultrastructural features of skeletal muscle differentiation such as Z lines (Hildebrand and Biserte 1978).

Biologic Features

Natural History. Malignant fibrous histiocytomas are usually locally aggressive tumors which infiltrate the subcutaneous and deep tissues as well as adjacent organs. These neoplasms usually cause the death of the animal or necessitate its killing as a result of the local effects, particularly when there is extensive tumor necrosis and ulceration of the overlying skin. Anemia, neutrophilia, and elevated levels of gamma globulins may be seen in association with these late changes (Greaves and Faccini 1981). Metastatic growth is observed, but this is seen less frequently than with histiocytic sarcomas (malignant histiocytoma).

Pathogenesis. The histogenesis of malignant fibrous histiocytomas occurring in humans has been controversial, but over recent years detailed immunocytochemical studies have all tended to indicate that most of these tumors are not of true histiocytic lineage but derived from a primitive extramedullary stem cell (Roholl et al. 1985; Lawson et al. 1987; Fletcher 1987). A similar conclosion has been reached in the case of rat malignant fibrous histiocytic neoplasms. These tumors develop in rats at the site of implantation of inert foreign bodies (Greaves et al. 1985). By the use of radiation and chimaeras it has been shown that neoplasms which develop in this model are derived from a local, primitive mesenchymal cell which is not derived from monocytes or bone marrow (Barnes et al. 1971). Katenkamp and Neupert (1982) have also demonstrated that neoplasms of fibrohistiocytic type develop in the rat following implantation of established fibrosarcoma cell lines but not of cell lines derived from monocytes. Tumors which develop from mono-

cyte or macrophage cell lines retain an appearance similar to the histiocytic sarcoma or malignant histiocytoma (Katenkamp and Neupert 1983). Thus, it seems probable that the malignant fibrous histiocytic phenotype is derived from a primitive mesenchymal stem cell, whereas the histiocytic sarcoma is probably of true histiocytic lineage.

Etiology. Although the etiology of malignant fibrous histiocytomas arising spontaneously in aged rats remains uncertain, neoplasms of identical type can be induced by the subcutaneous injection of certain plant extracts (Pradhan et al. 1974), 9.10-dimethyl-1.2-benzanthracene (Sakamoto 1986), or 4-(hydroxyamino)quinoline 1-oxide (Konishi et al. 1982), and subcutaneous implantation of nickel subsulphide (Lumb et al. 1987) or inert materials (Greaves et al. 1985). It is probable that sarcomas of similar type can be induced by other agents, but many models have not been evaluated in detail for fibrohistiocytic features.

Frequency. Small numbers of malignant fibrous histiocytomas occur spontaneously in aged rats, with a slightly greater prevalence in males than females. In a population of 3280 Sprague-Dawley rats of about 2 years of age, 19 pleomorphic and 23 spindle cell tumors were reported (Greaves and Faccini 1981). Of 25 males and 24 females of the same strain housed under similar conditions and implanted subcutaneously with Millipore filters, 17 males and 12 females developed malignant fibrous histiocytomas around the implants after a mean delay of 513 ± 119 days in males and 551 ± 109 days in females (Greaves et al. 1985).

Malignant fibrous histiocytomas induced by weekly injections of 4-(hydroxyamino)quinoline-1-oxide for 4 weeks occurred in 13 out of 15 (87%) of male F344 or Wistar rats between 16 and 48 weeks following the final injection (Konishi et al. 1982), although variation of the dosage regimen of this agent can undoubtedly influence the prevalance of these neoplasms (Mii et al. 1982). Two or three intra-articular injections of 9.10-dimethyl-1.2-benzanthracene at 4-weekly intervals in male Wistar rats produced malignant fibrous histiocytomas in nearly all injected rats 5–28 weeks after the final injection (Sakamoto 1986).

Comparison with Other Species

The term fibrosarcoma has been used for many years to encompass a wide spectrum of histological appearances found in rat sarcomas. These appearances range from monomorphic spindle cell neoplasms to those with a highly pleomorphic cellular pattern (Carter 1973). This situation contrasts strongly with soft tissue sarcomas reported in humans, in which fibrosarcomas are considered to be a fairly uncommon, *monomorphic* spindle cell neoplasm characterized by cells arranged in interlacing fascicles, often referred to as a herringbone pattern (Enterline 1981). In humans, it is now the malignant fibrous histiocytoma which has become the most commonly reported soft tissue sarcoma of adults (Weiss and Enzinger 1978; Enjoji et al. 1980). However, over the last few years, it has become increasingly evident that the apparent differences between experimental sarcomas and those found in humans are often a result of variations in classification rather than fundamental differences in cell types or biology. As early as 1974, it was noted that some mesenchymal tumors induced in rats by the subcutaneous injection of certain plant extracts were similar to fibrous malignant neoplasms found in humans (Pradhan et al. 1974). In a detailed study of rat sarcomas induced by subcutaneous injection of methylcholanthrene, Katenkamp and Stiller (1975) remarked upon a number of structural and cytochemical characteristics which were common to both the induced sarcomas and malignant fibrous histiocytomas found in humans.

Subsequently, a number of different studies have shown structural, cytochemical, and biological similarities of many sarcomas found spontaneously or induced in the rat to malignant fibrous histiocytomas found in man (Greaves and Faccini 1981; Greaves et al. 1982; Mii et al. 1982; Konishi et al. 1982; Greaves et al. 1985; Sakamoto 1986).

The recognition of this similarity between human and rat now extends to other species, including dog, cat, horse (Ford et al. 1975; Gleiser et al. 1979; Renlund and Pritzker 1984), and mouse (Stewart 1979). Indeed, some neoplasms developing from mouse fibrosarcoma cell lines, which are widely used as prototypes for malignant cells in experimental studies, also possess histological and ultrastructural appearances of malignant fibrous histiocytomas (Becker et al. 1982).

The importance of the recognition of the malignant fibrous histiocytomas in the rat and other species is that it may provide a firmer basis from which to interpret the revelance of certain experimental sarcoma models for human neoplastic disease.

References

Barnes DWH, Evans EP, Loutit JF (1971) Local origin of fibroblasts deduced from sarcomas induced in chimaeras by implants of pliable disks. Nature 233: 267–268

Becker FF, Nevares D, Mackay B (1982) Transplantable lines of spontaneous mouse fibrosarcomas. Vet Pathol 19: 206–209

Carter RL (1973) Tumours of the soft tissues. In: Turusov VS (ed) Pathology of tumours in laboratory animals. I. Tumours of the rat, pt I. IARC, Lyon, pp 151–167

Enjoji M, Hashimoto H, Tsuneyoshi M, Iwasaki H (1980) Malignant fibrous histiocytoma. A clinicopathologic study of 130 cases. Acta Pathol Jpn 30: 727–741

Enterline HT (1981) Histopathology of sarcomas. Semin Oncol 8: 133–155

Fletcher CDM (1987) Malignant fibrous histiocytoma? Histopathology 11: 433–437

Ford GH, Empson RN Jr, Plopper CG, Brown PH (1975) Giant cell tumor of soft parts: a report of an equine and a feline case. Vet Pathol 12: 428–433

Gleiser CA, Raulston GL, Jardine JH, Gray KN (1979) Malignant fibrous histiocytoma in dogs and cats. Vet Pathol 16: 199–208

Greaves P, Faccini JM (1981) Spontaneous fibrous histiocytic neoplasms in rats. Br J Cancer 43: 402–411

Greaves P, Martin JM, Masson MT (1982) Spontaneous rat malignant tumors of fibrohistiocytic origin: an ultrastructural study. Vet Pathol 19: 497–505

Greaves P, Martin JM, Rabemampianina Y (1985) Malignant fibrous histiocytoma in rats in sites of implanted millipore filters. Am J Pathol 120: 207–214

Hildebrand HF, Biserte G (1978) Ultrastructural investigation of a Ni_3-S_2-induced rhabdomyosarcoma in Wistar rats. Comparative study with emphasis on myofibrillar differentiation and ciliar formation. Cancer 42: 528–554

Katenkamp D, Neupert G (1982) Experimental tumors with features of malignant fibrous histiocytomas. Light microscopic and electron microscopic investigations on tumors produced by cell transplantation of an established fibrosarcoma cell line. Exp Pathol 22: 11–27

Katenkamp D, Neupert G (1983) Experimental tumors with features of malignant histiocytomas. Morphological studies on neoplasms produced by inoculation of an established macrophage-like cell line (WEHI-3). Exp Pathol 24: 143–153

Katenkamp D, Stiller D (1975) Structural pattern and histological behaviour of experimental sarcomas. I. General considerations, histology and histochemistry. Exp Pathol 11: 182–189

Konishi Y, Maruyama H, Mii Y, Miyauchi Y, Yokose Y, Masuhara K (1982) Malignant fibrous histiocytomas induced by 4-(hydroxyamino)quinoline 1-oxide in rats. JNCI 68: 859–865

Lawson CW, Fisher C, Gatter KC (1987) An immunohistochemical study of differentiation in malignant fibrous histiocytoma. Histopathology 11: 375–383

Lumb GD, Sunderman FW, Schneider HP, Chou RH (1987) Histogenesis of subcutaneous malignant tumors resulting from nickel subsulfide implantation. Ann Clin Lab Sci 17: 286–299

Mii Y, Maruayama H, Miyauchi Y, Yokose Y, Masuhara K, Konishi Y (1982) Experimental studies on malignant fibrous histiocytomas in rats. I. Production of malignant fibrous histiocytomas by 4-hydroxyaminoquinoline 1-oxide in bone of Fischer 344 strain rats. Cancer 50: 2057–2065

Pradhan SN, Chung EB, Ghosh B, Paul BD, Kapadia GJ (1974) Pontential carcinogens. I. Carcinogenicity of some plant extracts and their tannin-containing fractions in rats. JNCI 52: 1579–1582

Renlund RC, Pritzker KPH (1984) Malignant fibrous histiocytoma involving the digit in a cat. Vet Pathol 21: 442–444

Roholl PJM, Kleijne J, Van Basten CDH, Van der Putte SCJ, Van Unnik JAM (1985) A study to analyze the origin of tumor cells in malignant fibrous histiocytoma. A multiparametric characterization. Cancer 56: 2809–2815

Sakamoto K (1986) Malignant fibrous histiocytoma induced by intra-articular injection of 9.10-dimethyl-1.2-benzanthracene in the rat. Pathological and enzyme histochemical studies. Cancer 57: 2313–2322

Squire RA, Brinkhous KM, Peiper SC, Firminger HI, Mann RB, Strandberg JD (1981) Histiocytic sarcoma with a granulome-like component occuring in a large colony of Sprague-Dawley rats. Am J Pathol 105: 21–30

Stewart HL (1979) Tumors of the soft tissues. In: Turusov VS (ed) Pathology of tumours in laboratory animals. II. Tumours of the mouse, chap. 23. IARC, Lyon, pp 487–525

Weiss WS, Enzinger FM (1978) Malignant fibrous histiocytoma. An analysis of 200 cases. Cancer 41: 2250–2266

Mast Cell Tumor, Skin, Mouse

Michihito Takahashi and Yoshifumi Miyakawa

Synonyms. Mastocytoma; cutaneous mastocytoma.

Gross Appearance

Mast cell tumor is not usually detected with the naked eye, although the tumor may become large and appear as a yellowish-white, opaque, soft mass underneath the epidermis.

Microscopic Features

Mast cell tumors principally involve the corium but occasionally extend into subcutaneous tissue and rarely include the muscular layer. Tumors are composed of nonencapsulated, well-circumscribed sheets of discrete cuboidal or rhomboid cells (Figs. 144 and 145) (Bogovski 1979). The tumor cells are distinctive. The nucleus is centrally located and round or slightly oval. The nuclear chromatin is lighter than that of normal mast cells. Mitotic figures are rare. The cytoplasm is agranular, or very faintly granular, with H & E stain (Fig. 145). However, in sections stained with toluidine blue or Giemsa's stain, the metachromatic granules in the cytoplasm are clearly visible (Fig. 146).

Unlike the granules in normal mast cells, the granules in tumor cells vary in size (Fig. 147). Cutaneous mast cell tumors in the mouse consist of densely packed mast cells in a delicate stroma consistently composed of a fine reticulum and blood vessels (Ohmori et al. 1981).

We observed one mast cell tumor, $2.0 \times 1.0 \times 0.5$ cm in size, with deep infiltration of the subcutaneous tissue but without metastasis (Fig. 148). In the tumor cells one could see atypia, mitotic figures, and metachromatic granules of various size, shape, and number (Fig. 149).

Ultrastructure

In almost all tumor cells electronmicroscopic examination confirms the presence of intracytoplasmic granules, which are electron-dense bodies with irregular shapes and sizes. Compared with normal mast cells, granules are small, few, and vary considerably in both density and morphology. Tumor cells are densely packed; however, cell processes, which are numerous in normal mast cells, are not usually observed in tumor cells (Fig. 150).

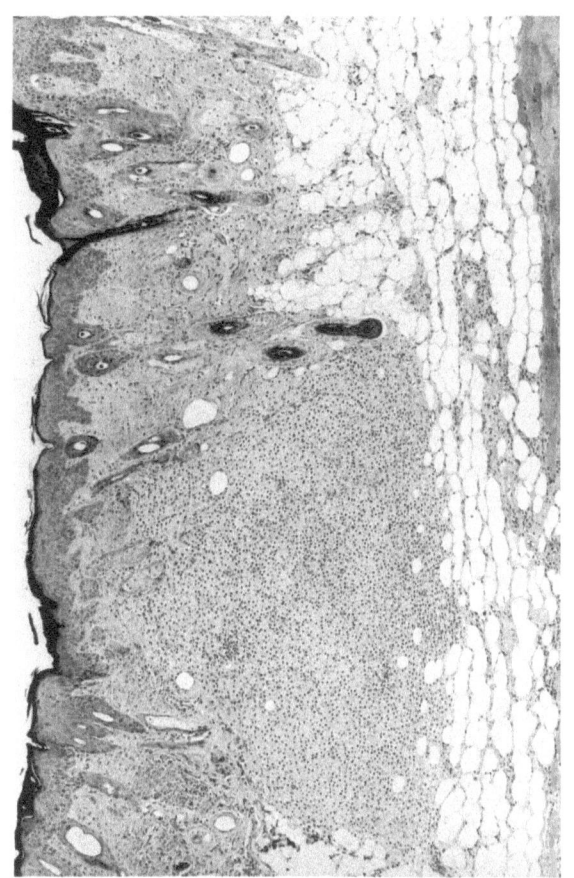

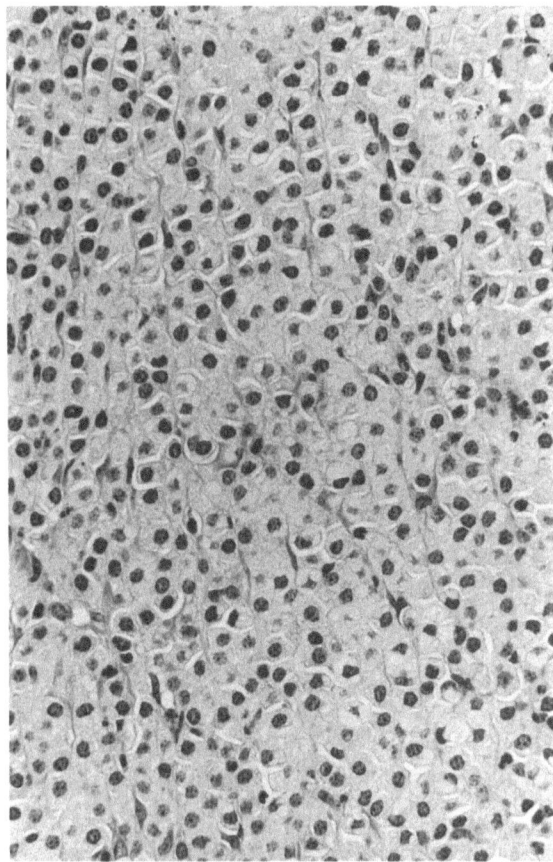

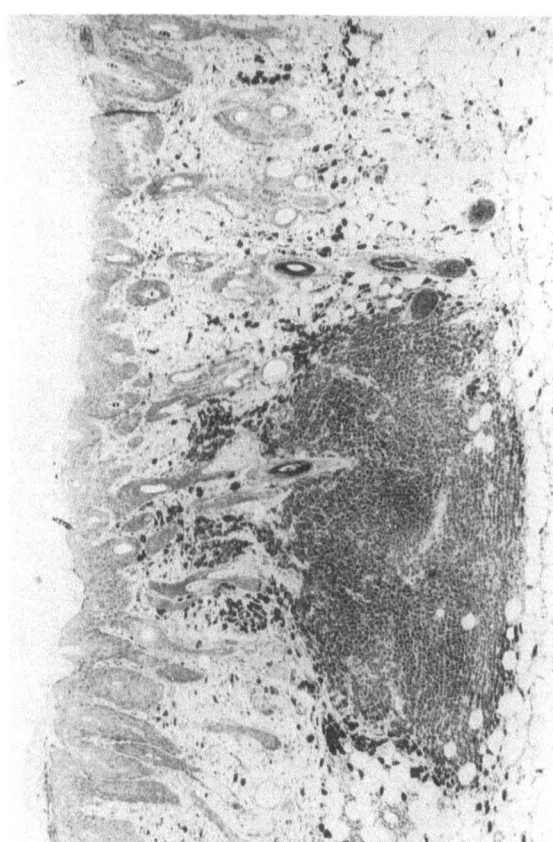

Fig. 144 *(upper left)*. Mast cell tumor induced in female BDF1 mouse treated with MNNG followed by TPA. Note the nonencapsulated, well-circumscribed tumor mass, epidermal hyperplasia, and dermal fibrosis. H and E, ×50

Fig. 145 *(upper right)*. Higher magnification of Fig. 144. Note the sheets of discrete cuboidal or rhomboid cells. H and E, ×300

Fig. 146 *(lower right)*. Section adjacent of Fig. 144. Metachromatic staining clearly distinguishes the cytoplasm of tumor cells. Toluidine blue, ×150

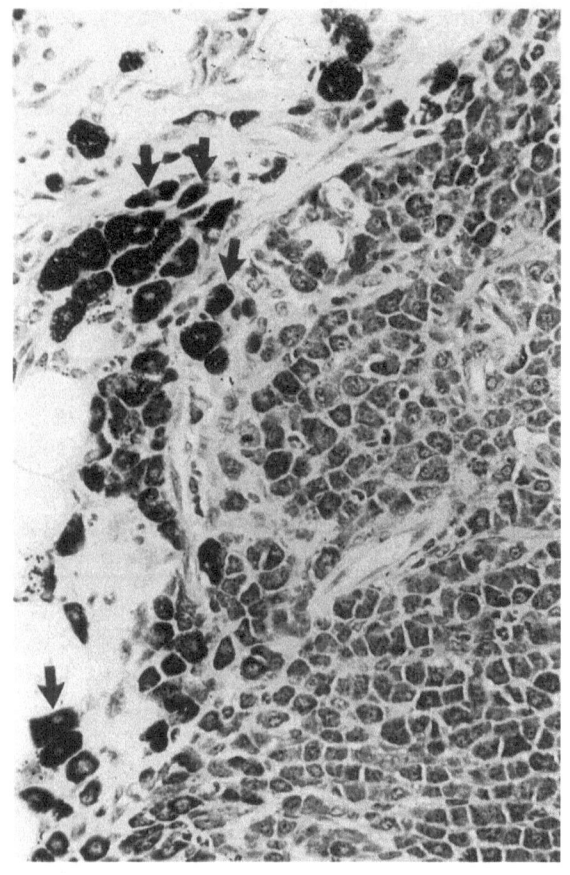

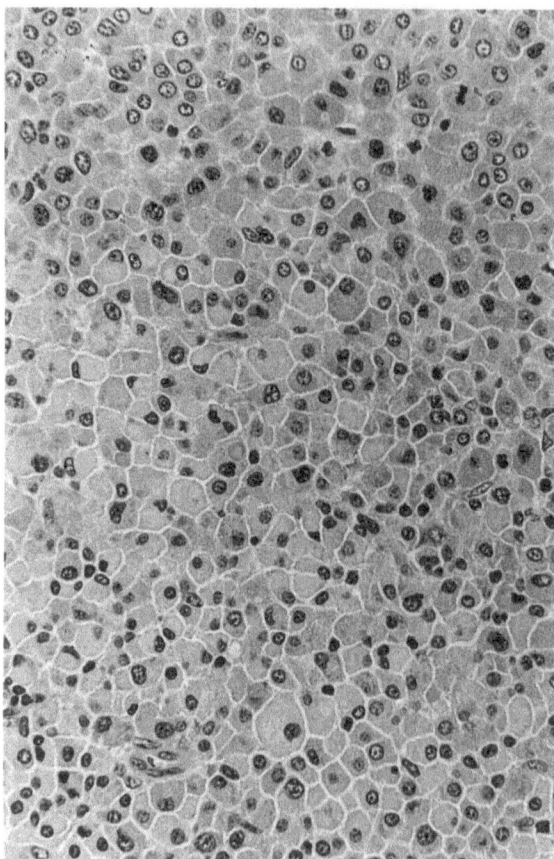

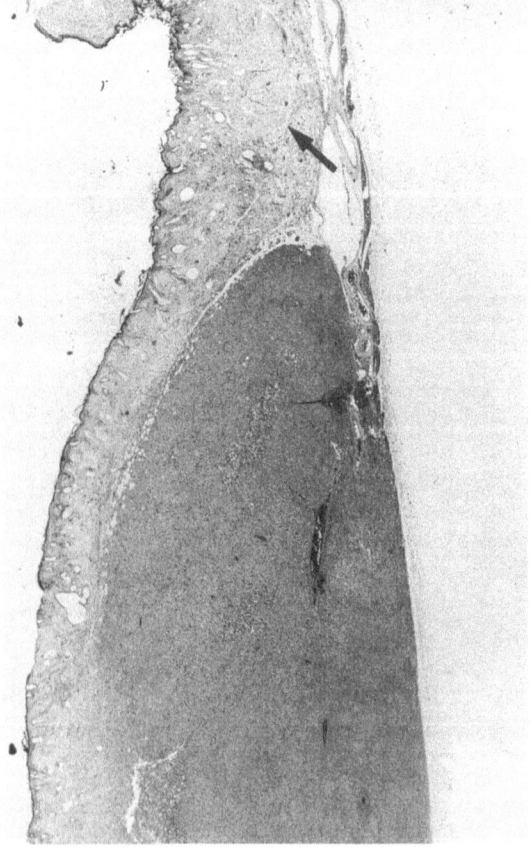

Fig. 147 *(upper left).* Higher magnification of Fig. 146. Tumor cells are smaller than normal cells *(arrows),* and cytoplasmic granules are smaller in number than those of normal mast cells. Toluidine blue, × 300

Fig. 148 *(lower left).* Malignant mast cell tumor induced in female DBA/2 mouse treated with MNNG followed by TPA. Note the deep infiltration. Benign mast cell tumor is also observed *(arrow).* H and E, × 15

Fig. 149 *(upper right).* Higher magnification of Fig. 148. Note the pleomorphism and mitotic figures. H and E, × 300

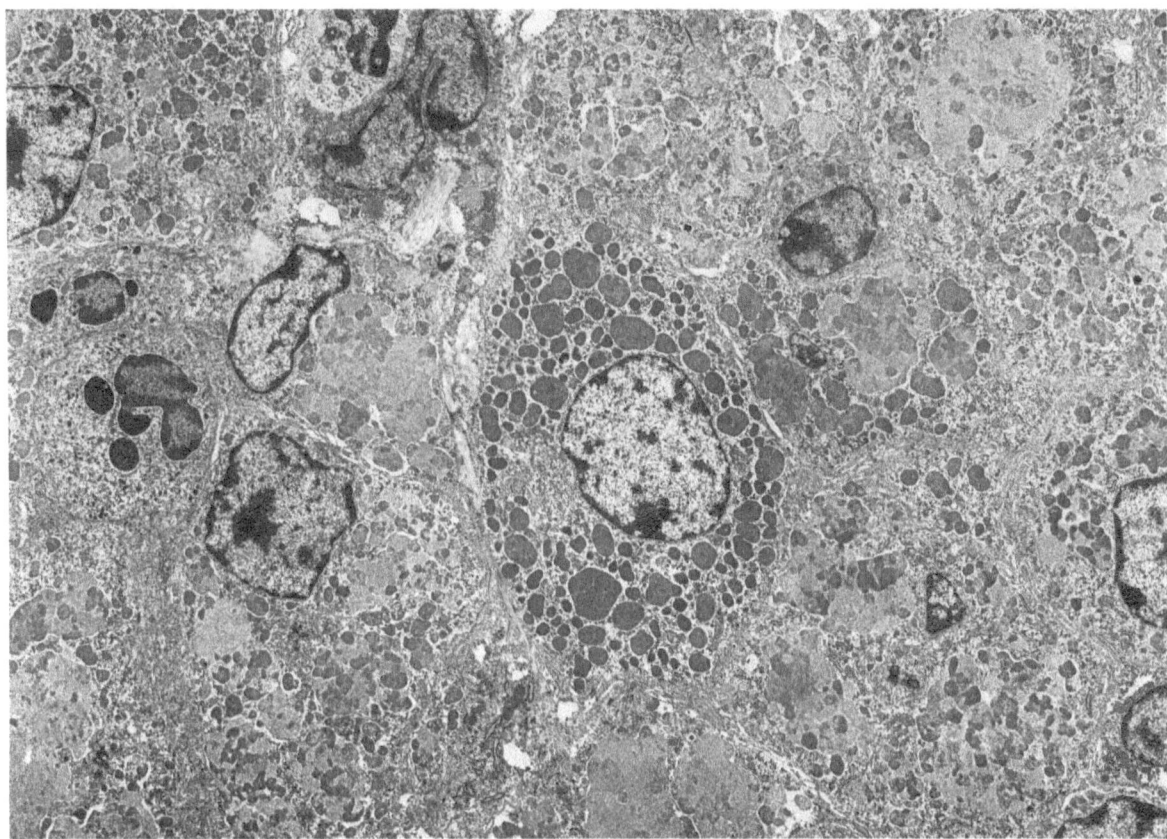

Fig. 150. Tumor mast cells. Note the variation in both density and morphology of intracytoplasmic granules. TEM from the formalin-fixed material after refixation with glutaraldehyde and OsO_4, × 3900

Differential Diagnosis

Mast cell tumor should be distinguished from local, diffuse, dermal mast cell infiltration or hyperplasia of mast cells observed in the skin following painting with carcinogens, cigarette tar, X-irradiation, or in any area of inflammation (Figs. 151 and 152). Table 7 lists morphological differences between diffuse dermal mast cell infiltration and mast cell tumor (Ohmori et al. 1981).

Biologic Features

Spontaneous mast cell tumors occur infrequently in mice. They can manifest as two distinct types: cutaneous tumors or systemic neoplasms with cutaneous involvement. Primary cutaneous mast cell tumors are very rare in mice (Deringer and Dunn 1947; Holland and Fry 1982; Rask-Nielsen and Christensen 1963). Chemically induced mast cell tumors have been reported in the al-tered dermis as a result of skin painting with coal tar (Schreuss 1923; Twort and Twort 1930), cigarette tar (Ohmori et al. 1981), or other chemicals such as 3-methylcholanthrene (Cramer and Simpson 1944) or 7.12-dimethylbenz[a]anthracene (Rizzi and Fiore-Donati 1962). We also observed a significant incidence of induced mast cell tumors in two-stage skin carcinogenesis with N-methyl-N'-nitro-N-nitrosoguanidine as an initiator and 12,0-tetradecanoylphorbol-13-acetate as a promoter.

The tumors have a slow growth rate with no tumor-related clinical symptoms and are therefore usually identified at autopsy or by microscopic examination. A transplantable mast cell tumor line has been developed from a DBA/2 mouse treated repeatedly with 3-methylcholanthrene (Dunn and Potter 1957). This line has been used extensively in immunological studies. The cells of this line secrete serotonin and histamine.

Table 7. Morphological differences between diffuse dermal mast cell infiltration (DDMI) and mast cell tumor

	DDMI	Mast cell tumor
Histological features		
Cellularity	Poorly cellular	Densely packed with tumor cells
Pattern of location	Local diffuse infiltration in the superficial part of the dermis	Nodular and well-circumscribed in the corium and subcutaneous tissue
Connective tissue	Bundles of connective tissue separating mast cells	No connective tissue between tumor cells except blood vessels
Reticulin network	Lack of proper reticulin network	Presence of fine and well-elaborated reticulin network
Cytological features		
Cytoplasmic granules	Usually rich in cytoplasmic metachromatic granules by toluidine blue stain	Lower quantity of cytoplasmic metachromatic granules or totally degranulated by toluidine blue stain
Cell atypia	Lacking	Rarely to frequently present
Nucleolus	Poorly visible nucleolus (masked by the granules)	Well-seen nucleolus
Chromatin	Regular	Lighter than that of normal mast cells
N/C ratio	Normal	Higher than that of normal mast cells
Mitosis	Absent	Rare to frequent mitosis
Ultrastructural feature		
Intracytoplasmic granules	Large round granules filling the cytoplasm	Small in size and in number compared with normal mast cells

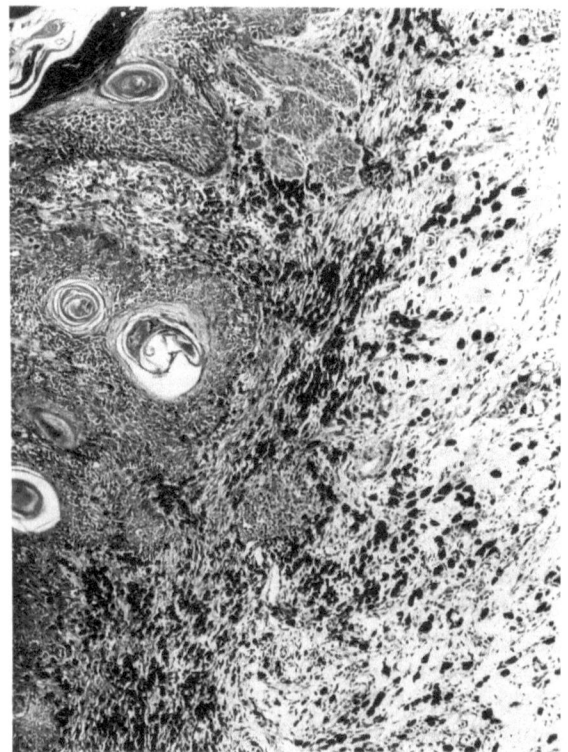

Fig. 151. Dermal mast cell infiltration in a female DBA/2 mouse treated with MNNG followed by TPA. Note the diffuse mast cell infiltration of the dermis below a squamous cell papilloma. Toluidine blue, × 75

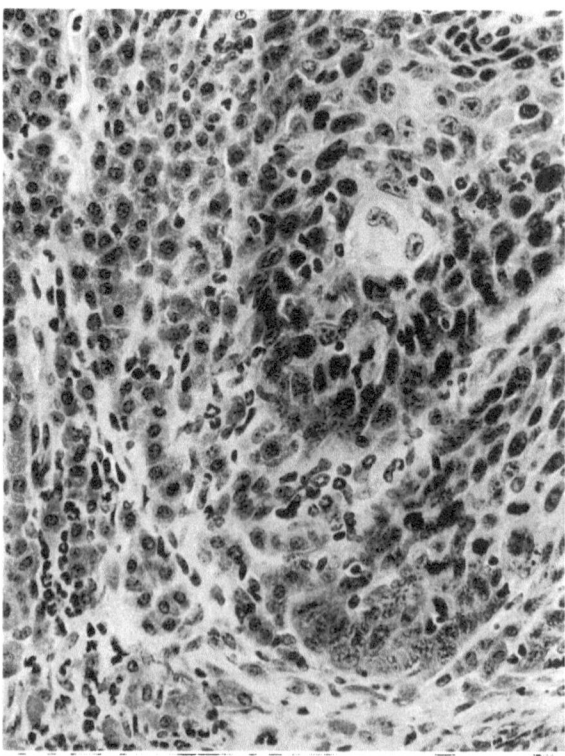

Fig. 152. Diffuse dermal mast cell infiltration in a female CDF1 mouse treated with DMBA followed by TPA. Note the mast cells and polymorphonuclear leukocytes adjacent to cells of an early stage of a squamous cell carcinoma. H and E, × 240

Comparison with Other Species

Mast cell tumor is one of the most common skin tumors in the dog. It has been reported that mast cell tumors represent 6% of all tumors in the dog (Lombard et al. 1963) and 13% of all skin tumors in the dog (Orkin and Schwarzman 1959). The histological appearance of mast cell tumor of the dog is similar to that of the mouse. In canine mast cell tumor, however, the presence of eosinophils in the tumor tissue is fairly characteristic, and the tumor cells are usually loosely arranged and rarely occur in sheets or in cords between collagen fibers or in large nests separated by collagen. In about one-third of the canine mast cell tumors, focal collagen necrosis and hyalinization of the vessel walls are present (Hottendorf and Nielsen 1966).

In the dog, aside from the direct effects of mast cell tumor, due to replacement of tissue, several side effects may develop, including gastric and duodenal ulcers, focal glomerulitis, defects in the immunologic response, and defective coagulation. These may be related to the release of histamine (Howard et al. 1969) and heparin (Hottendorf et al. 1965) by the tumor cells. Hottendorf and Nielsen (1968) suggested that an autoimmune reaction may be induced with mast cell tumor.

In cats, mast cell tumors account for approximately 2%-3% of all forms of cutaneous tumors (Cotchin 1961; Head 1958). The histopathology of feline mast cell tumors is similar to that of the dog. However, the presence of eosinophils and collagen denaturation is rare in felines (Wilcock et al. 1986). Sometimes, tumors are associated with a significant amount of inflammation. Also normal mast cells may accumulate in areas of chronic inflammation.

Head (1958) estimated that mast cell tumors represent about 3% of the cutaneous and subcutaneous tumors in cattle. In addition to cattle, domesticated animals with mast cell tumors include pigs, sheep, and horses (Stannard and Pulley 1978). In humans, mastocytomas are related to the skin disease urticaria pigmentosa (Cheville 1979).

References

Bogovski P (1979) Tumours of the skin. In: Turusov VS (ed) Pathology of tumours in laboratory animals, vol. II. Tumours of the mouse. IARC, Lyon, pp 1-42 (IARC Sci Publ no 23)

Cheville NF (1979) Urticaria pigmentosa. In: Andrews EJ, Ward BC, Altman NH (eds) Spontaneous animal models of human disease, vol. 2. Academic, New York, pp 41-44

Cotchin E (1961) Skin tumours of cats. Res Vet Sci 2: 353-361

Cramer W, Simpson WL (1944) Mast cell in experimental skin carcinogenesis. Cancer Res 4: 601-616

Deringer MK, Dunn TB (1947) Mast-cell neoplasia in mice. JNCI 7: 289-298

Dunn TB, Potter M (1957) A transplantable mast-cell neoplasm in the mouse. JNCI 18: 587-601

Head KW (1958) Cutaneous mast cell tumours in the dog, cat, and ox. Br J Dermatol 70: 389-408

Holland JM, Fry RJM (1982) Neoplasms of the integumentary system and Harderian gland. In: Foster HL, Small JD, Fox JG (eds) The mouse in biomedical research, vol 4. Experimental biology and oncology. Academic, New York, pp 513-528

Hottendorf GH, Nielsen SW (1966) Collagen necrosis in canine mastocytomas. Am J Pathol 49: 501-513

Hottendorf GH, Nielsen SW (1968) Pathological report of 29 necropsies on dogs with mastocytoma. Pathol Vet 5: 102-121

Hottendorf GH, Nielsen SW, Kenyon AJ (1965) Canine mastocytoma. I. Blood coagulation time in dogs with mastocytoma. Pathol Vet 2: 129-141

Howard EB, Sawa TR, Nielsen SW, Kenyon AJ (1969) Mastocytoma and gastroduodenal ulceration. Pathol Vet 6: 146-158

Lombard LS, Moloney JB, Rickard CG (1963) Transmissible canine mastocytoma. Ann N Y Acad Sci 108: 1086-1105

Ohmori T, Mori H, Rivenson A (1981) A study of tobacco carcinogenesis. XX. Mastocytoma induction in mice by cigarette smoke particulates (cigarette tar). Am J Pathol 102: 381-387

Orkin M, Schwarzman RM (1959) A comparative study of canine and human dermatology. II. Cutaneous tumors: the mast cell and canine mastocytoma. J Invest Dermatol 32: 451-466

Rask-Nielsen R, Christensen HE (1963) Studies on a transplantable mastocytoma in mice. I. Origin and general morphology. JNCI 30: 743-761

Rizzi I, Fiore-Donati L (1962) A morphological study of mast cell reaction in chemical skin carcinogenesis of mouse. In: The morphological precursors of cancer. Proceedings of an international conference held at the University of Perugia, June 26-30, 1961. Division of Cancer Research, Perugia, pp 515-526

Schreuss HT (1923) Über einen Mastzellen-Tumor bei der weißen Maus nach Teerpinselung. Dermatologische Zeitschrift 40: 9-14

Stannard AA, Pulley LT (1978) Tumors of the skin and soft tissue. In: Moulten JE (ed) Tumors in domestic animals. University of California Press, Berkeley, pp 16-74

Twort CC, Twort JM (1930) Classification of four thousand experimental oil and tar skin tumours of mice. Lanceti: 1331-1335

Wilcock BP, Yager JA, Zink MC (1986) The morphology and behavior of feline cutaneous mastocytomas. Vet Pathol 23: 320-324

Clitoral Gland Tumors, Mouse

Vladimir S. Turusov

Synonyms. Adenoma; adenoacanthoma; adeno-carcinoma; papilloma; keratoacanthoma; squa-mous cell carcinoma; mixed tumors.

Gross Appearance

The tumors of the clitoral gland appear as subcu-taneous nodules in the location specific for this gland. The small nodules are easily movable, the big ones frequently become firmly attached to the surrounding tissue, and the skin may undergo ulceration. The consistency of the tumor varies from rather soft or elastic to firm. On the cut sur-face, tumors are frequently formes of soft, yel-lowish tissue or contain cysts filled with necrotic masses or thick, purulent material.

Microscopic Features

Normal Structure. The clitoral glands, homolo-gous to the preputial glands of males, are paired, of sebaceous type, and located in the subcutane-ous adipose tissue at each side of the clitoris. Each gland is surrounded by a connective tissue capsule from which trabeculae penetrate the pa-renchyma, subdividing it into lobules. Acini are composed of large, pale, foamy cells with small dark nuclei; at the periphery of the acinus, flat, elongated basal cells are seen (Figs. 153 and 154). The excretory ducts are lined with squamous epi-thelium continuous with that of the clitoral fossa, and hair follicles can be seen (Hummel et al. 1966).
The tumors described here were induced in var-ious strains of mice with 1.2-dimethylhydrazine (DMH). Duct epithelium hyperplasia, areas of squamous metaplasia of acini, increased number of dark basal cells, and inflammatory changes in the gland and surrounding tissues were observed in early lesions.

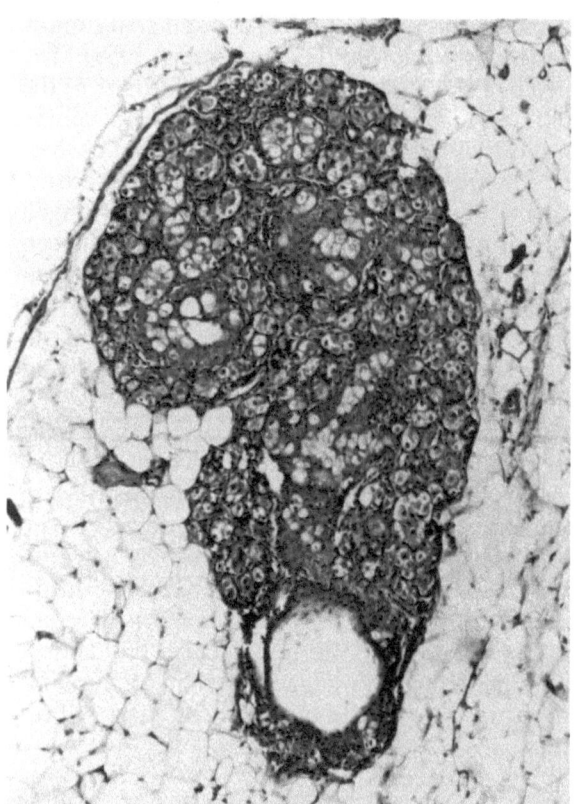

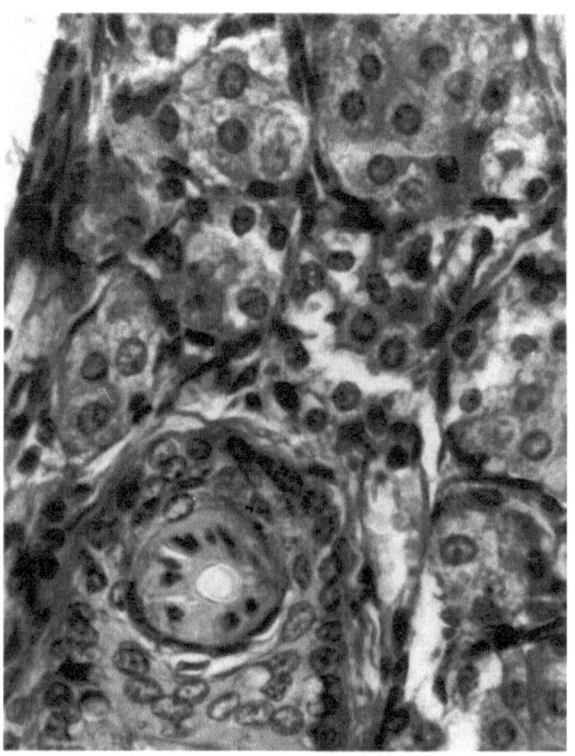

Fig. 153 *(above).* Clitoral gland of an 18-month-old CBA ▶ female mouse. Lobular structure, dilated duct, and squa-mous cell nests. H and E, × 90

Fig. 154 *(below).* Higher magnification of Fig. 153. Acini with sebocytes and dark flat basal cells at the periphery. Hair follicle *(lower left).* H and E, × 560

Tumors – whether benign or malignant – in general consisted of sebaceous (acinar) cells (sebocytes), basal cells, squamous cells, or a mixture of these cells. Depending on the predominant cell type, adenomas (adenocarcinomas), squamous cell papillomas, and carcinomas or basal cell tumors could be distinguished. The term "adenoacanthoma" was used for the tumors in which both adenomatous and squamous cell components were integral parts of the neoplasm. One or both glands in the same animal could be involved, and various structural patterns (solid, cystic, papillary) might be present in one tumor.

Small adenomas are generally of solid structure and may occupy only a part of the gland. They consist of groups of sebocytes surrounded by dark basal cells (Fig. 155). These are distinguished from normal glands by the lack of orderly arrangement and the increased number of dark cells. In larger tumors, ducts may become dilated, and the neoplasm acquires a cystic appearance.

Adenocarcinomas are distinguished by marked cell and nuclear polymorphism, high mitotic activity, and invasive growth into the capsule (Fig. 156). Central parts of large tumors are frequently necrotic so that only a narrow rim of viable tissue remains at the periphery (Figs. 157 and 158). Calcium deposits may be seen in the necrotic mass. Andenocarcinomas frequently mimic the structure and the holocrine secretion of the normal gland in that their main structural elements are sheets of sebocytes (acinar cells) surrounded by several layers of basal cells. Sebocytes undergo holocrine breakdown, and the elimination of the necrotic material leaves a peculiar cystic-papillary structure which gives the tumor a spongy appearance under low magnification (Figs. 159 and 160).

Adenoacanthomas – whether benign or malignant – are organoid tumors in which both adenomatous and squamous cell components are intimately intermingled (Figs. 161–163). Squamous cell papilloma and squamous cell carcinoma, which most likely develop from the duct epithelium, have the disarranged squamous structure typical for this type of tumor (Figs. 164 and 165).

In a few instances, poorly differentiated carcinomas (Fig. 166) with high mitotic activity were found in which only single, scattered sebaceous cells could be seen.

The tumor illustrated in Figs. 167 and 168 was composed mainly of dark basal cells; signs of squamous and sebaceous differentiation were also present.

Only a few tumors were of a pure adenomatous, basal cell, or squamous cell type. Most neoplasms contained all these elements in various proportions. Thus, in the tumor illustrated in Fig. 169, rather large areas were composed exclusively of cells of basal type while in other parts sebaceous and squamous cell differentiation were pronounced.

No tumors of hair follicle or mesenchymal cells were observed.

Differential Diagnosis

DMH not only induces clitoral gland tumors but also produces tumors of the skin, including sebaceous glands, in the anal region. Two types of sebaceous glands occur in this area. Ordinary sebaceous glands are those connected with hair follicles and located in the upper dermis, similar to sebaceous glands in other parts of the body. The distinction between tumors arising from these sebaceous glands and those of the clitoral glands is not difficult, at least at early stages, due to the superficial position of tumors of the sebaceous glands. The other type of sebaceous glands in this area is that located deep between the muscles of the anal sphincter and connected with a few huge hair follicles. Tumors arising from these sebaceous glands are located deep under the skin. The early tumors from these glands can be distinguished histologically, by their specific location between the sphincter muscles, but the origin of large tumors cannot be established with certainty (Turusov 1980).

Skin papillomas (warts) in the anal region, due to their development on the skin surface, cannot be confused (at least at their early stages) with squamous cell tumors of the clitoral glands. If the tumor has not been followed macroscopically from the very beginning of its appearance, establishing its origin when it reaches a large size and infiltrates surrounding tissues becomes practically impossible.

Another neoplasm from which the clitoral gland tumor should be differentiated is mammary gland carcinoma. This also develops in subcutaneous tissue and may have the same location and consistency; macroscopically both tumors are practically indistinguishable. Histologically, the distinction between the two does not present great difficulty in the majority of cases due to the highly characteristic structure of either tumor.

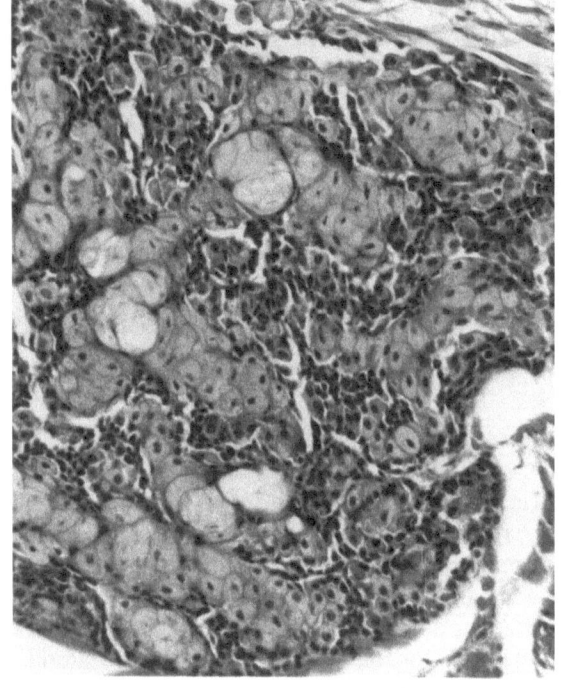

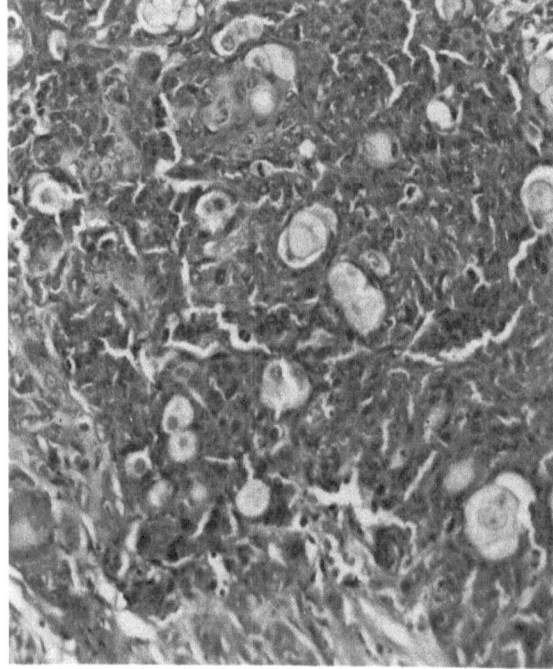

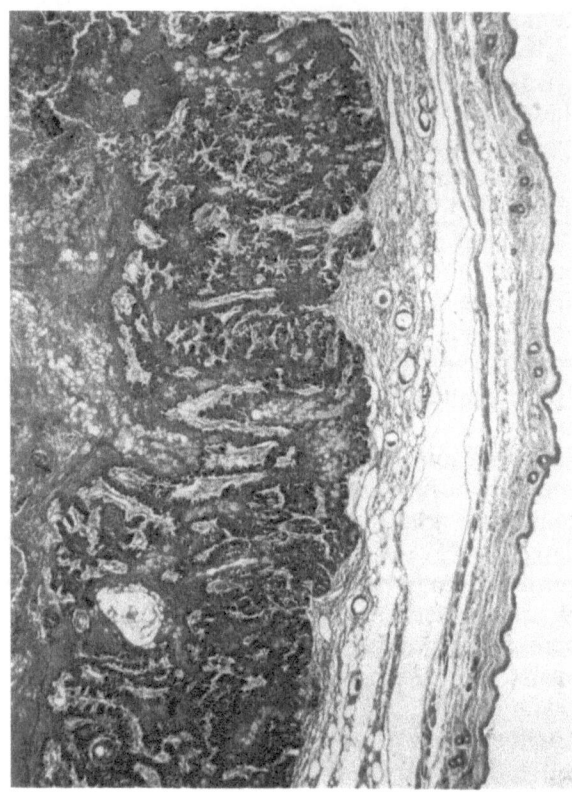

Fig. 155 *(upper left).* Clitoral gland adenoma, solid type. Clusters of sebocytes (acinar cells) intermingled with rather numerous, dark, basal cells. H and E, ×220

Fig. 156 *(lower left).* Carcinoma of the clitoral gland with infiltrative growth into the capsule. H and E, ×220

Fig. 157 *(upper right).* Clitoral gland adenocarcinoma. Central part of the tumor is necrotic with calcium deposits *(upper left).* In the tumor tissue, narrow spaces (pseudoducts) are seen which open into the central necrotic mass. H and E, ×35

Even the most poorly differentiated clitoral gland carcinomas do not resemble mouse mammary carcinoma (Squartini 1979). In some strains of mice (for example, BALB/c) adenoacanthomas of the mammary gland occur which consist of both squamous cell and glandular parts, which may be confused with clitoral gland tumors of the same type. Although the squamous cell part in both tumors is similar, the glandular component in mammary gland adenoacanthoma differs by consisting of specific acinar structures lined by simple columnar epithelium; the clitoral tumor glands are made up of solid nests of sebaceous cells.

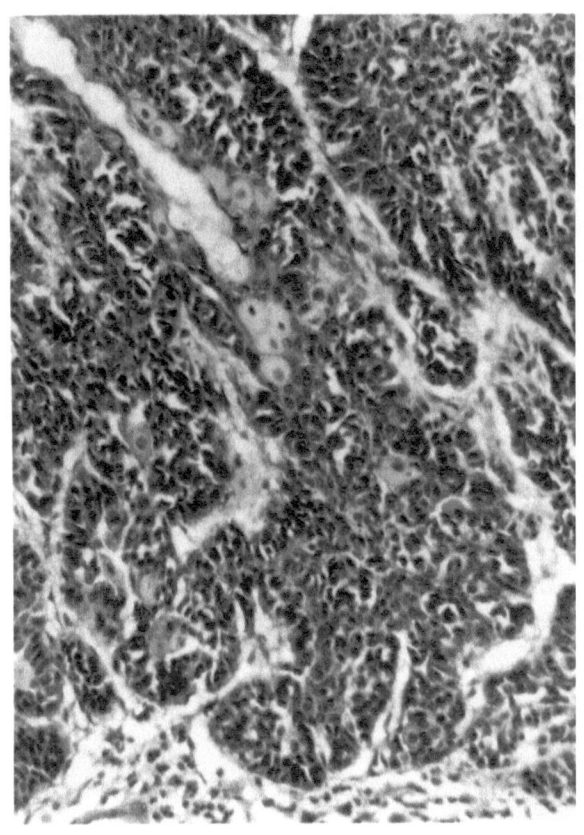

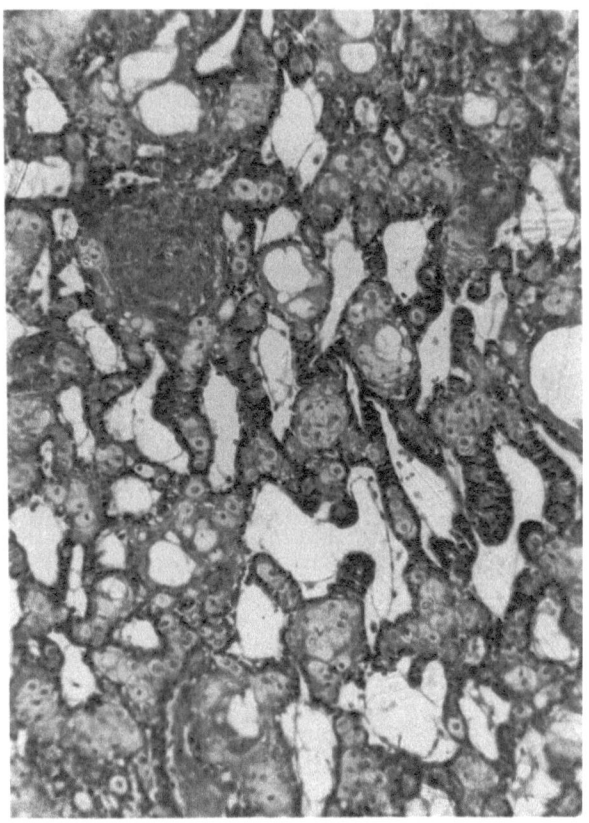

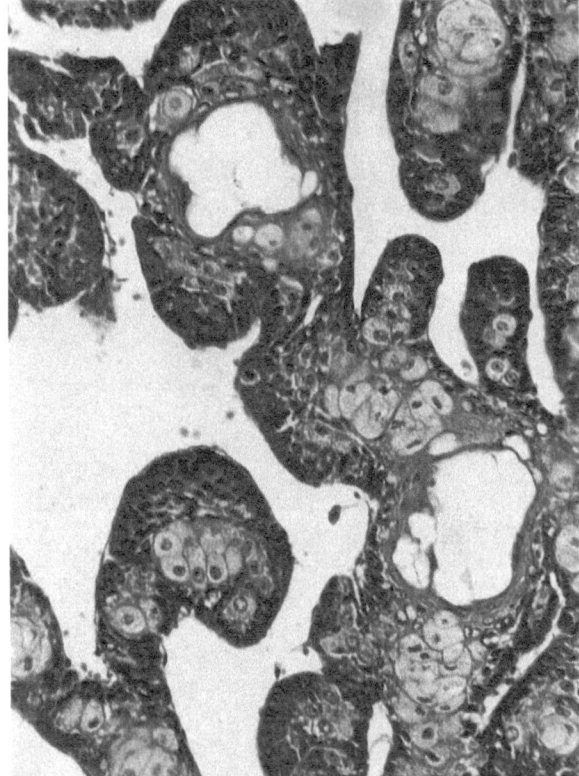

Fig. 158 *(upper left)*. Higher magnification of Fig. 157. Lobulated structure with the lumens into which dying acinar cells are released. H and E, × 220

Fig. 159 *(upper right)*. Adenoma with a cystic trabecular pattern. H and E, × 140

Fig. 160 *(lower right)*. Higher magnification of Fig. 159. Every trabecula represents a caricaturized normal acinus: sebocytes in the central part, basal cells at the periphery, and fibroblasts lining the spaces between trabeculae. Two cysts are formed within trabeculae. H and E, × 220

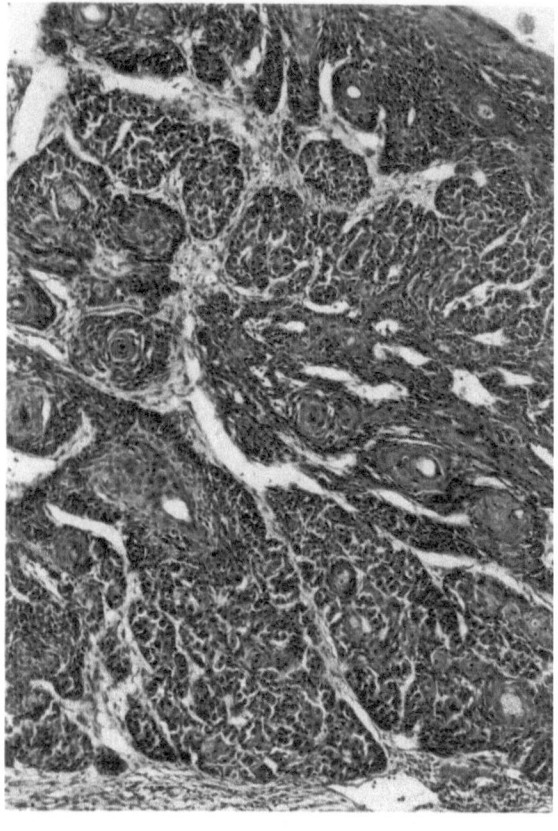

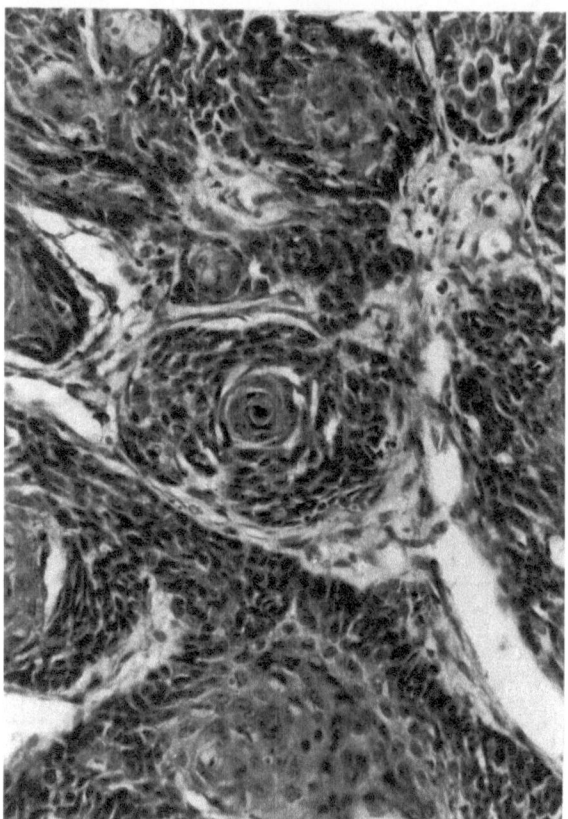

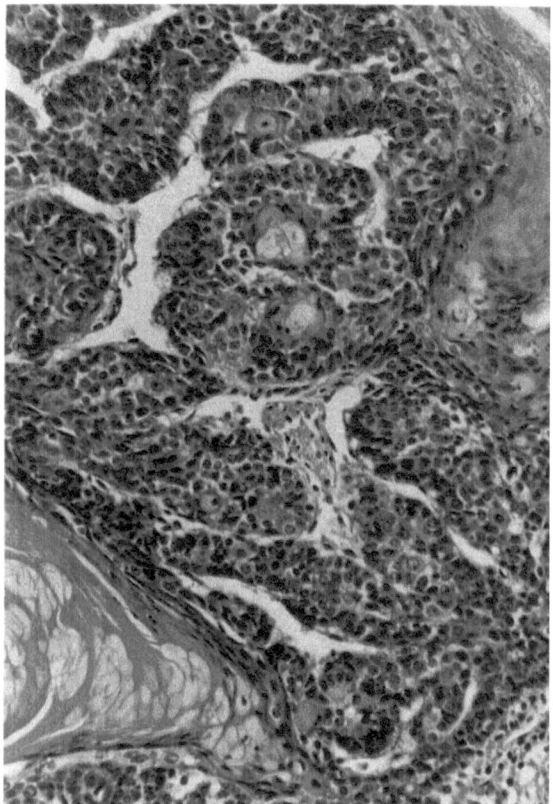

Fig. 161 *(upper left).* Malignant adenoacanthoma (mixed cell carcinoma). H and E, ×90

Fig. 162 *(lower left).* Higher magnification of Fig. 161. Predominantly adenocarcinomatous area. H and E, ×220

Fig. 163 *(upper right).* Same area as Fig. 161. Predominantly squamous differentiation although small groups of sebocytes (acinar cells) are also seen. H and E, ×220

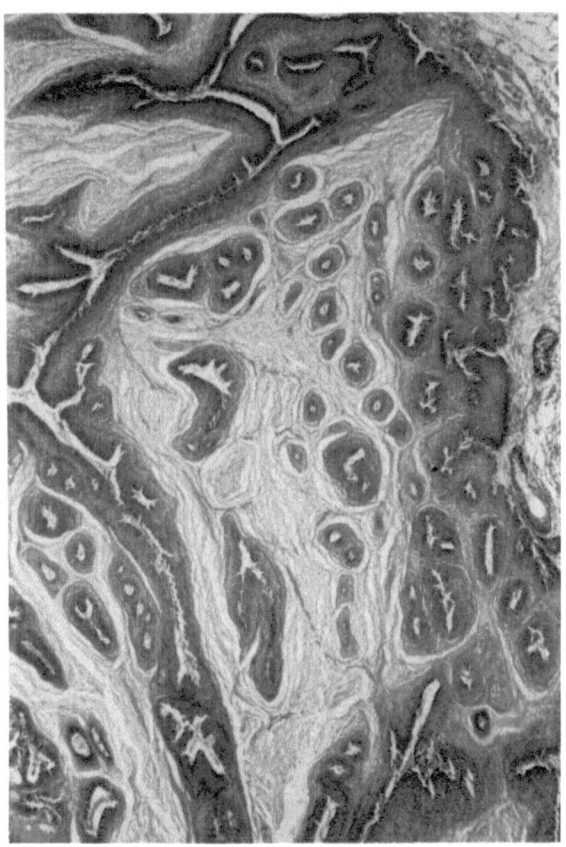

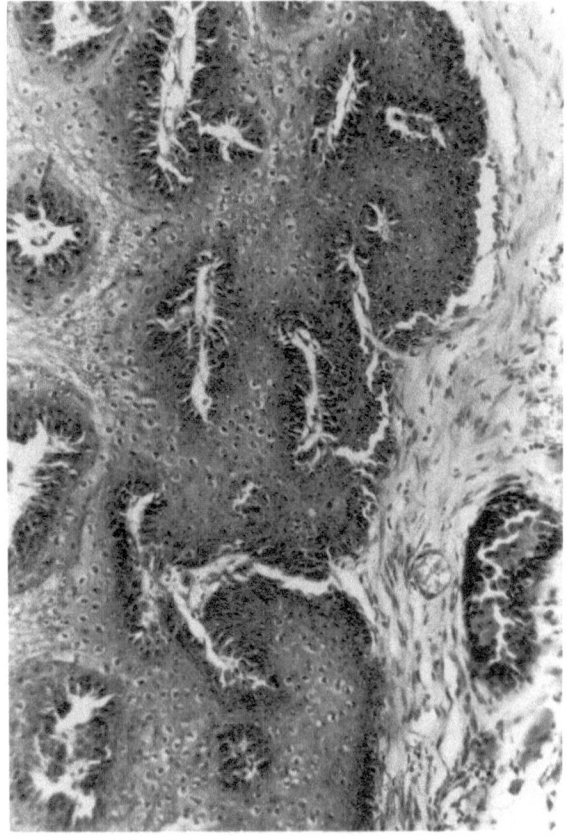

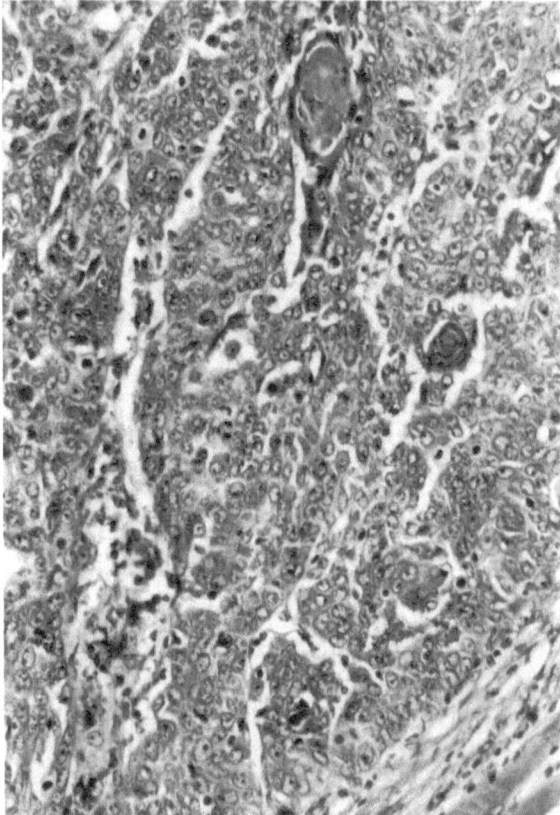

Fig. 164 *(upper left).* Squamous cell carcinoma, clitoral gland, mouse, with signs of invasion into the surrounding tissue. H and E, × 35

Fig. 165 *(upper right).* Higher magnification of Fig. 164. H and E, × 140

Fig. 166 *(lower right).* Anaplastic carcinoma, clitoral gland, mouse, with a high rate of mitoses and squamous cell nests. H and E, × 220

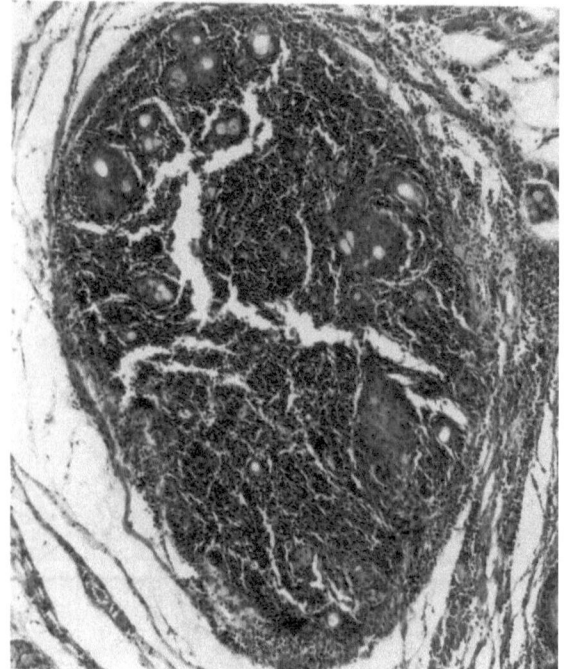

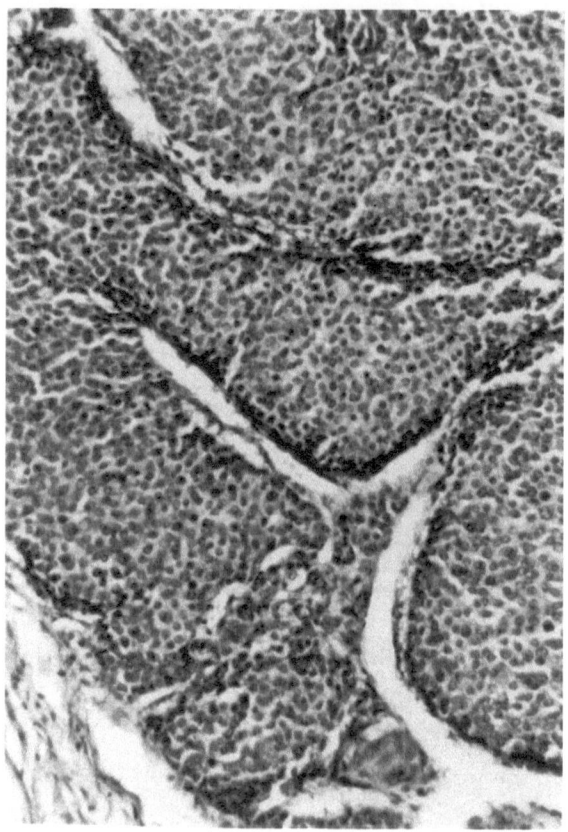

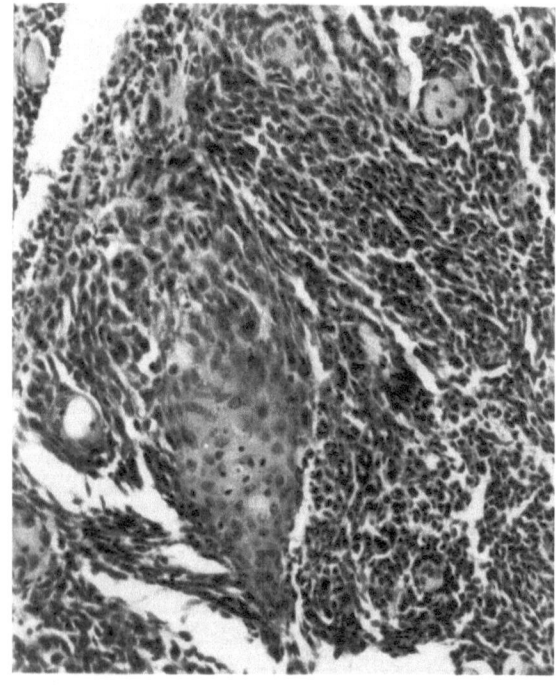

Fig. 167 *(upper left)*. Tumor occupying whole clitoral gland, mouse. H and E, × 90

Fig. 168 *(lower left)*. Detail of Fig. 167. Tumor is formed mainly of basal cells with some sebaceous and squamous cell differentiation. H and E, × 220

Fig. 169 *(upper right)*. Tumor, clitoral gland, mouse, formed of cells of basal type. In other parts of this tumor, differentiation into sebaceous and squamous cells was evident. H and E, × 220

Biologic Features

Some tumors of the clitoral gland grow very rapidly and reach 1–2 cm within 2–3 weeks; other grow very slowly and attain the same size within 2–3 months. Even large tumors may retain benign morphological properties and are surrounded by a fibrous capsule. In rare cases, the content of an ulcerated tumor is released, and the tumor shrinks, but complete regression does not occur. The malignant nature of many tumors is evident by structural and cellular anaplasia, numerous mitoses, and invasion of surrounding tissue. Metastasis, however, was observed in one case only, and it retained a structure typical of the primary tumor (Fig. 170).

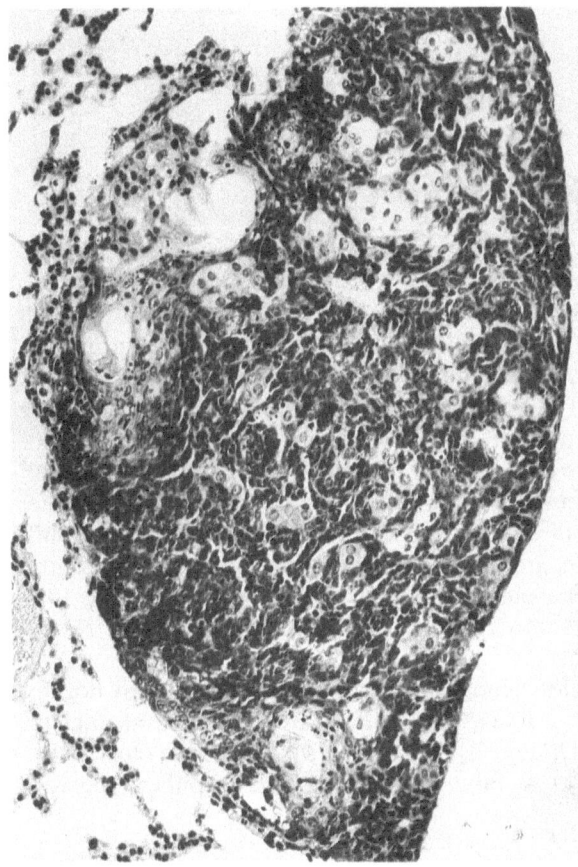

Fig. 170. Clitoral gland, adenocarcinoma, mouse. Metastasis to the lung. Acinar structure, even though distorted, is still preserved: groups of sebocytes surrounded by basal dark cells. H and E, × 220

Etiology and Frequency. DMH seems to be the only carcinogen which can induce these tumors regularly and with a high incidence (up to 50%) in various strains of mice (CBA, C57BL, C3H, C3HA, DBA). In CBA mice, on which most experiments have been carried out, these tumors start to appear approximately 20 weeks after weekly injections of DMH at the dose of 8 mg/ kg body weight regardless of the route of administration – subcutaneous, intraperitoneal, or oral. In C3HA mice estradiol dipropionate administered concurrently with DMH inhibited the induction of clitoral gland tumors, but no such effect was observed in CBA mice (Turusov et al. 1982).

Ten per cent of random bred Swiss mice treated with *N*-n-butyl-*N*-formylhydrazine developed clitoral gland tumors, and 12% of those treated with acetaldehyde methylformylhydrazone had similar tumors. These tumors were described as

squamous cell papillomas, keratoacanthomas, and carcinoma (Toth et al. 1980, 1981).

As far as I know, no spontaneous tumors of the mouse clitoral gland have been reported.

Comparison with Other Species

A number of clitoral gland tumors – spontaneous and carcinogen-induced – have been reported in the F344 rat. Spontaneous incidence ranged from 4% to 16% while the range in carcinogen-treated rats was between 0% and 28%. Four substances (5-nitroacenaphthene; 2.4-diaminoanisole sulfate; 5-nitro-*o*-anisidine; and 1.5-naphthalenediamine) were carcinogenic for the preputial or clitoral gland. Histologically, the rat clitoral gland tumors are very similar to the mouse tumors and were subdivided into adenomas, adenocarcinomas, and squamous cell tumors originating from duct cells. Among clitoral gland adenocarcinomas, mixed cell type was distinguished consisting of both squamous cells and acinar cells (Reznik and Ward 1981).

As far as I know, no clitoral gland tumors have been reported in other than mouse and rat species. The presumed human counterpart of clitoral gland tumors is reported by Reznik and Ward (1981).

References

Hummel KP, Richardson FL, Fekete E (1966) Anatomy. In: Green EL (ed) Biology of the laboratory mouse, 2nd edn. McGraw-Hill, New York, pp 247–308
Reznik G, Ward JM (1981) Morphology of neoplastic lesions in the clitoral and preputial gland of the F334 rat. J Cancer Res Clin Oncol 101: 249–263
Squartini F (1979) Tumours of the mammary gland. In: Turusov VS (ed) Pathology of tumours in laboratory animals, vol 2. Tumours of the mouse. IARC, Lyon, pp 43–90 (IARC Sci Publ no 23)
Toth B, Nagel D, Patil K (1980) Tumorigenic action of N-n-butyl-N-formylhydrazine in mice. Carcinogenesis 1: 589–593
Toth B, Smith JW, Patil KD (1981) Cancer induction in mice with acetaldehyde methylformylhydrazone of the false morel mushroom. JNCI 67: 881–887
Turusov VS (1980) Morphology and histogenesis of anal region and clitoral gland tumours induced in mice by 1,2-dimethylhydrazine. JNCI 64: 1161–1167
Turusov VS, Lanko NS, Krutovskikh VA, Parfenov YD (1982) Strain differences in susceptibility of female mice to 1,2-dimethylhydrazine. Carcinogenesis 3: 603–608

Hibernoma, Rat

Gerald L. Coleman

Synonyms. Hypernoma; brown fat tumor; brown fat lipoma.

Gross Appearance

Hibernomas are tan to dark brown with areas of gray to yellow where necrotic. The neoplasm is lobulated, giving a bosselated appearance to the surface (Fig. 171). In the rat the neoplasm may reach 40 mm in each dimension. The cut surface (Fig. 172) varies in color (as does the outside surface), may have areas of hemorrhage, and is somewhat greasy in texture. The neoplasm will float in formalin fixative similar to a lipoma. Lipid from the tumor may be seen on the surface of the fixative.

Microscopic Features

A relatively thick connective tissue capsule gives rise to thinner septae which enclose grapelike clusters of lipid-laden cells. The predominate cell type is a round to polygonal cell 15–20 μm in diameter containing medium-sized, round nuclei. The cytoplasm contains small to large, single or multiple, round vacuoles which occupy most of the cytoplasm. The remaining cytoplasm is a dull pink to faint brown color with eosin counter stain. A second cell type contains an eosinophilic, granular cytoplasm with a central or eccentric nucleus. It is similar in size to the first (Fig. 173). A third, usually less common, cell closely resembles the normal lipocyte in that it has a large, single vacuole and scanty cytoplasm, often not appreciable, and a small, oval, peripheral nucleus. These cells are arranged in grapelike clusters upon a faint to indiscernible capillary network

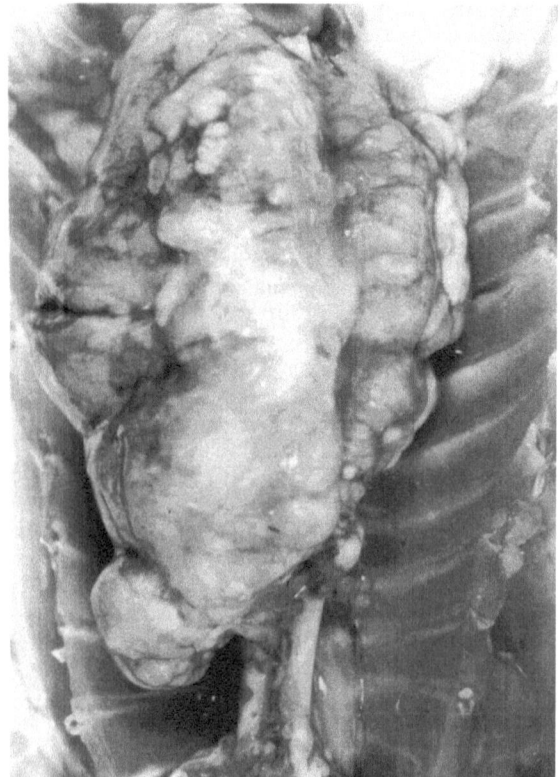

Fig. 171. Intrathoracic hibernoma, rat, in situ

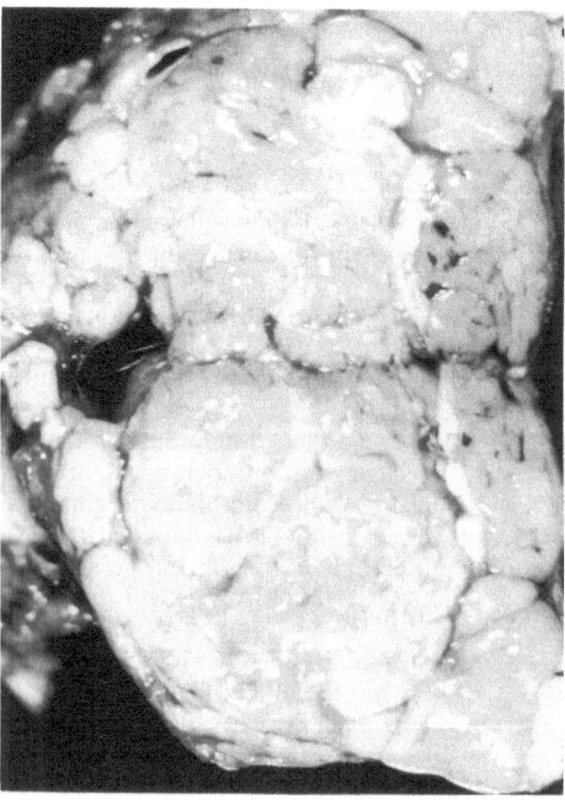

Fig. 172. Cut surface of hibernoma, rat

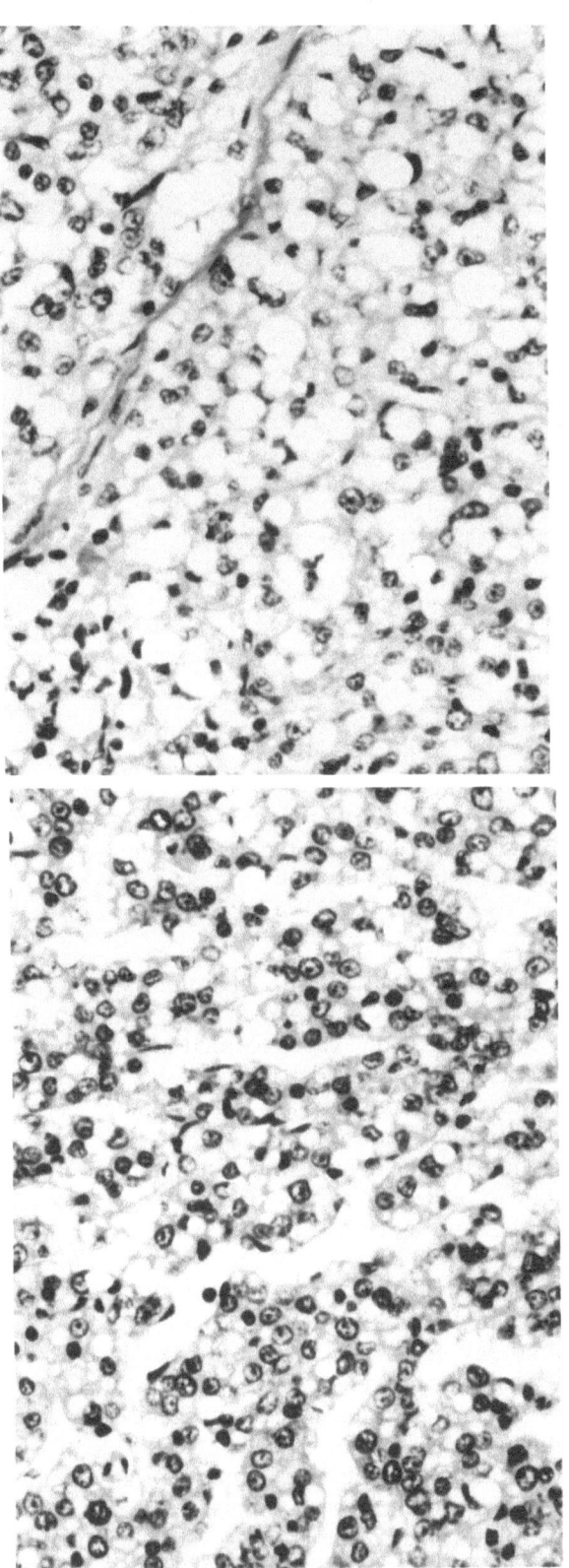

(Fig.174). The clusters are separated by thin connective tissue septae sometimes containing macrophages laden with brown granular material, some of which is PAS-positive. Thicker septae enclose several clusters of cells to give the lobulated appearance seen grossly. The free surfaces of the neoplasm are enclosed in a somewhat thicker connective tissue capsule covered by pleura or peritoneum in the thoracic or abdominal locations. Cells containing lipochrome pigment granules may be found within the clusters of brown fat cells as well as within the septae, giving rise to the brown color seen grossly (Sutherland et al. 1952). Areas of necrosis with little associated inflammation are common features of these neoplasms.

Ultrastructure

Levine (1972) and Gaffney et al. (1983) have described the neoplasm in humans, and Al Zubaidy and Finn (1983) have reported the neoplasm in the rat. The cells have distinct basal laminae enclosing fat vacuoles of variable size. Mitochondria are pleomorphic and vary in number inversely with the size of the fat vacuoles. Smooth endoplasmic reticulum is abundant, but rough endoplasmic reticulum glycogen, and lysosomes are scanty. Plasmalemmal invaginations or pinocytotic vesicles are frequently found, as are lipofuscin granules.

The description by Port et al. (1979) differs in that they failed to see lipofuscin granules and the cells had poorly developed or no basal lamina.

Differential Diagnosis

Although rare in occurrence, the diagnosis of hibernoma is not difficult. The location of a tan to brown, greasy mass in the thoracic or abdominal cavities or in the interscapular subcutis should be the first clue. Microscopically, there are similarities to adrenocortical carcinoma, but the presence of numerous septae, lipofuscin granules, and large fat vacuoles along with the gross color and location should be sufficient to preclude this error. Gross color and septate pattern with abundant capillary network serves to exclude lipoma. Some atypical lipomas could be mistaken for hibernoma (Port et al. 1979; Shuman 1971). However, the gross color and location as well as the microscopic features should allow differentiation. Although the total numbers

Fig. 173 *(above)*. Hibernoma, rat. Note area of necrosis, thin septum, and vacuolated cells. H and E, ×220

Fig. 174 *(below)*. Hibernoma, rat. Note capillary network, vacuolated cells, and a few granular cells. H and E, ×220

reported in rats are small, all but one of the rats (Port et al. 1979) was 66 weeks of age or older. Port et al. (1979) described the gross and light microscopic appearance of an atypical liposarcoma in a 21-week-old rat and then based the diagnosis of hibernoma on electron microscopic features which were lacking in two respects, i. e., few lysosomes and scanty basal laminae. In light of the more extensive data now at hand, it is likely that this first diagnosis of liposarcoma was the correct one.

Biologic Features

Brown fat differs from other fatty tissue in that it has a lower lipid content and a higher lipochrome content, and its somewhat smaller cells contain small, multiple, fat vacuoles (Brines and Johnson 1949) and a higher phospholipid and glycogen content (Novy and Wilson 1956). Brown fat is found in the "hibernating gland" of animals such as woodchucks and in the interscapular gland and ventral vertebral fat body (Fig. 175) of rodents (Brines and Johnson 1949). Neoplasms of brown fat have these same features and an abundant capillary network (Angervall et al. 1964).

Little is know about the biological features of these neoplasms in rodents due to their rarity. The neoplasms arise from the brown fat of the interscapular area or ventral to the thoracic vertebrae. In rats, most have occurred in the latter site. With the exception of that described by Port et al. (1979), all of those reported have been in older rats (Table 8) and have either been found incidentally or after death induced by the tumor. Signs of illness reported are weakness or paralysis of the hind limbs, dyspnea, generalized weakness, and piloerection; these signs may be present for as long as 46 weeks. From this one may infer that at least some hibernomas are slow-growing. The cause of these neoplasms is unknown, and no reports exist of their experimental induction.

Comparison with Other Species

Other than the rat, nearly all descriptions of hibernoma are of the neoplasm in humans. Valerio et al. (1968) mentioned the diagnosis of two hibernomas in the rhesus monkey, but no other information was provided. Ochoa (1972) reported on a case in the omentum of 9-month-old, male Labrador dog. This small (20 mm) neoplasm was

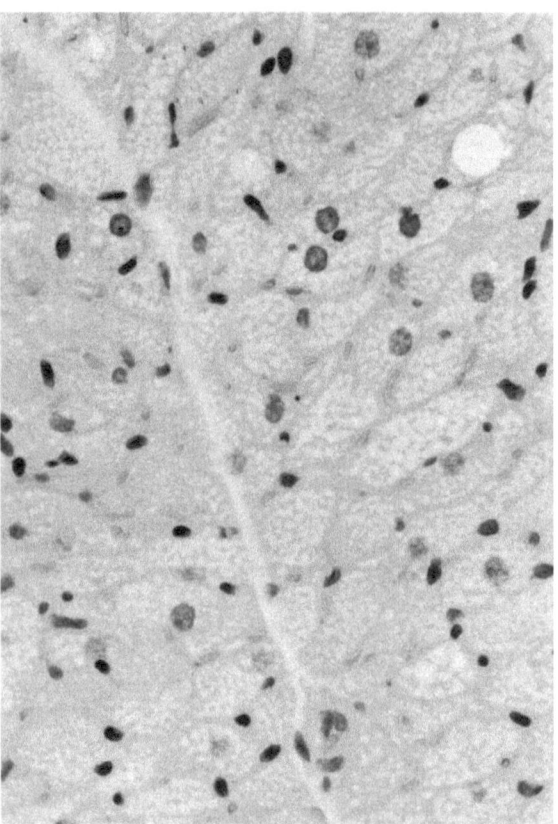

Fig. 175. Normal brown fat in the dorsal thoracic cavity of young rat. H and E, × 220

found incidentally during laparotomy for an undescended testis. The Armed Forces Institute of Pathology has one case recorded in the dog (accession #1037518, Pletcher, personal communication, 1987) and the case in the Fischer 344 rat cited in this manuscript.

In humans, the neoplasm has been located in the joint capsule (Sieber and Heller 1952), scapula, axilla, and back (Brines and Johnson 1949), shoulder and back (Novy and Wilson 1956), thoracic cavity (Kittle et al. 1950), mesentery (Kovalev and Popova 1964), and chest wall or thigh (Gaffney et al. 1983). In most cases in humans the neoplasms were diagnosed from either biopsy or surgical specimens. With few exceptions they were considered to be benign. While the reports of the neoplasm in humans are much more numerous than those in animals, it is still a rare neoplasm; many of the papers describe only one or two cases.

Table 8. Cases of hibernoma in rats

Strain	Anatomical location	Age at discovery	Number examined	Benign	Clinical signs	Reference
SD	Post mediast	94 wk	1000	Yes	Yes	Al Zubaidy and Finn 1983
Wistar	Post mediast	92 wk	800	Yes	Yes	Al Zubaidy and Finn 1983
Wistar	Interscapular	119 wk	800	Yes	Yes	Al Zubaidy and Finn 1983
SD	Post mediast	66 wk	9036	Yes	Yes	Coleman 1980
SD	Post mediast	79 wk	9036	Yes	Yes	Coleman 1980
SD	Post mediast	92 wk	9036	No	Yes	Coleman 1980
SD	Post mediast	117 wk	9036	Yes	No	Coleman 1980
Fischer	Post mediast	63 wk	115000	No	Yes	Stefanski et al. 1987
Fischer	NA	NA	115000	NA	NA	Stefanski et al. 1987
Fischer	NA	NA	115000	NA	NA	Stefanski et al. 1987
NA	NA	NA	NA	NA	NA	Carter 1973
SD	Dorsal subcutaneous	21 wk	NA	NA	NA	Port et al. 1979

SD, Sprague-Dawley; NA, not available or not recorded; Post mediast, posterior mediastinum.

References

Al Zubaidy AJ, Finn JP (1983) Brown fat tumours (hibernomas) in rats: histopathological and ultrastructural study. Lab Anim 17: 13–17

Angervall L, Nilsson L, Stener B (1964) Microangiographic and histological studies in two cases of hibernoma. Cancer 17: 685–692

Brines OA, Johnson MH (1949) Hibernoma, a special fatty tumor. Report of a case. Am J Pathol 25: 467–497

Carter RL (1973) Tumours of the soft tissues. In: Turusov VS (ed) Pathology of tumours in laboratory animals, vol I. Tumours of the rat, pc 1. (IARC Sci Publ no 5) IARC, Lyon, pp 151–168.

Coleman GL (1980) Four intrathroracic hibernomas in rats. Vet Pathol 17: 634–637

Gaffney EF, Hargreaves HK, Semple E (1983) Hibernoma: distinctive light and electron microscopic features and relationship to brown adipose tissue. Hum Pathol 14: 677–687

Kittle CF, Boley JO, Schafer PW (1950) Resection of an intrathoracic "hibernoma". J Thorac Cardivasc Surg 19: 830–836

Kovalev MM, Popova TI (1964) Malignant hybernoma of the mesentery. Arkh Patol 26: 51–53 (in Russian)

Levine GL (1972) Hibernoma: an electron microscopic study. Hum Pathol 3: 351–359

Novy FG Jr, Wilson WJ (1956) Hibernomas, brown fat tumors. Arch Dermatol 73: 149–157

Ochoa R (1972) Hibernoma in a dog. Report of a case. Cornell Vet 62: 130–144

Port CD, Nunez C, Battifora H (1979) An unusual neoplasm of adipose tissue in a rat. Lab Anim Sci 29: 214–217

Shuman R (1971) Mesenchymal tumors of soft tissues. In: Anderson WAD (ed) Pathology, vol I, 6th edn. Mosby, St Louis, pp 562–568

Sieber WK, Heller EL (1952) Hibernoma. Unusual location in popliteal space. Am J Clin Pathol 22: 977–980

Stefanski SA, Elwell MR, Yoshitomi K (1987) Malignant hibernoma in a Fischer 344 rat. Lab Anim Sci 37: 347–350

Sutherland JC, Callahan WP Jr, Campbell GL (1952) Hibernoma: a tumor of brown fat. Cancer 5: 364–368

Valerio M, Landon JC, Innes JRM (1968) Neoplastic diseases in simians. JNCI 40: 751–756

Epidermal Inclusion Cyst, Skin, Rat

Stephen G. Lake, Laura Hart-Elcock, Robert E. Mueller, and Barry P. Stuart

Synonyms. Keratinaceous cyst; epidermal cyst; pilar cyst; follicular cyst.

Gross Appearance

Epidermal inclusion cysts in rodents are intradermal or subcutaneous nodules, usually less than 0.5 cm in diameter. Grossly, they appear as a raised, smooth, round nodule in the skin. They may be attached to the skin and move with it, or be located under the skin and move independently (Figs. 176 and 177). Upon excision, the nodule may consist of single or multiple cysts containing gray to white desiccated material (Weiss and Frese 1974). At necropsy, an epidermal inclusion cyst can be confused with neoplastic lesions of the skin. In the rat, epidermal inclusion cysts have been reported along the dorsal midline of the back (Burek 1978) and have been observed in the tail and hindleg at our laboratory, but most references fail to state where these cysts are located.

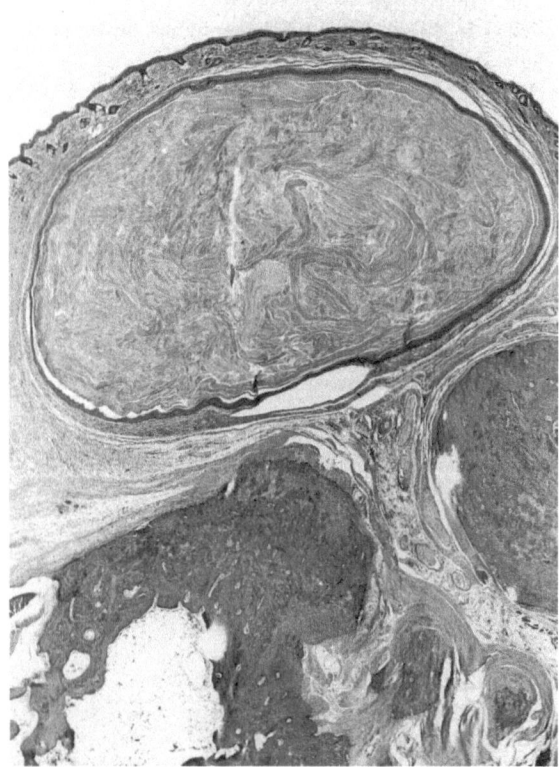

Fig. 176. Epidermal inclusion cyst from the left hindleg of a 22-month-old Fischer 344 rat. H and E, × 20

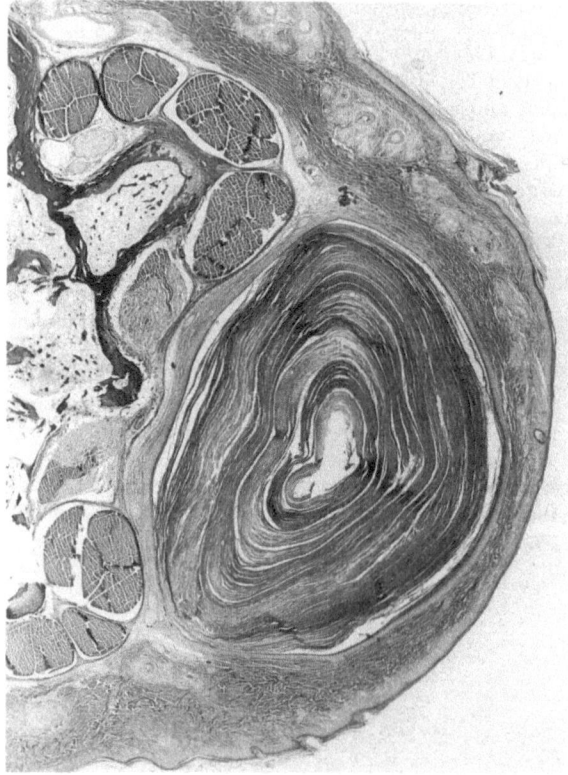

Fig. 177. Epidermal inclusion cyst from the tail of a 24-month-old Fischer 344 rat. H and E, × 15

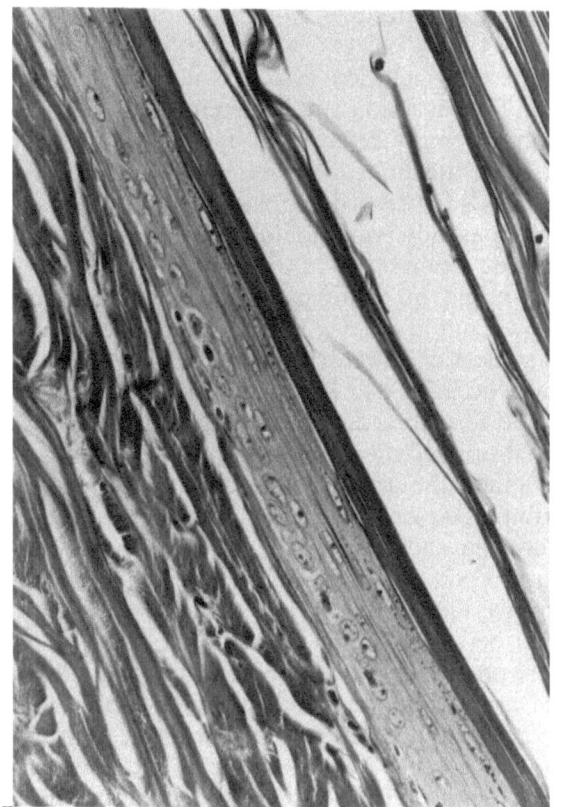

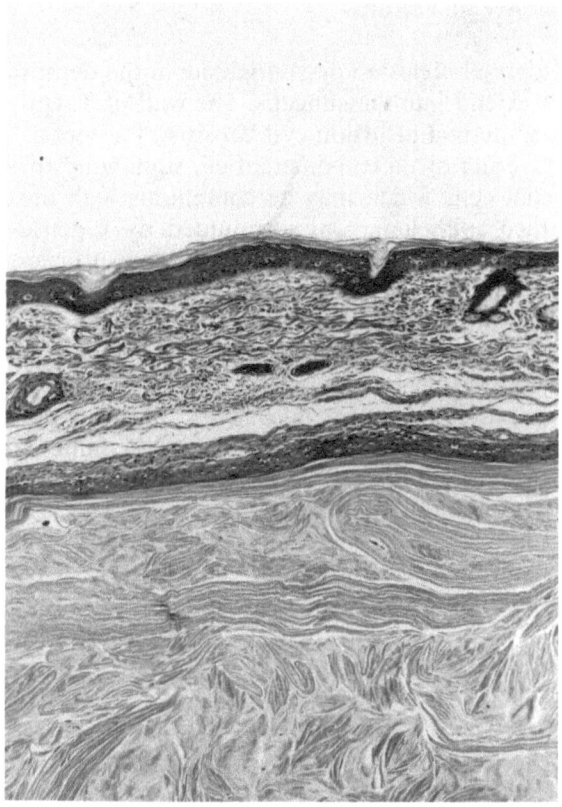

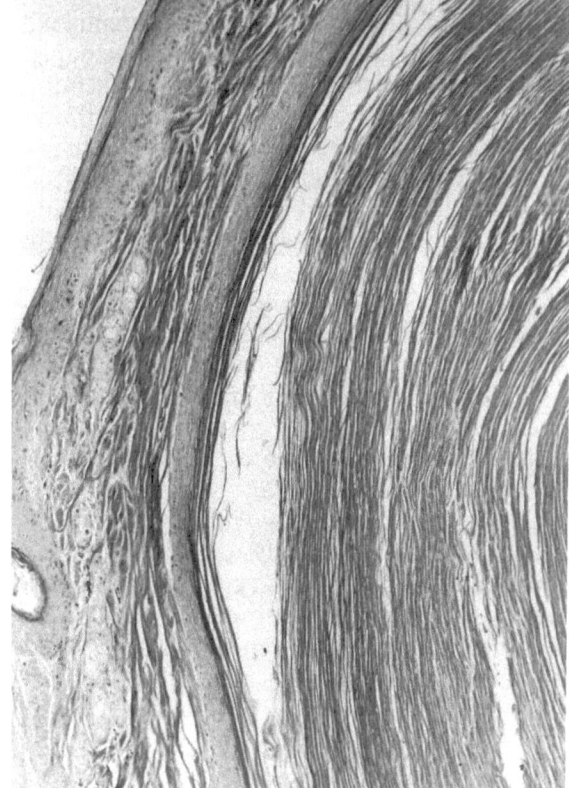

Fig. 178 *(upper left)*. Wall of epidermal inclusion cyst. Note flattened, stratified, squamous epithelial cells. H and E, ×340

Fig. 179 *(upper right)*. Epidermal inclusion cyst from the left hindleg of a Fischer 344 rat. Note the irregular layers of keratin. H and E, ×80

Fig. 180 *(lower right)*. Epidermal inclusion cyst from the tail of a Fischer 344 rat. Note the concentric layers of keratin. H and E, ×75

132   Stephen G. Lake, Laura Hart-Elcock, Robert E. Mueller, and Barry P. Stuart

Microscopic Features

Epidermal inclusion cysts originate in the dermis and extend into the subcutis. The wall of a typical epidermal inclusion cyst consists of an orderly layering of flattened, stratified, squamous epithelial cells which may be continuous with the surface epithelium and surrounded by a dense collagenous capsule (Fig. 178). No adnexal structures are present in the cyst wall. Occasionally, more complex cysts occur with thickened, irregularly folded walls of stratified squamous epithelial cells (Holland and Fry 1982).

Concentric and/or irregular layers or accumulations of keratinaceous debris start at the luminal surface and fill the cyst (Figs. 179 and 180). Calcification and inflammation are not normally associated with epidermal inclusion cysts, but if the cyst ruptures, a significant, foreign-body pyogranulomatous reaction can result. Since some cysts originate from an obstructed hair follicle, remnants of hair shafts may also be noted (Holland and Fry 1982).

Differential Diagnosis

Epidermal inclusion cysts must be differentiated from cystic neoplastic dermal lesions, including intracutaneous calcifying epitheliomas (keratoacanthoma), epidermoid cysts (dermoid cyst), trichoepitheliomas, lipomas, and inverted papillomas. Important distinguishing characteristics of epidermal inclusion cysts are the absence of adnexal structures in the wall and the lack of abnormal proliferation of basal cells.

The intracutaneous calcifying epithelioma (keratoacanthoma) is a benign cystic tumor lined by a complex wall of basal cells and keratin production. Epidermoid cysts (dermoid cyst) are developmental defects lined by a complex wall of basal cells with adnexal structures. Trichoepitheliomas, in an attempt at hair shaft formation, consist of nests of basal cells with central keratinization. Lipomas may grossly resemble an inclusion cyst and must be excised or evaluated histologically for identification. Inverted papillomas grow down into the dermis and can form a shallow cavity full of keratin and debris (Burek 1978).

Biologic Features

Epidermal inclusion cyst is a more descriptive term for this lesion and is therefore the preferred term. In most references, epidermal inclusion cysts are mentioned only briefly as a differential diagnosis for dermal neoplasia. Epidermal inclusion cysts, however, should not be considered neoplastic lesions.

The origin of epidermal inclusion cysts is not known, but in the dog and rat some may develop as a result of an obstructed hair follicle (Greaves and Faccini 1984; Jones and Hunt 1983). This would lead to a dilated infundibulum and slow expansion of the cyst due to desquamation of keratin by the stratified squamous epithelim.

Information on the frequency of occurrence of epidermal inclusion cysts in rodents is minimal. Burek (1978) reported epidermal inclusion cysts in three female BN/Bi rats out of 236 examined (1%) between 23 and 34 months of age. These were present in the subcutaneous tissue along the dorsal midline of the back. Goodman et al. (1979) reported epidermal inclusion cysts in 11 male Fischer 344 rats out of 1794 (0.6%) and 3 females out of 1754 (0.2%) in a 2-year oncogenicity study. Coleman et al. (1977) reported epidermal inclusion cysts in male Fischer 344 rats at a rate of 1 out of 37 (2.7%) between 18 and 24 months of age and 4 out of 46 (8.7%) between 24 and 30 months of age, for a total of 5 out of 140 (3.6%) animals up to 33 months of age. Dodd et al. (1987) reported epidermal inclusion cysts in 5 out of 120 (4.1%) control CD Sprague-Dawley rats. No cysts were reported in 120 control females. Port et al. (1987) reported epidermal inclusion cysts in 2 out of 128 (1.6%) control CD1 mice. No cysts were reported in 120 control females.

In our laboratory, epidermal inclusion cysts were reported in 13 out of 150 (8.7%) male and in 2 out of 150 (1.3%) female control Fischer 344 rats. Most of these cysts were located on the tail or hindleg. No epidermal inclusion cysts were reported in 150 male and 150 female control CD1 mice used in our studies.

Hairless, bald, or nude mutant mice and rats are used in some research laboratories. These rodents with genetic skin problems have various types of age-related cyst development (Inazu and Sakaguchi 1984). In any event, the incidence of epidermal inclusion cysts in rodents appears to be low and associated with age.

Comparison with Other Species

Epidermal inclusion cysts have been reported in man (Robbins and Cotran 1979), primates (baboons; Squire et al. 1978), dogs (Jones and Hunt 1983; Muller and Kirk 1976; Squire et al. 1978), cats (Muller and Kirk 1983), sheep (Yager and Scott 1985), mice (Holland and Fry 1982), and rats (Burek 1978; Greaves and Faccini 1984). The incidence is relatively low and generally considered in the differential diagnosis of dermal neoplasia. The basic description of an epidermal inclusion cyst applies across species. Some species (dogs and sheep) may have a higher tendency to cysts when compared with other species (Yager and Scott 1985).

References

Burek JD (1978) Pathology of aging rats. CRC, West Palm Beach, pp 161–162 (Age-associated pathology of skin and subcutaneous tissues)

Coleman GL, Barthold SW, Osbaldiston GW, Foster SJ, Jonas AM (1977) Pathological changes during aging in barrier-reared Fisher 344 male rats. J Gerontol 32: 258–278

Dodd DC, Port CD, Deslex P, Regnier B, Sanders P, Indacochea-Redmond N (1987) Two-year evaluation of misoprostol for carcinogenicity in CD Sprague-Dawley rats. Toxicol Pathol 15: 125–133

Goodman DG, Ward JM, Squire RA, Chu KC, Linhart MS (1979) Neoplastic and non-neoplastic lesions in aging F344 rats. Toxicol Appl Pharmacol 48: 237–240

Greaves P, Faccini JM (1984) Rat histopathology: a glossary for use in toxicity and carcinogenicity studies. Elsevier, Amsterdam, pp 1–3 (Integumentary system)

Holland JM, Fry RJM (1982) Neoplasms of the integumentary system and harderian gland. In: Foster HL, Small JD, Fox JG (eds) The mouse in biomedical research – experimental biology and oncology, vol IV. Academic, New York, pp 516–522

Inazu M, Sakaguchi T (1984) Morphologic characteristics of the skin of bald mutant rats. Lab Anin Sci 34 (6): 584–587

Jones TC, Hunt RD (1983) Veterinary pathology. Lea and Febiger, Philadelpia, pp 1102–1118 (The skin and its appendages)

Muller GH, Kirk RW (1976) Small animal dermatology, 2nd edn. Saunders, Philadelphia, pp 607–610

Muller GH, Kirk RW (1983) Small animal dermatology, 3rd edn. Saunders, Philadelphia, pp 607–610

Port CD, Dodd DC, Deslex P, Regnier B Sanders P, Indacochea-Redmond N (1987) Twenty-one-month evaluation of misoprostol for carcinogenicity in CD1 mice. Toxicol Pathol 15 (2): 134–142

Robbins SL, Cotran RS (1979) Pathologic basis of disease, 2nd edn. Saunders, Philadelphia, p 1422

Squire RA, Goodman DG, Valerio MG, Frederickson T, Strandberg JD, Levitt MH, Lingeman CH, Harshburger JC, Dawe CJ (1978) Tumors – integumentary system. In: Benirschke K, Garner FM, Jones TC (eds) Pathology of laboratory animals, vol II. Springer, Berlin Heidelberg New York, pp 1059–1062

Weiss E, Frese K (1974) Tumors of the skin. In: WHO Bull 50: 79–100

Yager JA, Scott DW (1985) Ectodermal neoplasms. In: Jubb KVF, Kennedy PC, Palmer N (eds) Pathology of domestic animals, vol 1. Academic, New York, pp 506–516

Alopecia, Rat and Mouse

Klaus Militzer and Moritz A. Konerding

Synonyms. Alopecia areata; alopecia circumscripta; psychogenic alopecia; self-inflicted dermatosis; trichotillomania; hair loss; hair pulling; hair barbering; whisker trimming.

Gross Appearance

In rats, sharply defined alopecic foci, either free from hair or covered with bristles, are preferentially seen in the lateral neck region. These areas are often crescent-shaped with the convex border positioned caudally. Other sites of variable shape may be located in the flank medial to the femur and, less frequently, in the scapular region. These changes in the fur coat are usually bilaterally symmetrical.

In mice, focal loss or sheared appearance of hair are most often seen in the muzzle region, around the orbit, and between the eyes and ears. Tactile and fur hairs may be affected either equally or to varied extents (Strozik and Festing 1981). Extensive hairless or sparsely haired regions may be seen along the back, extending from the neck to the sacrum. As in the rat, occasional, sharply defined lesions in the fur are also found on the flanks. The sides of the abdomen are seldom affected (Militzer and Wecker 1986). In contrast to the rat, the position and appearance of alopecia are more varied in the mouse. Mice with complete loss of hair may be seen, with only demarcated regions of the skin possessing longer hairs. Typically, in both species, the skin is initially unaffected, but continued existence of alopecia, secondary inflammation, and ulceration may appear. In animals with a black-pigmented coat, white or only partially pigmented lighter hairs frequently regrow in the periphery of active lesions or replace all of the hair in healed regions (Thornburg et al. 1973).

In general, hairless skin of normal appearance in alopecic regions often contains irregularly shaped but distinctly defined dark areas due to melanin pigmentation of the growing hair bulbs. These alterations resemble the normal active hair growth areas in the rat and mouse during anagen (mosaic pattern of the hair cycle). Long-term alopecia with secondary dermatitis leads to severe scar formation in the mouse. Contracted scars may arise in the extremities, leading to immobilization (Csiza and McMartin 1976; Kunstyr et al. 1980; Stowe et al. 1971).

Microscopic Features

Characteristically, there is a wide variability in the findings in the epidermis and corium. Depending on the sampling site chosen, unaltered skin regions up to highly ulcerated and inflamed areas can be observed in individual animals.

The epidermis undergoes only slight hyperplasia in the majority of cases. The hyperplasia is manifest by an increase in the number of cell layers from the basal to the granular layer, normally 1–2 to 3–5, in alopecia (trunk region). The degree

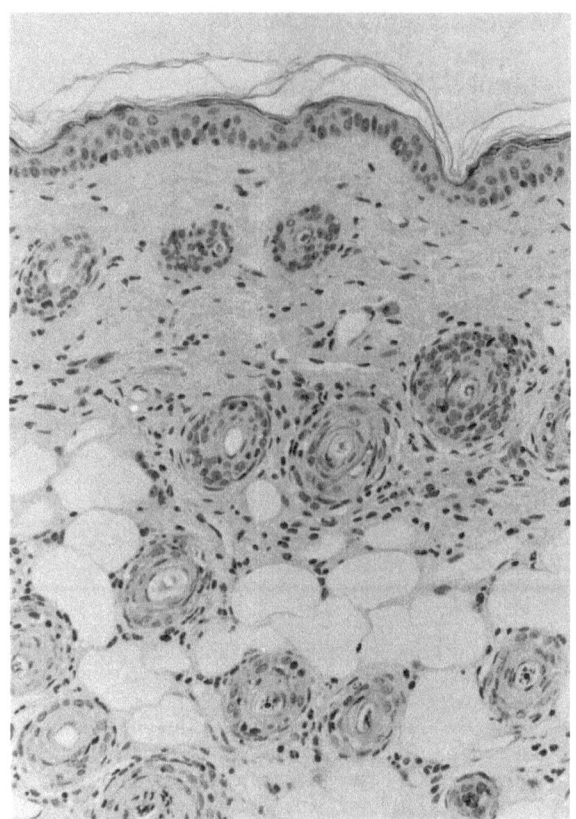

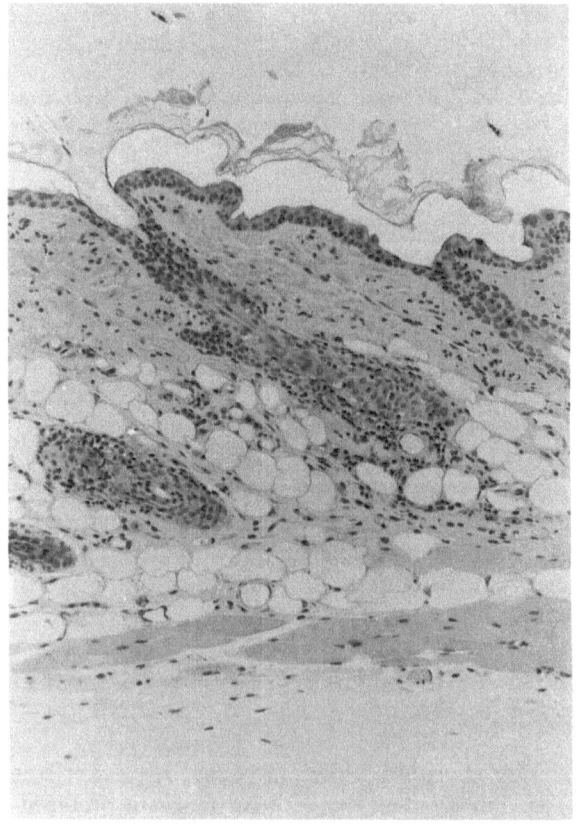

Fig. 181 *(above)*. Alopecia areata, skin from the back, ▶ mouse. Slight epidermal hyperplasia and hyperkeratosis in the periphery of lesions, moderate infiltration by mononuclear cells and leukocytes surrounding the hair bulbs. Active growing hair follicles, cut parallel to the hair rows. Epoxy resin, semithin section. H and E, × 128

Fig. 182 *(below)*. Alopecia areata, mouse. Longitudinal section of resting hair follicles in the center of alopecic lesion. Note the irregular structure of the corneal layer and the unequal distribution of inflammatory cells along the hair bulb. Epoxy resin, semithin section. H and E, × 80

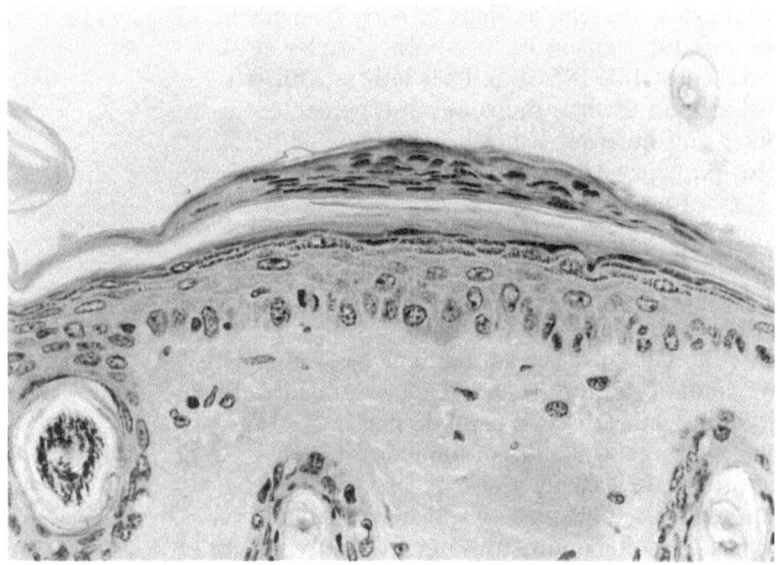

Fig. 183. Alopecia areata, skin from shoulder region, mouse. Hyperkeratosis, parakeratosis, and scar formation in an epidermal area with allogrooming-induced erosion. Note the low degree of intercellular edema (spongiosis). Epoxy resin, semithin section. H and E, × 320

of keratinization in the surface cell layers is also increased (Fig. 181). In some cases, the extent of lamination in the corneal layer increases and the scales have an irregular appearance.

Individual hairs in the follicles are indicative, with unclearly defined ends with a broken appearance, varying shaft diameters, and irregular growth (cyst formation, cork-borer, and tangled formations). In these regions, foreign body type granulomas have also been described (Thornburg et al. 1973). Similar changes have also been observed in the skin with inflammatory lesions of different etiology. At the center of the alopecic sites, the number of hair follicles is markedly reduced (Fig. 182).

Telogenic and atrophic hair follicles predominate. At the periphery of the lesions, however, the follicles are frequently found in anagen (Fig. 181). Apparently, new hair growth cycles are induced peripherally due to the inflammatory processes in the center.

Epidermal sites with enhanced hyperplasia, in particular around erosions and ulcerations, undergo parakeratosis and scar formation (Fig. 183). Based on histological sections, the number of hairs cut in cross section in the alopecic regions is decreased. This criterion for a semiquantitative assessment of hair deficiency is suitable for sections made parallel to the hair rows.

Mononuclear cells, in particular lymphocytes and monocytes as well as polymorphonuclear

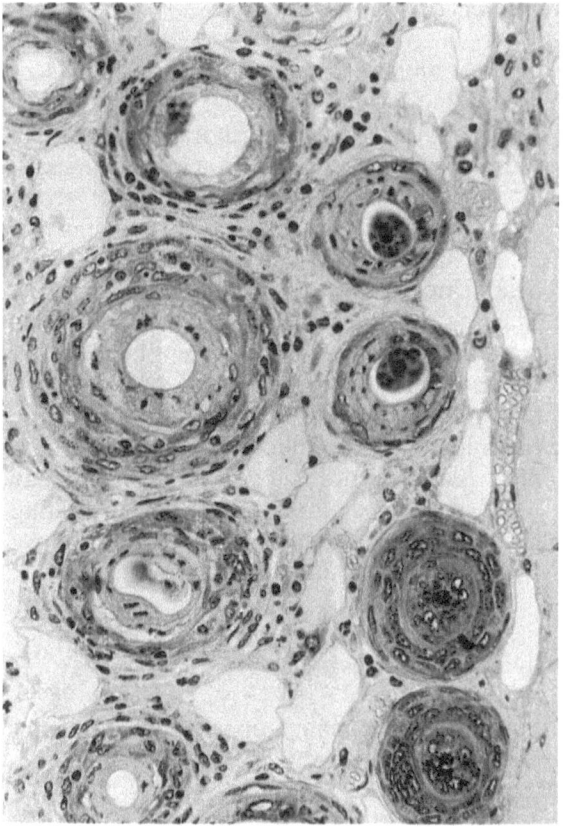

Fig. 184. Alopecia areata, same mouse as shown in Fig. 183. Infiltrates in the middle of the bulbs. Note the stasis in the small skin vessels. H and H, × 200

leukocytes, are seen as signs of early changes in the inferior segment of hair bulbs (Muller et al. 1983) (Figs. 181, 182, 184). They infiltrate the dermis around the hair bulbs but also penetrate the outer and inner root sheath of the hair follicles. The papillary layer and skin muscle are only rarely affected in the early stages. Stasis in the small skin vessels (Fig. 184), particularly those distal to the skin muscle, is apparent in the corium.

Inflammatory changes in all skin layers come to the fore with increasing continuance of alopecia, and leukocytic infiltrates then predominate. In addition, microabscesses and dermal necrosis are observed independently of the hair follicles. Later, proliferative changes also occur in the connective tissue, and lymphocytes, histiocytes, and fibroblasts are more numerous in chronically affected animals. A deep, moist dermatitis with scar formation in the corium then prevails (Kunstyr et al. 1980; Stowe et al. 1971).

Ultrastructure

In cases of alopecia, scanning electron microscopy is suitable for demonstrating the skin surface (Fig. 185). This appears more scaly and with a less uniform contour than in normal animals. The majority of hair bundles, consisting of strong terminal and fine intermediate hairs which pierce the skin, have broken and split ends above the follicle orifice. The short stumps of hair have irregular, jagged scales of the hair cortex. The fine intermediate hairs within a hair bundle are either often completely broken, or only single hairs exist (Fig. 186). The hair medulla is not uniformly opened, in contrast to the shaved, unaltered hair. Longer hairs extending over the surface may have an irregular diameter (Fig. 185). Infiltrating cells are attracted externally to the bulb above the "critical" level (Auber's line).

Differential Diagnosis

Primary or psychogenic alopecia is to be distinguished from other forms of hair loss, which occur as signs of existing basic disease. However, only very few details of the alopecic rodent skin are specific enough to permit this distinction. The clearly defined shape of alopecia areata, the typical predilection sites in the rat or mouse, and the lack of relationship to the regional hair cycle pattern are indicative of primary alopecia. Meta-

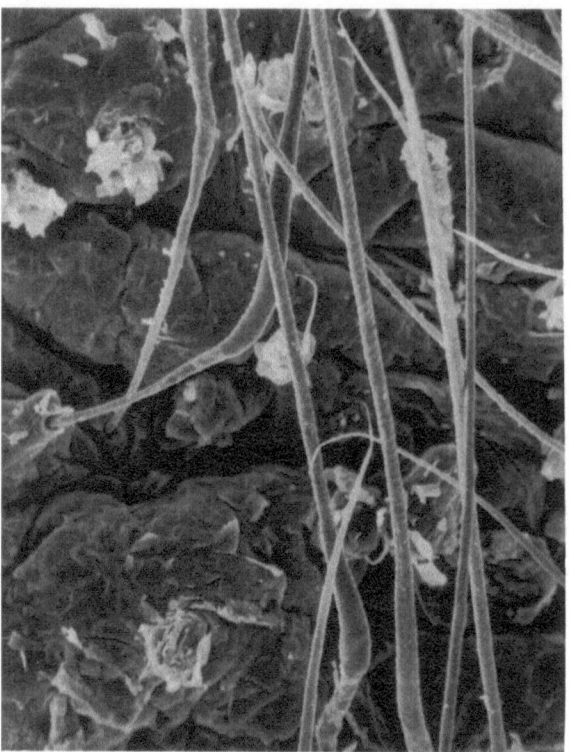

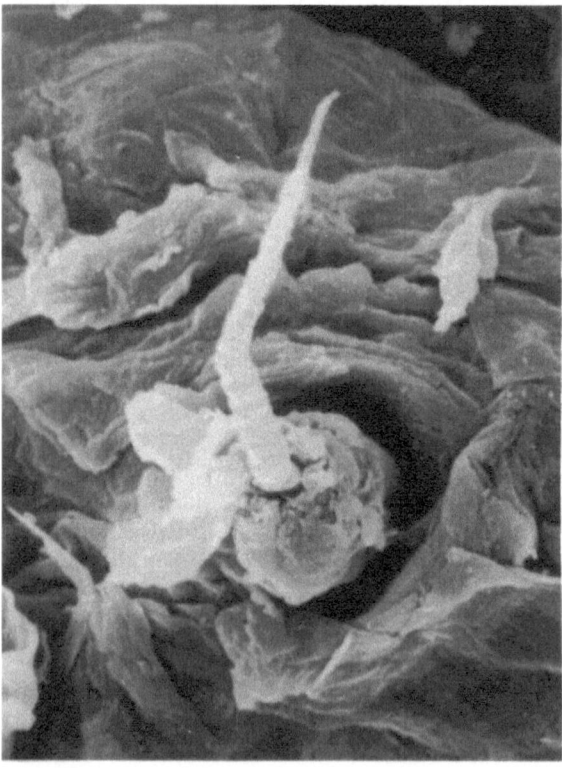

Fig. 185 *(above)*. Alopecia areata, mouse, same situation as in Fig. 181. Hair bundles with split ends above the orifice, few hairs with irregular diameters. SEM, × 260

Fig. 186 *(below)*. Center of an alopecic area, mouse. Hair bundle with only one, single, intermediate hair; others have been gnawed off. SEM, × 900

bolic disturbances and other factors such as ecto-parasites or mycoses must be ruled out. The split hair ends observed under the scanning electron microscope must be considered typical of this self-inflicted dermatosis. If the external stimuli affecting the animals's behavior are eliminated, e. g., through isolation of individual animals, primary alopecic lesions will heal without any kind of therapy. Hair regrowth will take at least 60 days in young mice (Strozik and Festing 1981).

For safety evaluation of drugs and chemicals the diagnosis primary or secondary alopecia needs to be made particularly carefully. After all, a spontaneous psychogenic alopecia can imitate a specific dermotoxic chemical effect. To what extent the described alopecic defects on the rat skin are indeed exclusively due to feeding of rapeseed oil (Hulan et al. 1976) and exposure to phenyl glycidyl ether (Lee et al. 1977) remains unclear in the published reports. However, pharmaceuticals can also cause alopecic lesions by activating a stereotype behavior (excessive grooming after doses of dopamine agonists or codeinone (Hartgraves and Randall 1986; Isaacson et al. 1987). However, this does not indicate a direct dermatologic activity of the test substances.

Biologic Features

Almost without exception, hair loss in rats and mice has been described by the term "alopecia." In humans, alopecia means a partial or total loss of hair. This is primarily noninflammatory and temporary. In small animals one generally refers to alopecia when hair is missing at those sites normally found to contain some (Muller et al. 1983). As a rule, alopecia arises secondarily in connection with other unequivocally diagnosable basic diseases. In the rat and mouse, these include infections due to viruses, bacteria, and fungi (Stowe et al. 1971), infestation with ectoparasites (Csiza and McMartin 1976; Weisbroth et al. 1976), and resorption of toxic substances (Hulan et al. 1976; Lee et al. 1977). Furthermore, genetic and immunologic (Thornburg et al. 1973; Furukawa et al. 1984) as well as endocrinologic factors responsible for the occurrence of alopecia in laboratory rodents have been discussed. Whereas mast cell proliferation does not influence the initiation, it does affect the regrowth of alopecia areata in mice (Tanii et al. 1985). In all such cases the diagnosis of the appropriate basic disease must take priority.

Often, however, the cause of disease cannot be identified. Rather, certain animal behavioral patterns must be considered as the cause of hair loss. These types are thus described as primary alopecia, sometimes also as psychogenic alopecia (Muller et al. 1983). In small laboratory rodents, these include hair pulling, barbering, or trimming (Strozik and Festing 1981; Bresnahan et al. 1983), alopecia after muzzle poking through ventilation holes (Litterst 1974), and other forms of behavior-associated alopecia areata (Beare-Rogers and McGowan 1973; Militzer and Wecker 1986). If it can be shown that alopecia arises from a certain type of behavior in the animals, the description "selfinflicted dermatosis" is justified. Compared with humans, it can also be referred to as trichotillomania. The initiation of this alopecia is dependent on a large number of predisposing factors.

Hair loss thus usually occurs at random and applies to specific housing situations, animal grouping, and strains. Thus, the primary alopecia in rats and mice is very difficult to assess by systematic and experimental studies.

Etiology and Frequency. For the majority of investigators, the etiology of alopecia areata in rats and mice is still unclear, although several have suggested hyperactive grooming behavior to be the cause (Long 1972; Beare-Rogers and McGowan 1973; Thornburg et al. 1973; Strozik and Festing 1981; Bresnahan et al. 1983). The above-described primary form of alopecia areata occurs exclusively in rats and mice kept in groups. The fur defects affect typical grooming regions in both species. Since dominant mice carry out a more intensive allogrooming of lower ranking ones, the distribution of lesions within a cage group is unequal. In addition, subordinate mice increase their self-grooming (Benton and Brain 1979). Therefore, low-ranking C57B1 mice (Long 1972; Reinhardt and Militzer 1979; Strozik and Festing 1981) and Fischer 344 rats (Bresnahan et al. 1983) have been shown to exhibit status-dependent alopecia and whisker loss. The degree of hair loss has even been attributed to sex differences in C57B1 mice. The more severe changes are found in male animals kept in breeding groups together with females (Long 1972). By means of time-lapse cinematography it has been shown that excessive grooming activity of the female mouse was the initiating factor (Militzer and Wecker 1986).

The stimulus for the excessive grooming activity in rats and mice has not yet been exactly determined. Nevertheless, each longer lasting type of anxiety, social tension in the group, stress, disturbances, and noise in animal rooms can considerably increase the grooming activity. Thus, alopecia areata can arise either spontaneously or randomly in susceptible animal collections. The incidence and extent of these skin defects correlated with the length of time the animals are kept in the animal group. In breeding groups, 18% of male C57B1 mice less than 9 months of age had alopecia whereas 93% of males over 1 year had similar lesions (Militzer and Wecker 1986). If initiating stimuli are not eliminated or the animals are not separated, frequently a fatal, deep, and disfiguring dermatitis can arise from bacterial contamination (Kunstyr et al. 1980; Stowe et al. 1971).

The relatively high frequency of alopecia in C57B1 mice may be because lesions are more obvious in this black-haired strain. In principle, when referring to the frequency of alopecia in different strains of rats and mice from the literature, it must be taken into consideration whether the strains predominate in use today or not.

Comparison with Other Species

In humans, the trichotillomania or traumatic alopecia is described as self-inflicted dermatosis. Trichotillomania is defined as a nonscarring alopecia resulting from a compulsion to pluck out one's own hair. In a pediatric psychiatric setting its prevalence is less than 1%; girls and women are more frequently affected than men. Trichotillomania is considered to be a "neurotic" disease, which can be initiated by stressful life situations (Gupta et al. 1987). Trichotillomania is a multidetermined condition. Its psychodynamics have been related primarily to emotional deprivation or frustration of the child's needs (Galski 1983). In the related syndrome in humans, alopecia areata, strong psychogenic factors are implicated (Koblenzer 1983).

In rhesus monkeys, hair pulling from one's own or from a partner's coat has been reported. In 96% of observations, it was performed by a dominant monkey (Reinhardt et al. 1986). The feline psychogenic alopecia has been described as an anxiety neurosis. Hair loss arises by means of hair pulling and breaking; later, severe irritation and excoriation occurs (Muller et al. 1983). Whether the alopecia described in calves and ewes (Pritchard et al. 1983; Morgan et al. 1986) is also behavior associated is presently still unsolved.

References

Beare-Rogers JL, McGowan JE (1973) Alopecia in rats housed in groups. Lab Anim 7: 237–238

Benton D, Brain PF (1979) Behavioural comparisons of isolated, dominant and subordinate mice. Behav Proc 4: 211–219

Bresnahan JF, Kitchell BB, Wildman MF (1983) Facial hair barbering in rats. Lab Anim Sci 33: 290–291

Csiza CK, McMartin DN (1976) Apparent acaridal dermatitis in a C57BL/6 Nya mouse colony. Lab Anim Sci 26: 781–787

Furukawa F, Tanaka H, Sekita K, Nakamura T, Horiguci Y, Hamashima Y (1984) Dermatopathological studies on skin lesions of MRL mice. Arch Dermatol Res 276: 186–194

Galski T (1983) Hair pulling (trichotillomania). Psychoanal Rev 70: 331–346

Gupta MA, Gupta AK, Haberman HF (1987) The self-inflicted dermatoses: a critical review. Gen Hosp Psychiatry 9: 45–52

Hartgraves SL, Randall PK (1986) Dopamine agonist-induced stereotypic grooming and self-mutilation following striatal dopamine depletion. Psychopharmacology (Berlin) 90: 358–363

Hulan HW, Hunsaker WG, Kramer JK, Mahadevan S (1976) The development of dermal lesions and alopecia in male rats fed rapeseed oil. Can J Physiol Pharmacol 54: 1–6

Isaacson RL, Hardy CA, Hannigan JH (1987) Age- and sex-related induction of excessive grooming and "wet-dog" shakes by the codeinone RX 336-M in the rat. Behav Neural Biol 47: 250–261

Koblenzer CS (1983) Psychosomatic concepts in dermatology. A dermatologist and psychoanalyst viewpoint. Arch Dermatol 119: 501–512

Kunstyr I, Heimann W, Matthiesen T, Militzer K (1980) Dermatomykosen bei Versuchstieren unter der besonderen Berücksichtigung von Differential-Diagnose, Prophylaxe und Therapie. Berl Münch Tierärztl Wochenschr 93: 347–350 (Engl. abstr)

Lee KP, Terrill JB, Henry NW III (1977) Alopecia induced by inhalation exposure to phenyl glycidyl ether. J Toxicol Environ Health 3: 859–869

Litterst CL (1974) Mechanically self-induced muzzle alopecia in mice. Lab Anim Sci 24: 806–809

Long SY (1972) Hair-nibbling and whisker-trimming as indicators of social hierarchy in mice. Anim Behav 20: 10–12

Militzer K, Wecker E (1986) Behaviour-associated alopecia areata in mice. Lab Anim 20: 9–13

Morgan KL, Brown PJ, Wright AI, Steele FC, Baker AS (1986) An investigation into the aetiology of "wool slip": alopecia in ewes which are housed and shorn in winter. Vet Rec 119: 621–625

Muller GH, Kirk RW, Scott DW (1983) Small animal dermatology, 3rd edn, chap. 11, 16. Saunders, Philadelpia

Pritchard GC (1983) Alopecia in calves associated with milk substitute feeding. Vet Rec 112: 435–436

Reinhardt V, Reinhardt A, Houser D (1986) Hair pulling and eating in captive rhesus monkey tropps. Folia Primatol (Basel) 47: 158–164

Reinhardt W, Militzer K (1979) "Schnurrbartbeissen" (whiskertrimming) und socialer Rang bei Mäusen. Z Versuchstierkd 21: 83-91 (In German with English abstr)

Stowe HD, Wagner JL, Pick JR (1971) A debilitating fatal murine dermatitis. Lab Anim Sci 21: 892-897

Strozik E, Festing MFW (1981) Whisker trimming in mice. Lab Anim 15: 309-312

Tanii T, Okada T, Fukai K, Nakagawa K, Hamada T (1985) Increase of mast cells in the alopecia lesion of mice. Acta Derm Venereol (Stockh) 65: 64-66

Thornburg LP, Stowe HD, Pick JR (1973) The pathogenesis of the alopecia due to hair-chewing in mice. Lab Anim Sci 23: 843-850

Weisbroth SH, Friedman S, Scher S (1976) The parasitic ecology of the rodent mite, *Myobia musculi*. III. Lesions in certain host strains. Lab Anim Sci 26: 725-735

Cutaneous Sensitization, Experimental, Mouse, Hamster, Rat

Pierre Duprat

Introduction

Skin sensitization (contact dermatitis or cutaneous delayed-type hypersensitivity, DTH) in experimental animals can be used for different purposes depending on the scientist's uses and needs:

1. For the immunologist, it is the model for studying reproducible changes and their mechanism (role of Langerhans' cells, T-cell population, T suppressor cells, etc., as discussed later) as well as their down regulation (suppression, tolerance, desensitization).
2. For the pharmacologist, it is a model for screening potential therapeutic agents for antiinflammatory or immunosuppressive properties (Dietrich and Hess 1970) and for estimating the immunotoxicity of chemicals (Descotes et al. 1985).
3. For the therapist, it is a potential model of human pathology registering flare-up reactions at a second provocationa and then aiding further development of a method for desensitization.
4. For the toxicologist, it is a biologic tool used to assess the sensitizing potential of drugs and chemicals.

Testing for allergic contact dermatitis is an ethical and legal requirement (TOSCA 1976; OECD 1981, 1986), to determine from animal studies the sensitization risk for a human population when exposed to a particular agent. This predictive testing can be performed in various laboratory animals with more or less simple techniques which include two phases, induction (achieved by intradermal injections and/or epicutaneous applications) and challenge, approximately 10 to 14 days apart. The response is delayed (from 1 to 3 or 4 days) and is T-cell mediated. Guinea pigs are the most widely used animals in a list of 15 predictive tests (Andersen and Maibach 1985; Andersen 1987) which have been extensively studied, validated, and criticized (Marzulli and Maibach 1974, 1980; Maurer et al. 1978; Buehler 1982, 1985; Marzulli and Maguire 1987). Guinea pigs are the traditional experimental animal of choice in contact dermatitis testing (Möller 1984); however, mice are also extensively used in immunologic studies because they are easily sensitized by various agents. Use of mice in testing of contact dermatitis has two end points: predictive testing (use of mice as an alternate species to guinea pigs) and better understanding of the pathogenesis of experimental skin sensitization.

The Mouse

Development of the Mouse as an Alternate Species to the Guinea Pig

Crowle (Crowle 1959a, b, 1975; Crowle and Crowle 1961) demonstrated that cutaneous delayed-type hypersensitivity (DTH) could be elicited in mice; oxazolone, among several compounds, is used as a positive reference substance in mice [as was dinitrochlorobenzene (DNCB) in guinea pig skin sensitization tests]. Simple methodologies for quantitative measurement of cutaneous hypersensitivity in mice are used.

For example, Asherson and Ptak (1968) sensitized mice by a single flank application of the test compound followed 5-6 days later by a topical challenge on one ear pinna by application of a lower concentration (and volume). The thickness of both ears is measured using a calliper at different time intervals. In addition, animals are sequentially killed, and the ear pinnas weighed. Plotted results of challenged sites usually show a peak at 24 h which persists up to 72 h. However, a minimal reaction is always present in control sites as stressed by Gad et al. (1986) and persists less than that of the positive challenged sites.

Because of a need for standardized methodologies in safety testing, Gad et al. (1986) developed and validated an alternative dermal sensitization test: the mouse ear swelling test (MEST). They studied intrinsic (strain, age, sex) as well as extrinsic (type of induction: route, timing, vehicle, use of an adjuvant; type of challenge: timing, vehicle, interval between induction and challenge) factors which may affect the outcome of the test. They found good correlation between guinea pig tests, MEST, and human data of 72 compounds and sufficient accuracy to consider the MEST sensitive in screening chemicals. The optimal design of the MEST is summarized as follows:

Sensitization period (day 0 to day 3)
Day 0: Intradermal injection of Freund's complete adjuvant into abdominal skin clipped free of hair, and epicutaneous application of the test compound at a minimally irritating concentration (100 µl pure or diluted in a suitable vehicle) on tape-stripped skin
Days 1, 2, 3: Same epicutaneous application on tape-stripped skin

Rest period (day 4 to day 9)

Challenge period (day 10 to day 12)
Day 10: Topical application of 20 µl of test compound at a nonirritating concentration (pure or diluted in a vehicle) on one ear, the contralateral one receiving 20 µl of either a negative control substance or the vehicle
Days 11, 12: Calliper measurement thickness of both ears

This optimized MEST technique uses a control group of mice treated as the sensitized animals except that on days 0, 1, 2, and 3, the test compound is omitted. In addition, Gad et al. (1986) recommend measurement of the ear the day before the challenge to avoid spontaneous differences.

The above study design represents a miniature of protocols used in guinea pigs with several advantages over this species as stressed by Gad et al. (1986):

1. Less labor intensive
2. Less expensive animals
3. Quantitative end point (and statistical analysis can be performed if large enough groups of animals are used) with easier assessment of the change (swelling) with the naked eye or a calliper than in guinea pig skin
4. Shorter test duration (14 days in mice versus 21 or 35 days in guinea pigs
5. Use of dose-response relationship (Stadler and Karol 1985)
6. In the literature there is an increasing amount of published data which correlates with results in guinea pigs [e.g., toluene diisocyanate in mice (Tanaka 1980) and in guinea pigs (Duprat et al. 1976)]

However, the response in mice does not persist as long (Tanaka 1980; Thorne et al. 1987) as in guinea pigs (Duprat et al. 1976), which could limit further cross-reactivity studies.

Additional parameters can be measured during this optimized MEST:

1. Weights of ear pinna
2. Diffusion of an intravenously injected dye followed by colorimetric measurement to assess better any modification of capillary permeability and facilitate observation of liminal responses
3. Histopathology (as proposed by Bäck and Groth 1983; Chapman et al. 1986) which consists of a comparison of histopathologic changes in compound- and control-challenged sites at termination of the test or at different sequential times to study the kinetics of the inflammatory response. Microscopically, early edema in the dermis and subcutis persists less than 24 h with a parallel inflammatory infiltrate persisting up to 72 h. Usually mononuclear cells represent more than 50% of the infiltrate, and the ratio of mononuclear to polymorphonuclear cells tends to increase with time
4. Detection of so-called weak sensitizers could be feasible because vitamin A-enriched diet enhances induction and elicitation of cutaneous hypersensitivity (Miller et al. 1984), which has not been demonstrated in guinea pigs.

Mechanism of Cutaneous Sensitization

Types of Cells and Their Histokinetics. The basic work of several immunologists constituted the foundation of the development of the MEST

(Gad et al. 1986); mice were the most favorable animals with which to study contact hypersensitivity elicitation and suppression, as reviewed by Oliver et al. (1986). Knight et al. (1985) used mice to study the importance of Langerhans' cells (dendritic cells, antigen-presenting cells) in the induction of delayed-type hypersensitivity. Langerhans' cells bear Fc, IgG, and C3 receptors and immune response-associated (Ia) antigen on their surface and are ATPase-positive-staining cells (Wolff and Winklemann 1967; MacKenzie and Squier 1975; Silberberg-Sinakin and Thorbecke 1980; Rowden 1981). Langerhans's cells are now considered a specialized set of cells of the skin-associated lymphoid tissue (Streilein 1985) which present antigens to lymphocytes (Rosenthal and Shevach 1973; Silberberg et al. 1976a). Recognition of these antigens in mice is dependent on the histocompatibility complex, as in humans (Silberberg et al. 1976a). Langerhans' cells found in the epidermis, dermal lymphatics, and lymph nodes (Silberberg et al. 1976b; Silberberg-Sirakin et al. 1980) play a key role in cutaneous sensitization, but it is still debated whether or not those found in lymph nodes originate from the epidermis (Silberberg-Sinakin et al. 1980) or from nodal dendritic cells (Sonada et al. 1985a). Dynamic changes of the dendritic cell population in the epidermis (Aiba et al. 1984) or lymph node (Sonoda et al. 1985a, b) corroborate previous information (Asherson et al. 1983) concerning multiple capabilities, namely, "rapid migration, antigen handling and presentation and selective susceptibility to ultraviolet B radiation" (Bergstresser et al. 1985). Suppressor cells also play a role in antigen handling (Asherson et al. 1980). The following additional information has also been gained using the mouse model:

1. The density of Langerhans' cells has apparently no direct influence in terms of magnitude of the response (Sauder and Katz 1983)
2. An increase in the numbers of Langerhans' cells is paralleled by one in cells containing Birbeck's granule in the paracortical area of the lymph nodes (Sonoda et al. 1985b)
3. Bergstresser et al. (1985) recognized and identified a new dendritic cell population with Thy-1 surface antigen (termed Thy-1[1] dEC) distinct from Langerhans' cells and in high density (as high as two-thirds of the number of Langerhans' cells) and having an antigen presentation capability. Most of these cells originate from bone marrow. They also play a role in down regulation, as do T lymphocytes, nat-

ural killer, and natural suppressor cells. T lymphocytes are involved in the cutaneous DTH as confirmed by analysis of the lymphocytic subpopulation (Dunn et al. 1984), with modulation by B lymphocytes (Katz 1980). This was shown by Turk et al. (1972) using cyclophosphamide; administered prior to sensitization, this substance destroys B cells and exacerbates the DTH reaction. The T cells responsible for cutaneous sensitization in mice have an antibody-mediated regulation (Mustain et al. 1986). The mechanism by which IgM antibodies limit the immunogenic response (lytic effect, modulating effect on antigen, or phagocytosis) is not yet established.

Tolerance and Desensitization. Down regulation of contact DTH is achieved by tolerance (exposure to antigen prior to sensitization), use of drugs [e.g., glucocorticoids (Bäck and Egelrud 1985) or reserpine (Mekori et al. 1985)] or desensitization (postsensitization treatment). The likely mechanisms of suppression of contact sensitivity on development of tolerance have been investigated. Administration of a test compound before sensitization, either intravenously (Yasumizu et al. 1985) or orally (Gautam and Battisto 1983), induces tolerance which is largely dependent on T suppressor efferent cells. Although this was known from studies performed a decade ago (Phanuphak et al. 1974), Yasumizu et al. (1985) demonstrated that tolerance could be induced in chimeric mice. The sequence of interactions between subpopulations of T cells during suppression of contact sensitivity was summarized by Marcinkiewicz (1983) using the picryl chloride model: the multiple T-cell subpopulations (T immune, T suppressor efferent, and T suppressor auxiliary cells), the macrophages (acting as antigen-presenting cells and also possibly supplying T auxiliary cell function), and the factors involved (T suppressor factor and macrophage suppressor factor) interact to elicit contact DTH suppression. Gautam and Battisto (1983) studied possible mechanisms by which hapten feeding causes suppression of T cell-mediated immune responses and concluded that different mechanisms are involved. More recently, Mekori and Claman (1986) demonstrated that haptenated mouse spleen cells induced immediate desensitization and tolerance to dinitrofluorobenzene by a suppressor mechanism. This is antigen specific as opposed to suppression by intravenous administration of antigen, which is antigen nonspecific and does not involve suppressor cells.

Ultraviolet B irradiation (280–320 nm) also suppresses contact sensitization in mice by acting on Langerhans' cells (Elmets et al. 1983). This effect is partially abolished when the animals are treated with an efficient sunscreen prior to irradiation (Morison 1984) or with drugs: glucocorticoids (Bäck and Egelrud 1985; Tanaka et al. 1985 a, b) or reserpine (Mekori et al. 1985). It has been shown that ultraviolet B also induces suppressor T lymphocytes and that the mechanism of systemic suppression of contact DTH requires a soluble factor (Swartz 1984; Kripke and Morison 1986).

Photosensitization

Mice can be used in standardized photosensitization studies to elicit a cutaneous reaction, either for testing purposes (Harber 1981; Maguire and Kaidbey 1982; Keane et al. 1984; Guidici and Maguire 1985; Hawkins et al. 1986) or to study the mechanism of cutaneous reactions (Miyachi and Takigawa 1983; Miyachi et al. 1986).

For either purpose, similar induction and challenge methods are used with ultraviolet B irradiation required at times of both sensitization and challenge. Photosensitization appears to be T-cell mediated (Maguire and Kaidbey 1982). Miyachi et al. (1986) demonstrated that oxygen intermediates are formed by light absorption, creating photoallergens by reaction with biological substrates. Reactions are grossly visible at 24 h after challenge and then decline. Further investigations (e.g., cross reactivity testing, histopathology) can be performed as in the MEST sensitization test.

The Hamster

A literature search covering the past decade reveals that hamsters and rats have been much less often used in studies of contact dermatitis although these two species have epidermal Langerhans' cells which are theoretically present in sufficient numbers (Toews et al. 1980) and bear Ia surface antigens (Streilein and Bergstresser 1981). Few studies have been reported of contact sensitization in hamsters, possibly a reflection of the relatively limited use of this species in toxicity and immunology studies.

Hamsters have been used recently to confirm the need of functional Langerhans' cells in elicitation of DTH (Sullivan et al. 1985) using spontaneously (cheek pouch) or experimentally (ultraviolet) depleted Langerhans' cell preparations. It is of note that hamster cheek pouch contains 4–10 times fewer Langerhans' cells than other cutaneous or mucosal regions except the eye (Toews et al. 1980). This confirmed previous work of Streilein and Bergstresser (1981) who demonstrated that sensitization cannot be promoted in inbred hamsters (this unresponsiveness is probably mediated by T lymphocytes and can be transferred to naive hamsters) in areas deficient in Langerhans' cells, either naturally (cheek pouch) or artificially (after ultraviolet irradiation).

Usually hamsters are used to study other types of DTH (local or systemic) after viral, bacterial, or protozoal infections, to follow the development of the immune response, or after tumor graft to elucidate the mechanism of tumor rejection. In addition, because hamsters are used in inhalation toxicity studies (mainly intratracheal administration of a carcinogen), Stein-Streilein (1983) proposed inhalation as the route of entry of hapten for induction, followed by an aerosol challenge. Results using known sensitizers were compared with those of epicutaneous sensitizations. Positive reactions, as evidenced by ear swelling, were obtained with both routes of sensitization. Transfer of hypersensitivity to naive hamsters was made possible with splenic cells or macrophages obtained from bronchial lavage. Using monoclonal hamster-specific Ia reagent, Stein-Streilein (1983) demonstrated that the vast majority of cells present in the bronchial lavage fluid "expressed Ia determinants on their membrane (as do Langerhans' cells) and were morphologically indistinguishable from macrophages." Transferability and membrane-bound immunoglobulin a (Ia) determinants must be viewed as part of the validation of the sensitizing method. Because lungs are another possible route of entry of potential sensitizers, especially in occupational hygiene, this method is worth more attention by industrial toxicologists.

The Rat

Usually rats are used to study development, mechanism(s), and modulation (suppression, enhancement) of DTH in various organs (joint, brain, heart, etc.) induced by compounds, microorganisms, or a combination of both, or after tumor transplantation, or during tumor rejection. In some instances cellular-mediated immunity was studied (using BCG, ovalbumin), and positive skin tests were elicited in the absence of circulating antibodies. Rats (and hamsters) were used as an alternate species to compare data with those obtained in mice and place them in better perspective (e.g., Vernes et al. 1972, studying variations due to parasitic adaptation in the tested species). As is mice, cutaneous hypersensitivity can be elicited in rats by ear or skin challenge and modulated as well (Allwood and Asherson 1971; Asherson and Allwood 1971). However, very limited information is available in this species, probably because rats are judged to be low responders (Nakamura et al. 1977; Nakamura and Aizawa 1981). In a recent study of male F344 rats, Tanaka et al. (1985a) used double epicutaneous induction (first application on the tail followed 7 days later by a second dorsal one) and ear challenge (1 week later); the delayed onset of the ear response, the histology of the swollen ear, together with the successful passive transfer with lymphocytes were characteristic features of contact sensitization.

Recently Prop et al. (1986) showed that in the rat DTH reaction specific suppressor cells are also involved in the afferent phase of contact hypersensitivity. Studies in mice have already provided enormous amounts of information, but no comparable data are yet available in rats. The circadian rhythm of DTH in rat ear swelling (as well as in its suppression) observed by Pownall and Knapp (1979) using oxazolone does not seem a problem in standardized comparative or basic studies.

The use of a rat model for screening cutaneous sensitization might be of less advantage than the mouse model (MEST) in terms of labor and cost but remains faster than a guinea pig test.

Although guinea pigs are still used and often recommended (OECD 1981, 1986) in sensitization testing of chemicals, it is possible that tests in rodents, especially in mice, will replace them eventually because the test is shorter and has a well-defined, measurable end point. General acceptance of this alternative method by the scientific community and government authorities would be required to revise the OECD guideline. A rather lengthy and difficult updating procedure would need to be proposed by the national representatives of at least two member states.

References

Aiba S, Aizawa H, Obata M, Tagami H (1984) Dynamic changes in epidermal Ia-positive cells in allergic contact sensitivity reactions in mice. Br J Dermatol 111: 507-516

Allwood GG, Asherson GL (1971) Depression of delayed hypersensitivity by pretreatment with Freund-type adjuvants. II. Mechanism of the phenomenon. Clin Exp Immunol 9: 259-266

Andersen KE (1987) Testing for contact allergy in experimental animals. Pharmacol Toxicol 61: 1-8

Andersen KE, Maibach HI (1985) Guinea-pig allergy tests: an overview. Toxicol Ind Health 1: 43-66

Asherson GL, Allwood GG (1971) Depression of delayed hypersensitivity by pretreatment with Freund-type adjuvants. I. Description of the phenomenon. Clin Exp Immunol 9: 249-258

Asherson GL, Ptak W (1968) Contact and delayed hypersensitivity in the mouse. I. Active sensitization and passive transfer. Immunology 15: 405-416

Asherson GL, Zembala M, Thomas WR, Perera MACC (1980) Suppressor cells and the handling of antigen. Immunol Rev 50: 3-45

Asherson GL, Colizzi V, Watkins MC (1983) Immunogenic cells in the regional lymph nodes after painting with the contact sensitizers picryl chloride and oxazolone: evidence for the presence of IgM antibody on their surface. Immunology 48: 561-569

Bäck O, Groth O (1983) The cellular infiltrate of the contact sensitivity reaction to picryl chloride in the mouse. Acta Derm Venereol (Stockh) 63: 304-307

Bäck O, Egelrud T (1985) Topical glucocorticoids and suppression of contact sensitivity. A mouse bioassay of anti-inflammatory effects. Br J Dermatol 112: 539-545

Bergstresser PR, Sullivan S, Streilein JW, Tigelaar RE (1985) Origin and function of Thy-1 + dendritic epidermal cells in mice. J Invest Dermatol 85: 85s-90s

Buehler EV (1982) Comment on guinea-pig test methods. (letter) Food Chem Toxicol 20: 494-495

Buehler EV (1985) A rationale for the selection of occlusion to induce and elicit delayed contact hypersensitivity in the guinea pig. A prospective test. Curr Probl Dermatol 14: 39-58

Chapman JR, Ruben Z, Buchko GM (1986) Histology of and quantitative assays for oxazolone-induced allergic contact dermatitis in mice. Am J Dermatopathol 8: 130-138

Crowle AJ (1959a) Delayed hypersensitivity in mice: its detection by skin tests and its passive transfer. Science 130: 159-160

Crowle AJ (1959b) Delayed hypersensitivity in several strains of mice studied with six different tests. J Allergy 30: 442-459

Crowle AJ, Crowle CM (1961) Contact sensitivity in mice. J Allergy 32: 302-320

Crowle AJ (1975) Delayed hypersensitivity in the mouse. In: Dixon FJ, Kunkel HG (eds) Advances in immunology, vol 20. Academic, New York, pp 197-264

Descotes J, Tedone R, Evreux JCL (1985) Immunotoxicity screening of drugs and chemicals: value of contact hypersensitivity to picryl chloride in the mouse. Methods Find Exp Clin Pharmacol 7: 303-305

144   Pierre Duprat

Dietrich FM, Hess R (1970) Hypersensitivity in mice. I. Induction of contact sensitivity to oxazolone and inhibition by various chemical compounds. Int Arch Allergy Appl Immunol 38: 246-259

Dunn IS, Liberato DJ, Castagnoli N, Byers VS (1984) Induction of suppressor T cells for lymph node cell proliferation after contact sensitization of mice with a poison oak urushiol component. Immunology 51: 773-781

Duprat P, Gradiski D, Marignac B (1976) Pouvoir irritant et allergisant de deux isocyanates: toluène diisocyanate (TDI) et diphénylméthane diisocyanate (MDI). Eur J Toxicol Environ Hyg 9: 41-53

Elmets CA, Bergstresser PR, Tigelaar RE, Wood PJ, Streilein JW (1983) Analysis of the mechanism of unresponsiveness produced by haptens painted on skin exposed to low dose ultraviolet radiation. J Exp Med 158: 781-794

Gad SC, Dunn BJ, Dobbs DW, Reilly C, Walsh RD (1986) Development and validation of an alternative dermal sensitization test: the mouse ear swelling test (MEST). Toxicol Appl Pharmacol 84: 93-114

Gautam SC, Battisto JR (1983) Suppression of contact sensitivity and cell-mediated lympholysis by oral administration of Hapten is caused by different mechanisms. Cell Immunol 78: 295-304

Guidici PA, Maguire HC Jr (1985) Experimental photoallergy to systemic drugs. J Invest Dermatol 85: 207-211

Harber LC (1981) Current status of mammalian and human models for predicting drug photosensitivity. J Invest Dermatol 77: 65-70

Hawkins CW, Bickers DR, Mukhtar H, Elmets CA (1986) Cutaneous porphyrin photosensitization: murine ear swelling as a marker of the acute response. J Invest Dermatol 86: 638-642

Katz SI (1980) New aspects of delayed hypersensitivity. In: Drill VA (ed) Current concepts in cutaneous toxicity. Academic, New York

Keane JT, Pearson RW, Malkinson FD (1984) Nalidixic acid-induced photosensitivity in mice: a model for pseudoporphyria. J Invest Dermatol 82: 210-213

Knight SC, Bedford P, Hunt R (1985) The role of dendritic cells in the initiation of immune responses to contact sensitizers. II. Studies in nude mice. Cell Immunol 94: 435-439

Kripke M, Morison W (1986) Studies on the mechanism of systemic suppression of contact hypersensitivity by ultraviolet B radiation. Photodermatol 3: 4-14

MacKenzie IC, Squier CA (1975) Cytochemical identification of ATPase-positive Langerhans cells in EDTA-separated sheets of mouse epidermis. Br J Dermatol 92: 523-533

Maguire HC Jr, Kaidbey K (1982) Experimental photoallergic contact dermatitis: a mouse model. J Invest Dermatol 79: 147-152

Marcinkiewicz J (1983) Suppression of contact sensitivity to picryl chloride. Interaction between T suppressor auxiliary cells, suppressor factors and macrophages. Arch Immunol Ther Exp (Warsz) 31: 849-855

Marzulli FN, Maguire C (1987) Validation of guinea pig tests for skin hypersensitivity. In: Marzulli FN, Maibach HI (eds) Dermatotoxicology. Hemisphere, New York, pp 177-290

Marzulli FN, Maibach HI (1974) The use of graded concentrations in studying skin sensitizers: experimental contact sensitization in man. Food Cosmet Toxicol 12: 219-227

Marzulli FN, Maibach HI (1980) Further studies of effects of vehicles and elicitation concentration in experimental contact sensitization testing in humans. Contact Dematitis 6: 131-133

Maurer TP, Thomann DG, Weirich EH, Hess R (1978) Predictive evaluation in animals of the contact allergenic potential of medically important substances. I. Comparison of different methods of inducing and measuring cutaneous sensitization. Contact Dermatitis 4: 321-333

Mekori YA, Claman HN (1986) Desensitization of contact allergy to DNFB in mice. III. Characteristics of immediate densensitization induced by haptenated spleen cells. Cell Immunol 98: 279-288

Mekori YA, Weitzman GL, Galli SJ (1985) Reevaluation of reserpine-induced suppression of contact sensitivity. Evidence that reserpine interferes with T-lymphocyte function independently of an effect on mast cells. J Exp Med 162: 1935-1953

Miller K, Maisey J, Malkovsky M (1984) Enhancement of contact sensitization in mice fed a diet enriched in vitamin A acetate. Int Arch Allergy Appl Immunol 75: 120-125

Miyachi Y, Takigawa M (1983) Mechanisms of contact photosensitivity in mice. III. Predictive testing of chemicals with photoallergenic potential in mice. Arch Dermatol 119: 736-739

Miyachi Y, Imamura S, Niwa Y, Tokura Y, Takigawa M (1986) Mechanisms of contact photosensitivity in mice. VI. Oxygen intermediates are involved in contact photosensitization but not in ordinary contact sensitization. J Invest Dermatol 86: 26-28

Möller H (1984) Attempts to induce contact allergy to nickel in the mouse. Contact Dermatitis 10: 65-68

Morison WL (1984) The effect of a sunscreen containing paraaminobenzoic acid on the systemic immunologic alterations induced in mice by exposure to UVB radiation. J Invest Dermatol 83: 405-408

Mustain EL, Claman HN, Moorhead JW (1986) Antibody-mediated regulation of T cell responses. I. Characterization of a monoclonal antibody which specifically regulates contact hypersensitivity to DNFB in BALB/c mice. J Immunol 136 12: 4372-4378

Nakamura K, Aizawa M (1981) Studies on the genetic control of picryl chloride contact hypersensitivity reaction in inbred rats. Transplant Proc 13: 1400-1403

Nakamura K, Tada N, Aizawa M (1977) Genetic control of the contact sensitivity to picryl chloride in inbred rats. Proc Jpn Soc Immunol 7: 345-346

OECD: Organisation for Economic Cooperation and Development (1981 and 1986) Guidelines for testing of chemicals. Skin sensitization. Publications and Information Center, Washington and Paris

Oliver GJA, Botham PA, Kimber I (1986) Models for contact sensitization-novel approaches and future developments. Br J Dermatol 115 31: 53-62

Phanuphak M, Moorhead JW, Claman HN (1974) Tolerance and contact sensitivity to DNFB in mice. III. Transfer of tolerance with suppressor T cells. J Immunol 113: 1230

Pownall R, Knapp MS (1979) A circadian study of corticosteroid suppression of delayed hypersensitivity. Int J Immunopharmacol 1: 293–298

Prop J, Griffiths A, Hutchinson IV, Morris PJ (1986) Specific suppressor T cells in rats active in the afferent phase of contact hypersensitivity. Cell Immunol 99: 73–84

Rosenthal AS, Shevach EM (1973) The function of macrophages in antigen recognition by guinea pig T lymphocytes. I. Requirement for histocompatible macrophages and lymphocytes. J Exp Med 138: 1194–1212

Rowden G (1981) The Langerhans cell. CRC Crit Rev Immunol 3: 95–180

Sauder DN, Katz SI (1983) Strain variation in the induction of tolerance by epicutaneous application of trinitrochlorobenzene. J Invest Dermatol 80 5: 383–386

Silberberg I, Baer RL, Rosenthal SA (1976a) The role of Langerhans cells in allergic contact hypersensitivity. A review of findings in man and guinea pigs. J Invest Dermatol 66: 210–215

Silberberg I, Thorbecke GJ, Baer RL, Rosenthal SA, Berezowsky V (1976b) Antigen-bearing Langerhans cells in skin, dermal lymphatics and in lymph nodes. Cell Immunol 25: 137–151

Silberberg-Sinakin I, Thorbecke GJ (1980) Contact hypersensitivity and Langerhans cells. J Invest Dermatol 75: 61–67

Silberberg-Sinakin I, Gigli I, Baer RL, Thorbecke GJ (1980) Langerhans cells: role in contact hypersensitivity and relationship to lymphoid dendritic cells and to macrophages. Immunol Rev 53: 203–232

Sonoda Y, Asano S, Miyazaki T, Sagami S (1985a) Electron microscopic study on Langerhans cells and related cells in lymph nodes of DNCB-sensitive mice. Arch Dermatol Res 277: 44–54

Sonoda Y, Miyazaki T, Asano S, Sagami S (1985b) Increased Langerhans cells and related cells in mesenteric lymph nodes of DNCB-sensitive mice. Arch Dermatol Res 278: 68–73

Stadler JC, Karol MH (1985) Use of dose-response data to compare the skin sensitizing abilities of dicyclohexylmethane-4,4'-diisocyanate and picryl chloride in two animal species. Toxicol Appl Pharmacol 78: 445–450

Stein-Streilein J (1983) Allergic contact dermatitis induced by intratracheal administration of hapten. J Immunology 131 4: 1748–1753

Streilein JW (1985) Circuits and signals of the skin-associated lymphoid tissues (SALT). J Invest Dermatol 85: 10s–13s

Streilein JW, Bergstresser PR (1981) Langerhans cell function dictates induction of contact hypersensitivity or unresponsiveness to DNFB in Syrian hamsters. J Invest Dermatol 77: 272–277

Sullivan S, Bergstresser PR, Streilein JW (1985) Intravenously injected, TNP-derivatized, Langerhans cell-enriched epidermal cells induce contact hypersensitivty in Syrian hamsters. J Invest Dermatol 84: 249–252

Swartz RP (1984) Role of UVB-induced serum factors(s) in suppression of contact hypersensitivity in mice. J Invest Dermatol 83: 305–307

Tanaka K (1980) Contact sensitivity in mice induced by toluene diisocyanate (TDI). J Dermatol (Tokyo) 7: 277–280

Tanaka KI, Nagaya Y, Marui S, Okamoto Y, Hanada S (1985a) Contact sensitivity in rats induced by toluene diisocyanate (TDI). J Dermatol 12: 484–488

Tanaka KI, Takeoka A, Hanada S, Okamoto Y, Ino T, Okuizumi J, Kohno S (1985b) Additional findings on contact sensitivity on mice induced by toluene diisocyanate (TDI). Arerugi 34: 128–134

Thorne PS, Hillebrand JA, Lewis GR, Karol MH (1987) Contact sensitivity by diisocyanates: potencies and cross-reactivities. Toxicol Appl Pharmacol 87: 155–165

Toews GB, Bergstresser PR, Streilein JW (1980) Epidermal Langerhans cell density determines whether contact hypersensitivity or unresponsiveness follows skin painting with DNFB. J Immunol 124: 445–453

Tosca (1976) Toxic Substance Control Act USA Public Law 94–469 Oct 11

Turk JL, Parker D, Poulter LW (1972) Functional aspects of the selective depletion of lymphoid tissues by cyclophosphamide. Immunol 23: 493–501

Vernes A, Biguet J, Floc'h et al. (1972) Delayed hypersensitivity during experimental schistosomiasis with *Schistoma mansoni*. 2. study in the rat and golden hamster. Comparison with mice and results according to parasitic adaptation. Ann Inst Pasteur 123: 721–730

Wolff K, Winklemann RK (1967) Ultrastructural localization of nucleoside triphosphatase in Langerhans cells. J Invest Dermatol 48: 50–54

Yasumizu R, Onoe K, Iwabuchi K, Ogasawara M, Geng L, Morikawa K (1985) Analysis of contact sensitivity to 2,4-dinitrofluorobenzene (DNFB) in allogeneic bone marrow chimaera in mice. Immunology 54: 149–153

Steatitis, Subcutaneous and Generalized, Rat

Berry H. J. C. Danse

Synonym. Yellow fat disease.

Gross Appearance

The gross appearance of adipose tissue with steatitis at an early stage is characterized by focal, bright yellow spots scattered over the glossy white fat depots. Initially, these small focal lesions are visible in the gonadal fat. During progression of the disease, perirenal, mesenteric, and subcutaneous fat depots are successively involved. All fat depots eventually have a yellow discoloration. The affected adipose tissue retains the soft consistency of normal adipose tissue during all stages of the disease.

Microscopic Features

The earliest change of steatitis consists of a diffuse infiltration with solitary or clusters of lipofuscin-laden macrophages in the adipose tissue without visible injury to the adjacent fat cells (Fig. 187). The lipofuscin pigment is responsible for the typical gross yellow discoloration of adipose tissue in this disorder. This pigment contains mainly lipid peroxides with different degrees of polymerization, which are not soluble in the solvents used for histotechnical processing and therefore remain in the paraplast section. In hematoxylin and eosin (H and E) sections, the lipopigment is seen as fine basophilic foaminess or distinct yellow globules which may be considered the early ceroid-type of lipofuscin. This ceroid is acid fast, with bright yellow autofluorescence (Fig. 188) in unstained sections viewed with a fluorescence microscope (exciting filter BG 12, barrier filters 53 and 44). Infiltration of macrophages in some cases may be very extensive without any visible involvement of fat cells. Usually, however, rapid progression to the next inflammatory stage takes place, in which fat cells are affected. In this stage, scattered, degenerated fat cells are surrounded by a dense layer of inflammatory cells, consisting of lipofuscin-laden macrophages, neutrophilic granulocytes, and lymphocytes (Fig. 189). The vacuole in the affected fat cell is often irregularly shaped due to inflammatory cells penetrating the lipid mass.

Moreover, the vacuole often contains lipid material which, as a result of polymerization, is insoluble in lipid solvents. Focal areas with fat cell necrosis and only very sparse inflammatory reaction (steatosis) are now obvious. These necrotic fat cells have a swollen cytoplasmic rim which is irregularly demarcated from the fat vacuole (Fig. 190).

In H and E sections steatotic areas are often colorless, giving the impression of an inadequately stained section. Enzyme histochemistry reveals characteristic features of steatosis, e.g., high 5'-nucleotidase (EC 3.1.3.5) activity as a result of plasma membrane damage and high esterase activity indicating endogeneous lipolytic activity (Danse and Steenbergen-Botterweg 1978). The disorder progresses rapidly when a vitamin E-deficient diet is supplemented with linseed oil (unpublished observation), producing steatosis in large areas of the affected adipose tissue. Under these conditions, extensive calcification of necrotic fat cells is also observed. Since steatosis is only noticed in the advanced stage of the disease, following steatitis, it is thought to be secondary to diffusion of toxic metabolites from the steatitic area. Vascular defects as in panniculitis in humans are not observed.

Even in a final stage of steatitis with more than 50% of all fat cells affected in rats exposed to a steatitis-inducing diet for as long as 3 months after birth, substantial fibrosis in the inflamed fat depots have not been seen (Danse and Verschuren 1978a).

Fig. 187 *(upper left)*. Steatitis, rat. Early change consisting ▶ of clusters of lipofuscin-laden macrophages infiltrated in the adipose tissue. H and E, × 320

Fig. 188 *(lower left)*. Lipofuscin-laden macrophages in early steatitis, rat, autofluorescence. × 320

Fig. 189 *(upper right)*. Steatitis, rat. Note affected fat cells surrounded with a dense inflammatory reaction, consisting of macrophages, neutrophilic granulocytes, and lymphocytes. H and E, × 320

Fig. 190 *(lower right)*. Focal fat cell necrosis (steatosis), rat. Affected fat cells have a swollen cytoplasmic rim, which is irregularly demarcated from the fat vacuole, and only sparse inflammatory reaction. H and E, × 320

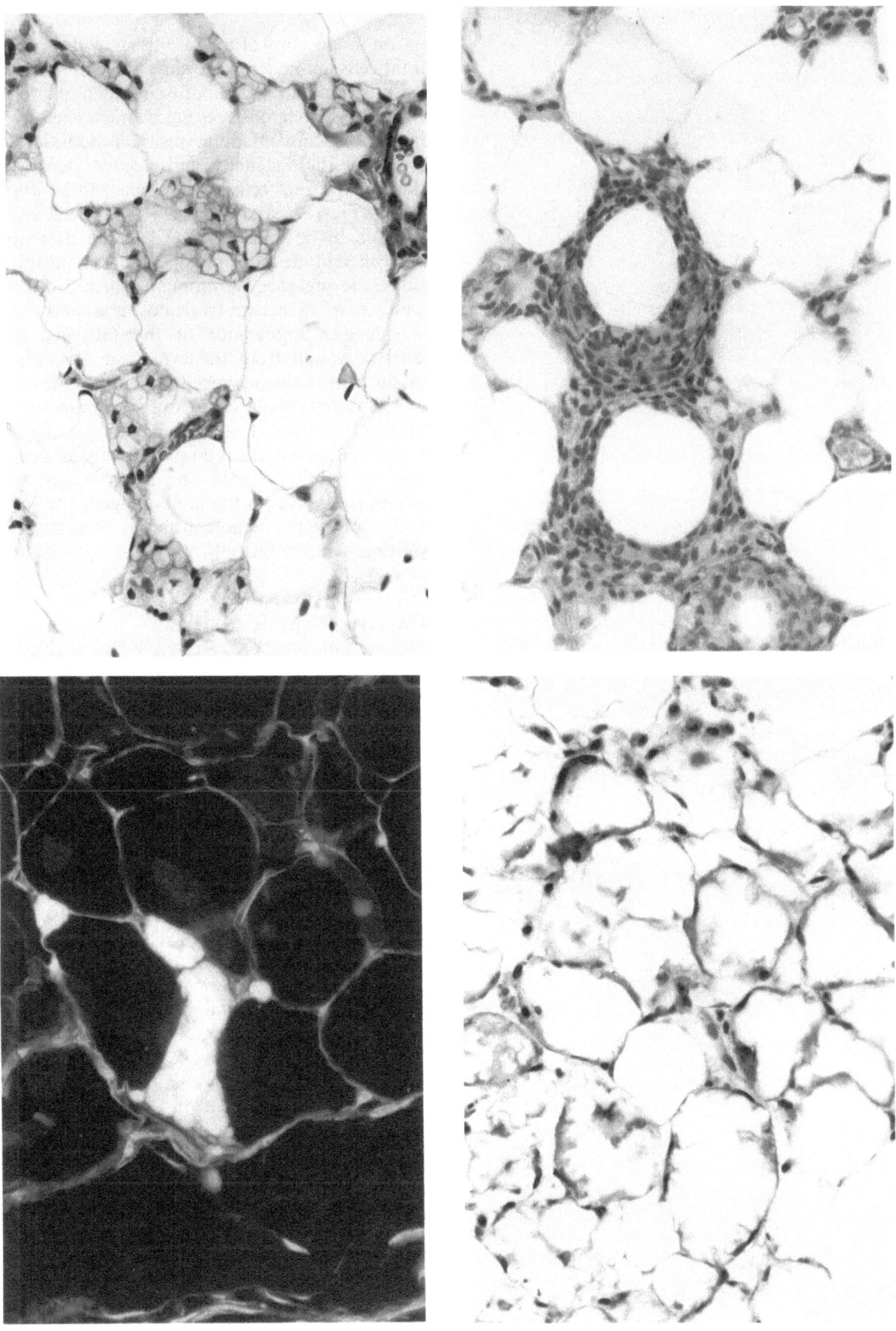

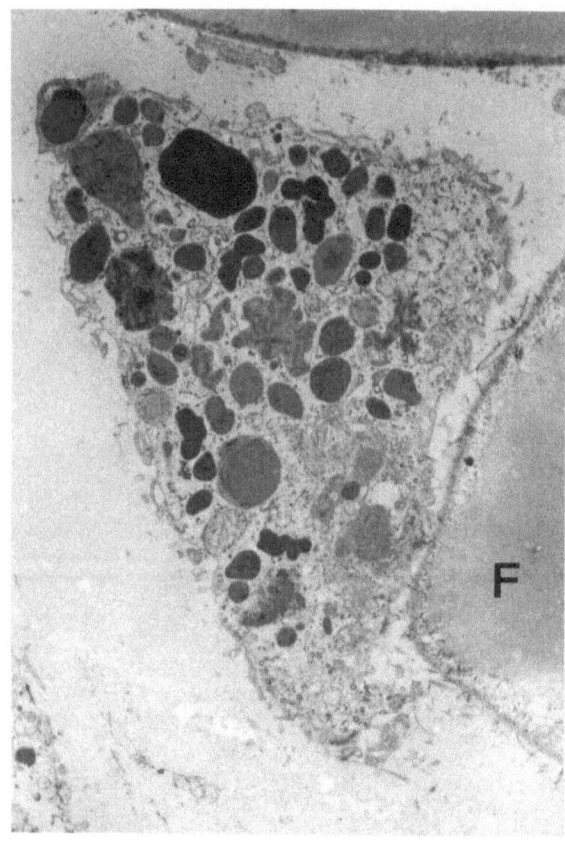

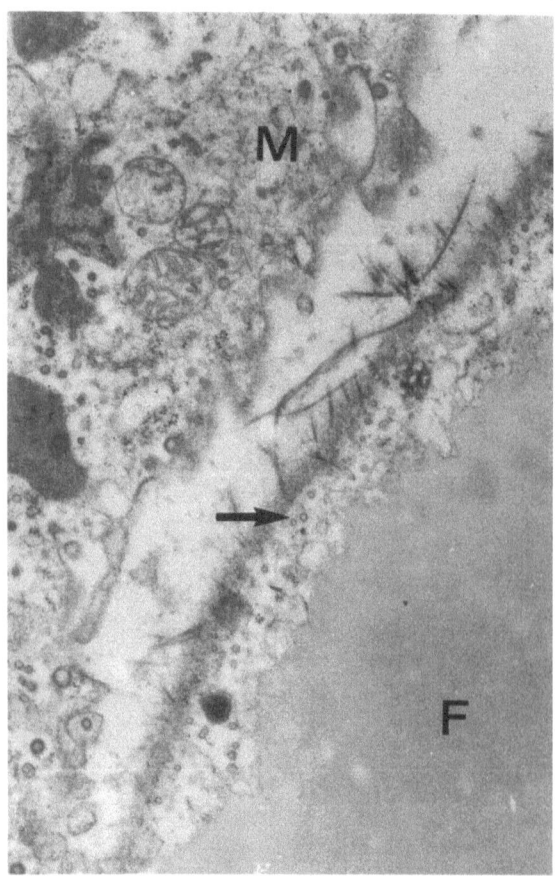

Ultrastructure

Electron microscopy of adipose tissue will reveal that fat cells are intact in the early stage of steatitis with accumulation of lipofuscin-laden macrophages. These macrophages are characterized by many lipofuscin-containing residual bodies of varying size, homogeneity, and electron density, and adjacent to fat cells which appear to be unaffected (Figs. 191 and 192). These fat cells are concluded to be intact, because of the normal plasma membrane with micropinocytotic invaginations, the presence of various unaltered cytoplasmic membranes and free ribosomes, and the homogeneous appearance of the fat vacuole clearly separated from the cytoplasm. In contrast, fat cells in the advanced stage of the disorder are invaded by various types of inflammatory cells (Fig. 193). The fat vacuole surrounding these penetrated cells has cleared up, probably as a result of exocytotic lipolysis. This lipolytic activity is one of the causes of the nonhomogeneous appearance of the fat vacuole, which is characteristic of degenerating fat cells.

Differential Diagnosis

Steatitis must be differentiated from steatosis which is often seen with (experimentally induced) acute pancreatitis. In most cases, steatosis is noticed in the visceral fat depots and on gross inspection appears as white dull foci in the adipose tissue, easily distinguishable from the bright yellow spots in steatitis. Under microscopic examination pancreas-associated steatosis is characterized by primary focal fat cell necrosis. Subsequently, a zone of inflammatory cells is formed around the necrotic area (Storck and Hansson 1972). Lipofuscin in macrophages or fat cells is not seen in this disorder.

In the pathogenesis of pancreas-associated steatosis, the close apposition of both tissues has been considered important, since the general

◀ **Fig. 191** *(above)*. Lipofuscin-laden macrophage lying close to infact fat cells *(F)* in the early stage of steatitis, rat. TEM, × 4500

Fig. 192 *(below)*. Detail from Fig. 191. Note the adipocytic cytoplasmic rim with a normal plasma membrane, micropinocytotic vesicles *(arrow)*, various cytoplasmic membranes, a homogenous fat vacuole *(F)*, and a lipofuscin-laden macrophage *(M)*. TEM, × 21000

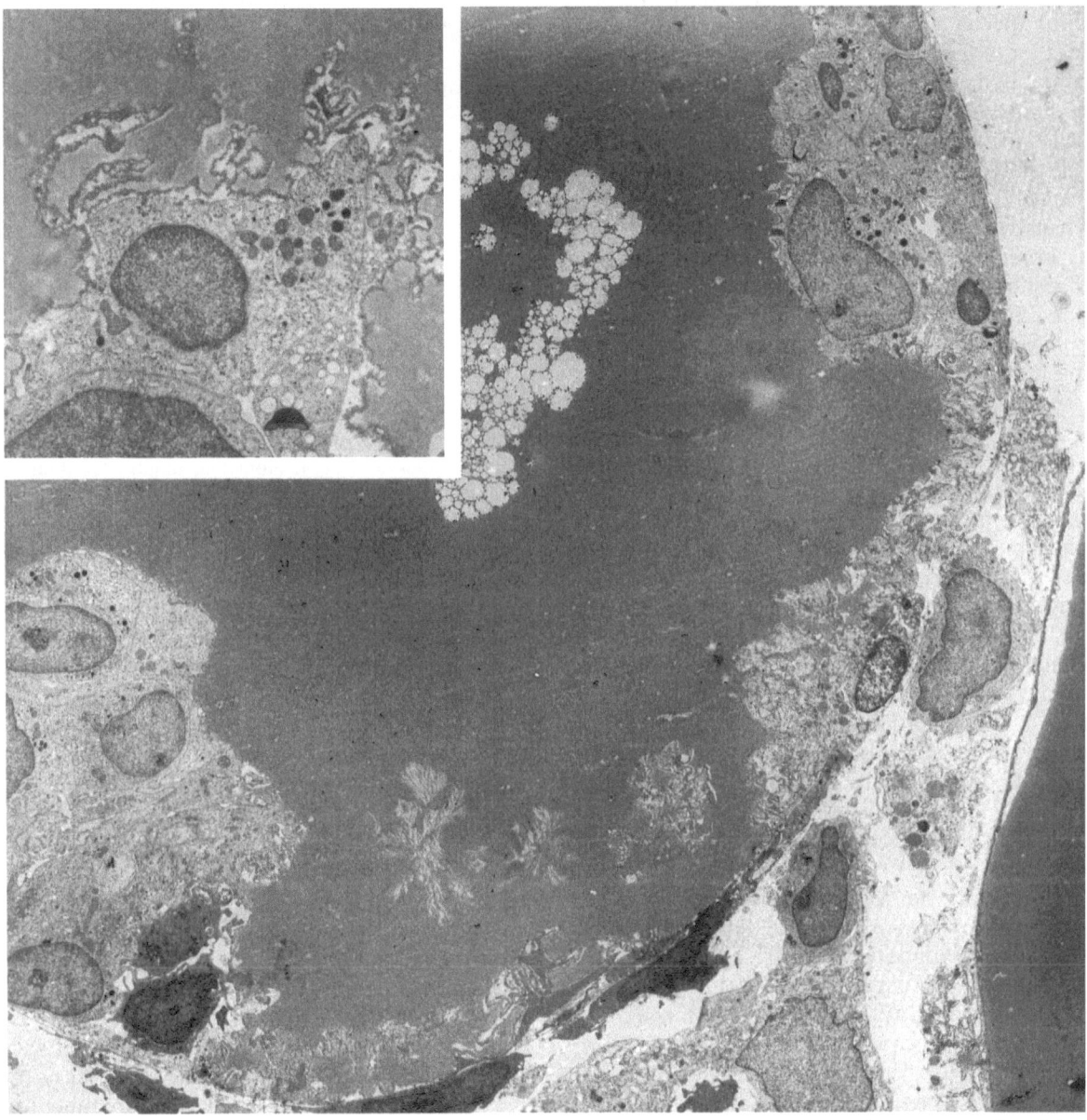

Fig. 193. Fat cell, rat, in an advanced stage of steatitis with invasion of inflammatory cells causing heterogeneity of the fat vacuole. *Inset,* detail of invading macrophage. Note clear zone in fat adjacent to projections of the plasma membrane. TEM, × 4400

opinion was that diffusion of pancreatic enzymes caused necrosis in the visceral adipose tissues. However, the finding of pancreas-associated steatosis in subcutaneous fat depots in humans (Reed et al. 1973) suggests that endogeneously activated lipolytic activity in adipose tissue may be the cause of necrosis in fat cells (Theve et al. 1973). In the rat, pancreas-associated steatosis has not been reported in other than visceral fat depots.

Biologic Features

Pathogenesis. The early changes of steatitis with infiltration of lipofuscin-laden macrophages are associated with lipofuscin storage in splenic macrophages and Kupffer's cells of the liver (Mason et al. 1946; Danse and Verschuren 1978a). This generalized lipofuscinosis of the mononuclear phagocyte system in a stage of the disorder in which adipocytes are not yet affected suggests that the pigment accumulation results from phagocytosis of blood-borne or interstitial reactive lipid species such as free radicals, hydroperoxides, or other pigment precursors. The weak lysosomal hydrolase activity of these macrophages as compared with those surrounding affected fat cells in an advanced stage of the disease supports this suggestion (Danse and Steenbergen-Botterweg 1978).

Phagocytosis of poorly digestible products such as lipids will induce less hydrolase activity than digestible substrates such as cell debris. Another possibility is that reactive lipid species such as peroxides may cause membrane damage, resulting in impaired enzyme protein synthesis.

The damage to fat cells which is manifest in the next stage of the disorder may be caused by the same extracellular reactive lipids which also provoked the initial macrophage reaction or by free radicals originating from the activated macrophages themselves (Nathan 1982). Once this process has started, its progression can be very rapid since the adipocytic vacuole content of rats with steatitis is always rich in unsaturated fatty acids, which are easily oxidized to yield reactive lipid peroxides. In this stage, affected fat cells are surrounded by a zone of inflammatory cells such as neutrophilic granulocytes, lymphocytes, and macrophages. In contrast to other species, fibrosis of adipose tissue is not seen in rats with steatitis. These differences in the inflammatory reaction may depend on the variety of lipids released from the affected fat cells. This was also observed when various lipids were injected subcutaneously (Abdulla et al. 1967). Fatty acid composition of fat depots in the rat parallels the dietary fat composition. In Table 9 can be seen the effect of dietary cod liver and linseed oil on the fatty acid composition of two fat depots in the rat. Characteristic fatty acids of cod liver oil are the highly unsaturated fatty acids eicosapentaenoate (20:5ω3), docosahexaenoate (22:6ω3), and the monounsaturated docosaenoate (22:1) which occur in concentrations of about 10% each. In linseed oil, the occurrence of a high amount (50%–60%) of linolenate (18:3ω3) is characteristic. Table 9 illustrates the clear differences in fat depot composition depending on dietary fat intake. Moreover, relative differences are evident between gonadal and subcutaneous fat after the same dietary conditioning, presumably due to a different metabolic rate. In the rat, the gonadal fat depot forms much faster and is metabolically more active than any other depot. Subcutaneous adipose tissue is therefore less active than gonadal fat, and a lower concentration

Table 9. Fatty acid composition of gonadal and subcutaneous adipose tissue of rats fed a diet supplemented with 15% cod liver or linseed oil for 8 weeks ($n=2$)

Fatty acid Cm:n[a]	Cod liver oil		Linseed oil	
	Gonad	Subcutis	Gonad	Subcutis
14:0	4.6	5.1	0.7	1.5
16:0	22.1	20.4	12.6	15.1
16:1	9.8	9.5	2.8	2.8
18:0	–	–	2.8	3.4
18:1	37.8	39.1	21.5	24.2
18:2ω6[b]	2.4	4.8	16.5	17.3
18:3ω3	–	–	43.1	35.7
20:5ω3	8.7	9.8	–	–
22:1	5.5	4.2	–	–
22:6ω3	7.0	4.4	–	–
rest	2.1	2.7	–	–

[a] Cm, number of carbon atoms; n, number of double bonds.

[b] ω, position of first double bond starting at methyl ending of fatty acid.

of certain incoming fatty acids (22:1, 22:6ω3; 18:3ω3) and a higher concentration of the pre-existing fatty acids such as oleate (18:1) and linoleate (18:2ω6) are present. These metabolic and compositional differences between fat depots can explain why in steatitis depots with different localization are not affected simultaneously or to the same degree.

Focal areas of steatosis are evident in the advanced stages of the disorder, when more than 30% of all fat cells are affected. The preferential appearance in this period indicates that these necrotic areas are associated with processes specifically occurring in this stage. Increased lipolytic activity is found in this affected adipose tissue (Danse and Verschuren 1978b) and results in a release of free fatty acids which have a damaging detergent effect on fat cell membranes. Increased lipolysis and release of free fatty acids are also important in the pathogenesis of fat cell necrosis in pancreatitis (Theve et al. 1973).

Etiology. Steatitis or yellow fat disease is considered an expression of vitamin E deficiency. Within this syndrome, though, steatitis only occurs when polyunsaturated fatty acids (PUFA) with at least three double bonds are present in the feed. In most of the studies, steatitis was induced with diets supplemented with fish oil or linseed oil. In these oils, the PUFA with three or more double bonds belong to a specific group (ω-3 family) with a specific position of the double bonds within the fatty acid molecule. It has been suggested that this structural specificity causes these particular lesions. However, steatitis was also induced in mice in an experiment with evening primrose oil (Danse and Nederbragt 1981) containing γ-linolenic acid (18: ω6). This fatty acid also has three double bonds but belongs to another structural group (ω-6 family). Thus, the induction of steatitis seems to depend on the presence of fatty acids with at least three double bonds, irrespective of the particular position of these bonds in the molecule.

Selenium is also an important etiological factor in the vitamin E deficiency syndrome. This is related to the integral position of selenium in the enzyme glutathione (GSH) peroxidase (EC 1.11.1.9), which catalyzes the degradation of lipid peroxides to nonreactive products. Therefore, many of the signs of vitamin E deficiency, such as myopathy, exudative diathesis, and dietary hepatosis, can be cured by administration of selenium. However, supplementation with selenium does not prevent or cure steatitis in spite of the presence of a substantial activity of selenium-dependent GSH-peroxidase in adipose tissue.

Frequency. Spontaneously occurring steatitis in rats is rare and as far as I know has not been reported. Rats have been found with initial changes of steatitis in toxicology studies in which rancid dietary fat or the test compound had affected the antioxidant supply of the feed (vitamin E, synthetic antioxidants). Young animals are affected preferentially, which can be explained by the effect of growth on tissue antioxidants. Even if the lesions are very slight, their value in monitoring the antioxidant status of the feed is important, since from experimental studies in which vitamin E deficiency was induced it is known that progression of the disease is generally very rapid. In experimentally induced steatitis in which fish, linseed, or evening primrose oil are given in the feed, all animals are affected by 2–4 weeks after the start of the experiment.

Comparison with Other Species

Generalized steatitis of fat depots as a sign of vitamin E deficiency is seen as a spontaneous disease in the horse, pig, mink, cat, and rabbit. Experimentally induced steatitis has been described in rat, rabbit, mouse, and mink (Danse and Verschuren 1978a). All monogastric mammals may develop this disorder when dietary PUFA are incorporated in the adipose tissue

without desaturation. In ruminants, on the other hand, dietary PUFA are desaturated in the rumen and therefore vitamin E-dependent steatitis is never seen.

The histopathologic characteristics of the inflammatory process in the above-mentioned susceptible species are the same as have been described in the rat. Extensive fibrosis is seen in the advanced stages of the disease in the horse and pig.

Although for some human adipose tissue disorders the etiology and pathogenesis are still unclear, a comparable disease of adipose tissue is not known. In lobular panniculitides in humans such as Weber-Christian disease, the infiltration of foam cells suggests similarity with yellow fat disease. However, the primary involvement of vascular elements in this disease is so dominating that some authors consider it more like vasculitis than a primary disorder affecting lipocytes (Reed et al. 1973).

Some cases of subcutaneous fat necrosis of the newborn or sclerema neonatorum have a certain pathogenetic similarity to yellow fat disease. In sclerema, an increased concentration of saturated fatty acids in fat depots was measured and suggested to induce a granulomatous reaction and fat cell necrosis (Horsfield and Yardley 1965). Although for the explanation of this increase of saturated fatty acids a defective desaturating enzyme system was suggested, another hypothesis might be a decrease of the amount of unsaturated fatty acids caused by peroxidation. Indeed, in linseed oil-induced yellow fat disease of rats, the total amount of PUFA (18:2ω6, 18:3ω3) in subcutaneous fat decreased from 53.0% (control value, Table 9) to 26.7% while the total amount of main saturated fatty acid (16:0, 18:0) increased from 18.5% (control value, Table 9) to 29.9% (unpublished observation). Regarding the inflammatory infiltrate, sclerema and yellow fat disease have many similar characteristics, and some cases of sclerema were recorded in which there was a generalized involvement of fat depots throughout the body. The presence of lipofuscin-laden macrophages in this human disease has not been reported, which implies a significant difference to yellow fat disease in animals.

References

Abdulla YH, Adams CW, Morgan RS (1967) Connective tissue reactions to implantation of purified sterol, sterol esters, phosphoglycerides, glycerides and free fatty acids. J Pathol Bacteriol 94: 63–71

Danse LHJC, Nederbragt H (1981) Tri-unsaturated fatty acids in the aetiology of yellow fat disease. Int J Vitam Nutr Res 51: 319

Danse LHJC, Steenbergen-Botterweg WA (1978) Fish oil-induced yellow fat disease in rats. II. Enzyme histochemistry of adipose tissue. Vet Pathol 15: 125–132

Danse LHJC, Verschuren PM (1978a) Fish oil-induced yellow fat disease in rats. I. Histological changes. Vet Pathol 15: 114–124

Danse LHJC, Verschuren PM (1978b) Fish oil-induced yellow fat disease in rats. III. Lipolysis in affected adipose tissue. Vet Pathol 15: 544–548

Horsfield GI, Yardley HJ (1965) Sclerema neonatorum. J Invest Dermatol 44: 326–332

Mason KE, Dam H, Granados H (1946) Histological changes in adipose tissue of rats fed a vitamin-E deficient diet high in cod liver oil. Anat Rec 94: 265–288

Nathan CF (1982) Secretion of oxygen intermediates: role in effector functions of activated macrophages. Fed Proc 41: 2206–2211

Reed RJ, Clark WH, Mihm MC (1973) Disorders of the panniculus adiposus. Hum Pathol 4: 219–229

Storck G, Hansson CG (1972) Experimental fat necrosis in the rat. II. A histopathological study. Acta Chir Scand 138: 165–169

Theve NO, Hallberg D, Carlström A (1973) Studies in fat necrosis. I. Lipolysis and calcium content in adipose tissue from rats with experimentally induced fat necrosis. Acta Chir Scand 139: 131–133

Follicular Hyperkeratosis, Induced, Rabbit Ear

Richard J. Kociba, David C. Keyes, and D. M. Williams

Synonyms. Chloracne rabbit ear bioassay; comedogenic rabbit ear bioassay; acnegenic rabbit ear bioassay; follicular dermatosis; acneform dermatitis.

Gross Appearance

The inner surface of the normal (untreated) albino rabbit ear pinna is covered by a smooth skin with numerous dark, slightly dimpled foci which, under magnification, seem to be the openings of the pilosebaceous units. The albino rabbit ear pinna is normally relatively thin adn pliable, with the pink coloration representative of its vascularity.

Gross examination is the basis for a grading scheme devised by Adams et al. (1941) which is used to evaluate the local response at the site of application to the inner surface of the ear pinna. The gross appearance of a follicular hyperkeratotic and comedogenic response is described according to the following grades:

Grade 0 – Within normal limits. The inner surface of the rabbit ear presenting the normal appearance of the albino rabbit ear pinna.

Grade 1 – Least detectable response. This response is manifest as an increased prominence of the hair follicles and pilosebaceous units, leading to their slight but perceptible enlargement that can be visualized and detected upon gentle palpation of the ear. This degree of response is commonly seen as part of a nonspecific, mild, and simple irritation which is maintained by the repeated applications of various substances. No particular significance is attached to this degree of response.

Grade 2 – Very slight response. This reaction appears on the inner surface of the ear pinna as a slight enlargement of the hair follicles and pilosebaceous units. Gross examination reveals a slightly roughened surface and a slight increase in thickness of the ear pinna. A very slight, scaly exfoliation may accompany this degree of response, but usually there is no detectable hyperemia or hair loss.

Grade 3 – Slight response. The ear pinna increases in thickness to approximately twice normal and feels stiffened and "leather-like." There is some hyperemia, scaly exfoliation, and hair loss. The hair follicles become slightly enlarged, raised, and hard.

Grade 4 – Moderate response. This reaction consists of a thickening of the ear that is 3–4 times normal. The ear becomes stiff and leathery. The hair follicles on the ear become moderately enlarged, raised, and hard, causing the surface of the ear pinna to feel like coarse sandpaper. The protruding nodules (comedones) can be expressed by gentle pressure or bending of the ear. A slight to moderate hyperemia is usually present. Exfoliation of a granular or scaly type is of moderate intensity. Hair loss is nearly complete. After several weeks the ear pinna is completely denuded of hair, slightly pitted, hyperemic, and possibly exhibiting exfoliation.

Grade 5 - Severe response. The ear pinna becomes thickened to many times normal and appears very stiff, hard, and heavy. Marked hyper-

emia and exfoliation are usually present. The enlarged hair follicles and pilosebaceous units are somewhat buried under the thickened surface. Large masses of keratin may be expressed, leaving pits that may reach 2-3 mm in width. By standard convention, a response of either grade 4 or 5 is considered indicative of a positive comedogenic response for that test substance in the rabbit ear bioassay. A response of grade 0-3 is considered indicative of a negative response.

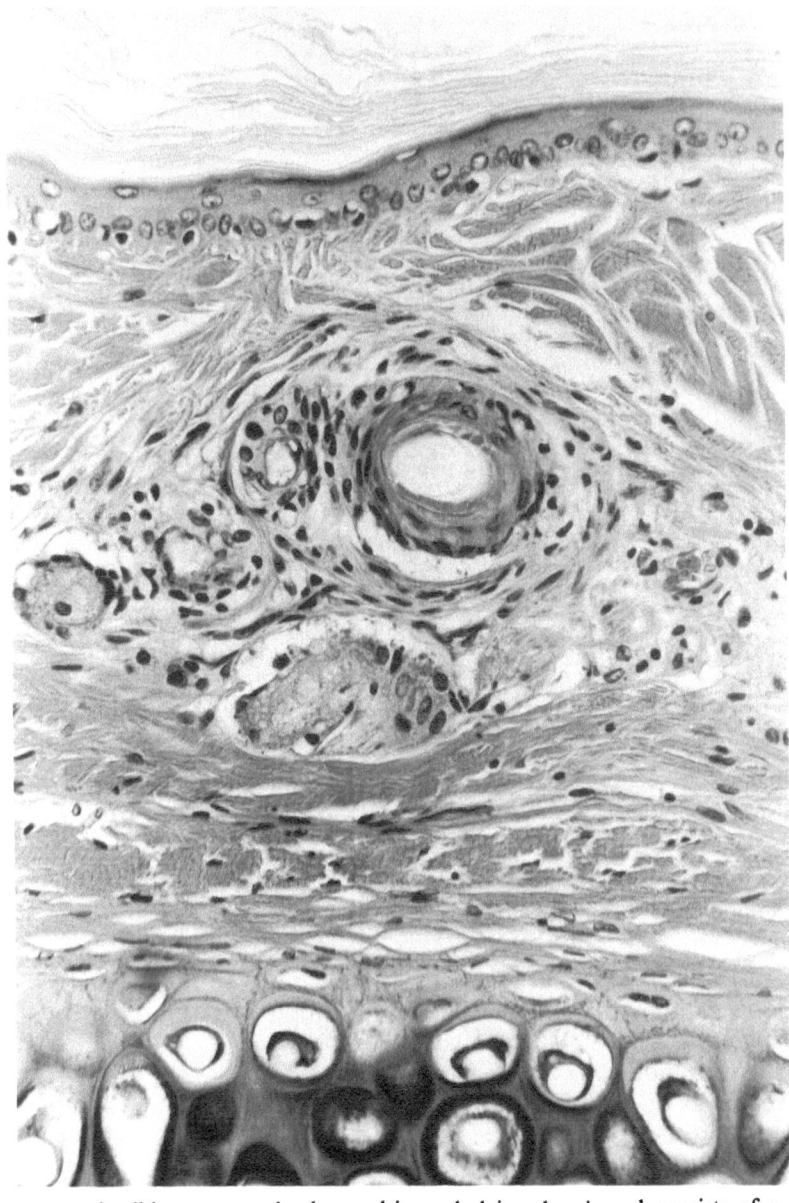

Fig. 194. Concave surface of normal, untreated, albino rabbit ear pinna. Normal thickness and appearance of epidermis, with no rete projections. Pilosebaceous appa-ratus is observed in underlying dermis and consists of a single hair shaft and follicle plus associated sebaceous glands. H and E, × 560

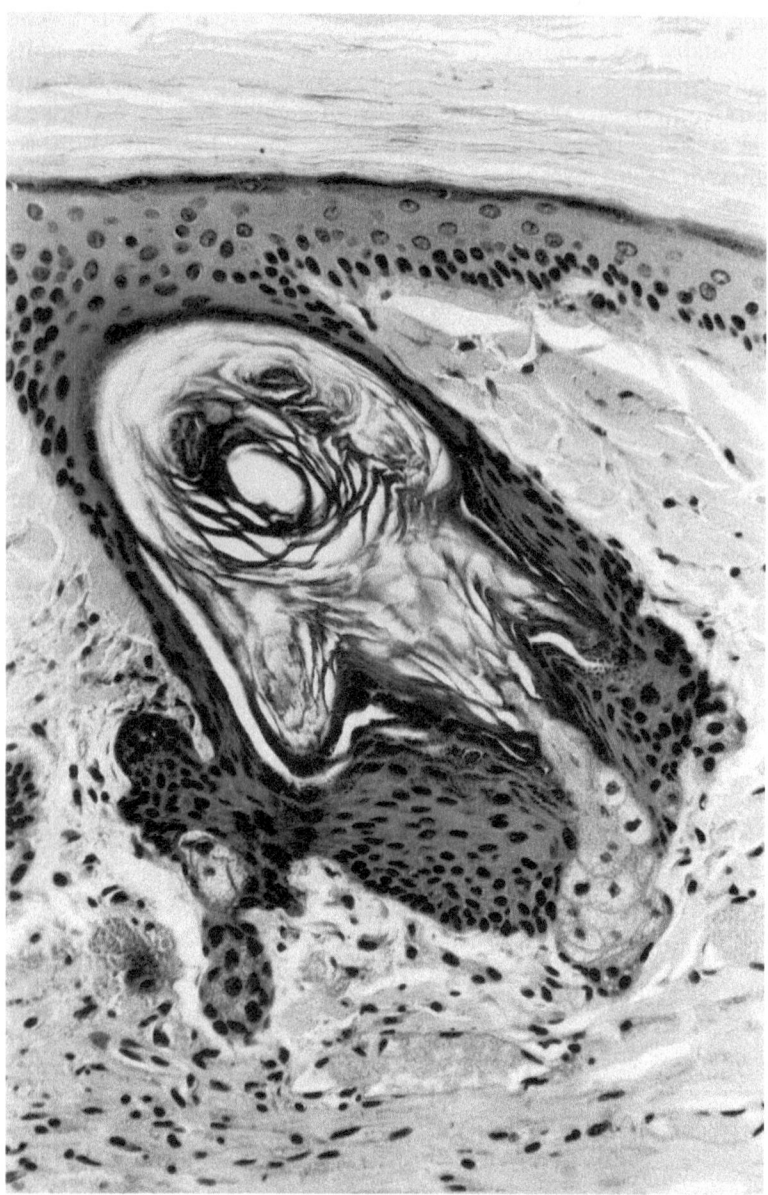

Fig. 195. Treated albino rabbit ear pinna. Depicts hyperplasia and hyperkeratosis occurring mainly in the hair follicle, leading to accumulation of keratotic material surrounding the hair shaft within the follicle. H and E, ×560

Microscopic Features

Normal Untreated Ear. The normal, untreated, albino rabbit ear pinna has on its inner surface an epidermis that is 4–8 cell layers thick, rests on a slightly undulating basement membrane, and is relatively devoid of downward projections of the rete (Fig. 194). The pilosebaceous apparatus is located within the dermis and does not extend into the dense layer of collagen located adjacent to the underlying cartilage. A single hair shaft projects from each follicle at an acute angle and

points caudally. This type of pilosebaceous apparatus which consists of a single hair in a follicle associated with large, complex, sebaceous glands contrasts with the anatomical arrangement of multiple hairs with minute sebaceous glands that are found on the furry skin covering other parts of the rabbit. There are no ceruminous (apocrine) glands in the skin covering the inner surface of the rabbit ear pinna. The sebaceous glands form a dense bed in the dermis surrounding each hair follicle. Multiple acini are located in a circular arrangement around the follicle. These acini

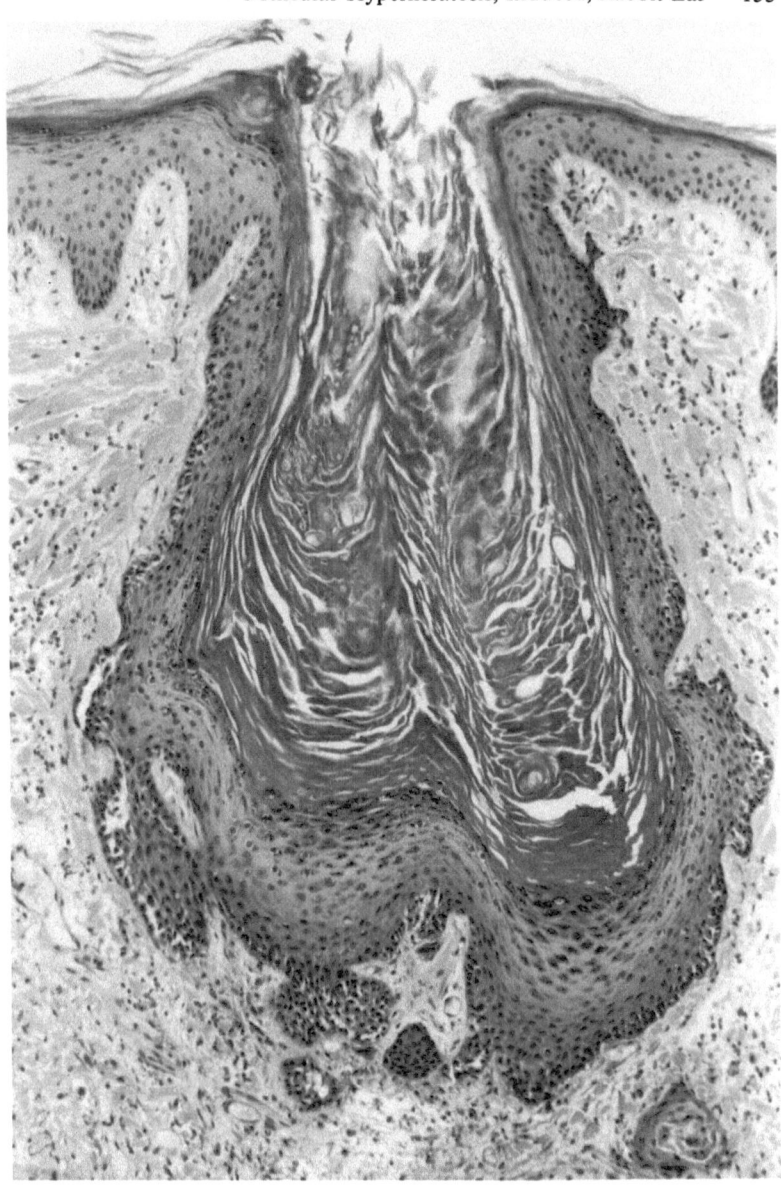

Fig. 196. Treated albino rabbit ear pinna. Depicts more advanced hyperkeratotic lesion leading to further accumulation of keratotic material within the follicle. Epidermal surface is also thickened, with creation of rete projections of hyperplastic epithelium. Dermis contains inflammatory infiltrate adjacent to affected follicle. H and E, ×265

empty into ducts which fuse to form 4 or 5 larger terminal sebaceous ducts which empty into the folicle or directly through the epidermis adjacent to the follicle (Figs. 194 and 195).

Ear Pinna Treated with Acnegenic Test Substance. After several daily applications of a test substance known to induce an acnegenic response, there is a slight thickening of the surface and follicular epithelium. There may be rete projections downward from the hyperplastic surface epithelium. The hyperplastic follicular epithelium spreads outward and downward, engulfing the hair follicle and sebaceous glands (Fig. 195). This epithelial hyperplasia may be accompanied by inflammatory changes in the dermis and subcutis, including congestion, edema, and leukocytic infiltration. The dermis may be slightly thickened, but the underlying cartilage is unchanged.

As the lesion progresses, the rate of hyperplastic proliferation of the surface and follicular epithe-

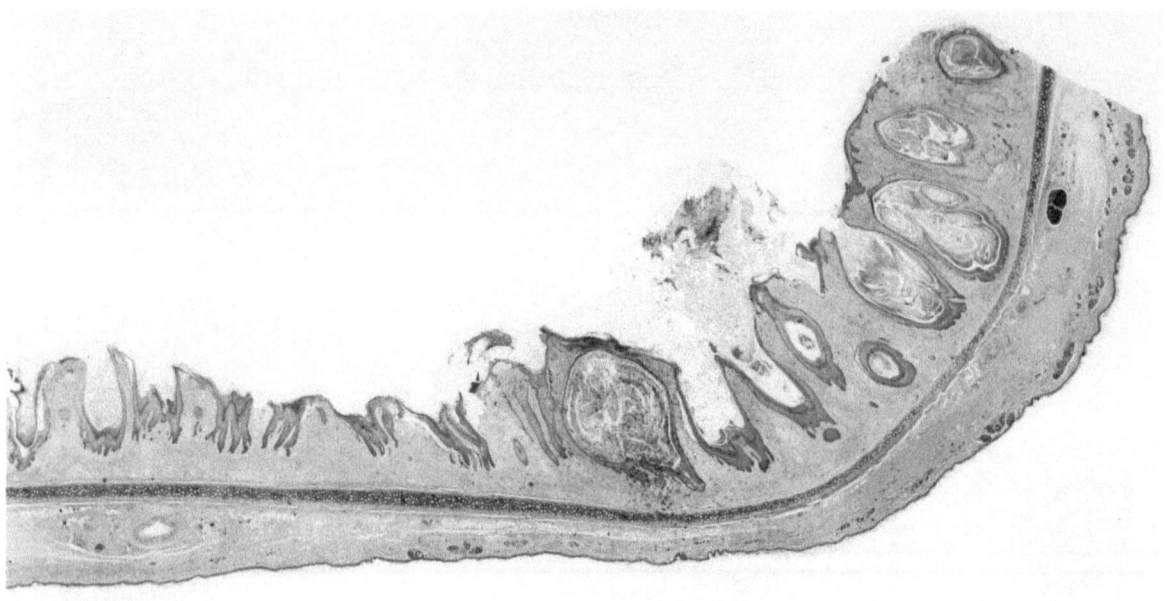

Fig. 197. Rabbit ear pinna, to whose concave surface a test material had been applied that induced a positive comedogenic response. Note the follicular hyperkeratosis and formation of comedones responsible for the roughened concave surface of the ear pinna. H and E, × 10

lium lessens while hyperkeratosis becomes the prevalent feature. The hyperkeratotic hair follicle becomes dilated and filled with a keratinous plug (comedo) Fig. 196. These keratinous plugs can be expressed onto the surface of the epidermis. There may be a diminution of sebaceous gland acini concomitant with the hyperkeratosis of the follicles and sebaceous gland ducts. An inflammatory response of varying degrees may be present, especially if some of the contents of the keratinized comedones has gained access into the adjacent dermis (Fig. 197).

In experiments in which treatment was discontinued, the surface epidermis, follicular epidermis, and sebaceous gland components of the pilosebaceous apparatus gradually returned to normal.

Biologic Features

Topical application of various irritants to the inner surface of the albino rabbit ear pinna can induce a follicular hyperkeratosis and keratinous cyst (comedo) formation that is readily discernible upon gross examination. This is the basis upon which the rabbit ear bioassay has been used as a laboratory animal model useful in the study of compounds known or suspected of inducing in humans a follicular hyperkeratosis described

clinically as an acneform dermatosis or chloracne. The clinical term chloracne was originally based on the historical observations made on industrial workers with excessive exposure to various chlorinated compounds, such as chloronaphthalenes and polychlorinated biphenyls.

The standard convention followed in the use of the rabbit ear bioassay involves the repeated inunction of the test substance (in an appropriate vehicle) directly onto the inner surface of the pinna of the rabbit ear, with the contralateral ear serving as a vehicle or untreated control site. A total of 20 applications are typically made five times weekly for 4 weeks, during which time the ear is examined for evidence of follicular hyperkeratosis and formation of comedones.

Comparison with Other Species

Follicular hyperkeratosis and formation of comedones by the pilosebaceous apparatus of the rabbit ear pinna has been used historically as a laboratory animal bioassay to detect the presence or absence of substances suspected of acnegenic activity in certain industrial work environments (Adams et al. 1941; Hambrick and Blank 1956). Some of these same substances have also been used in the experimental production of acne on the skin of humans (Shelley and Kligman 1957; Hambrick 1957). These comparative studies in rabbits and humans have indicated basic similarities in the formation of the follicular hyperkeratosis leading to comedo formation. The studies of Hambrick (1957) should be consulted for a specific discussion of the comparative aspects of the basic lesions in human skin and rabbit ear pinna.

The rhesus monkey can exhibit skin lesions, including folliculitis and acneform eruptions, after systemic treatment with certain chlorinated dioxins (McConnell et al. 1978). Distension of the meibomian glands of the eyelids has been reported to be a highly characteristic response. Hairless mice have also been reported to show hyperkeratosis of the skin following administration of certain chlorinated biphenyl compounds.

In cattle, a syndrome originally described by Olafson (1947) as "X disease" or bovine hyperkeratosis was experimentally produced with a chlorinated naphthalene (Sikes and Bridges 1952). This syndrome included a severe hyperkeratosis of the skin and hair follicles (Jones and Hunt 1983). Overall, the rabbit ear bioassay is considered the most useful and well-defined laboratory animal model for the assessment of the comedogenic potential of test materials.

References

Adams EM, Irish DD, Spencer HC, Rowe VK (1941) The response of rabbit skin to compounds reported to have caused acneform dermatitis. Indust Med 10: 1–4

Hambrick GW Jr, Blank MD (1956) A microanatomical study of the response of the pilosebaceous apparatus of the rabbit's ear canal. J Invest Dermatol 26: 185–200

Hambrick GW (1957) The effect of substituted naphthalenes on the pilosebaceous apparatus of rabbit and man. J Invest Dermatol 28: 89–103

Jones TC, Hunt RD (1983) Veterinary pathology, 5th edn. Lea and Febiger, Philadelphia, pp 901–1030

McConnell EE, Moore JA, Dalgard DW (1978) Toxicity of 2,3,7,8-tetrachlorodibenzo-p-dioxin in Rhesus monkeys (Macaca mulatta) following a single oral dose. Toxicol Appl Pharmacol 43: 175–187

Olafson P (1947) Hyperkeratosis (X-disease) of cattle. Cornell Vet 37: 279–291

Shelley WB, Kligman AM (1957) The experimental production of acne by penta- and hexachloronaphthalenes. Arch Dermatol 75: 689–695

Sikes D, Bridges ME (1952) Experimental production of hyperkeratosis ("X-disease") of cattle with a chlorinated naphthalene. Science 116: 506–507

Mousepox, Skin, Mouse

Anton M. Allen and Allan Lock

Synonym. Infectious ectromelia.

Gross Appearance

The principal route of ectromelia virus infection is through the broken skin at sites of abrasions. The virus replicates at the initial infection site and produces an erosive, encrusted lesion which becomes noticeable after 5-7 days. It is termed a primary lesion (Fenner 1947, 1948a) and is usually the first sign of infection. Such lesions may occur anywhere on the body but are more often observed on the head (Fig. 198) and feet. When present on an extremity, especially the foot, there may be severe cutaneous edema (Fig. 199). This occasionally leads to tissue ischemia, gangrene, and autoamputation; hence the use of the term "infectious ectromelia" by Marchal (1930), who first described the disease. The primary lesion provides the source of virus which infects the mouse internally, eventually leading to hematogenous dissemination and widespread development of secondary skin lesions. These lesions, which collectively are called the secondary rash or exanthem, become clearly visible on about the 10th or 11th day after infection. They resemble the primary lesions except that they develop a few days later and at many sites. Fenner (1948a) has shown that the rash may be detected as early as the 8th day in experimentally infected mice that are shaven. He states that the rash is "... first detected by feeling small lumps in the skin of the back when it is picked up between the index finger and the thumb." The rash then becomes visible as pale macules which quickly become papular and undergo ulceration (Figs. 200-202). The papules vary from a few millimeters in diameter to large coalescent ones.

Despite the seemingly predictable and characteristic appearance of the skin lesions, it should be realized that they can easily go unnoticed. The body rash may be hidden from view under the

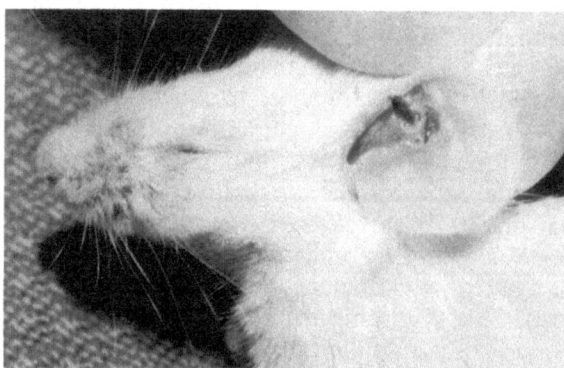

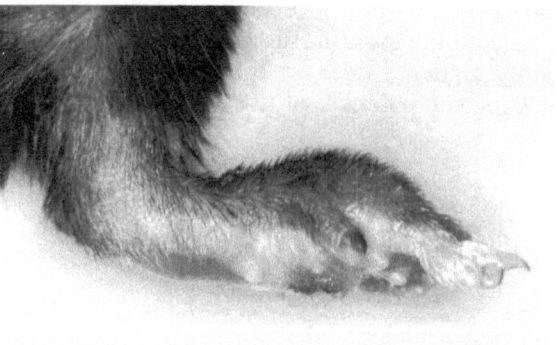

Fig. 198 *(above).* Primary skin lesion of mouse pox, ear, BALB/cAnN mouse; infection was acquired by contact exposure

Fig. 199 *(below).* Swollen rear foot of a C57/BL/6N mouse 11 days after inoculation of the footpad with ectromelia virus

hair (Fig. 201), and other more visible lesions on the head or extremities may be mistaken for bite wounds or other scabbed-over injuries. Also, certain of the more resistant strains of mice such as C57BL may fail to show a rash or any other clinical signs of illness (Wallace and Buller 1985; Jacoby and Bhatt 1987). Highly susceptible mice may die of acute infection before the appearance of the rash. When present, the skin lesions are more likely to signal mousepox if observed in

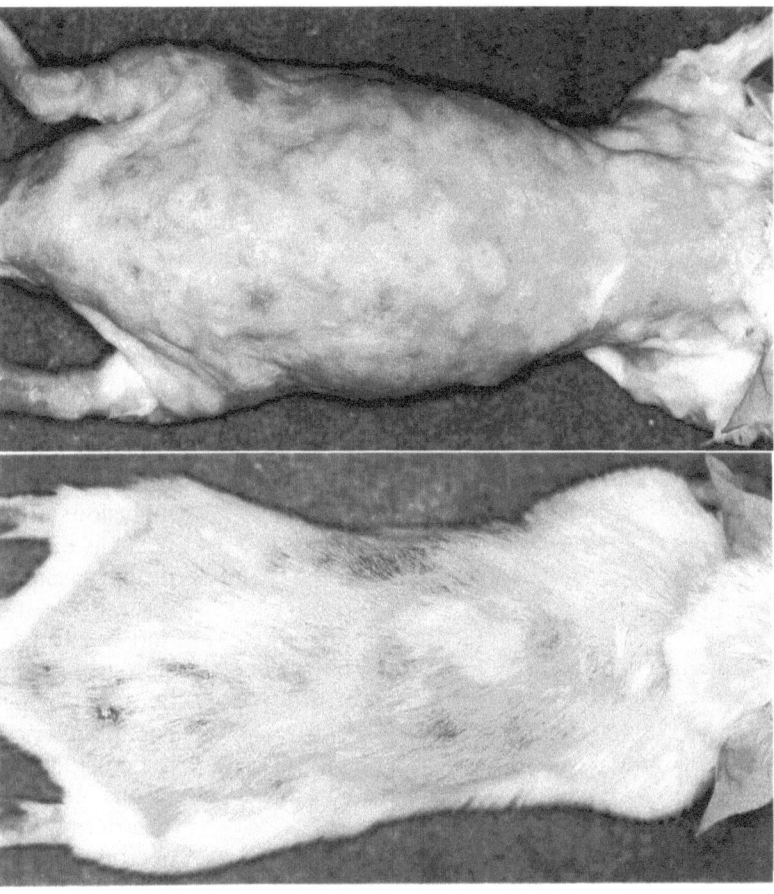

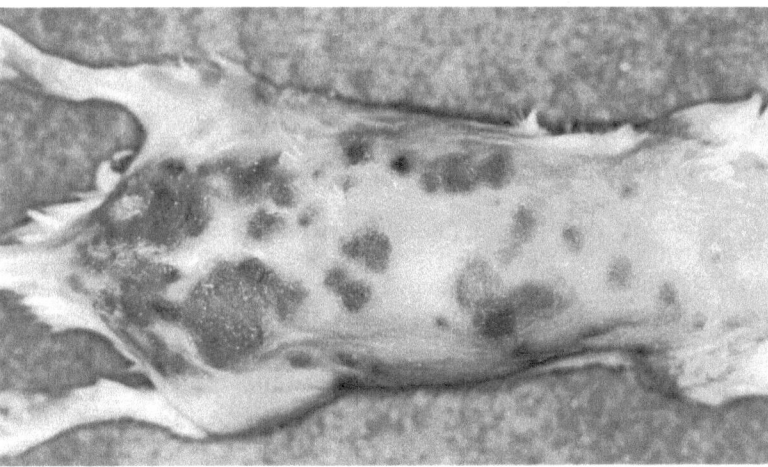

Fig. 200 *(above).* Secondary maculopapular lesions with beginning ulceration on the back of a N:GP(s) mouse 10 days after footpad inoculation of approximately 50 virions. Hair removed with a commercial depilatory agent.

Fig. 201 *(middle).* Secondary skin lesions on the back of a BALB/cAnN mouse as observed through partially clipped superficial hair

Fig. 202 *(below).* Same mouse as Fig. 201 after removal of the hair with a depilatory agent, revealing severe, ulcerative, maculopapular scarification of the lower back

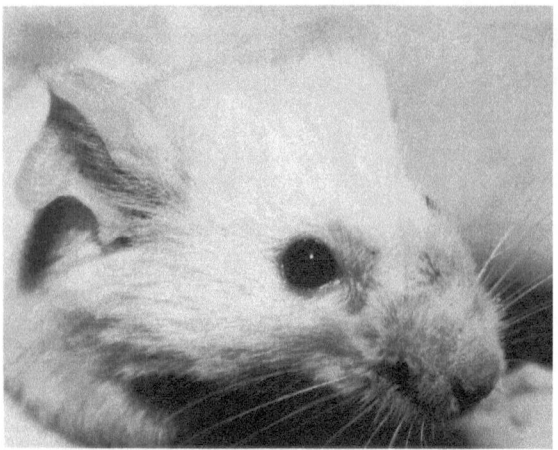

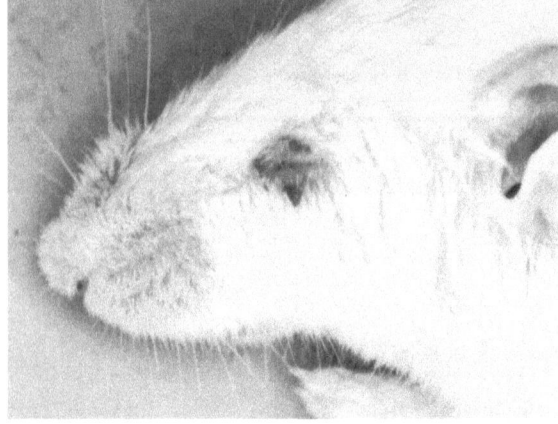

Fig. 203 *(above)*. Facial edema and exudative "sticky" conjunctivitis 11 days after inoculation with ectromelia virus by epidermal scarification of the lower back

Fig. 204 *(below)*. Focal periocular alopecia in a surviving BALB/cAnN mouse

concert with other signs such as increased mortality or morbidity characterized by lethargy, facial edema, and conjunctivitis (Fig. 203). In surviving mice, the lesions begin to heal within a few days. Scarring of the dermis at sites of more severe lesions sometimes leads to permanent, focal alopecia (Fig. 204) (Fenner 1948a, b).

Microscopic Features

In the experimentally infected mouse, the primary skin lesion begins as a few infected dermal and epidermal cells near the site of inoculation, as may be shown by immunofluorescent methods (Roberts 1962). The infected cells in the dermis appear to be macrophages and fibrocytes. Within a few days the number of infected dermal cells

increases dramatically while the epidermal infection extends slowly by lateral spread to contiguous cells. The dermis and adjacent subcutaneous tissues become edematous and increasingly infiltrated by lymphocytes and macrophages. The overlying epidermis increases in thickness due to swelling and/or hyperplasia of the epithelial cells. Many of the cells develop large eosinophilic cytoplasmic inclusion bodies (Marchal bodies) which Kato (1955) has designated as type A inclusions. They are also found in hair follicle epithelium and sebaceous gland cells after 2–3 days. On or about the 5th to 7th day after inoculation many of the infected epidermal cells become vacuolated and distended. The vacuoles merge to form a clear space in the cytoplasm around the inclusions. The epidermis then undergoes rapid necrosis and ulceration. It is at this stage that the primary lesions of either experimental or natural disease are more likely to be noticed clinically and examined histologically. The microscopic lesion usually seen is an epidermal erosion covered by a scab which overlies an area of necrotic and edematous dermis and subcutis. At the edges of the erosion, the epidermis is thickened, and a few of the cells usually contain type A inclusions. The dermis contains cellular debris, remnants of necrotic hair follicles and sebaceous glands, and many phagocytes. The affected area of the dermis is usually much larger than the epidermal lesion. However, there may be fairly extensive areas of epidermal hyperplasia adjacent to the erosions in which no inclusions or immunohistochemical evidence of viral antigen is present. According to Roberts (1962), "the hyperplasia in mouse epidermis resulting from ectromelia infection occurs in an annulus of normal cells just beyond the advancing margin of infected cells." In mice that survived the infection, the scab drops off, the epidermis repairs, and the dermal structures are largely replaced by scar tissue (Fenner 1948a, c).

In contrast to the primary lesions, the secondary lesions result from hematogenous spread of the

Fig. 205 *(above)*. Type A inclusions *(arrows)* in large, ▶ hydropic, "ballooned" cells of hyperplastic epidermis. H and E, ×850

Fig. 206 *(below)*. Secondary skin lesion, N:GP(s) mouse, showing extensive epidermal necrosis, beginning separation of the necrotic layer, and hyperplasia of the bordering epidermis. Despite necrosis of the hair follicles and sebaceous glands, there is only moderate inflammatory cell reaction in this dermis. H and E, ×250

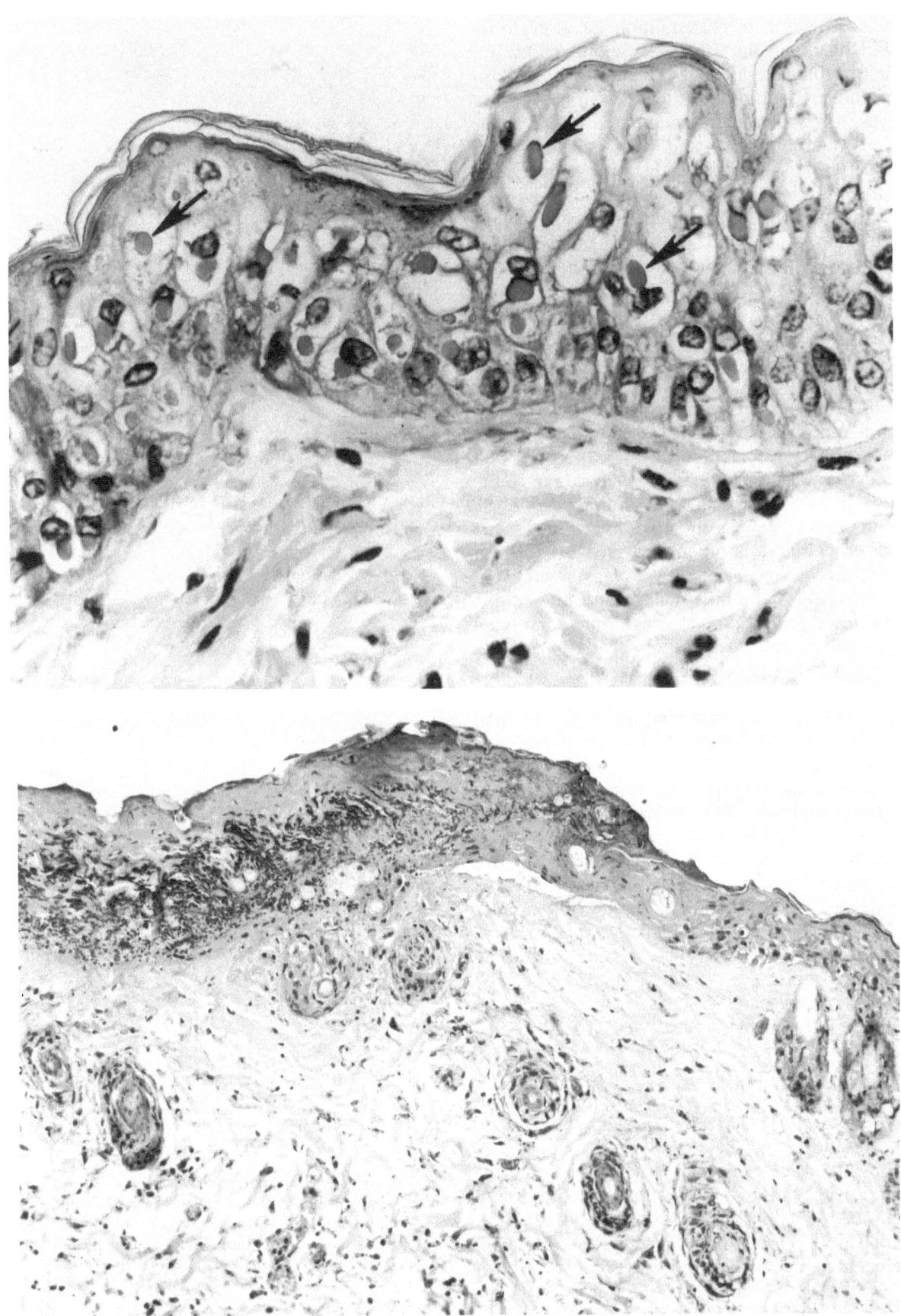

virus. The virus reaches multiple locations in the skin on about the 7th day after infection. The first histologic evidence is focal mild hyperplasia of the epidermis and slight swelling of basal cells, a few of which may contain type A inclusions. During the 8th and 9th days the areas of hyperplasia and edema become more widespread, and inclusion bodies extend to all noncornified layers of the epidermis and to cells of the hair follicles and sebaceous glands. Thickened areas of the epidermis correspond to the maculopapular rash observed clinically. Since different foci of infection are initiated in the skin over a 2–3 day period, various stages of lesion development may be observed at a given time. On about the 10th day many of the epidermal cells in these areas become distended and develop a zone of clear cytoplasm around the type A inclusion (Fig. 105). Shortly thereafter the cells undergo necrosis (Fig. 206). Necrosis may occur also in the epidermal cells prior to significant ballooning. The necrotic epidermis sloughs and the eroded area is quickly covered by a serous scab. According to Fenner (1948a, 1949) the dermis usually shows little change until the epidermal ulceration begins, at which time it becomes edematous and infiltrated by lymphocytes. In survivors, the epithelium grows back quickly under the scabs, and the dermis gradually returns to normal except that at sites of severe lesions; hair follicles and sebaceous glands are replaced by scar tissue.

In transmission studies following an outbreak of ectromelia at the National Institutes of Health in 1979, we found relatively mild inflammatory infiltrates in the dermis of 4–6-month-old BALB/c AnN and N:GP (s) mice, despite the presence of extensive necrosis (unpublished observations). The reactive cells were mixed and consisted mainly of mononuclear macrophages, small lymphocytes, and a few neutrophils. Small type A inclusions were found in some of the macrophages (Fig. 207) and in many fibrocytes (Fig. 208). Relatively large inclusions occurred in fibroblasts in areas of beginning fibroplasia. Viral antigen was readily demonstrated with the immunoperoxidase procedure (ABC method) in virtually all macrophages and in 50%–75% of fibrocytes at about the time epidermal structures became necrotic. The antigen usually appears as fine granular material either distributed throughout the cytoplasm or in small foci. The granules are considered to be individual virions. Because of their large size, pox virions may be observed with the light microscope if stained to contrast with the

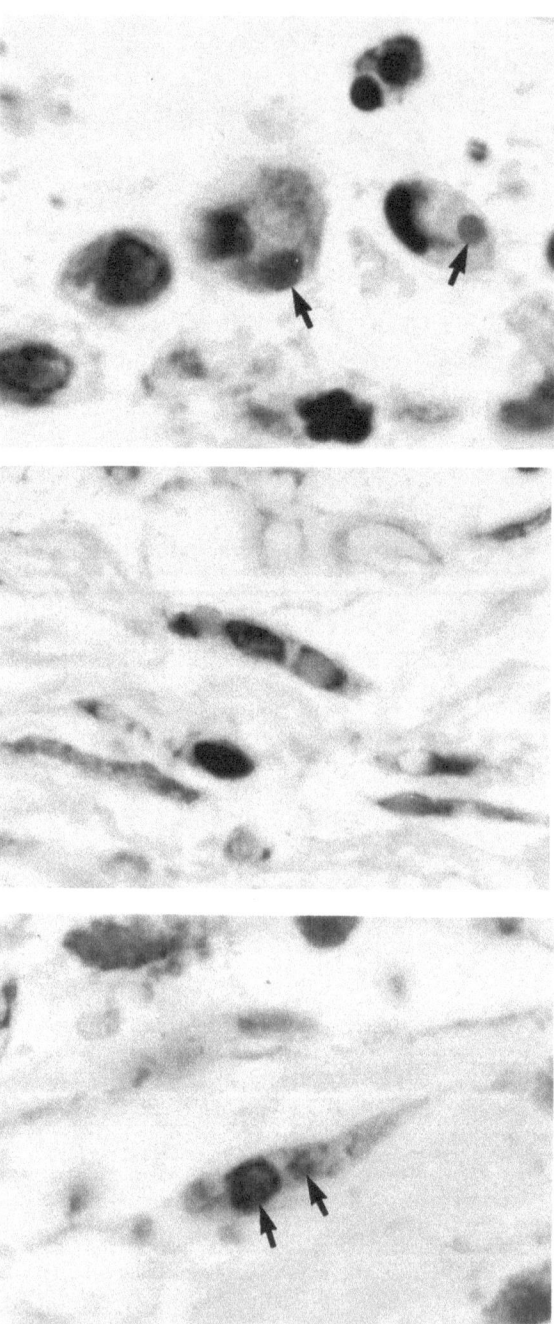

Fig. 207 (above). Two macrophages each containing a small type A inclusion (arrows). H and E, × 1800

Fig. 208 (middle). Fibrocyte containing two type A inclusions. H and E, × 1250

Fig. 209 (below). Circular aggregates (one large and one small, arrows) of ectromelia viral antigen corresponding to type B inclusions in the cytoplasm of a fibroblast. Avidin-biotin conjugate, immunoperoxidase method, × 1800

host cell cytoplasm. In fibrocytes, the granular antigen is occasionally in the form of circular aggregates (Fig. 209) similar to those that form around type B inclusions in ectromelia-infected hepatocytes (Allen et al. 1981). Small amounts of antigen are observed in endothelial cell cytoplasm in a few veins and capillaries. Mast cells in the edematous lesions often appear to be disrupted. Many of these changes in the dermal and subcutaneous tissues were described also by Marchal (1930) and Roberts (1962).

Two types of cytoplasmic inclusions are found. The type A inclusions already mentioned are brightly eosinophilic bodies with a glassy appearing texture. When fully formed they tend to be ovoid and measure up to 10×20 µm. They become especially prominent when cells begin to swell as the inclusions are surrounded by a clear space (Fig. 205). In contrast, the type B inclusions are small, indistinct, basophilic bodies which in our experience are very difficult to demonstrate in the basophilic cytoplasm of epidermal cells. They are more easily observed in cells with abundant acidophilic cytoplasm such as hepatocytes. There they appear as ill-defined basophilic foci, 2 to 6 µm in diameter, located randomly in the cytoplasm. With hematoxylin and eosin stain they may be rendered more distinct by doubling the hematoxylin staining time (Allen et al. 1981; Jacoby 1985). This procedure does not help to demonstrate type B inclusions in epidermal cells. However, small foci of viral antigen which are considered to be sites of the type B inclusions may be shown with immunohistochemical procedures. These foci are visible when the epidermal cells are first infected, before antigen is widely dispersed in the cytoplasm (Fig. 210). When hydropic vacuoles begin to develop in epidermal cells, much of the cytoplasm containing the antigen is compressed against the cell membrane (Fig. 211). This produces the clear space around the type A inclusions. A small amount of antigen is usually present on the surface of the type A inclusion and may also be found in slender threads of cytoplasm compressed between the expanding vacuoles. Ordinarily antigen is not found within the type A inclusions. An exception to this was described in studies of the Hampstead strain of ectromelia virus (Ichihashi and Matsumoto 1966).

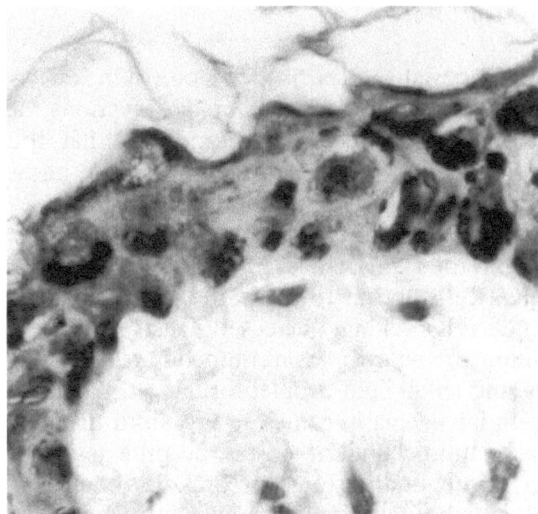

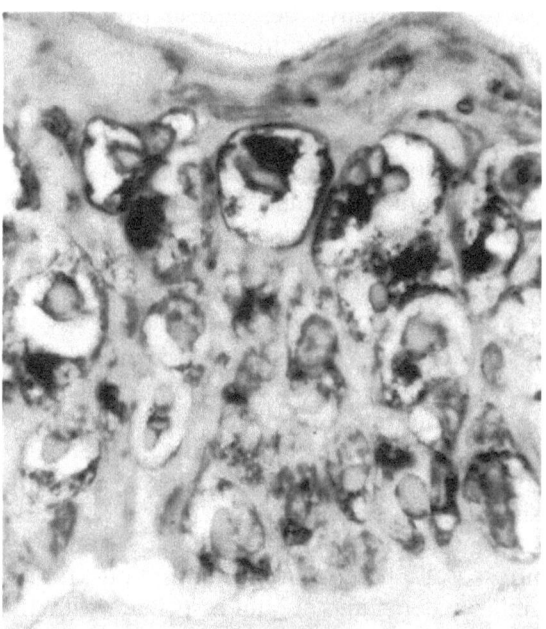

Fig. 210 *(above).* Dense foci of ectromelia viral antigen corresponding to type B inclusions in early infection of the epidermis. Avidin-biotin conjugate, immunoperoxidase method, × 1250

Fig. 211 *(below).* Hyperplastic epidermis with hydropic balloon cells. Ectromelia antigen is contained in the cytoplasm which is compressed against the cell membrane, and a small amount appears to be adherent to the surface of the type A inclusions. Avidin-biotin conjugate, immunoperoxidase method, × 1250

Ultrastructure

Ultrastructural studies of mousepox skin lesions have not been reported. Our observations of experimentally infected mice indicate that the principal targets in the epidermis are the basal and spinous cells. These cells undergo more severe infection and cellular changes than those closer to the skin surface. In fact, the keratinized corneal cells appear to be spared. Early changes include cell swelling, decreased density and vesiculation of the cytoplasm, mitochondrial dilatation, and small lipid droplet formation. Later, intracellular edema becomes severe, lipid droplets enlarge, mitochondrial cristae become less distinct, mitochondria fragment, and abnormal parallel membranous lamellae develop. There appears to be a relative decrease in cytoplasmic tonofilaments, and their normal perinuclear distribution is disrupted. Eventually the desmosomes separate and dissolve, the plasma membrane becomes discontinuous, and the basal cells detach from the underlying basal lamina. In addition, the nucleus contracts, the chromatin clumps and increases in density, and electron-dense debris accumulates in the nucleoplasm (Fig. 212).

As the cellular changes occur, type A and type B inclusions appear in the cytoplasm of infected keratinocytes. The type A inclusions, which are easily demonstrated by light microscopy, are even more obvious ultrastructurally. Infected keratinocytes contain single or multiple type A inclusions. The inclusions are generally ovoid, vary in size, and are not membrane bound. They are composed of a homogeneous, amorphous, finely granular material and are not associated with virus formation (Figs. 212 and 213).

In the skin, type B inclusions are visible only with electron microscopy and immunohistochemistry. The ultrastructural morphology of type B inclusions in keratocytes is consistent with their description in hepatocytes by Leduc and Bernhard (1962). Type B inclusions are usually smaller than type A inclusions. They vary greatly in shape and tend to have an irregular border. They are composed of a granular and fibrillar matrix mixed with ribosomes (Figs. 213 and 214). Various developmental stages of viral particles are found on the periphery of these matrices. Initially, C-shaped, trilaminar, membranous structures containing some matrix or viroplasm are formed. These structures develop into circular bodies filled with viroplasmic matrix (Figs. 213 and 214). Then the immature viral particle becomes ovoid, a portion of the viroplasm condenses, and an eccentric, electron-dense nucleoid develops. Finally, the membrane-bound nucleoid differentiates into a dense, biconcave, dumbbell-shaped, nuclear core that is characteristic of a mature poxvirus (Fig. 215). The mature virions are ovoid and approximately 262×162 nm. Our observations indicate that the developmental cycle of ectromelia virus in keratinocytes is similar to that reported for smallpox (Avakyan and Byckovsky 1965) and vaccinia viruses (Morgan 1976).

Additional cell types in the skin can be infected and exhibit degenerative changes. For example, smaller numbers of mature virions and smaller type A and type B inclusions are found in hair follicle and sebaceous gland epithelia. In the dermis many fibroblasts contain large type A inclusions, smaller type B inclusions, and small numbers of mature virions. The type A inclusions in fibrocytes tend to be smaller than those in fibroblasts. A few of the macrophages examined contain small type A inclusions and small numbers of mature virions. Several virions may be noted in the cytoplasm of mast cells and capillary endothelial cells; no inclusions are usually observed.

Although ultrastructural examination is useful, it is not essential for the diagnosis of ectromelia infection; it is, however, crucial for studying the cellular pathogenesis of the infection and the ontogenesis of the virus.

Differential Diagnosis

Several clinically observed skin lesions of mice must be distinguished from mousepox lesions. These include abrasions, bite wounds, and lesions associated with mite or fungal infections and exudative conjunctivitis. In no other spontaneous disease of mice are large epidermal type A inclusions found. The inclusions are observed also in affected conjunctiva and periocular skin, where infection is often so severe that permanent periocular alopecia results (in mice that survive). Any number of bacteria may infect the skin of the foot or tail of a mouse and result in acute swelling, and in rare instances cause necrosis and autoamputation, as occurs in 5%-10% of mousepox cases. Autoamputation has been observed in epizootic proportion in at least two ectromelia-free mouse colonies in which *Corynebacterium kutscheri* was repeatedly isolated from the infected limbs (Allen et al. 1981). Since

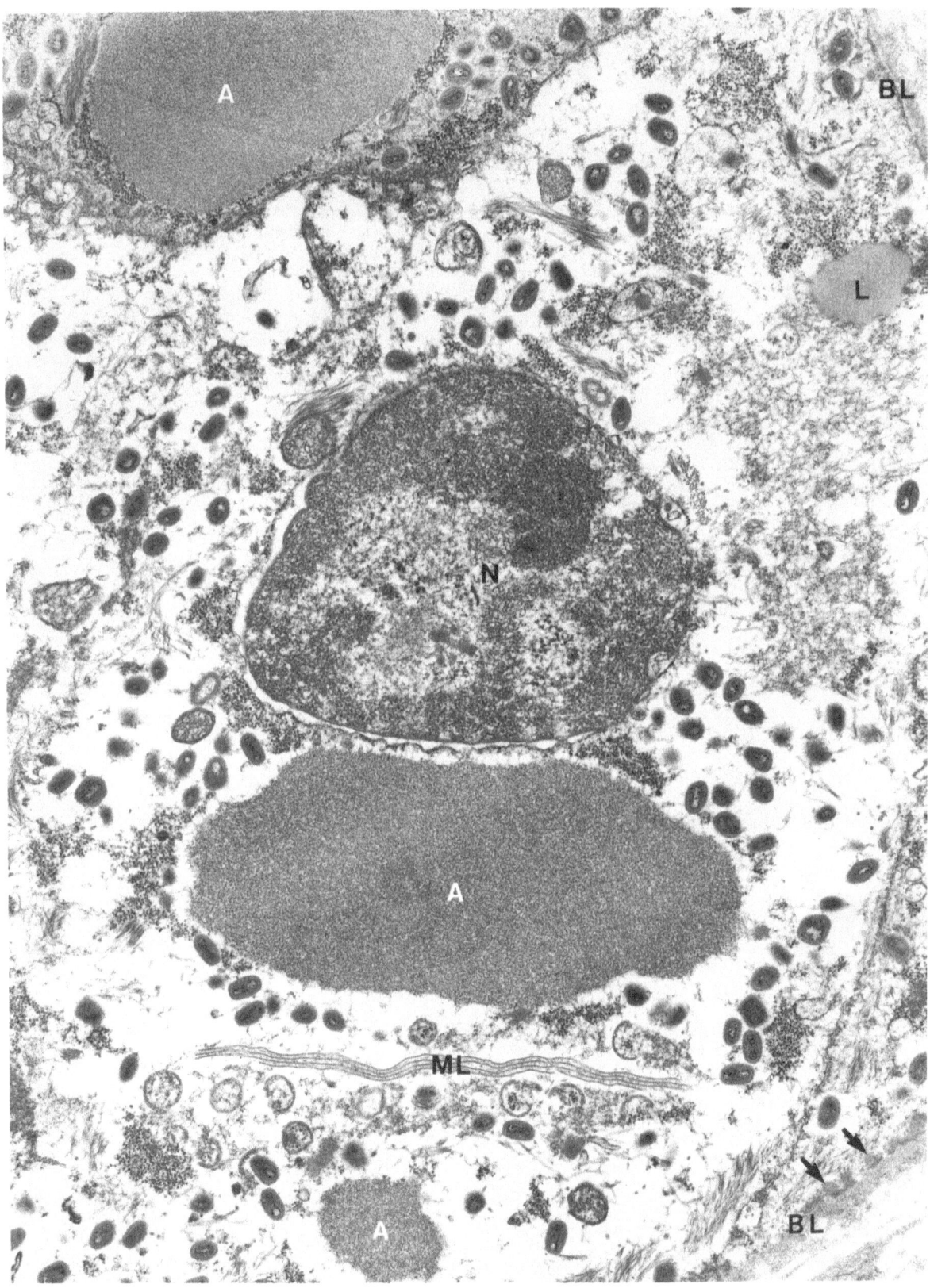

Fig. 212. Damaged ectromelia-infected basal cell. Note intracellular edema, sparse and widely scatterd tonofilaments, membranous lamellae *(ML)*, small lipid droplet *(L)*, dense nucleus *(N)*, and hemidesmosomes *(arrows)* attached to the basal lamina *(BL)*. Also note development stages of virus and type A inclusions *(A)*. TEM, ×19800

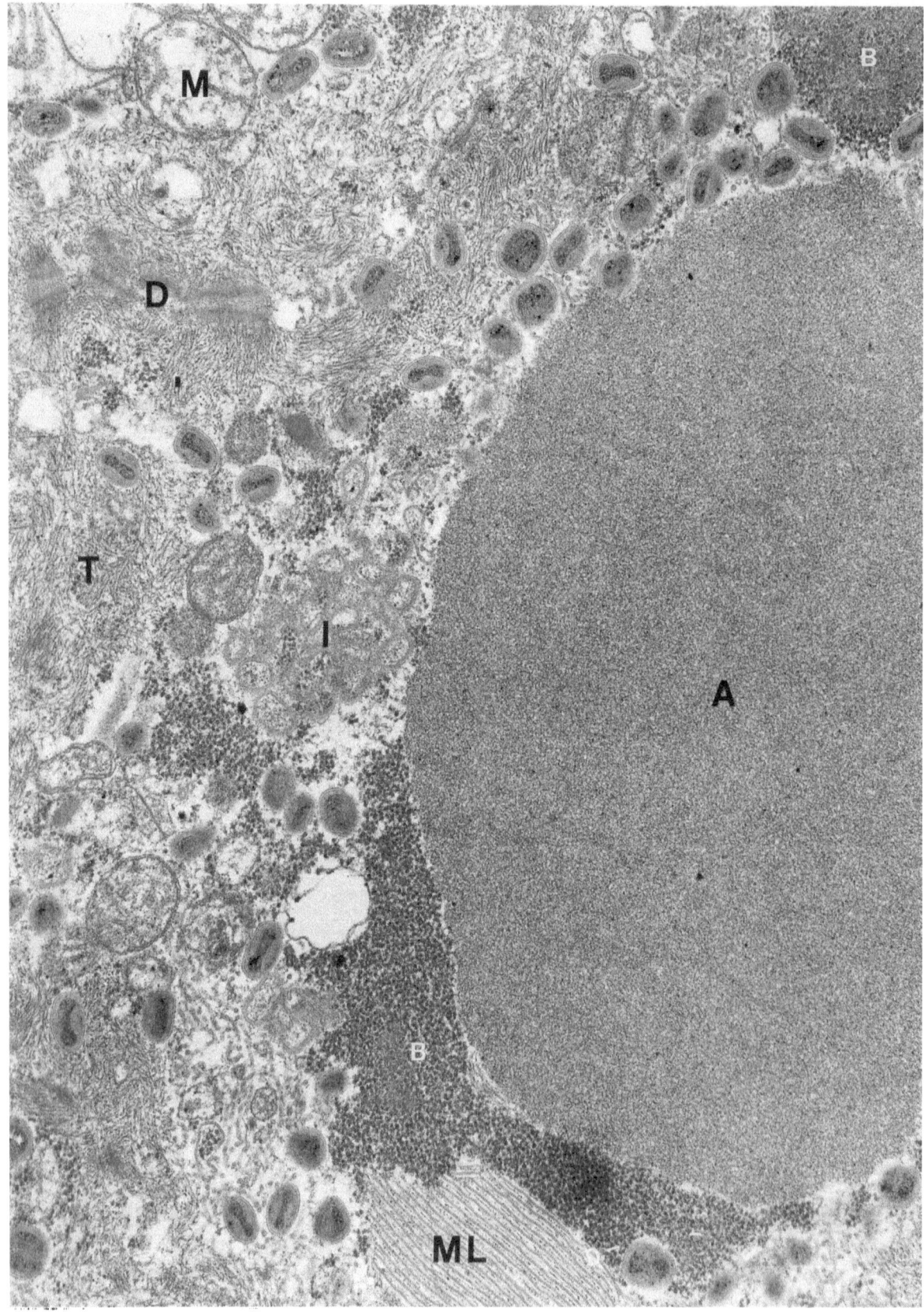

Fig. 213. Ectromelia-infected keratinocyte with large type A inclusion *(A)*, smaller type B inclusions *(B)*, immature viral particles *(I)*, and dispersed mature virions. Note membranous lamellae *(ML)*, swollen mitochondria *(M)*, tonofilaments *(T)*, and desmosomes *(D)*. TEM, ×36000

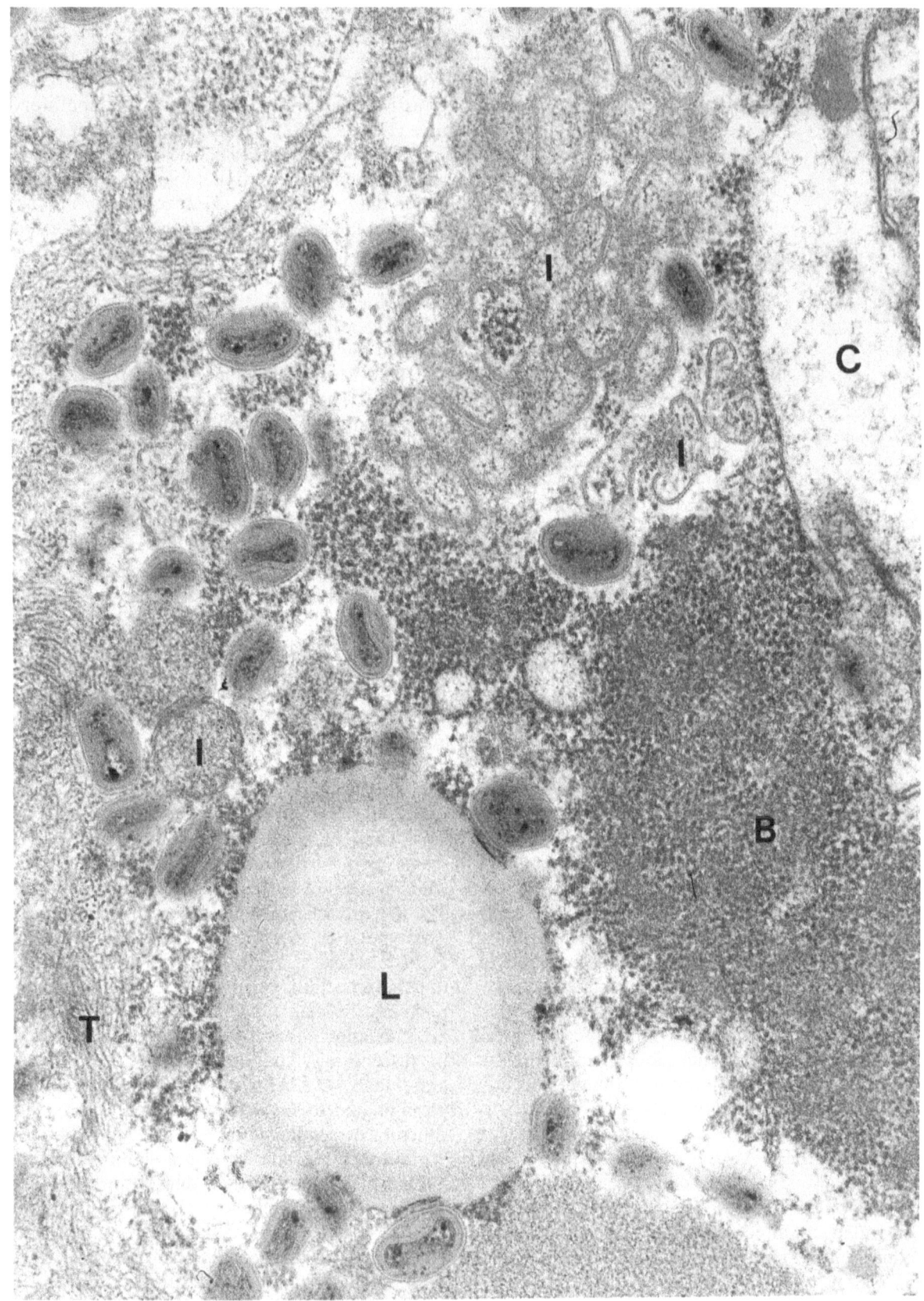

Fig. 214. Higher magnification of immature viral particles *(I)*, mature virions, and type B inclusion *(B)*, which is composed of a granular and reticular matrix with entrapped ribosomes. Note lipid droplet *(L)*, tonofilaments *(T)*, and dilated cisterna *(C)*. TEM, ×62000

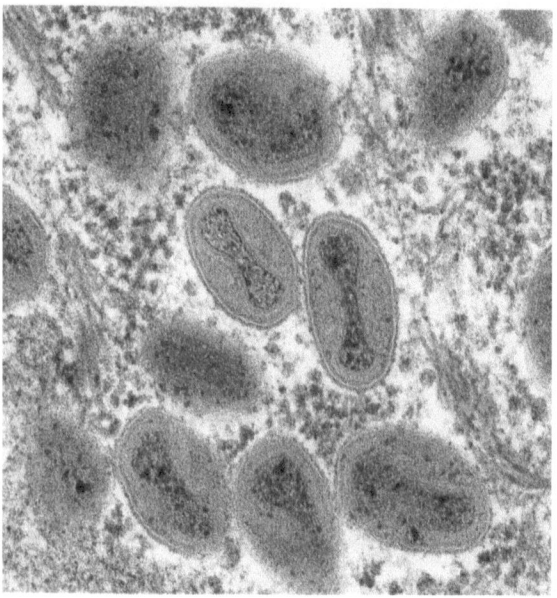

Fig. 215. Mature ectromelia virions with characteristic, electron-dense, biconcave, dumbbell-shaped nuclear core. TEM, × 78 000

loss of a limb occurs relatively late in the course of mousepox. the characteristic microscopic lesions with typical inclusions may no longer be present. Serologic testing is a more reliable means of diagnosis at this stage.

The hemagglutination inhibition (HI), enzyme-linked, immunosorbent assay (ELISA) and immunofluorescent antibody (IFA) tests are commonly used (Buller et al. 1983). Various other confirmatory diagnostic procedures are employed during the acute stages of the disease, depending on equipment and technical capabilities available. For example, the demonstration of severe splenic necrosis at necropsy gives strong presumptive evidence of mousepox. The histopathology of acute disease in susceptible strains of mice is usually diagnostic. The characteristic lesions include severe necrosis of lymph nodes, spleen, Peyer's patches, thymus, and often the liver as well as type A inclusions in epithelium of the skin, conjunctiva, intestines, vagina, and other locations. The large typical pox virion is easily demonstrated in acute stage lesions with electron microscopy. The virus can be isolated on the chorioallantoic membrane of hen's eggs and in a variety of cell cultures. Viral antigen can be demonstrated in affected tissues by immunohistochemical methods (Allen et al. 1981, 1986; Jacoby 1985).

Biologic Features

Mousepox is a disease of the laboratory mouse. However, it may occur in the wild house mouse in association with an outbreak in laboratory mice (Fenner 1982). Serologic evidence of infection in *Apodemus,* several voles, and woodmice has been reported (Gröppel 1962; Kaplan et al. 1980), but as noted by Fenner, these findings could be due to cross-reactions with other orthopoxviruses. Naturally occurring mousepox has been found in laboratory mice in many countries worldwide. Parodoxically, it has not been reported in Australia where much of the experimental work on the infection has been performed (Fenner 1982; Mims 1959, 1966; Blanden and Gardner 1976). The causative agent is ectromelia virus, a member of the genus orthopoxvirus, which includes variola, vaccinia, cowpox, and others.

In a series of classical studies published in the late 1940s, Fenner very accurately described the pathogenesis of mousepox in highly susceptible outbred mice. To summarize, the virus normally invades through the broken skin where it replicates and produces a primary skin lesion. The draining lymph node becomes infected, which seeds virus into its efferent lymphatics and into the bloodstream to produce a primary viremia. The virus is carried to lymph nodes systemically and to visceral organs, especially the spleen and liver, where it further replicates and causes organ necrosis. If the mouse survives this stage, a secondary viremia disseminates virus to the skin, resulting in the secondary skin rash and conjunctivitis. The extent of viral replication in the liver seems to be a significant factor in determining whether the mouse survives (Fenner 1949, 1982).

The lethality of mousepox varies with the mouse genotype. For example, the BALB/C, A, and DBA/2 strains are considered to be susceptible to lethal infection, whereas the C57BL strains are relatively resistant (Wallace et al. 1985). There are indications as well that substrain differences in susceptibility may exist (Buller 1985; Bhatt and Jacoby 1987a). Considerable evidence has accumulated to show that resistance is largely a function of cellular immunity and that antibody is produced too late to have a significant effect except in resisting lethal reinfection (Blanden and Gardner 1976; Tsuru et al. 1983). Buller et al. (1987a, b) have shown that survivability of infected mice is unaffected by procedures which inhibit production of neutralizing antibody.

Lethality of infection is affected also by the route of inoculation and dose of virus. Intraperitoneal inoculation with relatively high doses is most lethal (Fenner 1949; Jacoby and Bhatt 1987). Footpad inoculation is often used when the intent is to mimic natural infection. Intragastric inoculation results in longer incubation, lower mortality, and increased duration of virus shedding as compared with the footpad method (Wallace and Buller 1985). Fenner (1949) reported that the age of mice affects lethality of infection. Suckling mice and year-old adults were found to be more susceptible than 8-week-old mice. Fenner (1947) observed also that autoamputation occurs more frequently in young mice, 13–21 days old.

Transmission is accomplished by shedding of infected skin cells, debris, and sebum into the immediate environment (cages) where contact mice are infected through skin abrasions (Fenner 1947, 1949). Other probable sources of virus include excretions from the oropharynx, upper respiratory tract, genital tract, and intestines (Jacoby and Bhatt 1987). Biting, grooming, and cannibalism may result in significant transmission as well (Wallace and Buller 1985; Bhatt and Jacoby 1987b). Recent studies of the NIH-79 strain of virus indicate that mousepox is not highly contagious (Wallace et al. 1981; Wallace and Buller 1985; Bhatt and Jacoby 1987a, b) and that it is a self-limiting disease in colonies where the facilities and animal handling procedures are adequate. Fenner concluded early on that cage to cage spread is usually the result of improper animal handling techniques such as the pooling of mice from different cages for experimental manipulations or the use of a common holding receptacle when changing the bedding in a series of cages. Obviously the ever growing practice of exchanging genetically unique mice between laboratories may result in colony to colony spread. As noted by Fenner (1982), this can occur readily if mice from an enzootically infected colony are shipped at weanling age. Such mice may be infected but appear normal due to the partial protection afforded by maternal antibody. A similar situation may arise in shipping mice from a vaccinated colony. While immunization with vaccinia virus will prevent clinical expression of mousepox, infection and shedding of virus may still occur (Fenner and Fenner 1949; Buller and Wallace 1985). Indeed, the 1979 outbreak at NIH was caused by receipt of infected mice from a vaccinated colony (New 1981). Other more obvious ways include the shipment of infected mice of resistant strains that show little or no clinical manifestations, and exchange between laboratories of infected mouse specimens such as blood products, transplantable tumors and mouse-derived cells (Buller et al. 1981c).

Little is known about the nature of the type A inclusion except that it consists of an acidophilic protein which is soluble et pH 11.5, reprecipitates at pH 5.2, and appears to be antigenically unrelated to either virus or uninfected mouse cells used for virus culture (Ichihashi and Matsumoto 1966). Type B inclusions, which occur in the cytoplasm of cells infected with any poxvirus, have been shown to be sites of viral replication (Kato et al. 1959, 1963; Cairns 1960; Leduc and Bernhard 1962). They are described as foci of Feulgen-positive, basophilic material which when viewed with the electron microscope appear as a finely granular substance termed "matrix" material. Various stages of developing virions are found on the surface of the matrix areas. With immunohistochemical procedures, the type B inclusions appear either as dense foci of antigen or as circular aggregates. The latter configuration is probably the result of staining antigen in virions encircling the larger matrix areas. Infection by ectromelia virus characteristically produces focal hyperplasia of the mouse epidermis as well as the ectoderm of the chorioallantoic membrane of the embryonated hen's egg (Burnet and Lush 1936; Fenner 1949; Roberts 1962; Allen et al. 1981). The cause of the hyperplasia seems not to have been investigated. However, recent studies have shown that the closely related vaccinia virus in infected cell cultures produces a mitogenic polypeptide, vaccinia growth factor (VGF), which is structurally and functionally related to the epidermal growth factor (EGF) and transforming growth factor (TGF-alpha) (Blomquist et al. 1984; Brown et al. 1985; Reisner 1985). This finding led Brown to speculate that "production of EGF-like growth factors by virally infected cells could account for the proliferative diseases associated with members of the poxvirus family such as Shope fibroma virus, Yaba tumour virus, and molluscum contagiosum virus." Recently, experiments using vaccinia virus have determined that VGF is a virulence factor (Buller et al. 1988a) and contributes to cellular hyperplasia observed during infections of the chorioallantoic membrane of the chick embryo (Buller et al. 1988b). Whether the epidermal hyperplasia induced by ectromelia virus is caused by such a growth factor also remains to be determined.

For more comprehensive reviews of the biologic features of mousepox see Fenner (1982) and Jacoby (1985).

Comparison with Other Species

Fenner (1948c) used mousepox as a model to study acute viral exanthems of humans, especially smallpox (variola) and generalized vaccinia. He concluded that the rash produced in these infections was preceded by pathogenic processes analogous to those which occur in mousepox. In smallpox, however, the primary lesion is usually in the upper respiratory tract rather than in the skin. Histopathologically, variola, vaccinia, varicella zoster, and herpes simplex infections all produce skin lesions somewhat similar to those of ectromelia in that virus multiplication occurs in epidermal cells, leading to cellular edema and necrosis. It appears, however, that intraepithelial vesicle formation is a consistent feature of these exanthems, (Montgomery 1967; Lever and Schaumberg-Lever 1983) whereas in ectromelia infection clear-cut vesiculation is rare. This may be because the mouse epidermis is very thin, and attempts at vesicle formation are quickly thwarted by rupture of pockets of edema through the surface (Mims 1966). The "balloon cells" of ectromelia appear to be the result of hydropic vacuolation of epithelial cells throughout the thickness of the epidermis. Similar balloon cells are found in smallpox (Lever and Schaumberg-Lever 1983). In varicella zoster and herpes simplex lesions balloon cells are large, often multinucleated cells with abundant acidophilic cytoplasm (syncytial cells) which are usually located at the base of vesicles. In variola infections, only type B inclusions (Guarnieri's bodies) are found. In vaccinia infections, type B inclusions predominate, type A inclusions rarely being reported. Intranuclear inclusions are found in herpes infections.

It is not within the scope of this publication to compare in detail the lesions of all of the many epitheliotropic poxvirus infections of animals. However, it can be stated that in general, the exanthem-type lesions produced by poxviruses of humans (Fenner 1948c; Montgomery 1967; Lever and Schaumberg-Lever 1983; Mims 1966), monkeys (Sauer et al. 1960; Arita and Henderson 1968), rabbits (Maré 1974), camels, buffaloes and zoo animals (Baxby 1975; Zwart et al. 1971; Marennikova et al. 1977), and livestock (Jubb et al. 1985; Jones and Hunt 1983) have many similarities. Characteristic features, some or all of which may be found, include epidermal hyperplasia, cytoplasmic inclusions, intraepidermal edema leading to reticular degeneration and vesiculation, necrosis, and ulceration, often with secondary bacterial invasion and variable lesions of the underlying dermis and subcutis.

References

Allen AM, Clarke GL, Ganaway JR, Lock A, Werner RM (1981) Pathology and diagnosis of mousepox. Lab Anim Sci 31: 599–608
Allen AM, Collins MJ, Fenner F (1986) Ectromelia. In: Allen AM, Nomura T (eds) Manual of microbiologic monitoring of laboratory animals. US Gov-Printing, Washington DC, stock no 017-040-00500-8 (NIH pub no 86-2498)
Arita I, Henderson DA (1968) Smallpox and monkeypox in non-human primates. Bull WHO 39: 277–283
Avakyan AA, Byckovsky AF (1965) Ontogenesis of human smallpox virus. J Cell Biol 24: 337–347
Baxby D (1975) Identification and interrelationships of the variola/vaccinia subgroup of poxviruses. Prog Med Virol 19: 215–248
Bhat PN, Jacoby RO (1987a) Mousepox in inbred mice innately resistant or susceptible to lethal infection with ectromelia virus I. Clinical responses. Lab Anim Sci 37: 11–15
Bhatt PN, Jacoby RO (1987b) Mousepox in inbred mice innately resistant or susceptible to lethal infection with ectromelia virus III. Experimental transmission of infection and derivation of virus-free progeny from previously infected dams. Lab Anim Sci 37: 23–27
Blanden RV, Gardner ID (1976) The cell-mediated immune response to ectromelia virus infection I. Kinetics and characteristics of the primary effector T cell response in vivo. Cell Immunol 22: 271–282
Blomquist MC, Hunt LT, Barker WC (1984) Vaccinia virus 19-kilodalton protein: relationship to several mammalian proteins, including two growth factors. Proc Natl Acad Sci USA 81: 7363–7367
Brown JP, Twardzik DR, Marquardt H, Todaro GJ (1985) Vaccinia virus encodes a polypeptide homologous to epidermal growth factor and transforming growth factor. Nature 313: 491–492
Buller RML (1985) The BALB/c mouse as a model to study orthopoxviruses. In: Potter M (ed) Current topics in microbiology and immunology. Springer, Berlin Heidelberg New York, pp 148–153
Buller RML, Wallace GD (1985) Reexamination of the efficacy of vaccination against mousepox. Lab Anim Sci 35: 473–476
Buller RML, Bhatt PN, Wallace GD (1983) Evaluation of an enzymelinked immunosorbent assay for the detection of ectromelia (mousepox) antibody. J Clin Microbiol 18: 1220–1225
Buller RML, Yetter RA, Fredrickson TN, Morse HC III (1987a) Abrogation of resistance to severe mousepox in C57BL/6 mice infected with LP-BM5 murine leukemia viruses. J Virol 61: 383–387
Buller RML, Holmes KL, Hügin A, Fredrickson TN, Morse HC III (1987b) Induction of cytotoxic T-cell responses in vivo in the absence of CD4 helper cells. Nature 328: 77–79
Buller RML, Weinblatt AC, Hamburger AW, Wallace GD (1987c) Observation on the replication of ectromelia vi-

rus in mouse derived cell lines: implications for epidemiology of mousepox. Lab Anim Sci 37: 28-32

Buller RML, Chakrabarti S, Cooper JA, Twardzik DR, Moss B (1988a) Deletion of the vaccinia growth factor gene reduces virus virulence. J Virol 62: 866-874

Buller RML, Chakrabarti S, Moss B, Frederickson T (1988b) Cell proliferative response to vaccinia virus is mediated by VGF. Virology 164: 182-102

Burnet FM, Lush D (1936) The propagation of the virus of infectious ectromelia of mice in the developing egg. J Pathol Bacteriol 43: 105-120

Cairns J (1960) The initiation of vaccinia infection. Virology 11: 603-623

Fenner F (1947) Studies in infectious ectromelia in mice. II. Natural transmission: the portal of entry of the virus. Aust J Exp Biol Med Sci 25: 275-282

Fenner F (1948a) The clinical features and pathogenesis of mousepox (infectious ectromelia of mice). J Pathol Bacteriol 60: 529-552

Fenner F (1948b) The epizootic behavior of mouse-pox (infectious ectromelia). Br J Exp Pathol 29: 69-91

Fenner F (1948c) The pathogenesis of acute exanthems. An interpretation based on experimental investigations with mousepox (infectious ectromelia of mice). Lancet ii: 915-920

Fenner F (1949) Mouse-pox (infectious ectromelia of mice): a review. J Immunol 63: 341-373

Fenner F (1982) Mousepox. In: Foster HL, Small JD, Fox JG (eds) The mouse in biomedical research, chap 11. II. Diseases. Academic, New York

Fenner F, Fenner EMB (1949) Studies in mousepox (infectious ectromelia of mice). V. Closed epidemics in herds of normal and vaccinated mice. Aust J Exp Biol Med Sci 27: 19-30

Gröppel K-H (1962) Über das Vorkomen von Ektromelie (Mäusepocken) unter Wildmäusen. Arch Exp Veterinarmed 16: 243-278

Ichihashi Y, Matsumoto S (1966) Studies on the nature of Marchal bodies (A-type inclusion) during ectromelia virus infection. Virology 29: 264-275

Jacoby RO (1985) Mousepox, liver, mouse. In: Jones TC, Mohr U, Hunt RD (eds) Monographs on pathology of laboratory animals. Digestive system. Springer, Berlin Heidelberg New York, pp 145-151

Jacoby RO, Bhatt PN (1987) Mousepox in inbred mice innately resistant or susceptible to lethal infection with ectromelia virus II. Pathogenesis. Lab Anim Sci 37: 16-22

Jones TC, Hunt RD (1983) Veterinary pathology, chap 9. Lea and Febiger, Philadelphia

Jubb KVF, Kennedy PC, Palmer N (1985) Pathology of domestic animals, vol 1, chap 5. Academic, New York

Kaplan C, Healing TD, Evans N, Healing L, Prior A (1980) Evidence of infection by viruses in small british field rodents. J Hyg (Lond) 84: 285-294

Kato S (1955) Studies on the inclusion bodies of ectromelia virus propagated in the ascites tumor cells. Virus Ulrusu (Kyoto) 5: 111-118

Kato S, Takahashi M, Kameyama S, Kamahora J (1959) A study on the morphological and cyto-immunological relationship between the inclusions of variola, cowpox, rabbitpox, vaccinia (variola origin) and vaccinia IHD and a consideration of the term "Guarnieri body". Biken J 2: 353-363

Kato S, Aoyama Y, Kamahora J (1963) Autoradiography of the tissues of mice infected with ectromelia virus using 3H-thymidine. Biken J 6: 9-16

Leduc EH, Bernhard W (1962) Electron microscope study of mouse liver infected by ectromelia virus. J Ultrastruct Res 6: 466-488

Lever WF, Schaumberg-Lever G (1983) Histopathology of the skin. JB Lippincott, Philadelphia, chap 21

Marchal J (1930) Infectious ectromelia. A hitherto undescribed virus disease of mice. J Pathol Bacteriol 33: 713-728

Marennikova SS, Maltseva NN, Korneeva VI, Garanina NM (1977) Outbreak of pox disease among carnivora (Felidae) and Edentata. J Infect Dis 135: 358-366

Maré CJ (1974) Viral diseases. In: Weisbroth SH, Flatt RE, Kraus AL (eds) The biology of the laboratory rabbit. Academic, New York, chap 10

Mims CA (1959) The response of mice to large intravenous injections of ectromelia virus. II. The growth of the virus in the liver. Br J Exp Pathol 40: 543-550

Mims CA (1966) Pathogenesis of rashes in virus diseases. Bacteriol Rev 30: 739-760

Montgomery H (1967) Dermatopathology, vol I, chap 20. Hoeber Med Div, Harper and Row, New York

Morgan C (1976) Vaccinia virus reexamined: development and release. Virology 73: 43-58

New AE (1981) Ectromelia (mousepox) in the United States (preface). Lab Anim Sci 31: 552

Reisner AH (1985) Similarity between the vaccinia virus 19K early protein and epidermal growth factor. Nature 313: 801-803

Roberts JA (1962) Histopathogenesis of mousepox. II. Cutaneous infection. Br J Exp Pathol 43: 462-468

Sauer RM, Prier JE, Buchanan RS, Creamer AA, Fegley HC (1960) Studies on a pox disease of monkeys. I. Pathology. Am J Vet Res 21: 377-380

Tsuru S, Kitani H, Seno M, Abe M, Zinnaka Y, Nomoto K (1983) Mechanism of protection during the early phase of generalized viral infection. I. Contribution of phagocytes to protection against ectromelia virus. J Gen Virol 64: 2021-2026

Wallace GD, Werner RM, Golway PL, Hernandez DM, Alling DW, George DA (1981) Epizootiology of an outbreak of mousepox at the National Institutes of Health. Lab Anim Sci 31: 609-615

Wallace GD, Buller RML (1985) Kinetics of ectromelia virus (mousepox) transmission and clinical response in C57BL/6J, BALB/cByJ and AKR/J inbred mice. Lab Anim Sci 35: 41-46

Wallace GD, Buller RML, Morse HC III (1985) Genetic determinants of resistance to ectromelia (mousepox) virus-induced mortality. J Virol 55: 890-891

Zwart P, Gispen R, Peters JC (1971) Cowpox in okapis Okapia johnstoni at Rotterdam zoo. Br Vet J 127: 20-24

Papillomavirus Infection, Skin, Mouse

John P. Sundberg

Synonyms. Warts; papillomatosis; papillomas.

Gross Appearance

Adult European harvest mice *(Micromys minutis)* develop raised, firm, often hyperpigmented, verrucous masses on the haired skin, tail, and mucocutaneous junctions of the mouth (Fig. 216) and anus (Sundberg et al. 1987). The tumors are often round and less than 0.5 cm in diameter. Large conical masses, 0.5 cm wide and up to 1.5 cm in length, occasionally develop on the head.

Microscopic Features

A series of lesions have been identified in harvest mice. Although sequential time course studies of induced papillomas have not been done, it is likely that many of the lesions observed represent stages in the progression of the disease. Hyperplasia of the epidermis, without tumor formation, is associated with the presence of virus. In areas adjacent to epidermal hyperplasia, proliferation of epithelial cells of the hair follicles is evident. These areas are either solitary or form solid tumors (trichoepitheliomas) containing numerous, poorly formed hair follicles (Figs. 217 and 218). More typical squamous papillomas occasionally are contiguous with these or solitary and raised above the surface of the skin and consist of proliferation of the epidermis on thin fibrovascular stalks with various degrees of orthokeratosis (Fig. 219).

A variation is the cutaneous horn or hyperkeratotic papilloma. This has a papillomatous base and is covered by a large accumulation of laminated keratin, usually ten times or more the thickness of the viable epidermal cells of the papilloma. The affected epidermis contains epithelial pearls, and the cells have a high mitotic index (10-12 per high power field). The epidermal cells are not locally invasive. Another variation of the papilloma consists of lesions in which there is an invagination of the proliferating epithelial cells below the level of the normal epidermis (Fig. 219). Within this invagination, the epidermis forms papillary folds on thin fibrovascular stalks.

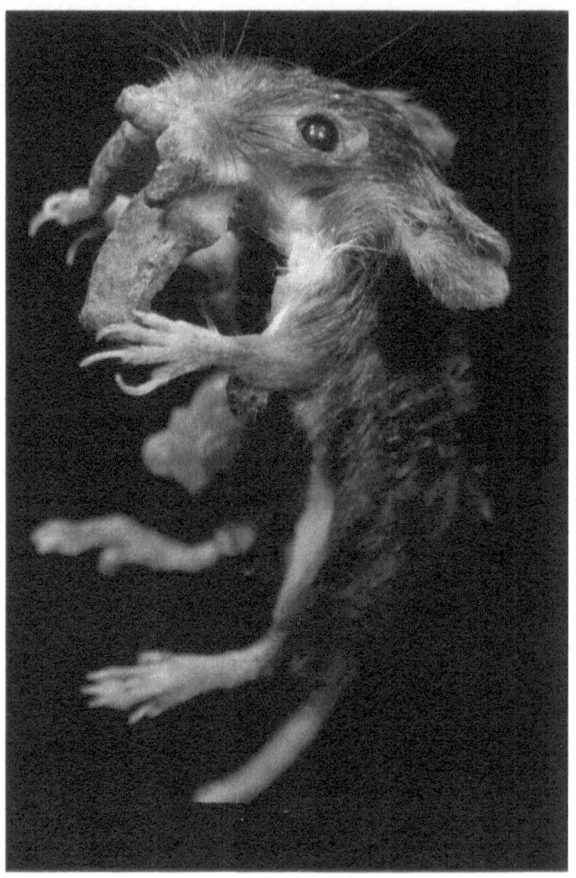

Fig. 216. Multiple cutaneous horns (hyperkeratotic papillomas) at the oral mucocutaneous junction. (Sundberg et al. 1988, courtesy of *Veterinary Pathology*)

This lesion is interpreted to be an inverted papilloma.

Solid tumors within the dermis consist of a uniform population of hyperchromatic cells with scant cytoplasm, high mitotic index, and a large nuclear to cytoplasmic ratio. Within these tumors are clusters or individual cells which have differentiated into sebaceous cells (Fig. 220). These are diagnosed as sebaceous carcinomas. One animal with this tumor on the haired skin of its head had multiple, gray, round masses in its lung. Microscopically, these were foci of squamous cells producing massive amounts of keratin (keratinaceous cysts) (Fig. 221). Viral DNA was detected in the squamous cells of this lesion by the Southern blot technique (Sundberg et al. 1987). Individual or clusters of cells in the stratum granulo-

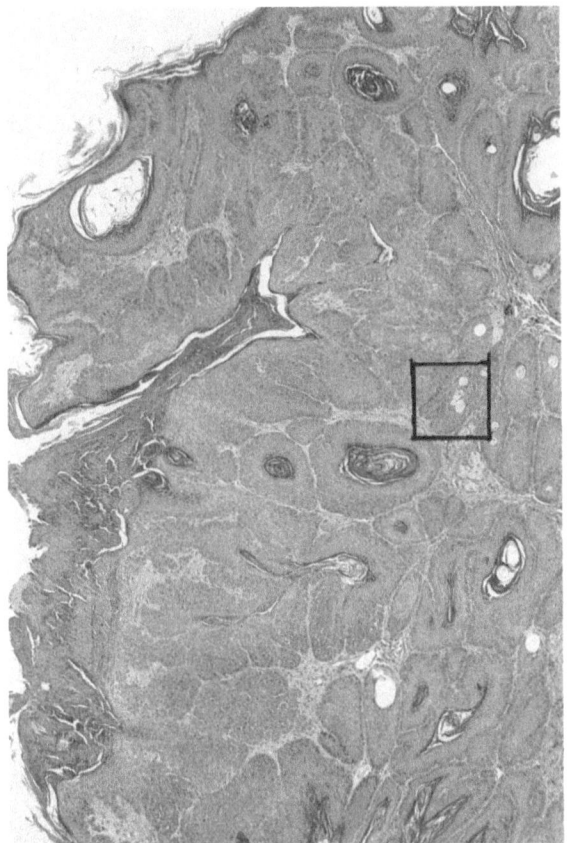

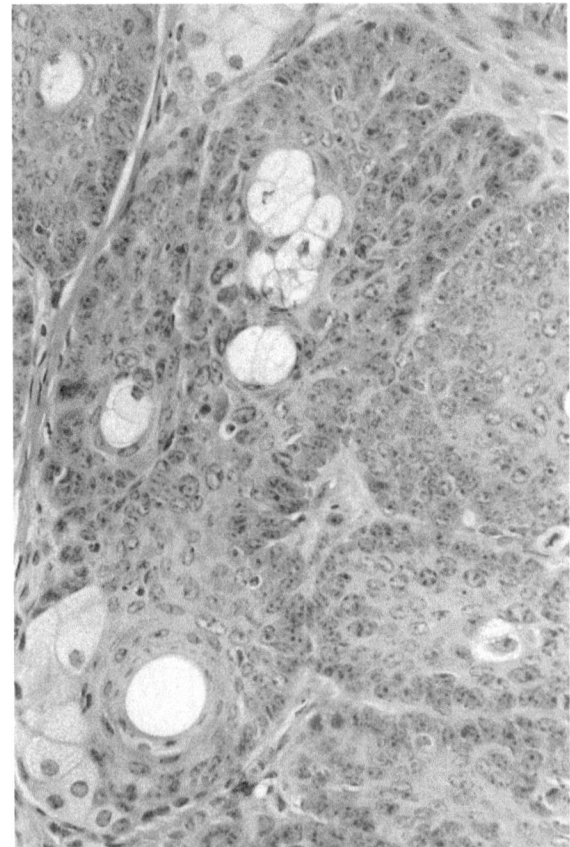

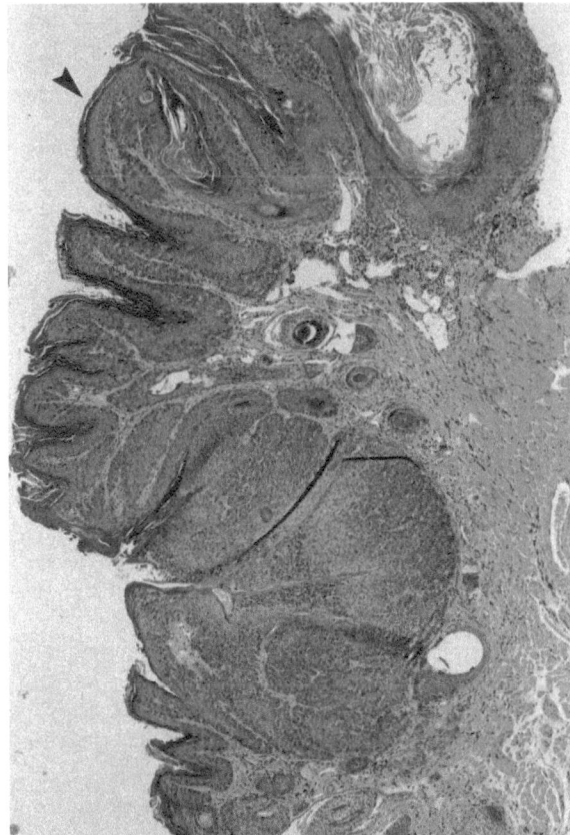

Fig. 217 *(upper left).* Numerous follicular structures at the base of a papilloma. H and E, × 40

Fig. 218 *(upper right).* Proliferation of cells of pilosebaceous structures from boxed area in Fig. 217. H and E, × 250

Fig. 219 *(lower right).* Normal epidermis *(bottom)* adjacent to interverted papilloma *(middle)* with exophytic papilloma *(arrowhead).* H and E, × 40

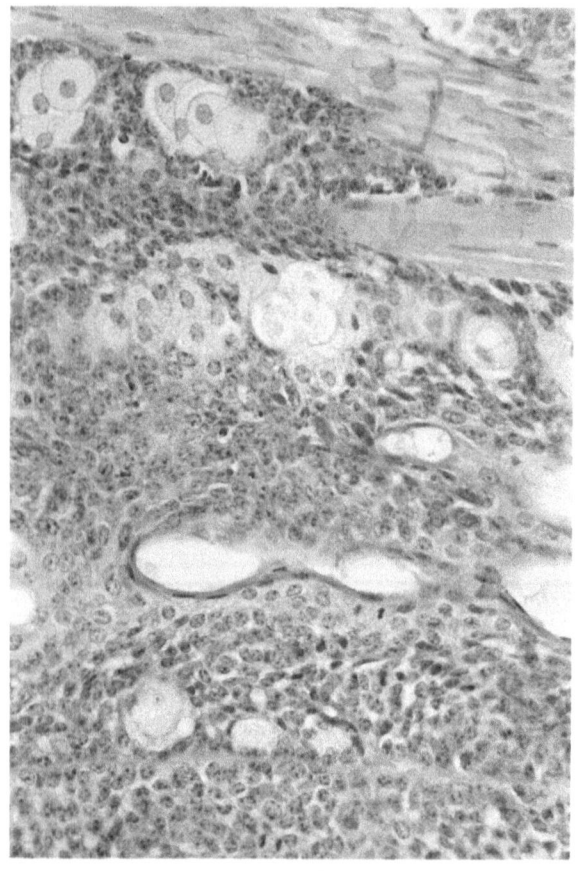

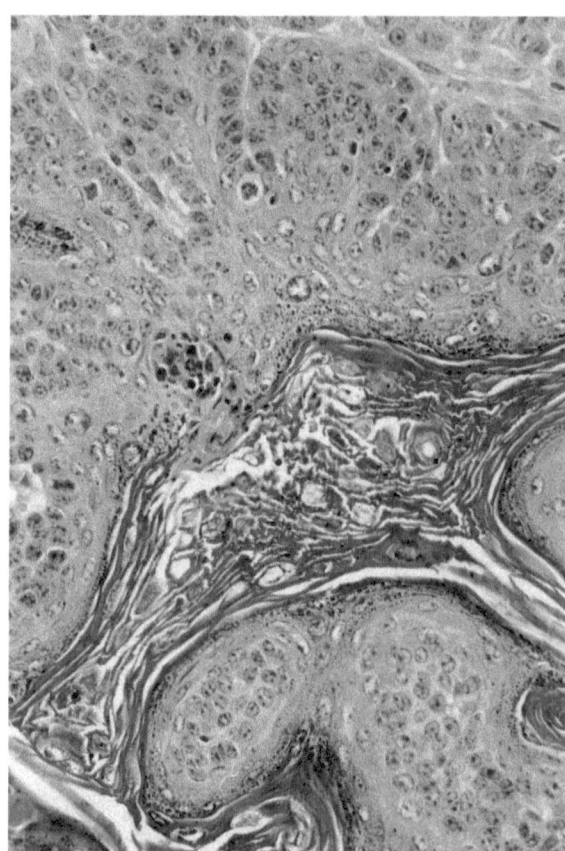

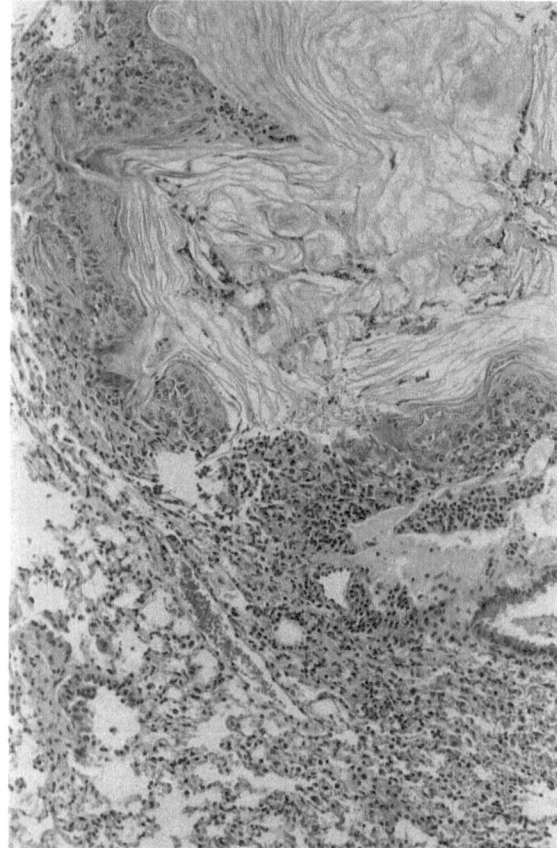

Fig. 220 *(upper left).* Sebaceous carcinoma with differentiated cells invading muscle. H and E, × 250

Fig. 221 *(lower left).* Lung, harvest mouse, keratinaceous cyst. H and E, × 100

Fig. 222 *(upper right).* Papilloma, skin, harvest mouse. Orthokeratosis and hypergranulosis. H and E, × 250

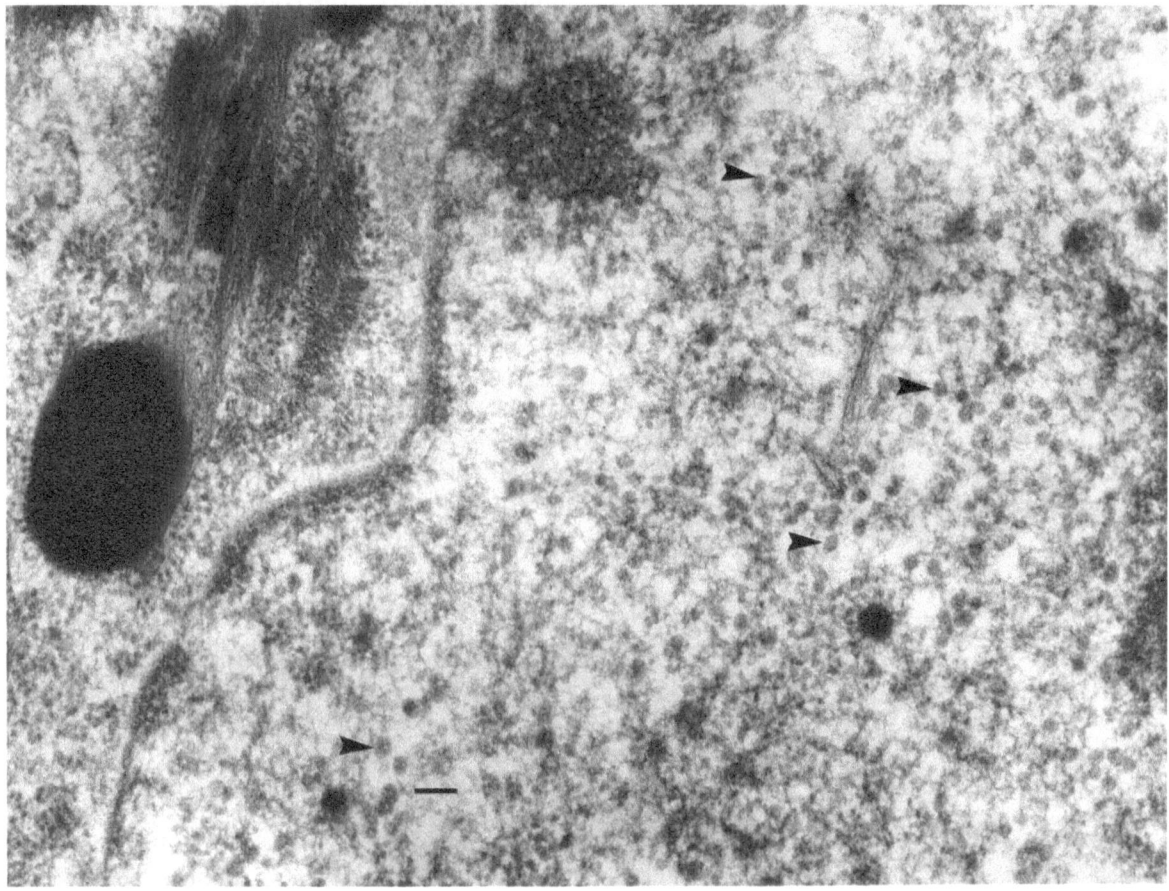

Fig. 223. Papilloma, harvest mouse, cell in the stratum granulosum. Intranuclear viral particles *(arrowheads).* *Bar*= 1 nm. (Sundberg et al. 1988, courtesy of *Veterinary Pathology*)

sum in which the cytoplasm was swollen stained poorly and contained large, darkly basophilic, keratohyalin granules of various sizes (Fig. 222). The nuclei were centrally located and stained positively for papillomavirus group-specific antigens by either the avidin-biotin or peroxidase-antiperoxidase techniques. Harvest mouse papillomavirus genomes could also be detected within these cells by in situ hybridization using a homologous cloned DNA probe under conditions of high stringency (Sundberg et al. 1988).

Ultrastructure

Nuclei within cells of the stratum granulosum contain small numbers of dispersed, circular, viral particles which average 35 nm in diameter (Fig. 223) (Sundberg et al. 1988). The stratum granulosum is thicker than normal and contains numerous, pleomorphic, electron-dense, keratohyalin-type granules (Fig. 224), typical of produc-

tive papillomavirus infection (Sundberg et al. 1985).

Differential Diagnosis

A variety of spontaneously occurring skin tumors or crusts forming over traumatized areas, particularly on the tail, may grossly resemble these lesions. Papillomas and squamous cell carcinomas of unknown etiology occur in inbred laboratory mice even under the best of husbandry conditions (Bogovski 1979). These tumors are rarely diagnosed in inbred strains and mutants of *Mus musculus,* and several studies have yielded no evidence of papillomavirus genomes in DNA extracted from the tumors (Lutzner et al. 1985; Sundberg, unpublished data). Since these tumors are morphologically similar, if not identical tumors, they cannot be readily differentiated at the gross level. Similar tumors have also been induced by chemical carcinogens. Preliminary

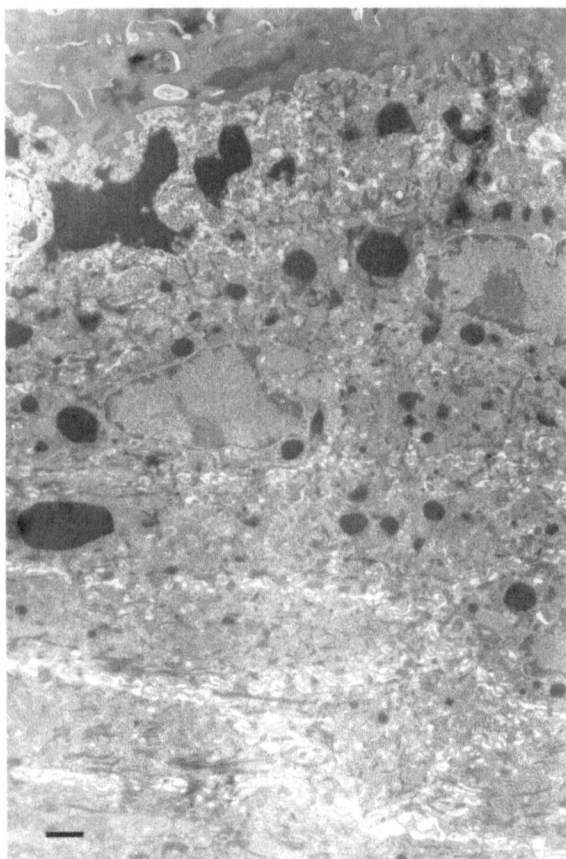

Fig. 224. Papilloma, skin, harvest mouse. Stratum granulosum contains numerous pleomorphic, electron-dense, keratohyalin granules. *Bar* = 100 nm

studies indicate that papillomaviruses are not involved in the pathogenesis of chemically induced papillomas (Sundberg and Maurer, unpublished data). Pigmented tumors such as melanomas will also resemble the superficially pigmented, papillomavirus-associated skin tumors.

Biologic Features

Natural History. A novel papillomavirus genome has been isolated from all cutaneous and pulmonary tumors removed from harvest mice (O'Banion et al. 1988). A small tumor developed at the injection site on the tail of one of two harvest mice but none of four immunocompetent inbred strains of *Mus musculus* or deer mice *(Peromyscus maniculatus)* (Sundberg et al. 1987). The method of natural infection is unknown.

Pathogenesis. Papillomavirus DNA was isolated from both normal tissues and tumors in all adult animals examined. The copy number of the viral genome was 100–1000 times higher in the tumors than in normal tissues (O'Banion et al. 1988). Although the pathogenesis has yet to be worked out, it is likely that this may be an endogenous virus in this species in which copy number increases in the skin (the target organ) with age and when it reaches a critical number, viral oncogene products cause transformation of the cells. This is based on similar observations in the multimammate rat *(Mastomys natalensis)* in which this appears to be the basic mechanism (Amtmann et al. 1984; Amtmann and Wayss 1987). In this species, several morphologically different tumors, including squamous cell carcinomas, develop (Rudolf and Thiel 1976).

Etiology. A 7.6-kilobase pair, double-stranded, supercoiled, circular DNA molecule was isolated from the squamous papillomas (O'Banion et al. 1988). This viral genome has been cloned in a pUC 18 vector at its single *Eco*RI site. The harvest mouse papillomavirus cross-hybridized with the genomes of human papillomavirus type 1a, rabbit oral papillomavirus, and *Mastomys natalensis* papillomavirus at Tm-33 °C (intermediate stringency). At lower stringency (TM-40 °C, less DNA homology) it hybridized with bovine papillomavirus types 2 and 6, human papillomavirus types 11, 16, and 18, white-tailed deer papillomavirus, European elk papillomavirus, and cottontail rabbit papillomavirus. No cross-hybridization was detected with equine cutaneous papillomavirus, canine oral papillomavirus, or bovine papillomavirus types 1, 4, and 5. Partial sequencing and computer comparisons with human papillomavirus type 1a confirmed the colinearity of this molecule, indicating that it is indeed a member of the genus papillomaviridae.

Frequency. All animals studied to date have originated from the same colony. Frequency data is not available. There have been no reports from other colonies.

Comparison with Other Species

This disease is similar in many respects to the papillomavirus-induced lesions in *Mastomys natalensis* as described above (Amtmann et al. 1984; Muller and Gissmann 1978; Rudolf and Thiel 1976) and epidermodysplasia verruciformis in humans (Orth 1987). Both of these appear to be caused by endogenous papillomaviruses. Many species of mammals are infected by one or more, spécies-specific papillomaviruses. The disease is usually easily transmitted horizontally by mechanical means. The animal papillomaviruses have been reviewed recently (Sundberg 1987; Sundberg and O'Banion 1989).

Spontaneous papillomas and squamous cell carcinomas have been described in the repeat epilation heterozygote (*Er*/+) mouse (Lutzner et al. 1985; p. 203, this volume). A viral etiology could not be determined even when bovine papillomavirus type 1 DNA was used as a molecular probe on Southern blots. Similar results have been obtained from hybridization studies using DNA extracted from papillomas and squamous cell carcinomas which occur spontaneously in other inbred strains and mutants (Sundberg, unpublished data).

References

Amtmann E, Volm M, Wayss K (1984) Tumor induction in the rodent *Mastomys natalensis* by activation of endogenous papilloma virus genomes. Nature 308: 291-292

Amtmann E, Wayss K (1987) Papillomaviruses and Carcinogenic Progression II: The *Mastomys Natalensis* Papillomavirus. In: Salzman NP, Howley PM (ed) The Papovaviridae, Vol II, The Papillomaviruses. Plenum Press, New York

Bogovski P (1979) Tumors of the skin. In: Turusov VS (ed) Pathology of tumours in laboratory animals, vol II. Tumours of the mouse. IARC, Lyon, pp 1-42 (IARC Sci Publ no 23)

Lutzner MA, Guenet JL, Breitburd F (1985) Multiple cutaneous papillomas and carcinomas that develop spontaneously in a mouse mutant, the repeated epilation heterozygote Er/+. JNCI 75: 161-166

Muller H, Gissmann L (1978) *Mastomys natalensis* papillomavirus (MnPV), the causative agent of epithelial proliferations: characterization of the virus particle. J Gen Virol 41: 315-323

O'Banion MK, Reichmann ME, Sundberg JP (1988) Cloning and characterization of a papillomavirus associated with papillomas and carcinomas in the European harvest mouse *(Micromys minutis).* J Virol 62: 226-233

Orth G (1987) Epidermodysplasia verruciformis. In: Salzman NP, Howley PM (eds) The Papovaviridae, vol II. The papillomaviruses. Plenum, New York

Rudolf R, Thiel W (1976) Pathologische Anatomie und Histologie von spontanen epithelialen Hauttumoren bei *Mastomys natalensis.* Zentralbl Veterinaermed [A] 23: 429-441 (In German with English abstr)

Sundberg JP (1987) Animal papillomavirus infections. In: Syrjanen K, Gissmann L, Koss L (eds) Papilloma viruses and human diseases. Springer, Berlin Heidelberg New York

Sundberg JP, O'Banion MK (1989) Animal papillomaviruses associated with malignant tumors. Adv Viral Oncol 8: 55-71

Sundberg JP, Hill DL, Williams ES, Nielsen SW (1985) Light and electron microscopic comparisons of cutaneous fibromas in whitetailed and mule deer. Am J Vet Res 46: 2200-2206

Sundberg JP, O'Banion MK, Reichmann ME (1987) Mouse papillomavirus: pathology and characterization of the virus. Cancer Cell 5: 373-379

Sundberg JP, O'Banion MK, Shima A, Knupp C, Reichmann ME (1988) Papillomas and carcinomas associated with a papillomavirus in European harvest mice *(Micromys minutus).* Vet Pathol 25: 356-361

INHERITED CONDITIONS

Obese Mutant Mice: Obese *(ob)* and Diabetes *(db)*

Douglas L. Coleman

Synonym. Obese mouse; obese hyperglycemic mouse; *ob/ob* mouse; diabetes mouse; diabetic mouse; *db/db* mouse.

Gross Appearance

Obese *(ob/ob)* and diabetes *(db/db)* mutant mice are phenotypically identical both being severely obese, adults weighing from 45-60 g compared with 25-30 g for normal littermates. Most of the excess body weight represents large stores of white adipose tissue located in the axial and inguinal regions. Both mutants have various degrees of glucose intolerance and diabetes, depending on the inbred background on which the mutant is maintained.

Microscopic Features

Aside from the massive accumulation of subcutaneous and intra-abdominal fat, the most striking histopathologic changes are observed in the pancreas. Early in the development of the condition, almost total degranulation of the beta cells of the islets of Langerhans are seen, followed by attempts at beta-cell regeneration (Coleman and Hummel 1967). Degranulation occurs as early as 28 days of age (Fig. 225 and 226) in mutants maintained on all backgrounds. The degree of adaptive compensation to the stress of the obesity-producing mutant gene depends on the inbred background on which the mutant is maintained.

Beta cells in the islets of both mutants maintained on the C57BL/Ks (BKs) background undergo initial abortive attempts at hypertrophy and regeneration, but between 2 and 3 months of age extensive beta-cell necrosis is evident in many of the islets (Fig. 227). In addition to degranulation and necrosis of beta cells, other degenerative changes are observed, including infiltration of the islet capsule by acinar cells of the exocrine pancreas, the appearance of proliferating intra-islet pancreatic ducts, and perturbations in the position and number of alpha, delta (D), and pancreatic polypeptide (PP) cells. A few granulated and functional beta cells remain within atrophic islets, usually adjacent to intra-islet ducts. Indeed, some of the epithelial cells of these dilated ducts appear to be undergoing transition to islet cells. Thus, it appears that in these mutants on the BKs background, disappearance of islet beta cells leads to the proliferation of intra-islet pancreatic ducts and beta-cell neogenesis from ductal epithelium. Evidence of beta cells incorporating [³H]thymidine establishes that a burst of beta-cell replication occurs early in these syndromes (Like and Chick 1970a). A reduction in the incorporation of [³H]thymidine occurs as the beta cell steadily decrease in number and become severely degranulated. Even so, insulin secretion remains enhanced and the atrophic, end-stage islets observed in older, severely diabetic mutants retain some functional beta cells capable of secreting normal to higher than normal amounts of insulin. In contrast, both mutations maintained on the C57BL/6J (B6) inbred background elicit many large islets granulated to various degrees with increased blood supply (Fig. 228). These morphological changes are indicative of hyperfunction and indeed are correlated with increased insulin synthesis and secretion. Remission from hyperglycemia is accompanied by sustained islet growth and eventual beta-cell regranulation.

Volume density changes in the beta cell mass (decrease on the BKs background and increase on the B6 background) lead to major shifts in the volume densities of the non-beta-cell islet endocrine types (Baetens et al. 1978; Berelowitz et al. 1980). Alpha-cell numbers are not increased in either syndrome on either background; however, D-cell numbers increase on the BKs background, whereas PP-cell hyperplasia is suggested on the

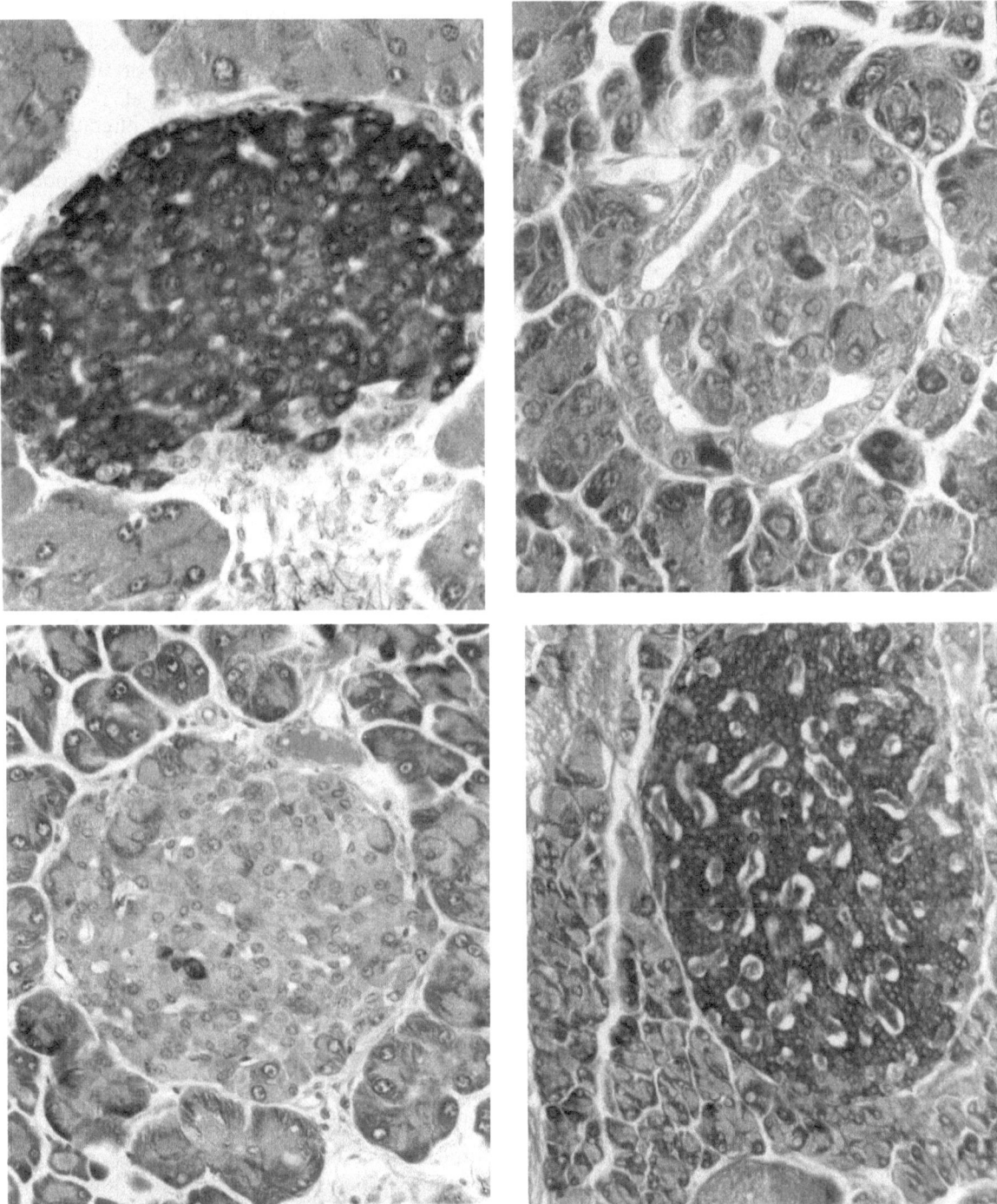

Fig. 225 *(upper left)*. Pancreas from BKs-+ / + normal female, 7 months of age. Note heavily granulated beta cells. Aldehyde fuchsin stain, × 400

Fig. 226 *(lower left)*. Pancreas from BKs-*ob/ob* male, 2 months of age. Note near normal size but almost total degranulation of beta cells. Aldehyde fuchsin stain, × 300

Fig. 227 *(upper right)*. Pancreas from BKs-*db/db*, 5 months of age with atrophied islet. Note large intra-islet

ducts and small numbers of aldehyde fuchsin-positive beta cells. Aldehyde fuchsin, × 400

Fig. 228 *(lower right)*. Pancreas from B6-*db/db* mouse. Note many granulated beta cells and enlarged sinusoids suggesting hyperactivity. Islet is much larger than normal (half the magnification is used here compared with the normal islet in Fig. 225). Aldehyde fuchsin stain, × 200

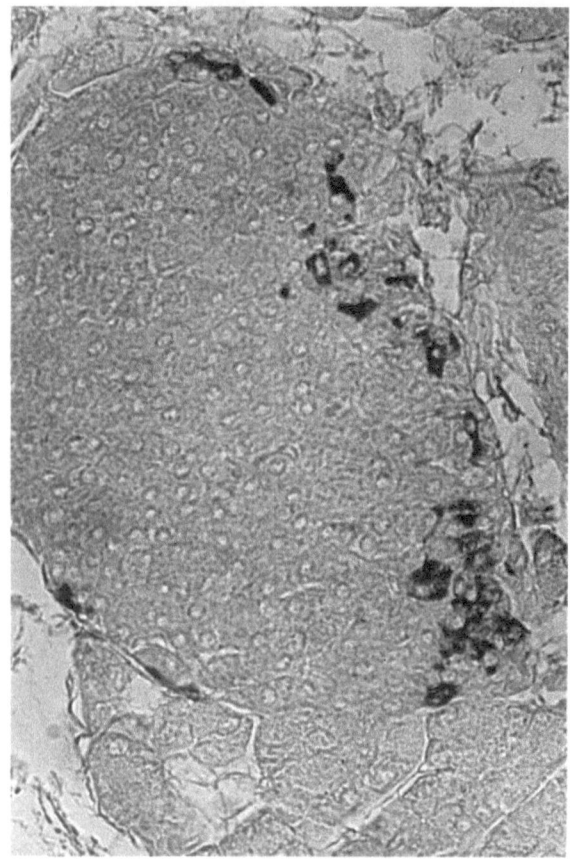

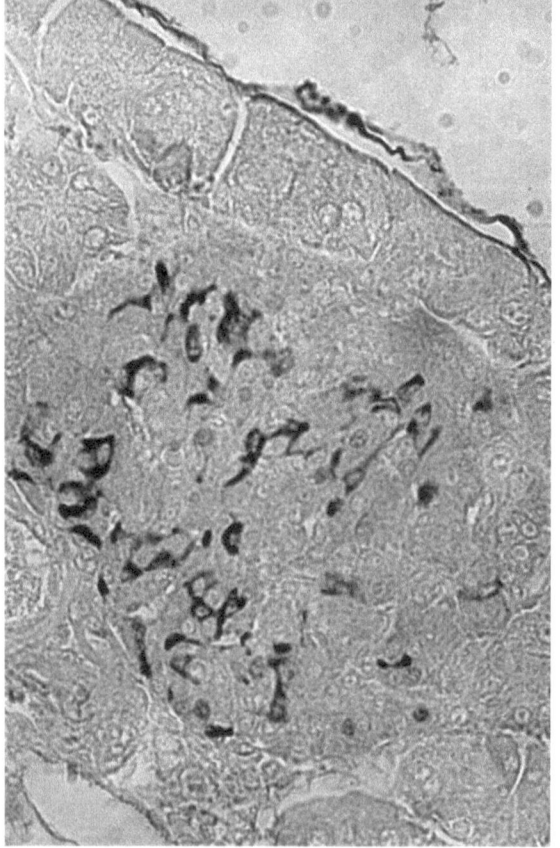

B6 background (Gapp et al. 1983). However, the normal distribution of the three non-beta cell types (Fig. 229) at the periphery of the cell is changed in BKs mutants (Leiter et al. 1979). Particularly striking is an inward migration of D cells into the beta-cell core; these interiorized D cells are characterized by extreme filipodial contacts with beta cells (Fig. 230).

A summary of the temporal changes that occur in blood sugar insulin concentration, islet cell type distribution, and relative volume density in 8Ks mutants is seen in Fig. 231. The early stages (up to 8–10 weeks in B6 mutants) are similar, if not identical, to those seen on the BKs background, but instead of increasing, blood glucose reaches a peak at 250–400 mg/dl and then declines to normal while the insulin concentration continues to rise sufficiently to maintain glucose homeostasis. Associated with these changes in B6 mutants is a marked increase in volume of the *db/db* islet due mainly to beta-cell hyperplasia with D-cell volume density exhibiting a transient increase during the initial phase pf beta-cell hyperplasia. A gradual reduction in volume density occurs later, until the average number and absolute volume of D cells per islet is comparable in *db/db* and in normal islets from older mice. In contrast PP-cell volume density remains stable throughout, suggesting that this cell type keeps pace with beta-cell hyperplasia. The volume density of alpha cells was reduced in contrast to all other cell types that responded positively although noncoordinately to the stimulus exerted by *db* gene expression (Gapp et al. 1983).

The livers of mutants are enlarged and contain increased amounts of both glycogen and lipid. Most of the hepatocytes are hypertrophied and filled with fat droplets, especially in areas surrounding the hepatic vein. In normal liver, glycogen is distributed uniformly throughout, whereas in mutants glycogen is massed in the cells surrounding the hepatic arteries and hepatic portal vein and reduced or lacking around the hepatic vein (Coleman and Hummel 1967).

◀ Fig. 229 *(above)*. Pancreatic islet from a normal 11-week-old female BKs-+/+ mouse with distribution of D cells at islet periphery. Immunoperoxidase stain for somatostatin, ×250

Fig. 230 *(below)*. Pancreatic islet, 11-week-old female BKs-*db/db* mouse (littermate of Fig. 229), demonstrating redistribution of D cells from peripheral location. D-cell filopodial extensions maximize surface contacts with beta cells. Immunperoxidase stain, ×250

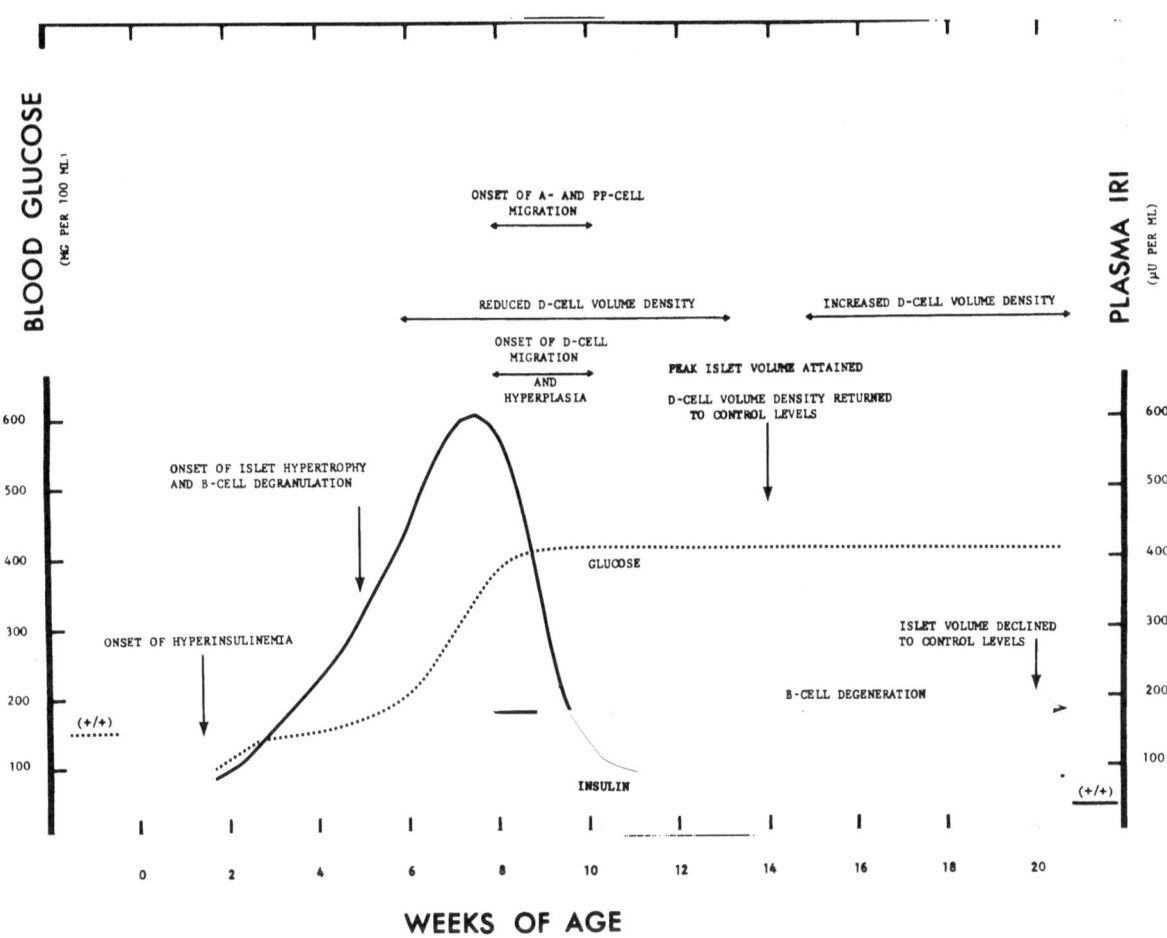

Fig. 231. Chart of temporal changes in blood sugar, plasma insulin concentration, and islet cell distribution in BKs-*db/db* mice

The ovaries, uteri, and mammary glands of mutants are atrophied, and the histologic appearance is that of a hypophysectomized mouse. In the ovaries, no follicles beyond the antrum stage and no corpora lutea or evidence of ovulation are seen. The uterus and mammary glands are juvenile in appearance. Testes are small and contain few tubules with active spermatogenesis, although males on some backgrounds are fertile. The adrenals and pituitary have no obvious abnormalities (Coleman and Hummel 1967). Transplantation of ovaries to normal hosts permits production of litters and if necessary can be used to increase the supply of either mutants or known heterozygotes. Reproductive failure in female *db/db* mice has been determined to be due to an inadequate release of gonadotropin-releasing hormone from the hypothalamus (Johnson and Sidman 1979).

Both mutants *(ob/ob* and *db/db)* maintained on the B6 inbred background have well-compensat-ed diabetes and remain free of most secondary complications associated with chronic hyperglycemia. However, when maintained on the BKs background, chronic hyperglycemia does produce some complications (Coleman 1982a). Several reports have demonstrated various degrees and types of peripheral neuropathies in hyperglycemic mice (Sima and Robertson 1978; Hanker et al. 1980; Moore et al. 1980). Disturbances in the sympathetic nervous system with regard to transport of norepinephrine in nerves of BKs-*db/db* mice have been described (Giachetti 1978, 1979). Microvascular lesions are characteristic of adult mice with long-standing diabetes (Bohlen and Niggl 1979a, b). Glomerular basement membrane thickening (Like et al. 1972), glomerular filtration hyperactivity (Gartner 1979), and deposition of immune complexes in the kidney (Bower et al. 1980; Meade et al. 1981) are also seen in BKs-*db/db* mice. Comparative studies on the incidence of secondary complications have not been completed systematically with both mutations maintained on different inbred backgrounds. Sexual dimorphism is observed in some inbred backgrounds; males being more severely diabetic (as in BKs) and females only obese (as in B6) would suggest that gender-associated background factors may be involved in producing BKs or B6 phenotypes, and any diabetic complications would be expected to be observed only in males.

The fact that the spleen and thymus of *db/db* mice and the spleen of *ob/ob* mice are smaller than normal suggests an immune deficiency (Bray and York 1979). Reduced cellular immunity has been demonstrated for both the *ob/ob* (Sheena and Meade 1978) and *db/db* mice (Fernandes et al. 1978; Mahmood et al. 1976). Allogenic skin grafts survive longer on both mutants. Although an abnormality in T-cell function has been suggested, it seems to be related to the environment in which the T cell resides and is not an intrinsic defect in the T cell itself. Recent studies (Leiter et al. 1987a) have demonstrated that bone marrow from +/+ mice did not prevent diabetes development in irradiated *db/db* recipients and marrow from *db/db* donors did not adoptively transfer diabetes in lethally irradiated normal recipients. These data show that intrinsic defects in the T cells cannot account for pathogenesis and also eliminate autoimmunity as the primary effector of beta-cell destruction.

Ultrastructure

Diabetes *(db/db)* or obese *(ob/ob)* mutants maintained on the BKs background develop severe hyperglycemia and also exhibit marked ultrastructural changes in the beta cells characteristic of the hypersecretory state. These include marked beta-cell degranulation, proliferation and dilation of tubular rough endoplasmic reticulum, and an increase in the size of the Golgi complex (Fig. 232). The Golgi elements are no longer compact organelles but become widely dispersed throughout the cell and frequently contain electron-opaque material and small granules within tubular and vesicular profiles (Like and Chick 1970b). In contrast to the uniformly small and slender mitochondria typical of normal mice, the mitochondria of mutants with established hyperglycemia are enlarged and polymorphic (Fig. 232). The number of beta granules are reduced and vary greatly in size and electron density, with a relative increase in small granules.

Prenecrotic beta cells have a moderate number of lysosomal structures and small myelin figures scattered amongst the cytoplasmic organelles. In necrotic beta cells, the lysosomes are larger, and many incorporate portions of the rough endoplasmic reticulum, small vesicles, and mitochondria.

Phagocytosis of necrotic debris is often observed. Ductal structures and differentiated acinar cells within the islet are often seen in severely affected diabetics. Beta cells of BKs mice can often be distinguished from those of B6 by their ability to express endogenous retrovirus (intracisternal type A particles, Leiter and Kuff 1984). Retroviral gene expression in BKs beta cells is glucose inducible, and thus increased numbers of the retroviral particles are observed in glucose-stressed beta cells from severely hyperglycemic BKs-*db/db* mice (Fig. 233).

Beta cells of the less severely affected B6 mutants have many of these same features early in the developing syndrome, including degranulation, increased area and volume of rough endoplasmic reticulum, and enlarged Golgi complex. Beta-cell necrosis is not seen. With the gradual reduction of the blood sugar concentration, regranulation occurs; as granulation becomes complete, normalization of the blood sugar concentration occurs. Individual, fully granulated beta cells cannot be distinguished, except by number and size, from those of normal mice. The increased extractable immunoreactive insulin correlates well with the hyperplasia and hypertrophy (Like and Chick 1970b).

Biologic Features

Obese *(ob)* and diabetes *(db)* are two, autosomal recessive, single gene mutations in the mouse

Fig. 232 *(above)*. Beta cell, male BKs-*db/db* mouse, ▶ 3 months of age. Note enlarged mitochondria *(m)*, reduced number of beta granules, and dilated endoplasmic reticulum (RER, *arrowhead*) and Golgi complex *(g)*. The pronounced dilatation of RER in the beta cell contrasts with the normal appearance of RER in an adjacent alpha cell *(arrow)*. TEM, ×7000

Fig. 233 *(below)*. Beta cell, C3H.SW/Lt-*db/db* male mouse, 7 weeks of age. Note the large number of intracisternal type A particles *(arrowheads)* within the dilated profiles of the endoplasmic reticulum (RER). TEM, ×2000. *Inset*, higher magnification of A particle *(arrow)* within an RER cisterna of a degranulated beta cell. TEM, ×45000

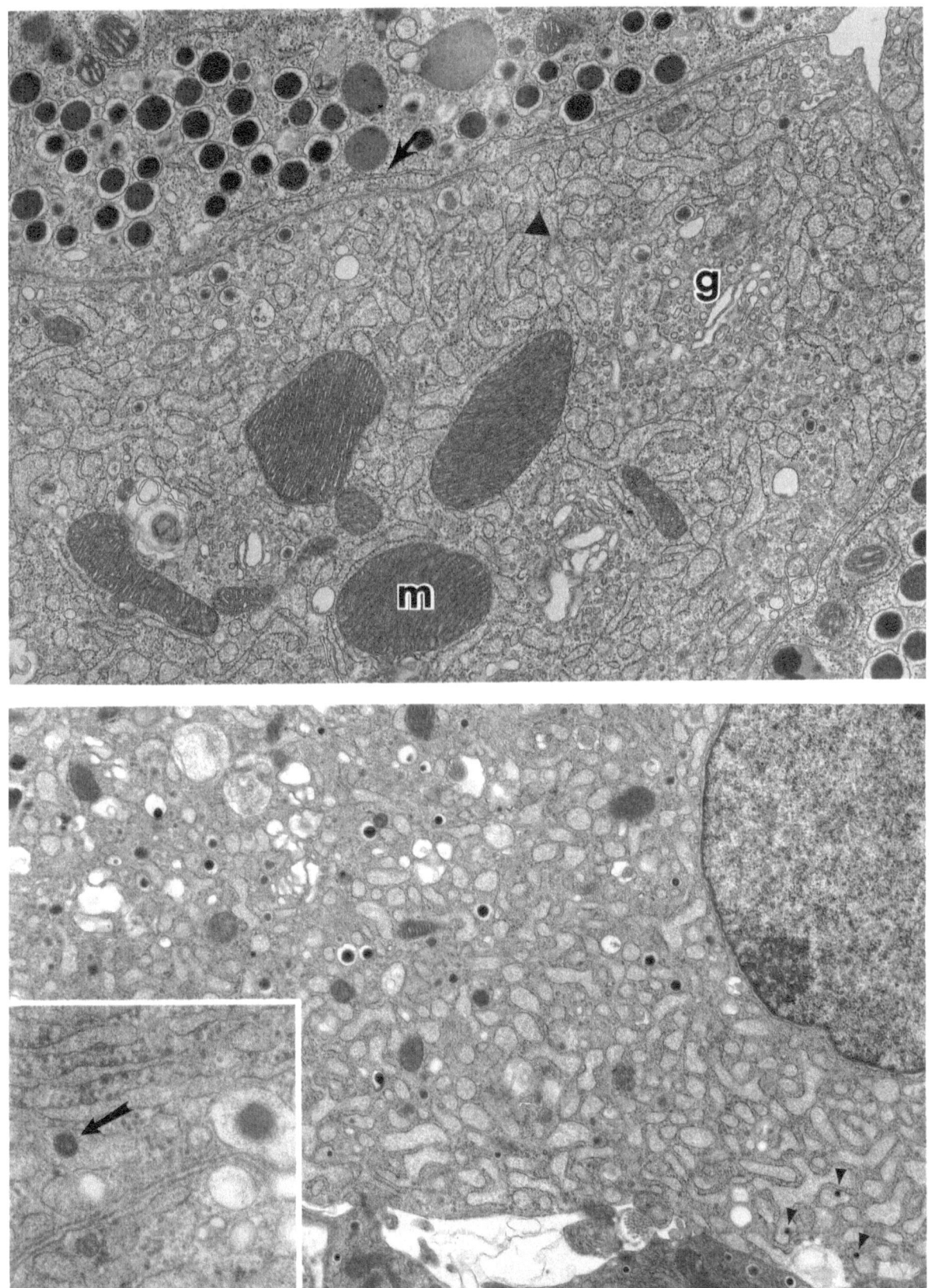

that cause similar, if not identical, diabetes-obesity syndromes. The obese gene is located on chromosome 6, whereas the diabetes gene is located on chromosome 4. Their localization on separate chromosomes suggests that two different primary defects are involved in producing the diabetes-obesity syndrome. The phenotype observed depends on the interaction of the mutation with unknown (not MHC, but gender related) modifiers (Leiter et al. 1981, 1987b) associated with the inbred background on which the mutation is maintained and not solely on the action of the mutant gene itself.

The early developmental stages of both mutations on any genetic background are similar (Coleman 1978, 1982a). The first defect, occurring at about 10 days after birth, is hyperinsulinemia associated with mild hypoglycemia. Both glucose and insulin concentrations increase at weaning (21 days) blood sugar is within the normal range, plasma insulin is elevated three- to fourfold, and insulin resistance is seen. Both plasma insulin and blood glucose continue to rise until 10–12 weeks of age, at which time on the BKs background blood glucose rapidly becomes maximal (400–500 mg/dl) and plasma insulin decreases (Fig. 231). Weight gain, mostly due to accretion of adipose tissue, is rapid in the early stage and slows at 10–16 weeks in association with increased insulin resistance and decreased circulating insulin. Weight loss occurs prior to premature death, usually at about 6–8 months. In contrast, on the B6 background, both mutants expand their insulin supply (sometimes reaching $50 \times$ normal), and the blood sugar concentration normalizes. The hyperglycemia is more pronounced and sustained longer in B6 males than in females. Fat accretion, marked hyperinsulinemia, and maintenance of normal blood glucose concentration persist throughout a near normal lifespan. The sequence of events that occur in the development of both syndromes is hyperinsulinemia, mild hypoglycemia, hyperphagia, increased stimulation of the beta cells, compensatory insulin resistance, and marked obesity with either severe diabetes and beta-cell necrosis or mild or transient diabetes associated with massive hypertrophy and hyperplasia of these beta cells, depending on the inbred background.

Diabetes (db) has been placed on several inbred backgrounds, and the diabetes observed on B6 and BKs appears to represent the extremes. In all backgrounds, males are affected more severely than females. This sexual dimorphism is accentu-

ated on some inbred backgrounds; on the CBA/J and C3HeB/FeJ backgrounds, only the males become severely diabetic and die prematurely, while females retain glycemic control and a near normal lifespan, although they become massively obese (Leiter et al. 1981).

The ob/ob mouse maintained on the B6 background is unique in that it has a hypertropic and hyperplastic type of obesity with both an enlargement and increase in number of the adipocytes contributing to the obesity (Johnson and Hirsch 1972). In contrast, BKs-db/db mice and most other nongenetic obesity conditions in rodents are characterized by adipocyte hypertrophy only. These differences may represent specific effects of the different mutations or may reflect aspects of the B6 background in which the maintenance of excessive plasma insulin concentrations throughout life may promote adipocyte proliferation. Comparative adipocyte studies with the individual mutations maintained on the same background have not been undertaken.

The diabetes-obesity conditions caused by each mutant gene are characterized by marked insulin resistance associated with decreased numbers of high affinity insulin receptors (down regulation) in liver, adipocytes, and lymphocytes (Kahn et al. 1973). Since manipulations (such as food restriction) which serve to reduce the hyperinsulinemia also improve insulin binding to its receptor, the reduced binding to plasma membrane receptors is most likely a reflection of the hyperinsulinemia and does not represent a primary lesion (Soll et al. 1975). However, insulin receptor number was not restored to normal by any treatment, and the relationship of receptor defect to primary defect remains unclear. Abnormalities in a variety of receptors or receptor-linked proteins as well as insulin have been demonstrated in diabetes mice. These include the vasopressin receptor (Assimacopoulos-Jeannet et al. 1983), the cholecystokinin receptor (Saito et al. 1981; Hays and Paul 1981), the guanine nucleotide receptor (Begin-Heick 1985), and the epidermal growth factor receptor (Blackshear et al. 1987). Most of these defects in receptor number or binding occur late into the developing syndrome and most likely represent secondary responses to the abnormal hormonal milieu.

Although many possible primary defects have been suggested for both the obese and diabetes conditions, the actual nature of each defect has not been established. Many of the abnormalities observed in each mutant (hyperphagia, hyperinsulinemia, infertility, and defects in thermoregulation) suggest a hypothalamic defect. Support for this comes from parabiosis studies of *db/db* with normal, *db/db* with *ob/ob*, and *ob/ob* with normal mice (Coleman 1978). These studies suggested that diabetes *(db/db)* mice lack a functional satiety center (presumably a defect in the hypothalamus), while obese *(ob/ob)* mice have a functional center but fail to produce satiety substances. It this is the case, both mutants would have either a nonfunctional or an unregulated satiety system and would be expected to develop identical syndromes when maintained on the same inbred background. The postulated lack of a factor in the obese mouse led to many studies attempting to identify the missing substances. Early studies suggested that it was pancreatic in origin (Strautz 1970), and as the gastroenteropancreatic hormones were identified, each in turn was suggested to be the missing factor. These include glucagon, somatostatin, pancreatic polypeptide, cholecystokinin, endorphins, enkephalins, and galanin (Woods et al. 1986). Longitudinal studies with each polypeptide during development have shown that these changes in most instances are common to both the obese and diabetes mutations and secondary to early hormonal abnormalities, especially hyperinsulinemia.

All diabetes-obesity mutants have the ability to utilize food more efficiently (Cox and Powley 1977; Coleman 1978). Even if fed half the amount of food eaten by a normal mouse on the same time schedule, the mutant mouse still becomes obese. This increment in metabolic efficiency has been suggested to relate to an inability of mutants to thermoregulate normally, and much controversy has developed over whether the deficiency in thermoregulation observed is sufficient to account for all the increased metabolic efficiency (Coleman 1982b, 1985). When mutants are pair fed with normal mice in a thermoneutral environment at 33 °C, conditions that would not require energy for thermoregulation and would prevent diet-induced thermogenesis, mutants still become obese. This suggests that any defect in thermogenesis seen under normal mouse husbandry conditions contributes to, but cannot account for, all of the increased metabolic efficiency. The identical increases in metabolic efficiency observed in both the obese *(ob/ob)* and the diabetes *(db/db)* mutants suggest that the increased efficiency is not primary but is probably secondary to mutant gene action. The hyperinsulinemia could increase metabolic efficiency by its anabolic action which in promoting synthesis and preventing normal synthesis-degradation cy-

cles could decrease normal metabolic energy expenditure considerably. Furthermore, the excess insulin in mutants would be antagonistic to catabolic hormones such as glucagon and catecholamines and prevent these hormones from activating both cold- and diet-induced thermogenesis. Critical studies in vivo regarding rates of metabolic cycling in normal and mutant mice are needed before the nature of any efficiency mechanisms can be delineated and quantified.

Carbohydrate metabolism in mutants is typical of that resulting from chronic exposure to high insulin concentrations and is characterized by increased glycolysis and increased glucose and glycogen turnover. Much of the carbohydrate metabolism is directed to lipid synthesis, and the rate of lipogenesis is greatly enhanced. In spite of the increased insulin concentration, gluconeogenesis which should be repressed remains maximally induced, while most other insulin-responsive pathways (lipogenesis and glycolysis) respond normally. Feeding the adrenal prohormone, dehydroepiandrosterone, and some of its metabolites prevents islet atrophy and the associated diabetes in BKs mutants (Coleman et al. 1984a, b) as well as decreasing the rate of weight gain in mutants maintained on the B6 background. Of the many metabolic pathways studied in steroid-treated mutants, only the anomalously high rate of gluconeogenesis appears changed, being normalized after as little as 24-48 h of treatment. This normalization in the rate of synthesis and release of new glucose by the liver may decrease the hyperglycemic stress sufficiently to preserve pancreatic beta-cell structure and function.

Comparison with Other Species

These single gene obesity conditions produce massive obesities that are not typically seen in humans. However, studies on the regulations of the metabolic efficiency mechanisms involved in exacerbating the obesity in mice could have major implications for the prevention and control of obesity in humans. With respect to diabetes, these mutants have some aspects of both noninsulin-dependent (type II) and insulin-dependent (type I) forms, and each has some application to studies of both. Varying the background and sex on which the mutation is maintained has profound effects on the type of diabetes produced. Investigators wishing to study a model of juvenile-onset hyperglycemia could choose either the diabetes *(db/db)* or obese *(ob/ob)* mutants on the BKs background, whereas those more interested in obesity without permanent hyperglycemia could choose these same mutants on the B6 background. An understanding of the mode of action of these modifying genes that change the course of the disease from a benign obesity to a condition of severe hyperglycemia coupled with massive beta-cell necrosis and islet atrophy would be an important contribution to the understanding of human diabetes variants.

Acknowledgments. I would like to thank Dr. David A. Gapp for some of the material used and format for Fig. 231 and Dr. E. H. Leiter for providing the photomicrographs used in Figs. 229, 230, 232 and 233 and for his careful critical review of the manuscript. The writing of this manuscript was supported by NIH grant DK14461.

References

Assimacopoulos-Jeannet F, Cantau B, Van de Werve G, Jard S, Jeanrenaud B (1983) Lack of vasopressin receptors in liver, but not in kidney, of *ob/ob* mice. Biochem J 216: 475-480

Baetens D, Stefan Y, Ravazzola M, Malaisse-Lagae F, Coleman DL, Orci L (1978) Alteration of islet cell populations in spontaneously diabetic mice. Diabetes 27: 1-7

Begin-Heick N (1985) Absence of the inhibitory effect of guanine nucleotides on adenate cyclase activity in white adipocyte membranes of the *ob/ob* mouse. Effect of the *ob* gene. J Biol Chem 260: 6187-6193

Berelowitz M, Coleman DL, Frohman LA (1980) Temporal relationship of tissue somatostatin-like immunoreactivity to metabolic changes in genetically obese and diabetic mice. Diabetes 29: 717-723

Blackshear PJ, Stumpo DJ, Kennington EA, Tuttle JS, Orth DN, Thompson KL, Hung M-C, Rosner MR (1987) Decreased levels of hepatic epidermal growth factor receptors in obese hyperglycemic rodents. J Biol Chem 22: 12356-12364

Bohlen HG, Niggl BA (1979a) Adult microvascular disturbances as a result of juvenile-onset diabetes in *db/db* mice. Blood Vessels 16: 269-276

Bohlen HG, Niggl BA (1979b) Arteriolar anatomical and functional abnormalities in juvenile mice with genetic or streptozotocin-induced diabetes mellitus. Circ Res 45: 390-396

Bower G, Brown DM, Steffes MW, Vernier RL, Mauers M (1980) Studies of the glomerular mesangium and the juxtaglomerular apparatus in the genetically diabetic mouse. Lab Invest 43: 333-341

Bray GA, York DA (1979) Hypothalamic and genetic obesity in experimental animals: an autonomic and endocrine hypothesis. Physiol Rev 59: 719-809

Coleman DL (1978) Obese and diabetes: two mutant genes causing diabetes obesity syndromes in mice. Diabetologia 14: 141-148

Coleman DL (1982a) Diabetes obesity snydromes in mice. Diabetes 31 (2) [Suppl I]: 1-6

Coleman DL (1982b) Thermogenesis in diabetes-obesity syndromes in mutant mice. Diabetologia 22: 205-211

Coleman DL (1985) Increased metabolic efficiency in obese mutant mice. Int J Obes 9 [Suppl 2]: 69-73

Coleman DL, Hummel KP (1967) Studies with the mutation, diabetes, in the mouse. Diabetologia 3: 238-248

Coleman DL, Leiter EH, Applezweig N (1984a) Therapeutic effects of dehydroepiandrosterone metabolites in diabetes mutant mice (C57BL/KsJ-*db/db*). Endocrinology 115: 239-243

Coleman DL, Schwizer RW, Leiter EH (1984b) Effect of genetic background on the therapeutic effects of dehydroepiandrosterone (DHEA) in diabetes-obesity mutants and in aged normal mice. Diabetes 33: 26-32

Cox JE, Powley TL (1977) Development of obesity in mice pair-fed with lean siblings. J Comp Physiol Psychol 91: 347-378

Fernandes G, Handwerger BS, Yunis EJ, Brown BM (1978) Immune response in the mutant diabetic C57BL/Ks-db+ mouse. Discrepancies between in vitro and in vivo immunological assays. J Clin Invest 61: 243-250

Gapp DA, Leiter EH, Coleman DL, Schwizer RW (1983) Temporal changes in pancreatic islet composition in C57BL/6J-*db/db* (diabetes) mice. Diabetologia 25: 439-443

Gartner K (1979) Glomerular hyperfiltration during the onset of diabetes mellitus in 2 strains of diabetic (C57BL/6J *db/db* and C57BL/KsJ *db/db*) mice. Diabetologia 15: 59-63

Giachetti A (1978) The functional state of sympathetic nerves in spontaneously diabetic mice. Diabetes 27: 969-974

Giachetti A (1979) Axoplasmic transport of noradreanlin in the sciatic nerves of spontaneously diabetic mice. Diabetologia 16: 191-194

Hanker JS, Ambrose WW, Yates PE, Koch GG, Carson KA (1980) Peripheral neuropathy in mouse hereditary diabetes mellitus I. Comparison of neurologic, histologic and morphometric parameters with dystonic mice. Acta Neuropathol (Berl) 51: 145-154

Hays SE, Paul SM (1981) Cholecystokinin receptors are increased in cerebral cortex of genetically obese mice. Eur J Pharmacol 70: 591-592

Johnson LM, Sidman RL (1979) A reproductive endocrine profile in the diabetes *(db/db)* mutant mouse. Biol Reprod 20: 552-559

Johnson PR, Hirsch J (1972) Cellularity of adipose deposits in six strains of genetically obese mice. J Lipid Res 13: 2-11

Kahn CR, Neville DM Jr, Roth J (1973) Insulin-receptor interaction in the obese-hyperglycemic mouse: a model of insulin resistance. J Biol Chem 248: 244-250

Leiter EH, Kuff EL (1984) Intracisternal type A particles in murine pancreatic B cells. Immunocytochemical demonstration of increased antigen in genetically diabetic mice. Am J Pathol 114: 46-55

Leiter EH, Gapp DA, Eppig JJ, Coleman DL (1979) Ultrastructural and morphometric studies of delta cells in pancreatic islets from C57BL/Ks diabetes mice. Diabetologia 17: 297–309

Leiter EH, Coleman DL, Hummel KP (1981) The influence of genetic background on the expression of mutations at the diabetes locus. III. Effect of *H-2* haplotype and sex. Diabetes 30: 1029–1034

Leiter EH, Prochazka M, Shultz LD (1987a) Effect of immunodeficiency on diabetogenesis in genetically diabetic *(db/db)* mice. J Immunol 138: 3224–3229

Leiter EH, Le PH, Coleman DL (1987b) Susceptibility to db gene and streptozotocin-induced diabetes in C57BL mice; control by gender associated, MHC unlinked traits. Immunogenetics 26: 6–13

Like AA, Chick WL (1970a) Studies in the diabetic mutant mouse I. Light microscopy and radioautography of pancreatic islets. Diabetologia 6: 207–215

Like AA, Chick WL (1970b) Studies in the diabetic mouse II. Electron microscopy of pancreatic islets. Diabetologia 6: 216–242

Like AA, Lavine RL, Poffenbarger PL, Chick WL (1972) Studies in the diabetic mutant mouse. VI. Evolution of glomerular lesions and associated proteinuria. Am J Pathol 66: 193–224

Mahmood AHF, Rodman HM, Mandel MA, Warren KS (1976) Induced and spontaneous diabetes mellitus and suppression of cell-mediated immunological response. Granuloma formation, delayed dermal activity and allograft rejection. J Clin Invest 57: 362–367

Meade OJ, Brandon DR, Smith W, Simmonds RG, Harris S, Sowter C (1981) The relationship between hyperglycemia and renal immune complex deposition in mice with inherited diabetes. Clin Exp Immunol 43: 109–120

Moore SA, Peterson RG, Felton DL, Cartwright TR, O'Connor BL (1980) Reduced sensory and motor conduction velocity in 25-week-old diabetic [C57BL/Js *(db/db)*] mice. Exp Neurol 70: 548–555

Saito A, Williams JA, Goldfine ID (1981) Alterations of brain cerebral cortex CCK receptors in the *ob/ob* mouse. Endocrinology 109: 984–986

Sheena J, Meade CJ (1978) Mice bearing *ob/ob* mutation have impaired immunity. Int Arch Allergy Appl Immunol 57: 263–268

Sima A, Robertson DM (1978) Peripheral neuropathy in the mutant diabetic mouse [C57BL/Ks *(db/db)*]. Acta Neuropathol (Berl) 41: 85–89

Soll AH, Kahn CR, Neville DM Jr (1975) Insulin binding to liver plasma membranes in the obese hyperglycemic *(ob/ob)* mouse. J Biol Chem 250: 4702–4707

Strautz RL (1970) Studies of hereditary obese mice *(ob/ob)* after implantation of pancreatic islets in millipore filter capsules. Diabetologia 6: 306–312

Woods SC, Tuborsky GI Jr, Porte D Jr (1986) Central nervous system control of nutrient homeostasis. In: Bloom FE (ed) Handbook of physiol sect 1, vol IV. Williams and Wilkins, Baltimore, pp 341–54 (American Physiological Society series)

The Skin of the Rhino Mouse

Lorraine H. Kligman and Albert M. Kligman

Gross Appearance

Surely one of the oddities of nature, the rhino mouse as it matures becomes "curiouser and curiouser." This recessive, single gene mutant of the house mouse was first described by Howard in 1940. During the first 2 weeks of life, the homozygous animal resembles its heterozygous and normal littermates. Born naked, it develops a full, darkly pigmented first pelage. Then, over the next 10–12 days, the hair is lost in a cephalad to caudal wave, leaving the animal once again quite naked. With the exception of a few hairs in an occasional animal, a second pelage never appears because of an aberration in the first catagen (Mann 1971). The dermal papilla fails to follow the contracting follicle and becomes isolated in the subcutaneous tissue. The two never rejoin, rendering the follicle permanently hairless. Shortly thereafter, the skin becomes progressively loose and redundant, falling increasingly into rhinoceroslike folds, flaps, and ridges (Fig. 234). This extraordinary expansion of the surface occurs because the empty follicles widen into ampulliform cavities or "utriculi" which become distended with retained horny cells. The horn-filled utriculi are not grossly apparent until the animal ages (Fig. 235), which it does prematurely in 6 months to 1 year. The mature rhino mouse usually weighs more than its haired littermates mainly because of the large masses of skin. Indeed, the muscles and subcutaneous tissue regress (Davies et al. 1971).

With time other unattractive features appear, viz, long, coiled nails and a waxy deposition which peels off in large flakes.

Microscopic Features

The most striking feature of rhino mouse skin is the close rows of horn-filled utriculi which occu-

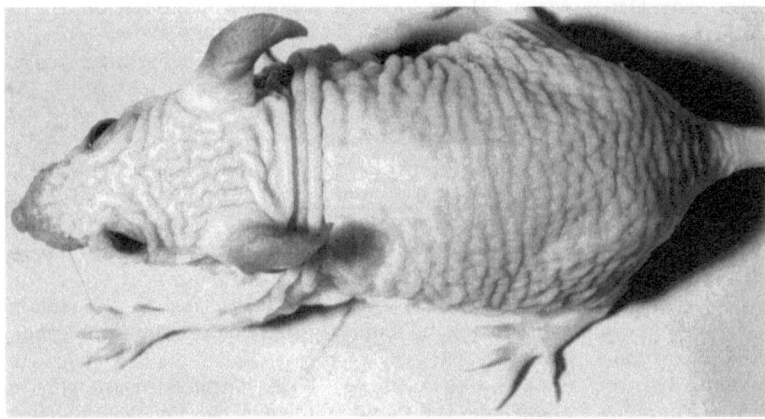

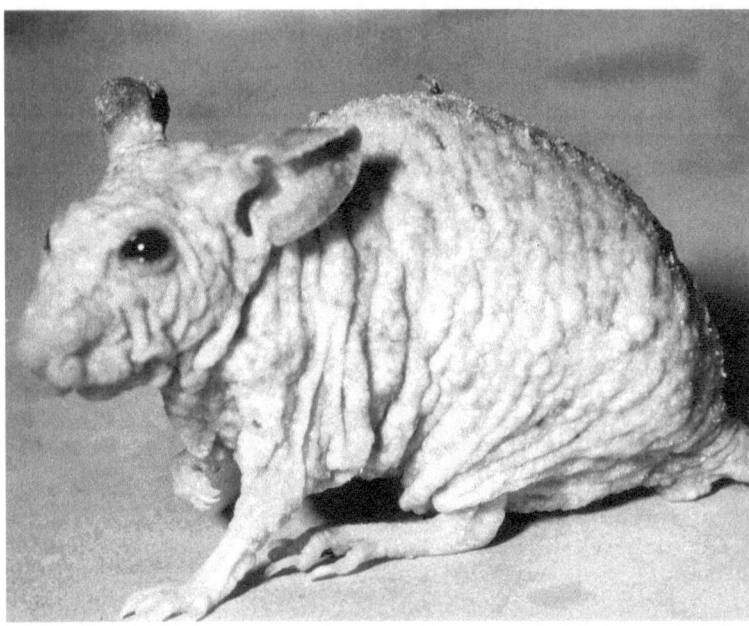

Fig. 234 *(above).* Rhino mouse, age 9 weeks. Skin surface is rugose and lies in thick folds in the head and neck region

Fig. 235 *(below).* Rhino mouse, age approximately 1 year. The horn-filled utriculi are visible on the surface as multiple nodules

py most of the upper dermis and strikingly resemble the open comedomes of human acne (Fig. 236). Sebaceous glands are regularly found at the base of the utriculi but are tiny, again analogous to human comedones. The scant interfollicular epidermis is 4–6 cells thick, including 2–3 layers of granular cells, while the stretched epithelial lining of the utriculi consists of 2–4 cell layers. The stratum corneum is thick but loosely organized. One to two rows of horn-filled cysts of variable size occupy the lower dermis (Fig. 236), derivatives from fragments of follicular epithelia segregated during catagen. These are similar to the cysts of the familiar hairless (Skh-hairless) mouse, a less deformed animal.

The high density of capacious utriculi reduces the volume of intervening connective tissue. Aside from the more densely packed collagen bundles, what can be visualized with histochemical stains resembles that reported for the regular hairless mouse (Kligman et al. 1982). Elastic fibers are thin and sparse (Fig. 237), and there is minimal ground substance.

Biochemical Features

The only biochemically defined feature of the rhino mouse is the skin lipids. Logani et al. (1975, 1977) have described two, unique, neutral,

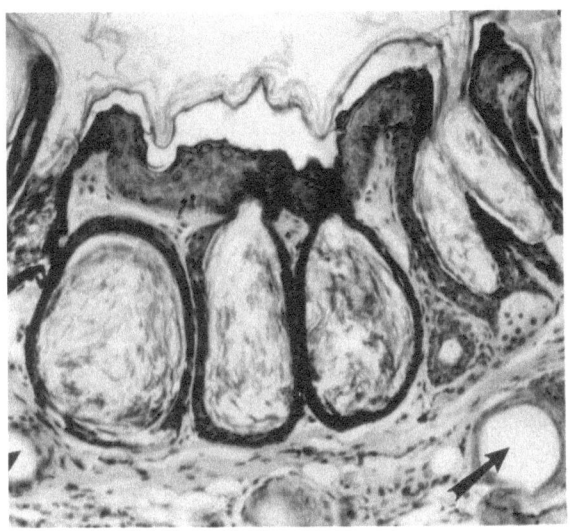

Fig. 236. Skin rhino mouse. Contiguous, horn-filled utri-culi fill the upper dermis and reduce the extent of inter-follicular epidermis. Small epithelial cysts *(arrows)* are present in the lower dermis. H and E, × 125

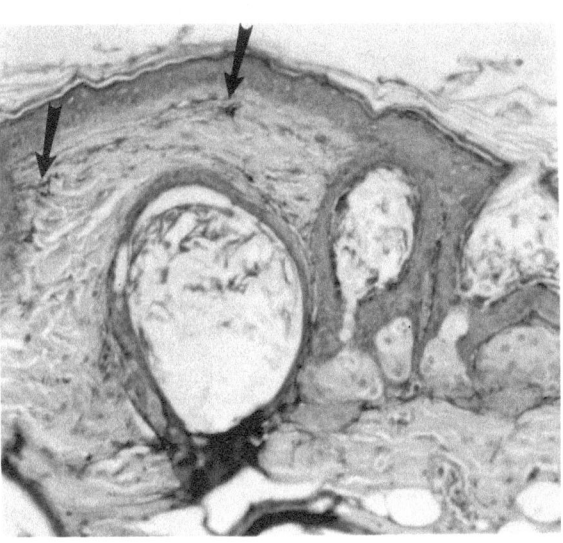

Fig. 237. Skin, rhino mouse. Elastic fibers *(arrows)* are thin and sparse. Luna's aldehyde fuchsin, × 125

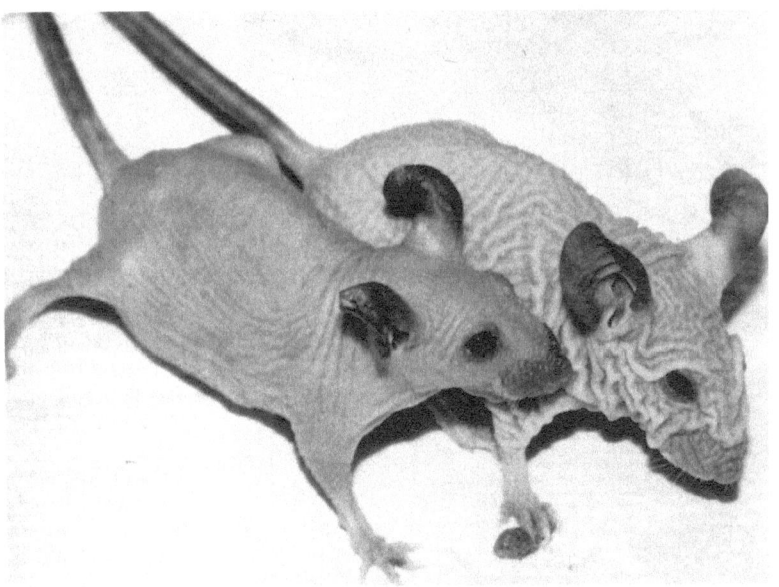

Fig. 238. Rhino mouse *(left)* treated with retinoic acid and its untreated littermate. Daily application of 0.05% retinoic acid for 3 weeks has virtually effaced the wrinkles and folds

triester isomeric waxes. These are composed of three structural units: nonhydroxylated fatty ac-ids, ω-hydroxy fatty acids, and 1–2 alkanediols. Like normal mice and a number of other ani-mals, rhino skin is deficient in triacylglycerol. This animal also lacks the adipose tissue stores of this triglyceride (Davies et al. 1971). On the other hand, large stores of lathosterol, a choles-terol precursor, are present. These findings point to gross abnormalities in lipid metabolism (Dav-ies et al. 1971). Because of the difficulties in separating the epidermis from the dermis, the lo-calization of these various lipids is uncertain, in that these could be either of epidermal or seba-ceous origin.

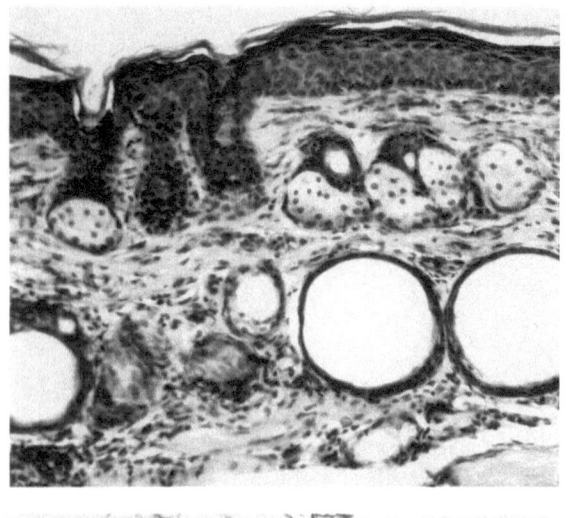

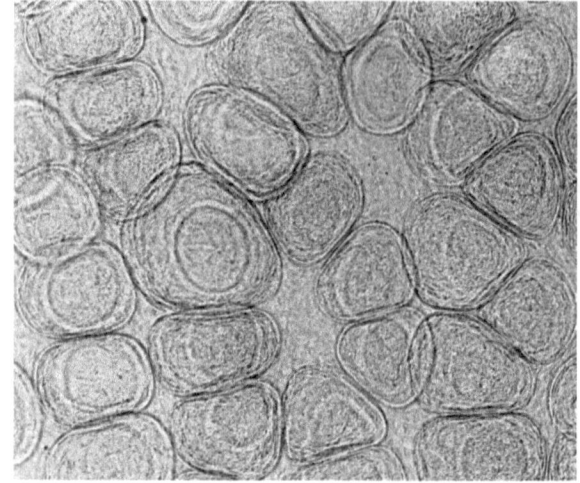

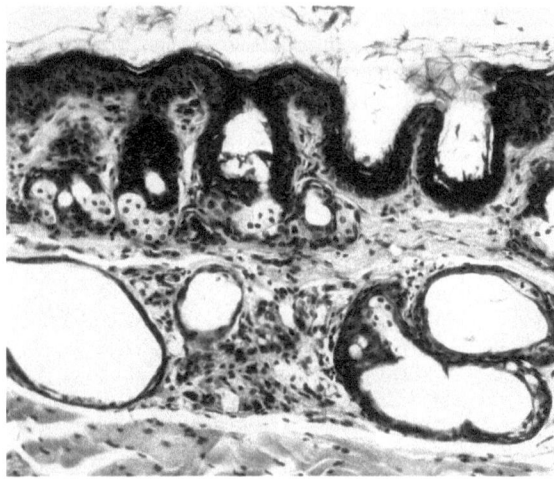

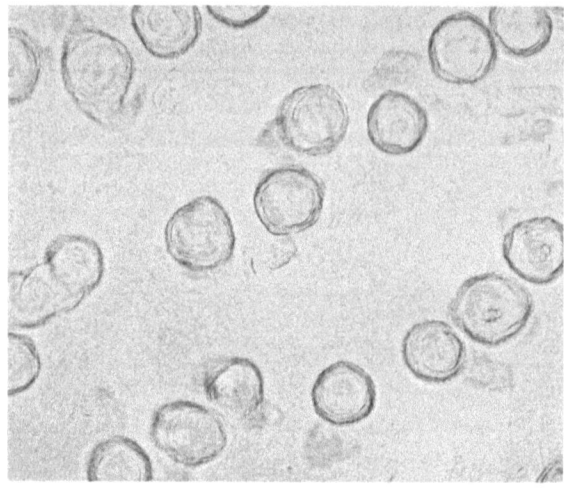

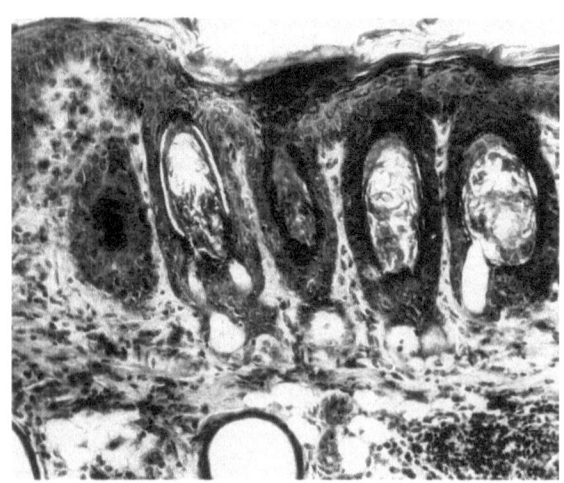

Fig. 239 *(upper left)*. Skin, rhino mouse. Topical 0.05% retinoic acid applied for 3 weeks. Utriculi have reverted to normal follicular architecture. Impacted horn has been expelled and interfollicular epidermis is more extensive. H and E, ×125

Fig. 240 *(middle left)*. Skin, rhino mouse. Topical 0.0005% retinoic acid applied for 3 weeks. Although this is close to threshold dose, the utriculi are nonetheless partially normalized. H and E, ×125

Fig. 241 *(lower left)*. Treatment with squalene for 3 weeks. Utriculi are narrowed but have hyperplastic epithelia and contain dense horn

Fig. 242 *(upper right)*. Rhino mouse, epidermis, whole mounts photographed from dermal surface. Untreated skin: utriculi are inflated spheres. Unstained, ×70

Fig. 243 *(lower right)*. Rhino mouse, epidermis, whole mounts photographed from dermal surface. 0.05% retinoic acid applied daily for 3 weeks: utricular diameters are greatly diminished. Unstained, ×70

Biologic Features

Experimental Usage. The rhino mouse is extremely sensitive to chemical carcinogens such as polycyclic hydrocarbons. Ultraviolet radiation readily induces tumors (Davies et al. 1971). However, it has not become a biological model for these purposes. The greatest value of this animal lies in its response to retinoids. Early studies by Fraser (1949) and Mauer (1961) using oral vitamin A were undertaken because the skin changes were thought to be similar to those of vitamin A-deficient animals. There is no evidence, however, that the rhino mouse suffers from such a deficiency (Davies et al. 1971). In fact, hypervitaminosis A is easily induced. Administration of vitamin A did not prevent hair loss. Surprisingly, the comedolike utriculi did not regress. Administration of vitamin A from birth did seem to limit formation of the dermal cysts.

In a preliminary study, Van Scott (1972) found that topical retinoic acid caused shrinkage of the horn-filled utriculi. This led us to examine this effect more systematically (Kligman and Kligman 1979). After only 3 weeks of topical application of 0.05% all-*trans*-retinoic acid to the backs of mice aged 6–8 weeks, the gross effect was stunning with virtual effacement of the redundant folds and wrinkles (Fig. 238). The involutional changes were striking. Utriculi reverted to normal follicular dimensions, free of horny impactions (Fig. 239). The interfollicular epidermis became broader and hyperplastic (7–10 cells) with a well-developed granular layer of 4–5 cells. These effects were strictly retinoid dose dependent. Moreover, even very low concentrations (0.0005%) caused partial regression of utriculi (Fig. 240).

Other agents are capable of modulating the peculiar skin of this animal. Halowax increases horny utriculi impaction (Van Scott 1972), while salicylic acid has a modest reducing effect (Kligman and Kligman 1979), Squalene and benzoyl peroxide (Fig. 241) cause the utriculi to elongate via follicular epithelial hyperplasia (Kligman and Kligman 1979), To date, only retinoids, including some of the newest ones, have been found capable of fully "normalizing" utriculi. Involution can be demonstrated either by oral or topical application.

A method for quantification of the degree of "normalization" has been described by Mezick et al. (1984). They first separated the epidermis with its attached utriculi by immersion of whole skin in 0.5% acetic acid. After passing it through a graded series of alcohols followed by xylene, the resulting whole mount allowed sharp visualization of the utriculi from the underside (Figs. 242 and 243). The diameters of utriculi can thus be determined with greater accuracy.

Comparison with Other Species

There are a number of hairless mutant mice available for experimental use and at least one type each of hairless rats, hamsters, guinea pigs, and dogs. Even hairless moles, rabbits, goats, horses, cattle, and humans have been reported (David 1931). None of these, however, possess horn-filled utriculi and redundant skin folds. To our knowledge, the only other rhino mutants described were three deer mice (Rigdon and Packchanian 1957) and a group of Norway rats (Robinson 1965). Both species became hairless, developed utriculi and dermal cysts, and became progressively wrinkled with age. These deer mice and Norway rats are currently not available as research animals. Thus, the rhino mouse maintains its uniqueness in the animal kingdom.

References

David LT (1931) Hairless mammals. Comparative histologic studies: preliminary report. Arch Dermatol Syphilol 24: 196–203

Davies RE, Austin WA, Logani MK (1971) The rhino mutant mouse as an experimental tool. Trans NY Acad Sci (series II) 33: 680–693

Fraser CF (1949) The effect of vitamin A on hereditary hyperkeratosis in the mouse. Can J Res 27 (D series): 179–185

Howard A (1940) "Rhino", an allele of hairless in the house mouse. J Hered 31: 467–470

Kligman LH, Kligman AM (1979) The effect on rhino mouse skin of agents which influence keratinization and exfoliation. J Invest Dermatol 73: 354–358

Kligman LH, Akin FJ, Kligman AM (1982) Prevention of ultraviolet damage to the dermis of hairless mice by sunscreens. J Invest Dermatol 78: 181–189

Logani MK, Austin WA, Nhari DB, Davies RE (1975) Neutral lipids from the skin of the rhino mutant mouse. Biochim Biophys Acta 380: 155–164

Logani MK, Nhari DB, Davies RE (1977) Composition of novel triesters from the skin of the rhino mutant mouse. Lipids 12: 283–287

Mann SJ (1971) Hair loss and cyst formation in hairless and rhino mutant mice. Anat Rec 170: 485–500

Mauer I (1961) The effect of vitamin A in hyperkeratotic mouse mutants. J Exp Zool 146: 181–207

Mezick JA, Bhatia MC, Capetola RJ (1984) Topical and systemic effects of retinoids on horn-filled utriculus size in the rhino mouse: a model to quantify "antikeratinizing" effects of retinoids. J Invest Dermatol 83: 110–113

Rigdon RH, Packchanian AA (1957) Histologic study of the skin of hairless American deer mice *(Peromyscus maniculatus gambeli)*. Arch Pathol 64: 210–221

Robinson R (1965) Pelage variations (chap 2). In: Robinson R (ed) Genetics of the Norway rat. Pergamon, New York, pp 39–52

Van Scott EJ (1972) Experimental animal integumental models for screening potential dermatologic drugs. In: Montagne WA, Van Scott EJ, Stoughton R (eds) Pharmacology of skin. Appleton-Century-Crofts, New York, pp 523–533

Hairless Mouse, HRS/J *hr/hr*

John P. Sundberg, Robert W. Dunstan, and John G. Compton

Gross Appearance

HRS/J mice, homozygous for the autosomal recessive gene "hairless" *(hr)*, develop a syndrome characterized by loss of hair after growth of the first pelage (Fig. 244), rudimentary mammary gland development, and susceptibility to lymphomas (Figs. 245 and 246) (Morrissey et al. 1980; Meier et al. 1969). At about 14 days of age, when the eyes open, *hr/hr* mice can be recognized by loss of hair on the upper eyelids (Snell 1931). Shedding begins under the jaw and on all four limbs then progresses to the base of the tail. During the 3rd week of life a wave of shedding spreads from these areas. The animal becomes essentially naked except for scattered hairs from tylotrich follicles (Mann and Straile 1961). The vibrissae become less numerous with age (Snell 1931). The skin of *hr/hr* animals appears wrinkled (Fig. 244); however, heterozygotes have similar wrinkling which is not apparent due to the presence of the normal hair coat (David 1934). The homozygotes also develop grotesquely curved nails (Crew and Mirskaia 1931) (Fig. 246). Normal haired males do not mate with the hairless females (Crew and Mirskaia 1931). HRS/J *hr/hr* mice have a 45% incidence of T-cell lymphoma by 8–10 months of age which increases to over 70% by 18 months, compared with 1% and 20%, respectively, for normal heterozygotes. Hairless mice with lymphoma are seen to have generalized lymphadenopathy associated with enlargement of the spleen, liver, and thymus (Figs. 245 and 246) (Meier et al. 1969).

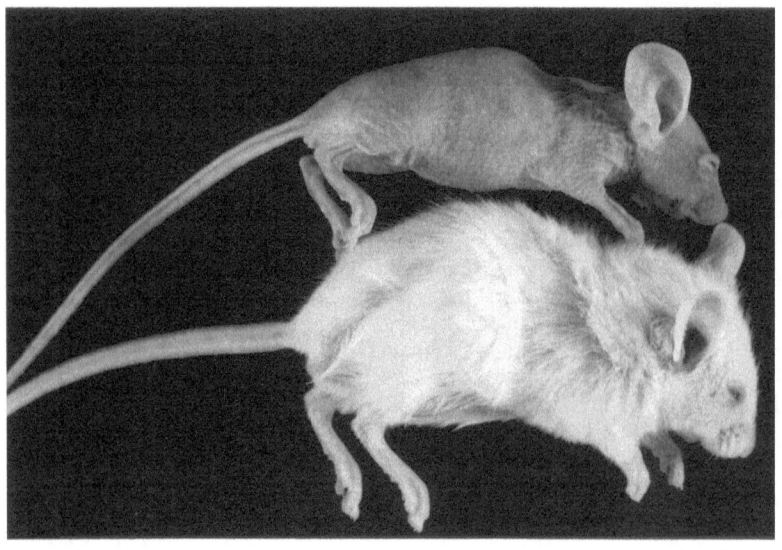

Fig. 244. Mice, 4-week-old males *(above)* HRS/J *hr/hr* and *(below) hr/+*

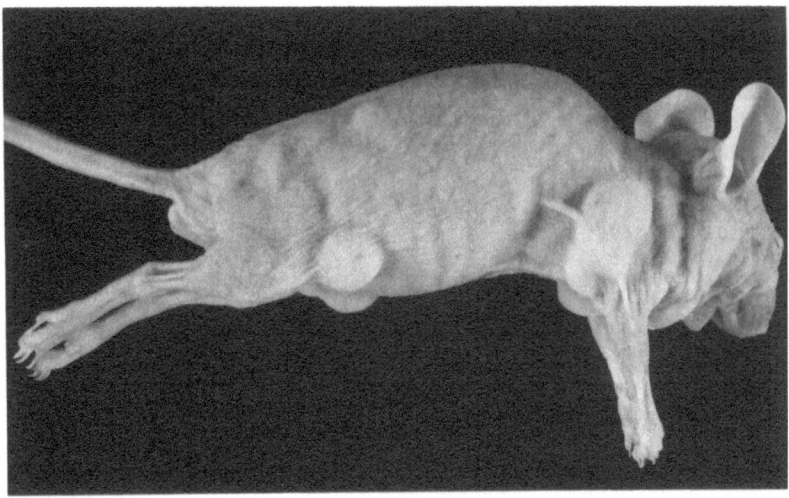

Fig. 245. Mouse, male HRS/J *hr/hr,* with peripheral lymphadenopathy due to T-cell lymphoma

Microscopic Features

Three features characterize the skin of HRS/J *hr/hr* mice: the formation of comedones (pilary cysts), the formation of dilated ducts of sebaceous glands, and granulomatous inflammation of the dermis associated with rupture of the follicles. Generalized acanthosis and orthokeratosis of the skin affect the entire body of these mice (Figs. 247 and 248). The comedones develop shortly after the first hair cycle. They are characterized by dilation of follicular infundibula which are filled with keratin and sebum (Figs. 249 and 250). The ducts of sebaceous glands consist of dilated, cystic structures lined by flattened epithelial cells with clear, finely vacuolated cytoplasm similar to cells in adjacent sebaceous glands (Figs. 248 and 251).

Sebaceous glands undergo hypertrophy at 30 days of age and atrophy after 1 year of age (Figs. 247–249) (Mann 1971). A nodular to diffuse, granulomatous, inflammatory cell infiltrate may be present in the dermis. A mixture of cells, consisting of macrophages and giant cells, surrounds keratin or hair shafts from ruptured dermal cysts (Fig. 252). Multiple cutaneous ulcers often develop due to fighting when males are housed together.

The lymphoma which develops in HRS/J *hr/hr* mice has been classified as a lymphoblastic lymphoma of the T cell type (Pattengale and Taylor 1983). The tumors consist of a homogeneous population of mitotically active, intermediate-sized, lymphoid cells with round to slightly irreg-

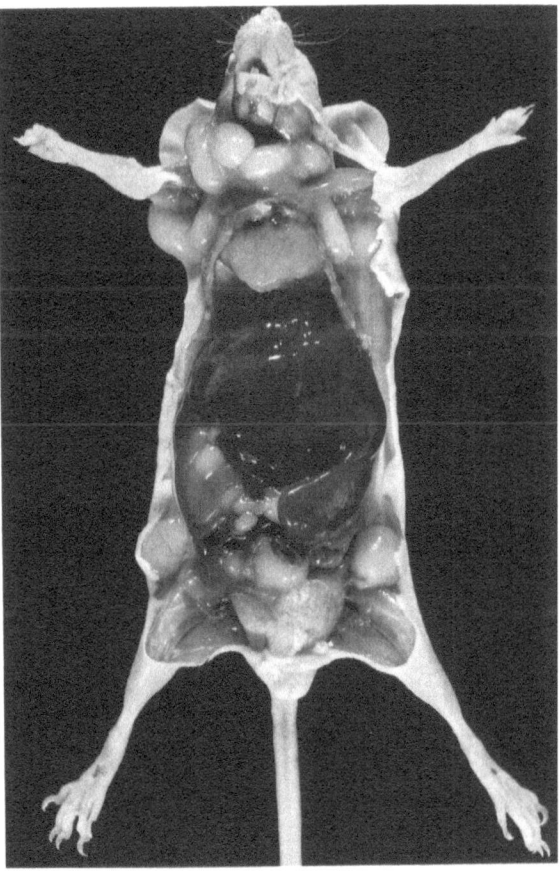

Fig. 246. Same male mouse (HRS/J *hr/hr*) as in Fig. 245: generalized lymphadenopathy and enlarged thymus, spleen, and liver

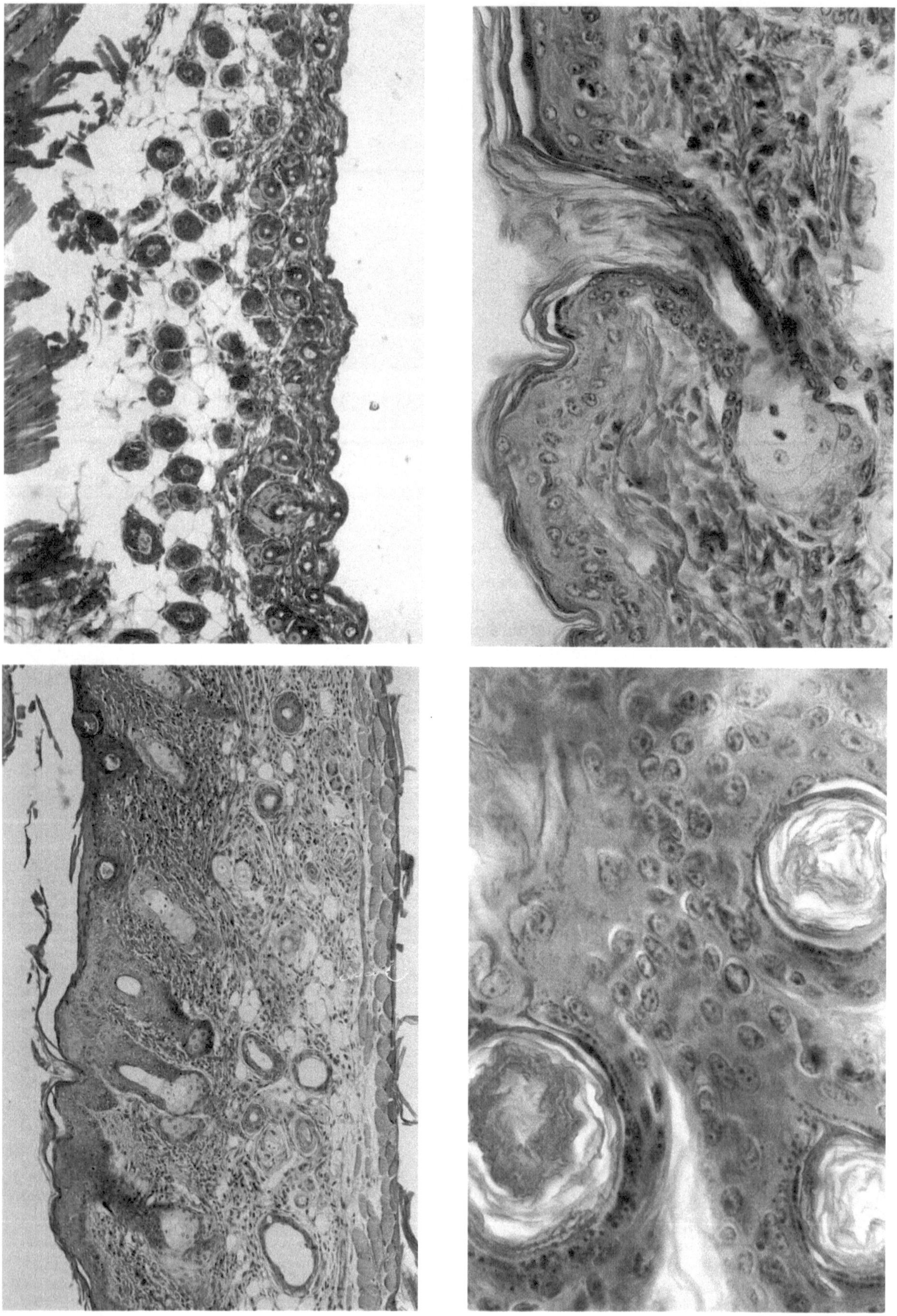

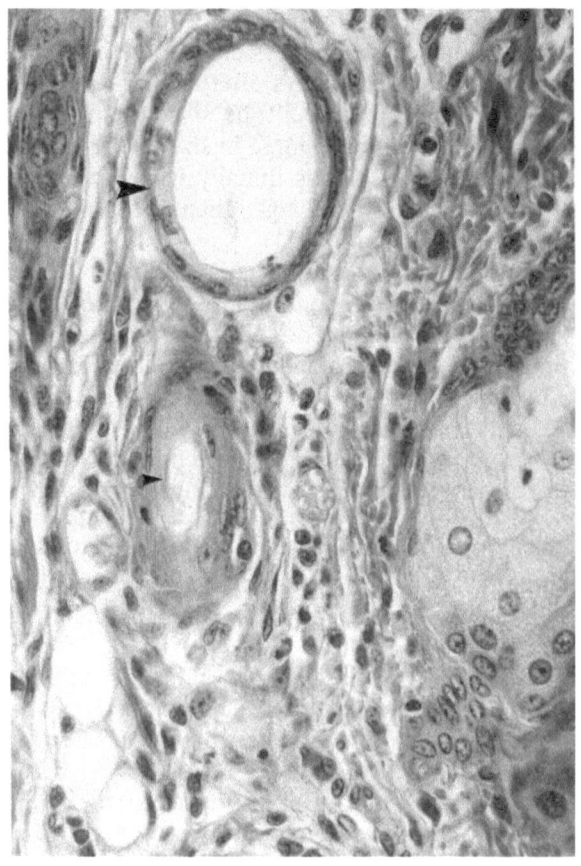

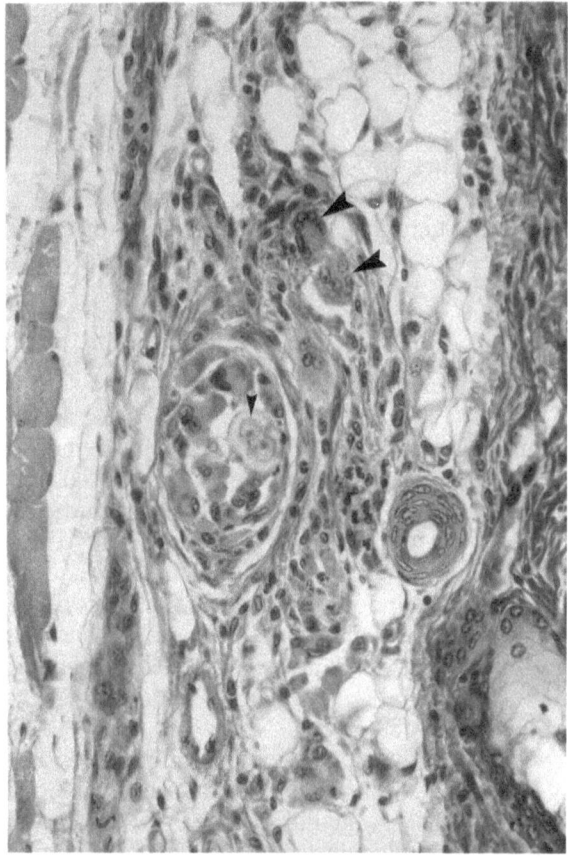

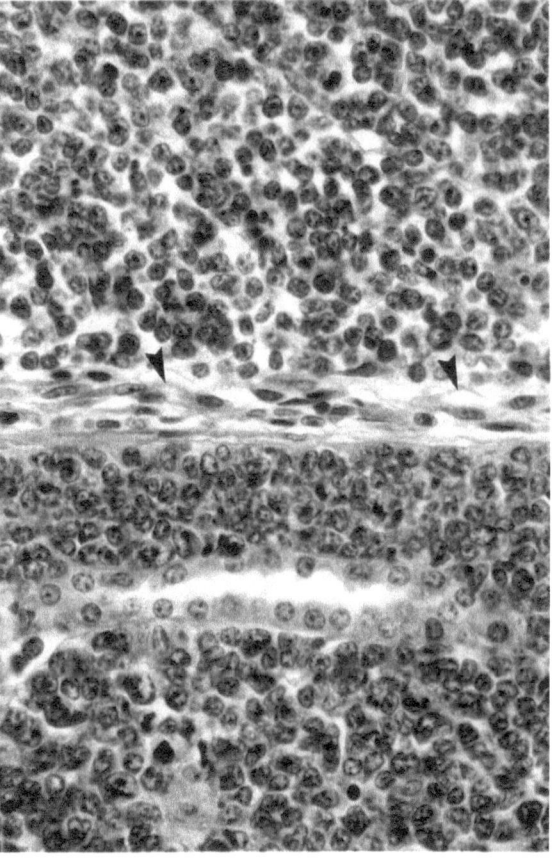

◀ **Fig. 247** *(upper left).* Normal skin of *hr/+* mouse. H and E, ×100

Fig. 248 *(lower left).* Skin of *hr/hr* mouse with severe acanthosis, mild orthokeratosis, dilated sebaceous gland ducts, fibrosis of the hypodermis, and hair shafts within a granuloma in the reticular dermis. H and E, ×150

Fig. 249 *(upper right).* Skin of *hr/hr* mouse with follicle packed with keratin from the surface to the entrance of the sebaceous gland. H and E, ×250

Fig. 250 *(lower right).* Skin, *hr/hr* mouse. Follicles are dilated with laminated keratin. H and E, ×500

Fig. 251 *(upper left).* Skin, *hr/hr* mouse. A small follicle ▶ *(small arrowhead)* is adjacent to a cyst lined by sebaceous cells *(large arrowhead)* below a normal sebaceous gland. H and E, ×400

Fig. 252 *(upper right).* Dermis, *hr/hr* mouse. Hair shaft *(small arrowhead)* surrounded by macrophages and multinucleated giant cells *(large arrowheads).* H and E, ×250

Fig. 253 *(lower right).* Kidney, *hr/hr* mouse. T-cell lymphoma surrounding and invading the kidney. Renal capsule *(arrowheads).* H and E, ×400

ular nuclei and delicate, finely dispersed, stippled chromatin (Fig. 253). The tumor cells stain positively for surface Thy-1.

Ultrastructure

No ultrastructural abnormalities of keratinization in the hairless mouse have been described (Raknerud et al. 1971; Raknerud 1974, 1975).

Differential Diagnosis

A number of other mutations occur in the house mouse *(Mus musculus)* in which generalized hair loss occurs. The most widely studied include the "nude" *(nu)*, "naked" *(N)*, and "rhino" *(hr^{rh})* mutants. With the exception of the rhino mutation, the other loci are on different chromosomes. The rhino mutation is allelic with hairless *(hr)* and is a more severe manifestation of the hairless mutation (Mann 1971). The rhino mutation is described on p. 187.

The skin of athymic nude mice is morphologically normal at birth except for poorly developed hair follicles. Follicular atrophy is associated with keratin plugging of follicular infundibula which contain curled and degenerate hairs and small, fragmented surface hairs (Rigdon and Packchanian 1974). In comparison with hairless, these are no cysts, less hyperkeratosis, and a population of follicles which can reenter anagen and produce hair under the influence of cyclosporin A (Sawada et al. 1987).

Mice heterozygous for the dominant naked *(N)* gene have hair follicles with few abnormalities except that hair is shed at the end of the growth cycle. The hairs break off when structurally abnormal regions of the hair shafts reach the surface. The animal remains bare until the next hair cycle. Few hairs erupt during the first hair cycle in homozygous *(N/N)* mice even though follicles are active. Abnormal hairs may erupt during subsequent cycles; however, most do not emerge from follicles (Raphael et al. 1982).

Biologic Features

Natural History. Male *hr/hr* mice are fecund; however, the female is infertile (Crew and Mirskaia 1931). The *hr/hr* and *hr/+* genotypes are therefore maintained by forced heterozygosis (Heiniger et al. 1974).

Pathogenesis. Pilary canals fill with keratin and sebum shortly after the loss of hair. Dermal cysts develop at about 40 days after birth and apparently originate from malformed components of hair follicles, which enlarge in size as the animal ages. Sebaceous glands initially undergo hypertrophy at 30 days of age, then atrophy after 1 year of age (Mann 1971).

The underlying mechanisms involved in the development of hair abnormalities in *hr/hr* mice are not well understood. Studies have centered on (a) abnormal catagen stages, (b) abnormal club hairs, (c) hair loss, and (d) cutaneous cysts. The first observable feature of catagen phase in *hr/hr* mice is the presence of tricholemmal keratinization around the terminal hair shaft prior to formation of the club (David 1934; Orwin et al. 1967). Elongation and keratinization of the presumptive club hair is restricted once the terminal hair shaft is encased within the external root sheath (Mann 1971).

Fraser (1946) suggests that hair loss resulted from abnormal widening and hyperkeratosis of the pilary canal since malformation of the club hairs is variable. However, Mann (1971) noted that widening of the pilary canal in the rhino mouse *(hr^{rh}hr^{rh})* resulted in retention of hairs within the infundibulum.

The cystic structures in the skin of the hairless mouse are generally lined by sebaceous cells. However, normal sebaceous glands may not be necessary for their formation since in doubly homozygous hairless and asebia *(hr/hr ab/ab)* mice similar cysts form as the animals age (Gates et al. 1969). The asebic mouse has defective differentiation of sebaceous glands and is not asebic as originally described (see p. 218). It appears that dermal cysts arise from epithelial units of disorganized hair follicles stranded within the dermis and pilary canal cysts, from widened and hyperplastic hair canals (Mann 1971).

Etiology. The hairless mutation is autosomal recessive. The *hr* locus is on chromosome 14 (Snell 1931).

The high incidence of lymphomas in *hr/hr* mice compared with *hr/+* animals is associated with expression of xenotropic and polytropic C-type RNA viruses in the *hr/hr* but not in the *hr/+* mice even though both have high titers of ecotropic viruses. This is similar to the situation in the AKR strain (Hiai et al. 1977).

Hereditary immunodeficiency in the hairless mouse has been implicated in the high incidence of spontaneous lymphomas (Heiniger et al.

1974). These mice express selective defects in T-cell functions, notably in T helper cells (Reske-Kunz et al. 1979; Morrissey et al. 1980) and in macrophages (Archinal and Wilder 1988).

Frequency. The *hr* gene has been placed on a variety of genetic backgrounds (Smith et al. 1982). Many are available from production colonies.

Comparison with Other Species

Congenital alopecia or alopecia associated with aging or hair color are documented in many mammalian species. Hair loss associated with the formation of comedones and follicular cysts has been recognized in humans and is called papular atrichia (Rook and Dawber 1982). A similar abnormality has been observed in the Chinese crested dog (Muller et al. 1983; Dunstan, unpublished data). Although the hairless mouse is currently being proposed as a model for studying hair growth-promoting compounds, it has little in common either clinically or histologically with male pattern baldness in humans (Lattanand and Johnson 1975).

References

Archinal WA, Wilder MS (1988) Susceptibility of HRS/J mice to listeriosis: dynamics of infection. Infect Immun 56: 607–612

Crew FAE, Mirskaia L (1931) The character "hairless" in the mouse. J Genet 25: 17–24

David LT (1934) Studies on the expression of genetic hairlessness in the house mouse *(Mus musculus)*. J Exp Zool 68: 501–518

Fraser F (1946) The expression and interaction of hereditary factors producing hypotrichosis in the mouse; histology and experimental results. Can J Res 24D: 10–25

Gates AH, Arundell FD, Karasek MA (1969) Hereditary defect of the pilosebaceous unit in a new double mutant mouse. J Invest Dermatol 52: 115–118

Heiniger HJ, Meier H, Kaliss N, Cherry M, Chen HW, Stoner RD (1974) Hereditary immunodeficiency and leukemogenesis in HRS/J mice. Cancer Res 34: 201–211

Hiai H, Morrissey P, Khiroya R, Schwartz RS (1977) Selective expression of xenotropic virus in congenic HRS/J (hairless) mice. Nature 270: 247–249

Lattanand A, Johnson WC (1975) Male pattern alopecia: a histopathologic and histochemical study. J Cutan Pathol 2: 58–70

Mann SJ (1971) Hair loss and cyst formation in hairless and rhino mutant mice. Anat Rec 170: 485–499

Mann SJ, Straile WE (1961) New observations on hair loss in the hairless mouse. Anat Rec 140: 97–101

Meier H, Myers DD, Huebner RJ (1969) Genetic control by the *hr*-locus of susceptibility and resistance to leukemia. Proc Natl Acid Sci USA 63: 759–766

Morrissey PJ, Parkinson DR, Schwartz RS, Waksal SD (1980) Immunologic abnormalities in HRS/J mice. I. Specific deficit in T lymphocyte helper function in a mutant mouse. J Immunol 125: 1558–1562

Muller GH, Kirk RW, Scott DW (1983) Small animal dermatology. Saunders, Philadelpia

Orwin DF, Chase HB, Silver AF (1967) Catagen in the hairless house mouse. Am J Anat 121: 489–507

Pattengale PK, Taylor CR (1983) Experimental models of lymphoproliferative disease. The mouse as a model for human non-Hodgkin's lymphomas and related leukemias. Am J Pathol 113: 237–265

Raknerud N (1974) The ultrastructure of the interfollicular epidermis of the hairless (hr/hr) mouse. II. Plasma membrane modifications during keratinization. Virchows Arch [B] 17: 113–135

Raknerud N (1975) The ultrastructure of the interfollicular epidermis of the hairless (hr/hr) mouse. III. Desmosomal transformation during keratinization. J Ultrastruct Res 52: 32–51

Raknerud N, Hovig L, Iverson OH (1971) The ultrastructure of the interfollicular epidermis of the hairless (hr/hr) mouse. I. Basal and granular layer. Virchows Arch [B] 8: 206–224

Raphael KA, Chapman RE, Frith PA, Pennycuic PR (1982) The structure of hair and follicles of mice carrying the naked (N) gene. Genet Res 39: 139–148

Reske-Kunz AB, Scheid MP, Boyse EA (1979) Disproportion in T-cell subpopulations in immunodeficient mutant *hr/hr* mice. J Exp Med 149: 228–233

Rigdon RH, Packchanian AA (1974) Histologic study of the skin of congenitally athymic "nude" mice. Tex Rep Biol Med 32: 711–723

Rook A, Dawber D (1982) Diseases of the hair and scalp. Mosby, St Louis

Sawada M, Terada N, Taniguchi H, Tateishi R, Mori Y (1987) Brief communication. Cyclosporin A stimulates hair growth in nude mice. Lab Invest 56: 684–686

Smith SM, Forbes PD, Linna TJ (1982) Immune responses in non-haired mice. Int Arch Allergy Appl Immunol 67: 254–261

Snell GD (1931) Inheritance in the house mouse, the linkage relations of short-ear, hairless, and naked. Genetics 16: 42–74

Skin of the Pupoid Fetus *(pf/pf)* Mutant Mouse

Chris Fisher

Gross Appearance

Mice homozygous for the pupoid fetus *(pf)* mutation have a typical gross appearance that includes stumpy limbs, snout, and tail, the absence of vibrissae, and a smooth, taut epidermis (Figs. 254 and 255). While all proximal skeletal elements of the stunted limbs are present and appear to be normal, the metacarpal and metatarsal bones are reduced, and the phalanges fail to form (Ede 1980). The absence of these skeletal elements suggests that the development of the limb is arrested at 12–13 days gestation (Rugh 1968) and supports the notion that the limb abnormalities are due to an interruption of the function of the apical ectodermal ridge since the *pf* gene appears to exert its affect primarily on the epidermis. The stunted forelimbs are fused to the flank, and the hindlimbs are fused with the tail. In addition, the oral cavity, nares, and anal canal are obscured due to the fusion of the epithelia lining in these cavities. Newborn animals die shortly after birth from suffocation. The pups are cannabalized by the mother.

Microscopic Features

The normal murine epidermis is fully differentiated by 18 days gestation. At this time the epidermis has spinous, granular, and cornified layers and has attained a thickness of approximately 40–50 μm (Fig. 256). The epidermis of animals homozygous for the *pf* mutation is considerably thickened by 18 days gestation, often ranging between 150 and 250 μm (Fig. 257). The *pf/pf* epidermis is also permeated throughout by a network of ectopic cells from the dermis that includes fibroblasts, blood vessels, and nerves (Fisher and Kollar 1985; Anderson et al. 1985). Perhaps the most striking effect of the mutation is the failure of epidermal differentiation in animals homozygous for *pf,* even by birth. The stratum corneum, the terminally differentiated cell layer of normal mice, is completely missing from the *pf/pf* epidermis. The granular layer of the newborn *pf/pf* epidermis is sparse and discontinuous but, when present, is generally found in the proper location 4–8 cell layers above the basal cells. The deeper cell layers generally tend to be

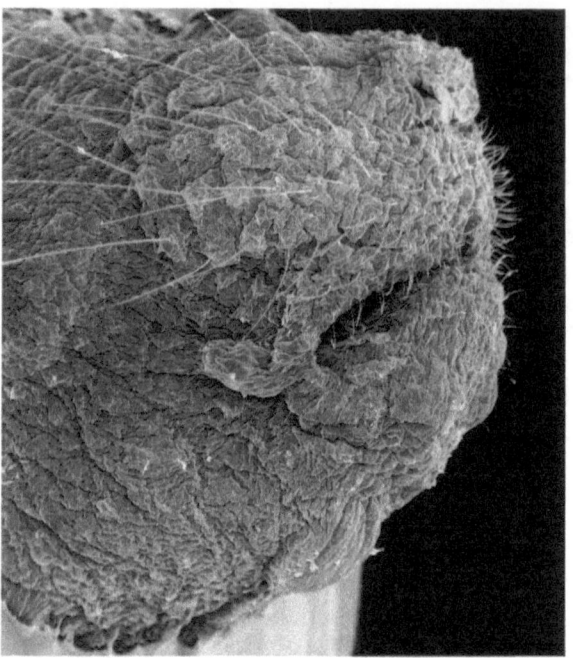

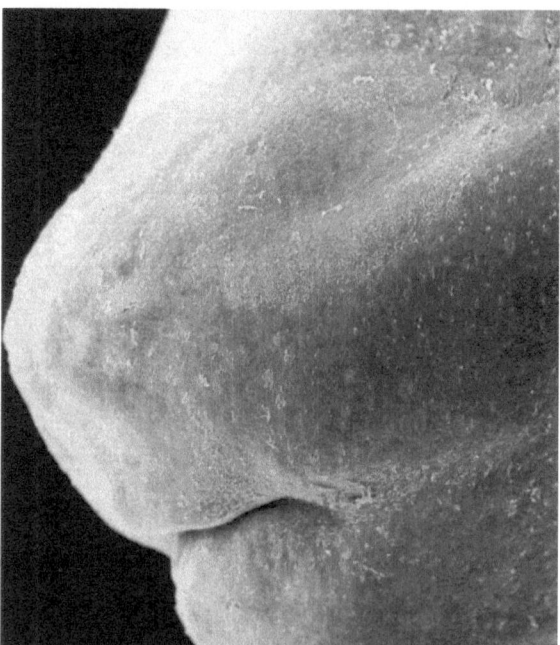

Fig. 254 *(above).* Profile of normal newborn mouse. Note vibrissae, nares and mouth. SEM, × 10

Fig. 255 *(below).* Profile of newborn *pf/pf* mutant. Note absence of vibrissae and nares, blunted snout, and smooth, taut epidermis. SEM, × 10

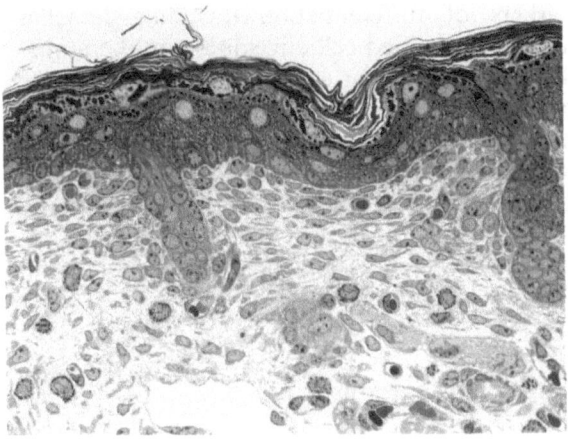

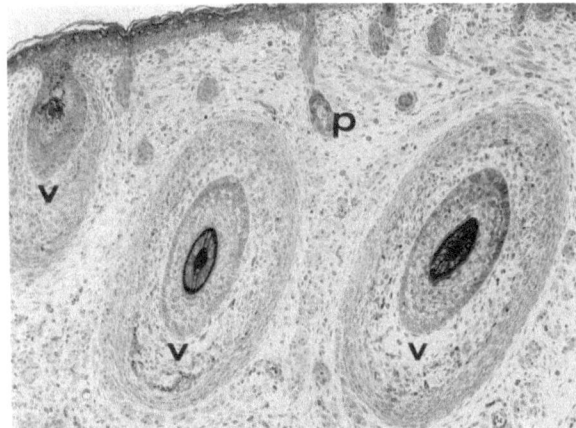

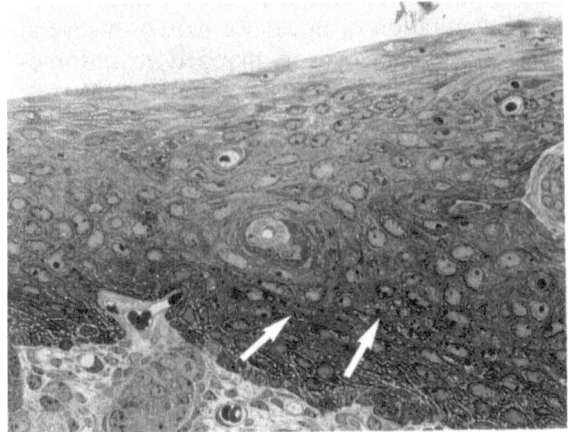

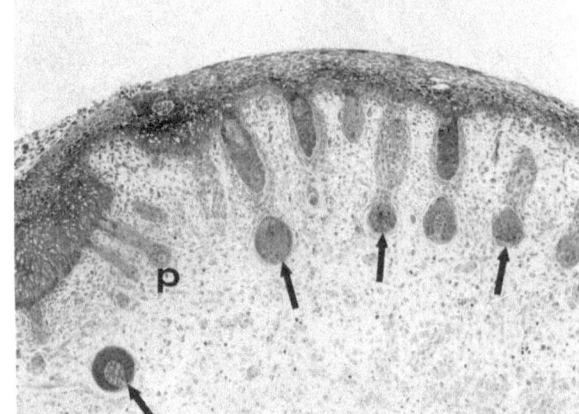

Fig. 256 *(upper left).* Newborn normal skin with fully differentiated epidermis and well-developed stratum corneum. Richardson's stain, × 320

Fig. 257 *(lower left).* Newborn *pf/pf* skin. The epidermis is not keratinized, contains networks of blood vessels and other elements from the dermis, and has a hypoplastic granular layer *(arrows).* Richardson's stain, × 320

Fig. 258 *(upper right).* Newborn normal mouse, 1-μm section through vibrissal region depicting nonkeratinized pelage follicles *(p)* and keratinized vibrissal follicles *(v).* Richardson's stain, × 125

Fig. 259 *(lower right).* Newborn *pf/pf* mutant mouse snout, 1-μm section through vibrissal region showing nonkeratinized pelage follicles *(p)* and larger, underdeveloped, nonkeratinized follicles that share some traits of vibrissal follicles *(arrows).* Large, keratinized vibrissal follicles are not detected. Richardson's stain, × 125

darker staining than the more superficial cell layers; differences between these layers have also been noted in expression of epidermal structural proteins (Fisher et al. 1984, 1987; Fisher and Kollar 1985; Fisher 1987).

Vibrissal follicle development is also affected in *pf/pf* mice. As revealed by scanning electron microscopy, vibrissae do not appear on the surface of 18-day gestation *pf/pf* mice, while normal littermates elaborate well-developed vibrissae by this stage (Fig. 254 and 255). Sections through the vibrissal pad of normal mice reveal fully developed and keratinized vibrissal follicles and nonkeratinized pelage follicles (Fig. 258). Similar sections through the vibrissal region of newborn

pf/pf mice demonstrate that vibrissal follicles are missing but that smaller, well-developed follicles, displaying some characteristics of vibrissal organization and morphology, are present (Fig. 259). It is unclear whether these *pf/pf* mutant follicles are actually vibrissa follicles whose development is retarded, or if they are pelage follicles that display some of the regional characteristics of a vibrissa follicle. The fact that the onset of development of vibrissal follicles occurs earlier (12 days gestation) than that of pelage follicles and closely correlates with the time of onset of the *pf/pf* phenotype may explain their selective perturbation in *pf/pf* mutants.

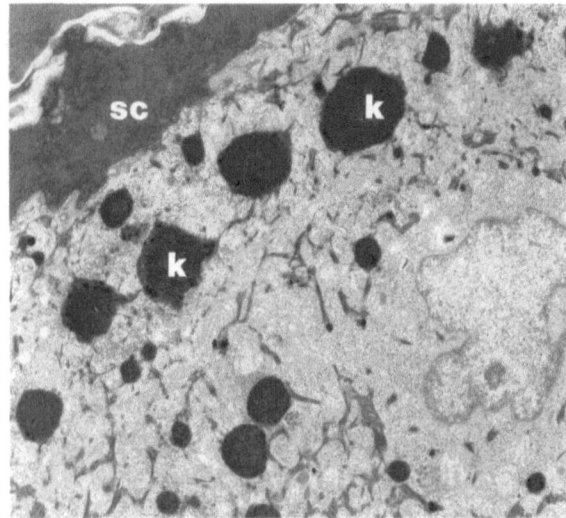

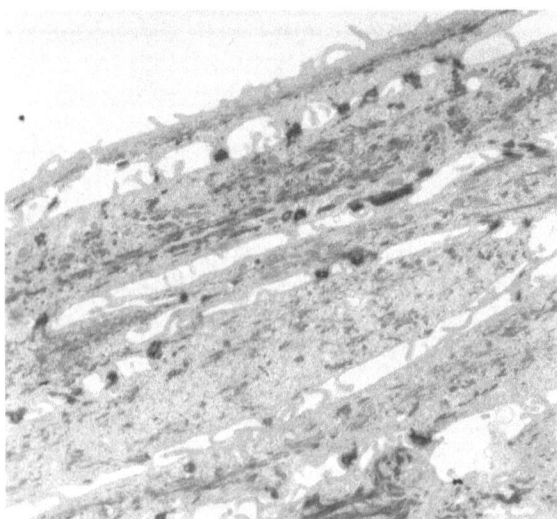

Fig. 260 *(above).* Newborn normal mouse epidermis. Note differentiated, superficial cells with keratohyalin granules *(k)* and cornified squames of the stratum corneum *(sc).* TEM, × 6000

Fig. 261 *(below).* Newborn *pf/pf* epidermis, superficial cells demonstrating a lack of keratinization. Note numerous desmosomes and bundles of keratin filaments. TEM, × 6000

Ultrastructure

The epidermis of newborn normal mice has the ultrastructural appearance of differentiated, keratinizing epithelium including cornified cell envelopes, lamellar granules, well-developed keratohyalin granules, and cornified cells with a typical "keratin pattern" (Fig. 260). In contrast, even the most superficial epidermal cells of newborn *pf/pf* animals appear viable but undifferentiated (Fig. 261). They are negative for ultrastructural

markers of differentiation including lamellar granules, cornified cell envelopes, and keratohyalin granules (Fisher et al. 1984) and also fail to express the well-characterized biochemical markers of differentiation, the differentiation-specific keratins (Fisher et al. 1987). The layers of the *pf/pf* epidermis that contain keratohyalin granules do not posses other structural indicators of differentiation such as lamellar granules or cornified cell envelopes.

Differential Diagnosis

The *pf* mutation is similar to the repeated epilation *(Er)* mutation of mice (see p. 203) in several respects: both have been mapped to chromosome 4 (Guenet 1977), are lethal in homozygotes, and result in epidermal hyperplasia and failure to keratinize (Guenet et al. 1979; Holbrook et al. 1982). Both mutations cause similar gross abnormalities including stumpy limbs and snout, and both the *pf/pf* and *Er/Er* phenotypes are first detectable at approx. 12 days gestation. The *Er/Er* mutant epidermis also exhibits many of the features of abnormal keratin expression and processing displayed by the *pf/pf* mutant and recovers the ability to differentiate when grafted or maintained in organ culture (Fisher 1987; Fisher et al. 1987; see p. 207, this volume). On the other hand the *pf* mutation behaves differently from the *Er* mutation in several respects. While *pf* is inherited as an autosomal recessive, *Er* behaves as an autosomal semidominant. The *pf/pf* epidermis has an underdeveloped granular layer, while the *Er/Er* epidermis elaborates a granular cell layer that is focally hyperplastic and produces abundant amounts of the keratohyalin protein, profilaggrin. In addition, the *Er/Er* epidermis does not exhibit the loss of epidermal integrity that is a hallmark of the *pf/pf* phenotype. Finally, while the *pf* and *Er* mutations have been mapped to the same region of the same chromosome and exhibit a significant number of similar biologic features, preliminary complementation tests indicate that these genes do not behave as alleles (Fisher 1987).

Biologic Features

The *pf* mutation is a radiation-induced, autosomal recessive mutation that has been mapped to chromosome 4 (Meredith 1964; Green 1981). Abnormalities in the skin of *pf/pf* mice are first de-

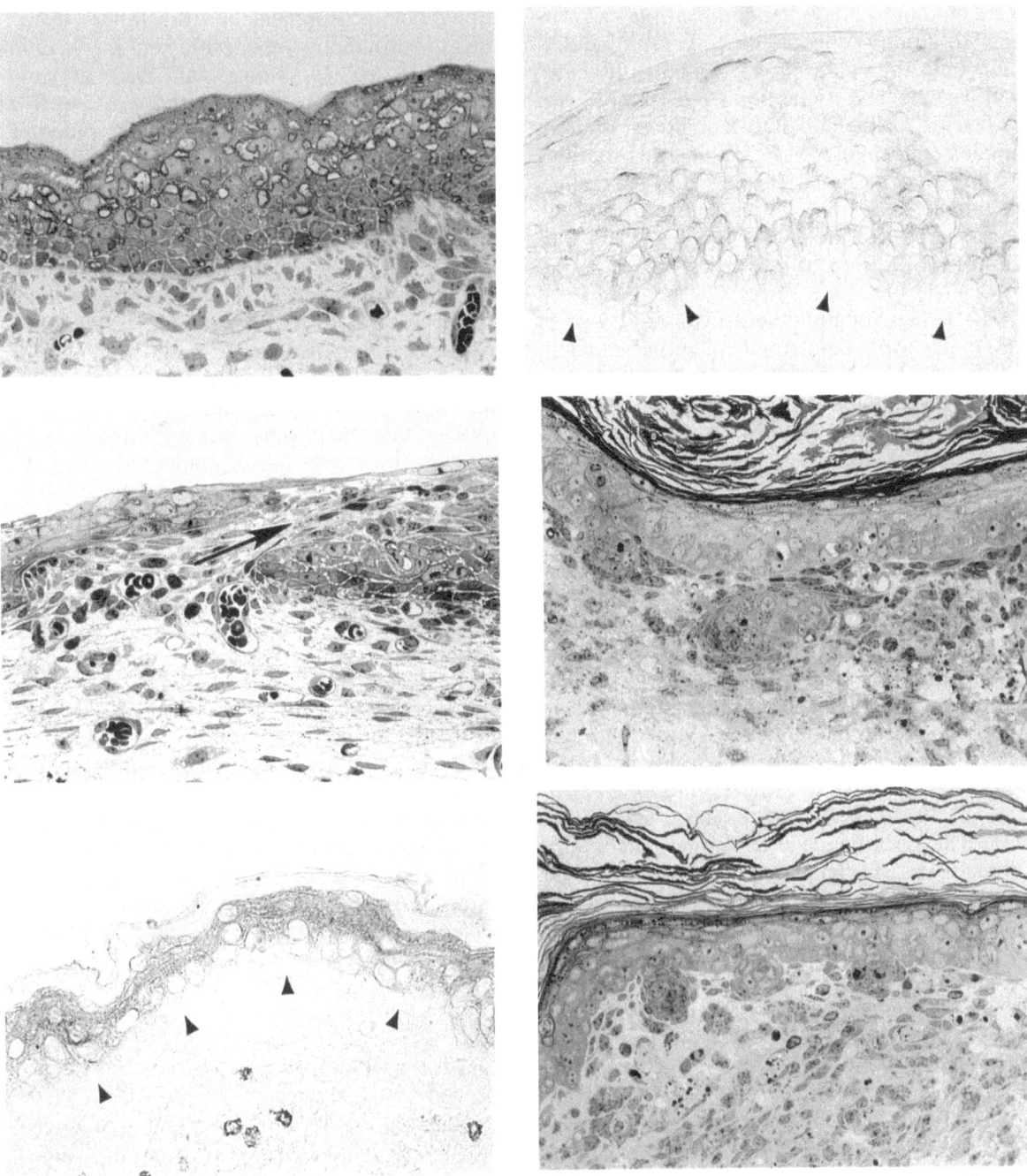

Fig. 262 *(upper left)*. Normal mouse epidermis at 16 days gestation prior to onset of keratinization. Richardson's stain, × 320

Fig. 263 *(middle left)*. Mutant mouse epidermis at 16 days gestation. Note absence of keratohyalin granules and dermal cells extending into the epidermis *(arrow)*. Richardson's stain, × 320

Fig. 264 *(lower left)*. Newborn normal mouse epidermis. Note the localization of binding of antibodies directed against a differentiation-specific keratin (K1). The antibody binds to the viable, suprabasal cells. *Arrowheads* indicate the basal cell layer. Richardson's stain, × 320

Fig. 265 *(upper right)*. Newborn *pf/pf* mutant epidermis. Note the abnormal distribution of the differentiation-specific keratins (K1). A deep suprabasal cell population is positive for K1 but the superficial cell layers are negative. *Arrowheads* indicate the basal cell layer. × 320

Fig. 266 *(middle right)*. Explant of normal 17-day-gestation epidermis following 6 days in organ culture, 1-μm section. Note well-keratinized epidermis. Richardson's stain, × 320

Fig. 267 *(lower right)*. Explant of *pf/pf* mutant skin at 17 days gestation following 6 days in organ culture, 1-μm section. Note well-keratinized epidermis. Richardson's stain, × 320

tected at about 12 days gestation, a time correlating with stratification of the embryonic epidermis. While the epidermis of normal littermates stratifies in an orderly fashion from a simple, two cell-layered epithelium into a multicell-layered, complex epithelium, the *pf/pf* epidermis stratifies in a disorderly fashion. Some areas of the epidermis remain quite thin and may appear to be degenerating while adjacent areas stratify into plaques up to ten cells thick (Fisher et al. 1984).

By 15–16 days gestation the structure of the *pf/pf* skin, in particular the dermal-epidermal junction, is disturbed. At this stage the normal epidermis is 5–8 cell layers thick and just beginning to accumulate keratohyalin granules in the superficial cell layers (Fig. 262). At 15 days gestation in *pf/pf* mice, cells from the dermis proliferate adjacent to the dermal-epidermal junction. Dermal structures, including blood vessels, fibroblasts, and nerves (Fisher and Kollar 1985; Fisher 1987), extend into and through the epidermis (Fig. 263). Ultrastructural studies and immunolocalization of basement membrane components at this stage demonstrate that wherever this ectopic population of dermal cells contacts the epidermis, even if that happens to be on the most superficial surface of the epidermis, a basement membrane is deposited separating it from the epidermis (Fisher et al. 1984; Fisher and Kollar 1985; Fisher 1987). This disturbance of epidermal polarity is a distinct feature of the *pf/pf* phenotype. It is clear that the integrity of the mutant epidermis is compromised at this particular stage of development, but the etiology remains unknown. The epidermis may be invaded by cells from the dermis, or these cells could passively enter following epidermal degeneration. By 18 days gestation the *pf/pf* epidermis overgrows the intrusive dermal elements which remain as a network of cells, including fibroblasts, blood vessels, and nerves, that extends throughout the hyperplastic epidermis (Fig. 255).

The failure of differentiation of the *pf/pf* epidermis may also be studied by following the expression of proteins known to participate in the keratinization process. The protein profilaggrin, thought to be the major component of keratohyalin, is greatly reduced in *pf/pf* epidermis (Fisher et al. 1984; Fisher 1987). The expression of keratins, the intermediate filament proteins of the epidermis, is also dramatically altered in *pf/pf* epidermis (Fisher et al. 1987). The most notable examples of abnormal keratin expression include the expression of the hyperproliferative keratins

throughout development and the failure to express the differentiation-specific keratins (keratin numbers 1 and 10, Moll et al. 1982) at early stages of development and in the most superficial cell layers of late gestation *pf/pf* epidermis (Fisher et al. 1987) (Figs. 264 and 265). In addition, while the differentiation-specific keratins undergo proteolytic processing during the formation of the stratum corneum, these keratins are not processed in the mutant epidermis. The abnormalities in expression and processing of these proteins known to participate in the keratinization process may explain, in part, the failure of morphological differentiation of the *pf/pf* epidermis. Grafting and organ culture studies indicate, however, that the *pf* gene does not directly interfere with the expression of epidermal structural proteins.

The mutant epidermis is capable of normal morphologic differentiation when whole skin is removed from the mutant animal and maintained either as a graft (Fisher et al. 1984, 1987; Fisher 1987) or in organ culture (Figs. 266 and 267). Ultrastructural, immunohistochemical, and biochemical studies indicate that grafted mutant skin recovers the ability to express a normal phenotype, including the normal complement of epidermal structural proteins, suggesting that the mutant gene is not primarily expressed in the skin and that abnormalities in the mutant epidermis arise secondary to a systemic expression of the *pf* gene. It is unclear what systemic substances are involved in the abnormal development of the *pf/pf* skin but growth factors, retinoids, and other modulators of epidermal differentiation are potential candidates for this role.

Comparison with Other Species

No other reported example of a failure of epidermal differentiation has been found in other mammalian species, but certain features of the *pf/pf* phenotype are exhibited in epidermal disorders in humans. For example, although no disease has been reported in humans resulting in failure of keratinization, there are many hyperproliferative disorders of humans including psoriasis, ichtheosis vulgaris, and neoplastic disorders that exhibit some of the traits of the *pf/pf* epidermis including expression of the hyperproliferative keratins (Weiss et al. 1984). In addition, the loss if epidermal integrity and the subsequent development of blood vessels throughout the *pf/pf* mutant epidermis are unusual defects making the *pf/pf* mutant a potential model with which to study the regulation of neovascularization, a process known to play an important role in tumor formation (Folkman 1982).

Acknowledgments. This work was supported by NIH grants HD-17664 and AR-07892. I thank Dr. K. A. Holbrook for her critical review of the manuscript and Dr. D. R. Roop for providing keratin-specific antibodies.

References

Anderson S, Ede DA, Watson PJ (1985) Embryonic development of the mouse mutant pupoid foetus (pf/pf). Anat Embryol (Berl) 172: 115–122

Ede DA (1980) Role of the ectoderm in limb development of normal and mutant mouse (disorganization, pupoid fetus) and fowl (talpid) embryos. In: Merker H, Nau H, Neubert D (eds) Teratology of the limbs. Fourth symposium on prenatal development. Gruyter, Berlin, pp 53–66

Fisher C (1987) Abnormal development in the skin of the pupoid fetus mutant mouse: abnormal keratinization, recovery of a normal phenotype, and relationship to the repeated epilation (Er/Er) mutant mouse. In: Sawyer RH (ed) Current topics in developmental biology, vol 22. Academic, New York

Fisher C, Kollar EJ (1985) Abnormal skin development in pupoid foetus (pf/pf) mutant mice. J Embryol Exp Morphol 87: 47–64

Fisher C, Dale BA, Kollar EJ (1984) Abnormal keratinization in pupoid fetus (pf/pf) mutant mice. Dev Biol 102: 290–299

Fisher C, Jones A, Roop DR (1987) Abnormal expression and processing of keratins in pupoid fetus (pf/pf) and repeated epilation (Er/Er) mutant mice. J Cell Biol 105: 1807–1819

Folkman J (1982) Angiogenesis: initiation and control. Ann NY Acad Sci 401: 212–227

Green MC (1981) Genetic variants and strains of the laboratory mouse for international committee on standardized genetic nomenclature for mice. Fischer, Stuttgart

Guenet J-L (1977) Communication. Mouse News Lett 56: 57

Guenet J-L, Salzgeber B, Tassin MT (1979) Repeated epilation: a genetic epidermal syndrome in mice. J Hered 70: 90–94

Holbrook KA, Dale BA, Brown KS (1982) Abnormal epidermal keratinization in the repeated epilation mutant mouse. J Cell Biol 92: 387–397

Meredith R (1964) Communication. Mouse News Lett 31: 25

Moll R, Franke WW, Scheller DL, Geiger B, Krepler R (1982) The catalog of human cytokeratins: patterns of expression in normal epithelia, tumors and cultured cells. Cell 31: 11–24

Rugh R (1968) The mouse: its reproduction and development. Burgess, Minneapolis

Weiss RA, Eichner R, Sun T-T (1984) Monoclonal antibody analysis of keratin expression in epidermal diseases: a 48- and 56-kdalton keratin as molecular markers for hyperproliferative keratinocytes. J Cell Biol 98: 1397–1406

Skin of the Repeated Epilation *(Er/Er)* Mutant Mouse

Chris Fisher

Gross Appearance

The *Er* mutation causes a pattern of repeated loss and regrowth of hair in heterozygous animals that otherwise display a normal gross morphology (Hunsicker 1960). Animals homozygous for the *Er* gene show many gross abnormalities that appear to be a less severe manifestation of the abnormalities displayed by the *pf* mutation (Figs. 268 and 269; see also p. 198). Limbs and snout are stunted, the tail is shortened, and the nares and oral, anal, and urogenital orifices are closed due to epithelial fusion (Guenet et al. 1979; Tassin et al. 1983). The forelimbs are fused to the flank epidermis and the hindlimbs are fused with the tail (Fig. 269). The digits of all limbs never separate although their bony elements are present, and the mutant digits never radiate. Claws are rarely found in *Er/Er* mice (Salzgeber and Guenet 1984).

Microscopic Features

While normal newborn epidermis is fully keratinized by 18 days gestation, the *Er/Er* epidermis remains, for the most part, nonkeratinized even at birth (Figs. 270 and 271) (Guenet et al. 1979; Holbrook et al. 1982). The newborn *Er/Er* epidermis is hyperplastic and of variable thickness (Fig. 271). A single basal cell layer and two to several spinous cell layers are generally present.

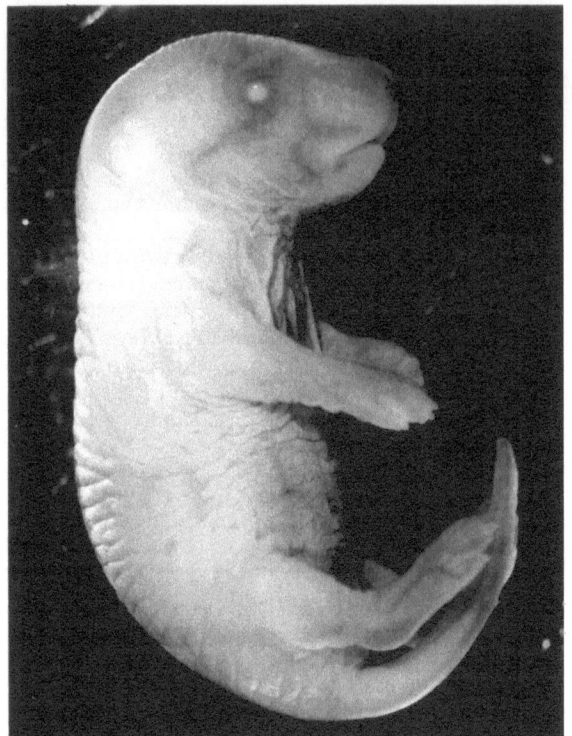

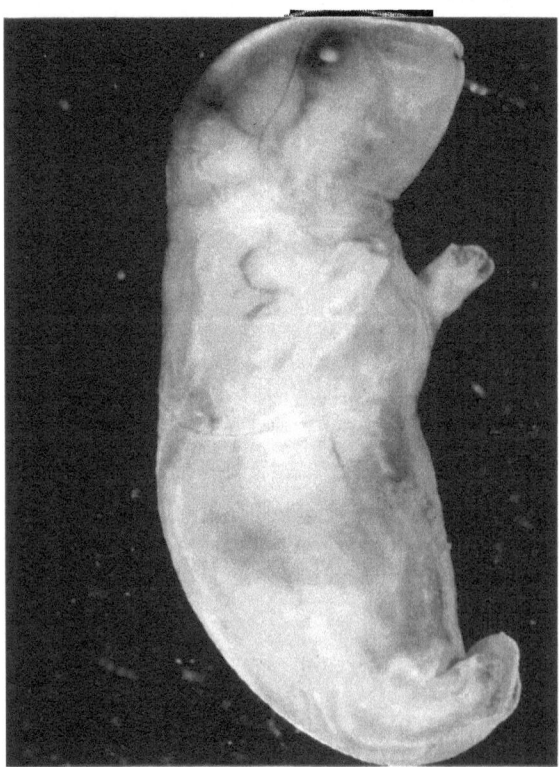

Fig. 268 *(above).* Newborn normal mouse. × 3.8 (Photograph provided by courtesy of Dr. K. A. Holbrook)

Fig. 269 *(below).* Newborn *Er/Er* mouse. Note stumpy limbs, snout, and tail, and fusion of hind limbs to tail. × 3.8 (Photograph provided by courtesy of Dr. K. A. Holbrook)

Considerable heterogeneity exists with respect to the granular cell layer, which may be lacking entirely or hyperplastic and is generally located in the more superficial regions of the thickened mutant epidermis (Holbrook et al. 1982) (Fig. 271). Zones of cornification may sometimes be detected within regions containing abundant keratohyalin granules, but the epidermis remains, for the most part, nonkeratinized (Holbrook et al. 1982).

Vibrissae are fully formed by 18 days gestation in normal mice (Fig. 272) (Davidson and Hardy 1952), but vibrissae are rare or missing entirely from newborn *Er/Er* mutants (Guenet et al. 1979; Holbrook et al. 1982). However, sections of the vibrissal region reveal that well-formed and keratinized vibrissal follicles are present in 18-day gestation *Er/Er* mice (Fig. 273). While the *Er/Er* vibrissal follicles appear to be hyperplastic with regard to those of normal littermates, they are readily distinguished from those of *pf/pf* mutants, in which vibrissal development is retarded. This observation distinguishes the *Er/Er* from *pf/pf* mutants, which appear to be lacking vibrissal follicles (see p. 199).

Ultrastructure

As reported by Holbrook et al. (1982), ultrastructural study of *Er/Er* epidermis reveals cells in various stages of partial keratinization in the more superficial regions (Fig. 274). Cornified cells may be found embedded in the granular cell layers. These cells generally display the ultrastructural markers of a differentiated epidermal cell including cornified cell envelopes, extruded lamellar granules, and depletion of most organelles. As suggested by light microscopy, much variability exists in the *Er/Er* epidermis with regard to keratohyalin granules. Small keratohyalin granules are often detected by electron microscopy in regions in which granules are undetectable by light microscopy. In addition, while keratohyalin granules of normal epidermis increase in size toward the cell surface, the granules of *Er/Er* epidermis are variable with respect to size and shape. A number of ultrastructural differences between *Er/Er* and normal mice have been noted in the basal cell layers as well (Holbrook et al. 1982). There are fewer desmosomes among basal cells of *Er/Er* mice, resulting in large intercellular spaces between the basal and lower spinous cells. Phagolysosomes as well as large, electron-opaque granules within mitochondria are com-

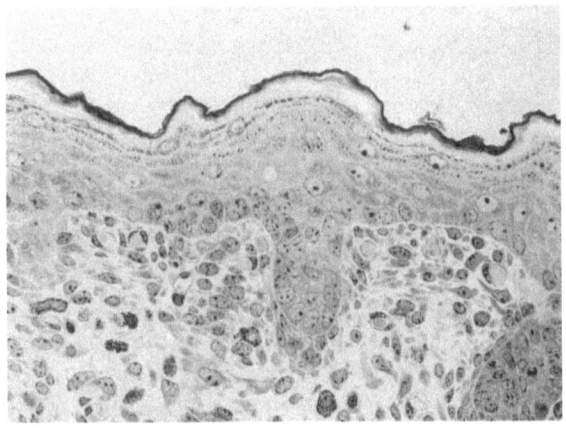

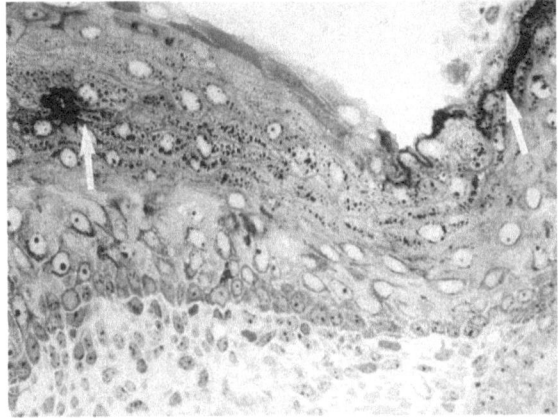

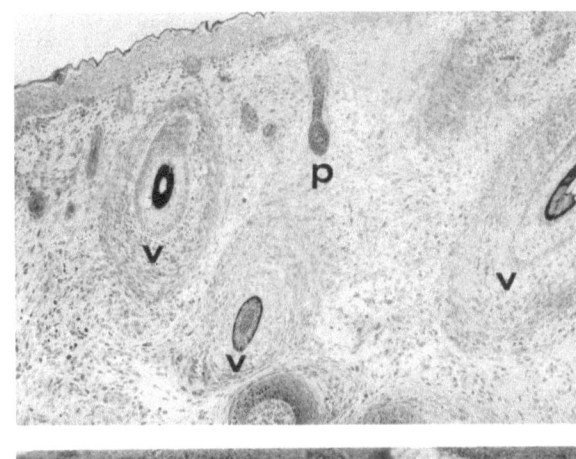

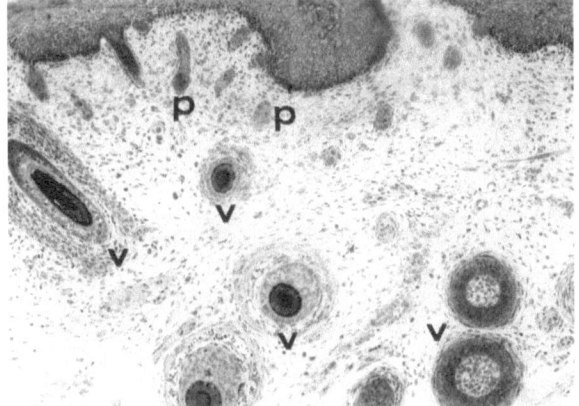

Fig. 270 *(upper left).* Normal mouse skin, 1-μm section, 18 days gestation. Richardson's stain, × 320

Fig. 271 *(lower left).* Skin, *Er/Er* mouse, 18 days gestation. Note abnormal granular layer and areas of keratinization *(arrows).* Richardson's stain, × 320

Fig. 272 *(upper right).* Skin, normal mouse. Section (1 μm) through vibrissa region at 18 days gestation demonstrat-

ing both pelage *(p)* and vibrissa *(v)* follicles. Richardson's stain, × 125

Fig. 273 *(lower right).* Skin, *Er/Er* mouse. Section of vibrissa region at 18 days gestation demonstrating both pelage *(p)* and vibrissa *(v)* type follicles. Note mesodermal tissue surrounding vibrissa follicles appears hypoplastic with respect to normal (Fig. 272). Richardson's stain, × 125

mon to these cell layers (Holbrook et al. 1982). It should be noted that many of these ultrastructural features including increased intercellular spaces, phagolysosomes, mitochondrial inclusions, and increased granules in cell layers are generally characteristic of hyperplastic epidermis (Argyris 1979; Bhisey and Satyavati 1977; Frei and Sheldon 1961; Raick 1973).

Differential Diagnosis

The *Er* mutation is quite similar to another mutation of mice known as pupoid fetus *(pf).* For a discussion of the similarities and dissimilarities between these two mutations, see p. 207. For a

comparison of these traits see Table 10 (Fisher et al. 1984; Fisher and Kollar 1985).

Biologic Features

The *Er* mutation has been mapped to chromosome 4 and is inherited as an autosomal, semidominant mutation with heterozygotes being distinguished from wild-type animals by a pattern of hair loss and regrowth beginning 2 weeks after birth (Eicher and Fox 1978; Guenet et al. 1979). Newborn *Er/+* mice are distinguishable from wild-type by a bloody, thickened tail tip. While no histologic features of the skin of the trunk of *Er/+* animals readily distinguish it from that of

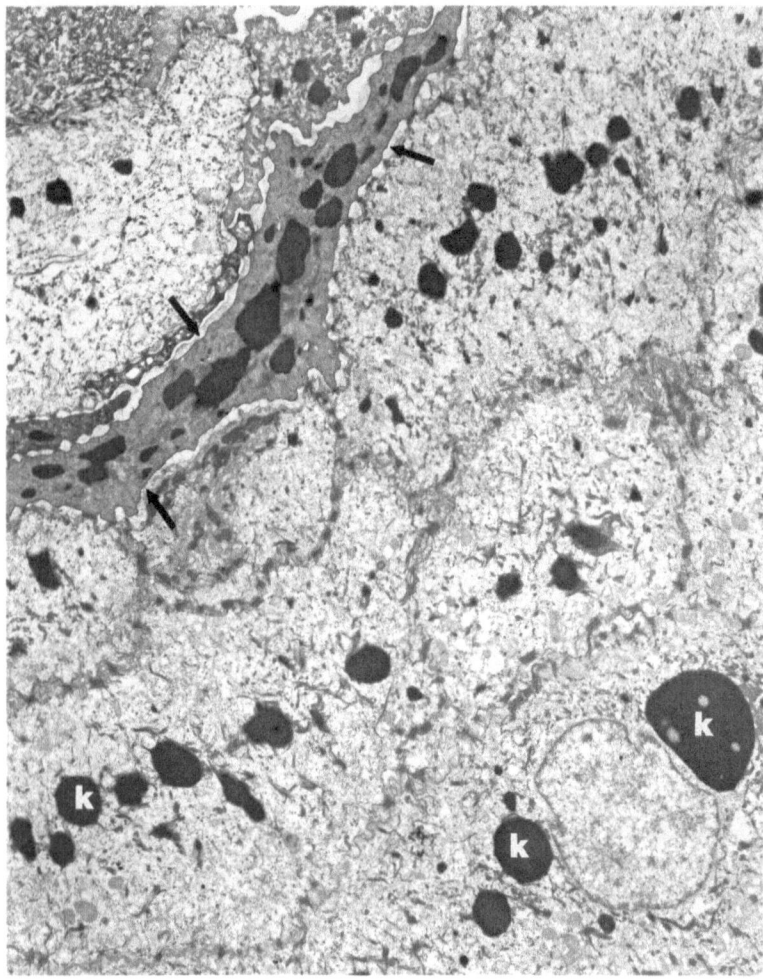

Fig. 274. Epidermis, *Er/Er* mouse, 19 days gestation, in various stages of keratinization. Note the isolated cornified cell surrounded by extruded lamellar granules *(ar-* *rows)* and keratohyalin granules *(k)*. TEM, × 4600 (Micrograph provided by courtesy of Dr. K. A. Holbrook)

wild-type, the epidermis of the head of *Er/+* animals is hyperplastic (Holbrook et al. 1982).

Animals homozygous for *Er* are first distinguished from wild-type and heterozygous littermates at about 12 days gestation because of their stumpy limbs and tail. It is at this time that the normal epidermis stratifies from a simple, two cell-layered epidermis having basal and peridermal cell layers into a complex, stratified epithelium with basal, peridermal, and intermediate cell layers. The *Er/Er* epidermis stratifies in a disorderly fashion and may vary from 2–7 cell layers (Holbrook et al. 1982). Ultrastructural studies demonstrate that wide spaces separate the epidermal cells at this stage and that a diffuse matrix material is deposited in the intercellular spaces (Holbrook et al. 1982). The mutant epidermis continues to thicken due to hyperplasia

of spinous and granular layers so that by birth the *Er/Er* epidermis is nonkeratinized and may be several times thicker than normal (Fig. 271).

The failure of keratinization in *Er/Er* epidermis is correlated with abnormalities in expression and processing of two different classes of epidermal proteins. Keratin expression is altered in several ways. The hyperproliferative keratins (keratins 6 and 16 from the terminology of Moll et al. 1982), which are not normally expressed in interfollicular epidermis, are expressed at high levels throughout the suprabasal cells of *Er/Er* epidermis, particularly in the more superficial cell layers (Fisher et al. 1987). The differentiation-specific keratins (keratins 1 and 10 from Moll et al. 1982), which are normally synthesized in all viable suprabasal cell layers (Fig. 275), are produced in the deeper suprabasal cell layers of *Er/*

Table 10. Summary and comparison of normal, *Er/Er,* and *pf/pf* skin traits

Normal	*Er/Er*	*pf/pf*
	Autosomal semi-dominant mutation, mapped to chromosome 4	Autosomal recessive mutation, mapped to chromosome 4
Vibrissal follicles formed by 18 days gestation	Vibrissal follicle develops and keratinizes	Vibrissal follicle development retarded
Epidermis keratinizes by 18 days gestation	Newborn epidermis hyperplastic and nonkeratinized, except for isolated cells	Newborn epidermis hyperplastic and nonkeratinized
Granular layer 3–4 cells thick	Hyperplastic, uneven granular layer	Hypoplastic granular layer
Profilaggrin-filaggrin produced in granular layer	Profilaggrin synthesized but not processed to filaggrin	Profilaggrin synthesis greatly reduced
Keratins 1 and 10 expressed in all viable suprabasal cells	Expression of keratins 1 and 10 limited to deeper epidermal cell layers	Expression of keratins 1 and 10 limited to deeper epidermal cell layers
Basal cell keratin expression (keratins 5 and 14) limited to basal cell layer	Basal cell keratins expressed throughout epidermis	Basal cell keratins expressed throughout epidermis
Hyperproliferative keratins (keratins 6 and 16) not normally produced in interfollicular epidermis	Abundant expression of keratins 6 and 16, particularly in superficial cell layers	Abundant expression of keratins 6 and 16, particularly in superficial cell layers

Summarized from Fisher et al. 1984; Fisher and Kollar 1985; Fisher 1987; Guenet et al. 1979; Holbrook et al. 1982; Salzgeber and Guenet 1984; Tassin et al. 1983.

Er epidermis (Fig. 276) (Fisher et al. 1987). Furthermore, the differentiation-specific keratins are not processed in *Er/Er* epidermis (Fisher 1987). The alteration in expression and processing of the differentiation-specific keratins may offer some insight into the failure of keratinization of the *Er/Er* epidermis since both of these occurrences are intimately associated with this process. In addition to the differentiation-specific keratins, the newborn *Er/Er* epidermis is also defi-

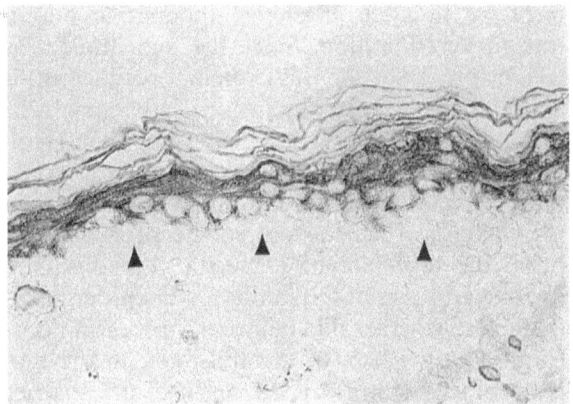

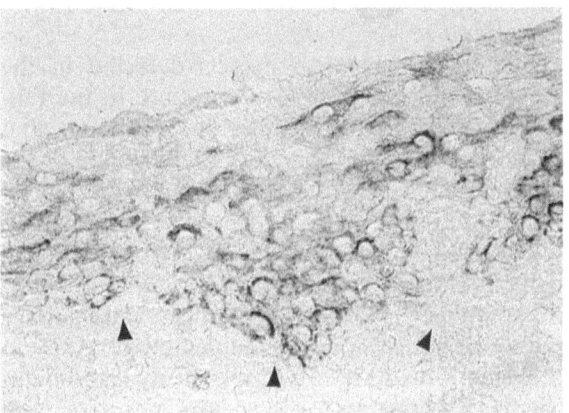

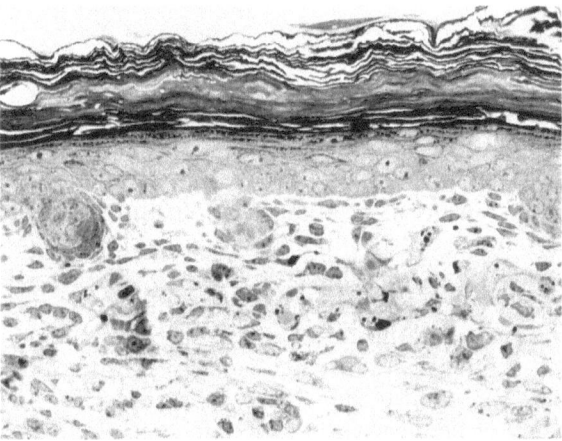

Fig. 275 *(above).* Skin, normal mouse, 18 days gestation. Note differentiation-specific keratin (K10) in the suprabasal cell layers of epidermis. *Arrowheads* indicate position of the basal cell layer. ×320 (Antibodies provided by courtesy of Dr. D. R. Roop)

Fig. 276 *(middle).* Skin, *Er/Er* mouse, 18 days gestation. Note localization of a differentiation-specific keratin (K10) in epidermis. Note negative superficial cell layers. *Arrowheads* indicate basal cell layers. ×320 (Antibodies provided by courtesy of Dr. D. R. Roop)

Fig. 277 *(below).* Epidermis, *Er/Er* mouse, 16-day-gestation *Er/Er* epidermis following 8 days in organ culture (compare with Fig. 271). Note the mutant epidermis is thinner and well-keratinized. Richardson's, ×320

cient for filaggrin, a protein thought to play a role in keratinization. Since the high molecular weight precursor for this protein, profilaggrin, is abundant in *Er/Er* epidermis, a deficiency in its proteolytic processing has been suggested (Holbrook et al. 1982). *Er/+* mice show an intermediate effect with regard to both filaggrin and profilaggrin. Thus the proteolytic processing of both the differentiation-specific keratins and profilaggrin is retarded in the *Er/Er* epidermis. It is unclear whether this failure of processing contributes to the lack of keratinization in the mutant epidermis or if it is the result of the absence of the hydrolytic environment associated with cornifying cells.

While the biochemical defects detected in the *Er/Er* epidermis certainly contribute to the failure of epidermal differentiation, it is likely that these defects occur secondary to the action of the mutant gene. The *Er/Er* epidermis is capable of normal differentiation as determined by morphological and biochemical means when mutant skin is maintained either as a graft (Fisher 1987) or in organ culture (Fig. 277). These observations have led to the conclusion that the mutant gene acts in a systemic manner. The most likely candidates for this factor are growth factors, retinoids, and other mediators of epidermal differentiation.

Comparison with Other Species

While there are no direct comparisons between the abnormalities of *Er/Er* mutant skin and known disorders of human skin, features such as epidermal hyperproliferation and thickening are exhibited in a number of human disorders. It should also be pointed out that *Er* heterozygotes exhibit a high incidence of spontaneous cutaneous papillomas and carcinomas, suggesting that the *Er/+* mice may serve as models for the study of predisposition to certain cancers.

Acknowledgements. This work was supported by NIH grants HD-17664 and AR-07892. I thank Dr. K.A. Holbrook for critical review of the manuscript.

References

Argyris TS (1979) Ribosome accumulation and the regulation of epidermal hyperplastic growth. Life Sci 24: 1137–1147

Bhisey RA, Satyavati SM (1977) Sequential ultrastructural alterations in the mouse epidermis after a single subcutaneous injection of 20-methylcholanthrene. Indian J Cancer 14: 18–23

Davidson P, Hardy MH (1952) The development of mouse vibrissae in vivo and in vitro. J Anat 86: 342–356

Eicher EM, Fox S (1978) Communication ('repeated epilation'). Mouse News Lett 58: 50

Fisher C (1987) Abnormal development in the skin of the pupoid fetus (pf/pf) mutant mouse: abnormal keratinization, recovery of a normal phenotype, and relationship to the repeated epilation (Er/Er) mutant mouse. In: Sawyer RH (ed) Current topics in developmental biology, vol 22. Academic, New York

Fisher C, Kollar EJ (1985) Abnormal skin development in pupoid fetus (pf/pf) mutant mice. J Embryol Exp Morphol 87: 47–64

Fisher C, Dale BA, Kollar EJ (1984) Abnormal keratinization in the pupoid fetus (pf/pf) mutant mouse epidermis. Dev Biol 102: 290–299

Frei JV, Sheldon H (1961) Corpus intra cristam: a dense body within mitochondria of cells in hyperplastic mouse epidermis. J Biophys Biochem Cytol 11: 724–729

Guenet J-L, Salzgeber B, Tassin MT (1979) Repeated epilation: a genetic epidermal syndrome in mice. J Hered 70: 90–94

Holbrook KA, Dale BA, Brown KS (1982) Abnormal epidermal keratinization in the repeated epilation mutant mouse. J Cell Biol 92: 387–397

Moll R, Franke WW, Schiller DL, Gieger B, Krepler R (1982) The catalog of human cytokeratins: patterns of expression in normal epithelia, tumors and cultured cells. Cell 31: 11–24

Raick AN (1973) Ultrastructural, histological and biochemical alterations produced by 12-O-tetradecanolphorbol-13-acetate on mouse epidermis and their relevance to skin tumor promotion. Cancer Res 33: 269–286

Salzgeber B, Guenet J-L (1984) Studies on 'repeated epilation' mouse mutant embryos. II. Development of limb, tail and skin defects. J Craniofac Genet Dev Biol 4: 95–114

Tassin MT, Salzgeber B, Guenet J-L (1983) Studies on "repeated epilation" mouse mutant embryos: I. Development of facial malformations. J Craniofac Genet Dev Biol 3: 289–307

The Tight Skin (TSK) Mouse

Sergio A. Jimenez and Reza I. Bashey

Synonyms. Dominant mutant TSK (mouse); progressive systemic sclerosis (PSS); scleroderma (human).

Gross Appearance

Skin and Subcutis. The characteristic hypertrophic changes in the loose connective tissue of the subdermal and subcutaneous regions of TSK/+ mice that are responsible for the thickening and firm attachment of skin to the underlying muscle were initially described by Green et al. (1976). The skin tightness was not apparent at birth but was recognizable by 7 days of age. At 2 months of age, prominent skin thickening, particularly in the interscapular region, results in a pronounced hump, and a hunched posture becomes apparent. At autopsy, the skin from affected animals is much more difficult to separate from the underlying muscular layers. Detailed study of the morphological and mechanical properties of TSK skin confirmed that the skin of TSK/+ animals is characteristically thickened and displays decreased pliability, increased stiffness, and a loss of the normal directional differences in skin tensile properties (Menton and Hess 1980; Menton et al. 1980). The increased skin thickness in affected animals was subsequently confirmed by other investigators (Jimenez et al. 1984; Osborn et al. 1983). The gross morphological and biomechanical alterations described above suggest that the TSK mutation causes quantitative and/or qualitative alterations in the content of skin connective tissue macromolecules as well as in the fibrous architecture of dermal collagen.

Visceral Involvement. In addition to the presence of generalized connective tissue hyperplasia in TSK/+ mice, the original studies of Green et al. (1976) showed that notable visceral involvement was found in the lungs and heart of mutants. Several investigators have subsequently confirmed these findings (Osborn and Bauer 1984; Rosenberg et al. 1984).

Pulmonary. The abnormalities in the lungs of TSK/+ mice result in very enlarged lungs and a distended chest cage.

Cardiac. Green et al. (1976) noted significant enlargement and increased weight of the heart in TSK/+ mice. A moderate increase in left and right ventricular weight (6.2% and 13.1%, respectively) and a marked increase in right and left auricular weight (25.6% and 27.8%, respectively) were described. Osborn and Bauer (1984) confirmed the increased cardiac weights in the TSK/+ mouse.

Microscopic Features

Skin and Subcutis. Detailed light microscopic studies of the skin and subcutaneous tissue of TSK/+ were performed by Green et al. (1976), who demonstrated marked hyperplasia of the loose connective tissue in the subdermis and subcutaneous tissue of TSK/+ mice. Extensive replacement of subcutaneous adipose tissue by thick fibrous tracts was observed both above and below the panniculus carnosus, resulting in a marked increase in total skin thickness. These changes are present in the dorsal, lateral, and ventral aspects of the thoracic and abdominal regions as well as in the tail and extremities, especially over the knees and elbows. Prominent changes were also found in the connective tissue surrounding the mammary glands, the brown interscapular fat, and the ventral side of the sternum. In our own studies (Fig. 278) we confirmed the marked hypertrophy of the loose connective tissue and the replacement of the subdermal adipose tissue by newly deposited, lightly staining, eosinophilic connective tissue. Histochemical studies demonstrate that the most abundant intercellular material is collagen, as shown by the presence of pale blue staining with Masson's trichrome stain (Fig. 279) (Jimenez et al. 1984).

Pulmonary. Histologically the changes in the lung resemble human emphysema with little evidence of fibrosis. The presence of markedly dilated alveolar spaces with thin, disrupted alveolar walls and of numerous subpleural cysts and bullae was described by Szapiel et al. (1981). A marked accumulation of inflammatory cells in the interstitium as well as in the alveolar spaces was also noticed.

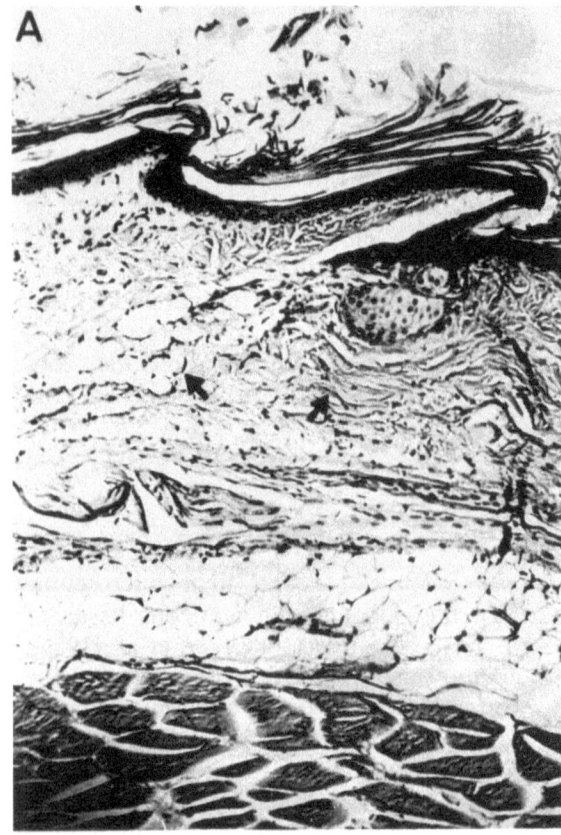

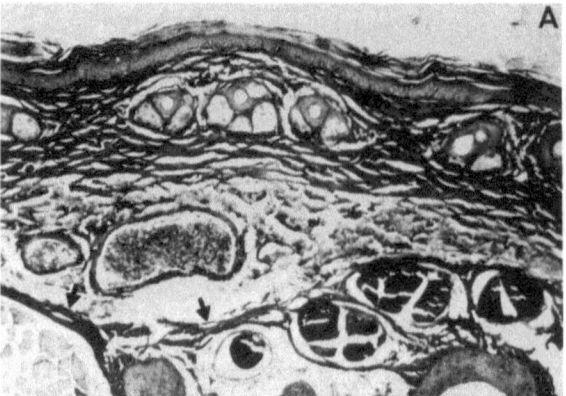

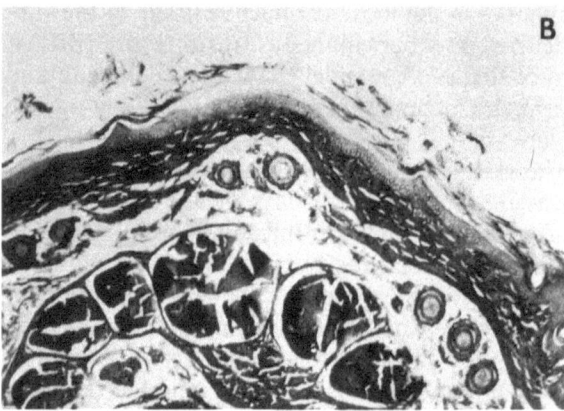

Fig. 279 A, B. Transverse sections of tail from TSK/+ (**A**) and normal (**B**) mice. Note thickening of dermis and subdermal tissues, replacement of loose adipose tissue by newly deposited collagen, and thickened peritendinous fascia *(arrow)*. Trichrome stain, × 600

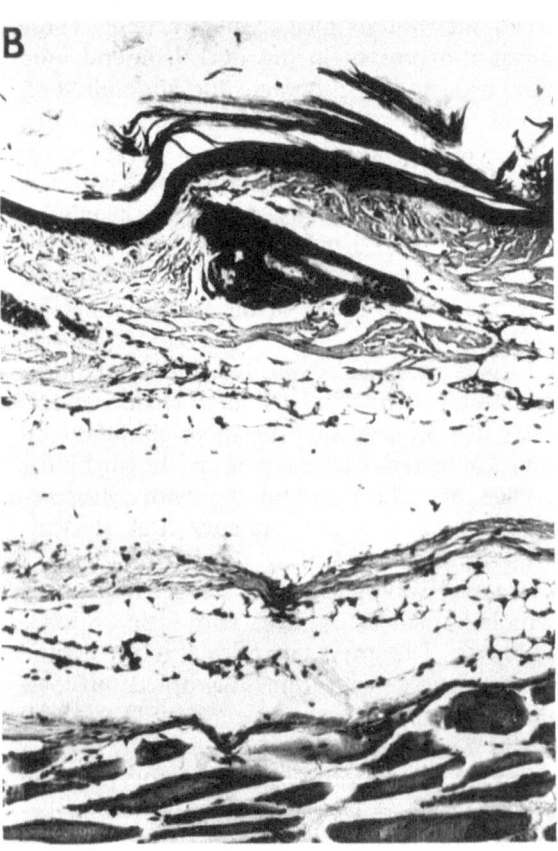

◀**Fig. 278 A, B.** Skin from TSK/+ (**A**) and normal mice (**B**). Dermal thickening and replacement of subcutaneous adipose tissue by homogeneously stained collagen are seen in the skin of TSK/+ mice. H and E, × 600

The presence of large numbers of inflammatory cells in the alveolar spaces and interstitium of affected animals suggests that these cells play a pathogenetic role in abnormalities of the alveolar wall described above. Rossi et al. (1984) found a significant increase of neutrophils in the alveolar walls, bronchi, and alveoli in TSK/+ mice without evidence of infection. Normal proportions of lung T and B lymphocytes were also found, suggesting that there was no gross abnormality in the cell-mediated immunity in the lungs.

Cardiac. Extensive accumulation of perivascular and interstitial edema, with areas of moderately increased amounts of collagen within interstitial sites were found histologically (Osborn and Bauer 1984).

Ultrastructure

It has been found by transmission electron microscopy that the reticular dermis of skin from TSK/+ mice is consistently thicker and more cellular and the network arrangement of collagen is frequently more disorganized (Green et al. 1976; Menton and Hess 1980).

Furthermore, TSK/+ fibroblasts often contain greatly distended cisternae of rough endoplasmic reticulum with clearly visible, electron-dense, flocculent material. In contrast, the rough endoplasmic reticulum in fibroblasts from normal mice skin were much less distended and contained little electron-dense material. These findings indicate substantially increased biosynthetic activity in TSK/+ fibroblasts.

Our own studies of the fine structure of collagen fibrils from the reticular dermis demonstrate a striking variability in fibril diameter in both TSK/+ and control mice. In both the diameter of the fibrils varies over a very wide range (30–500 nm) and numerous unusually large (300–500 nm) and irregular fibrils are present (unpublished data). These changes were, however, much more prominent in the mutants. In addition, the hypodermis of TSK/+ contained numerous disorganized fine filaments measuring 10–20 nm in diameter and lacking obvious periodicity.

Electron microscopic studies of the heart confirmed the increased accumulation of collagen. High magnification of individual collagen fibrils did not show structural differences between the cardiac collagen of TSK/+ and control mice. No inflammatory cells were observed in the cardiac interstitium.

Biologic Features

Natural History. The tight skin mouse (TSK) is a dominant mutant of the inbred BIO.D2(58N)/Sn mouse strain. It was isolated at the Jackson Research Laboratories by Bunker in 1967 and was first described by Green et al. (1976). The heterozygote animals (TSK/+) are characterized by the presence of a thickened skin which is firmly bound to the subcutaneous and deep muscular tissues and lacks the pliability and resiliency characteristic of normal skin. It has been described above that the increased skin thickness in affected animals is due to excessive accumulation of collagen in the dermis and subdermal tissues (Menton and Hess 1980; Menton et al. 1980; Jimenez et al. 1984; Osborn et al. 1983). In addition, increased collagen deposition and increased collagen content in some internal organs such as the heart has been documented (Green et al. 1976; Osborn and Bauer 1984).

Genetic Abnormality in the TSK Mutation. The primary biochemical defect caused by the TSK gene abnormality has not been identified, but the phenotypic effects of the mutation appear to be confined almost exclusively to the connective tissue. Genetic studies have indicated that the TSK gene is located in chromosome 2 and the mutation is transmitted in an autosomal dominant pattern (Green et al. 1976). The homozygous TSK/TSK mutation is lethal, and embryos carrying this genotype die in utero at about 8–10 days of gestation. The heterozygous TSK mice (TSK/+), however, are viable and do not appear to have a shortened life-span but do manifest marked thickening, induration, and tightness of the skin. These changes are particularly apparent in the dorsum and interscapular regions. The TSK mutant co-segregates with a mutation in fur color, and all the animals expressing the abnormal gene have black fur. Although the initial studies of Green et al. (1976) indicated that the phenotypic effects of the mutation became fully expressed at 2 months of age, biochemical studies have shown that a variety of abnormalities in connective tissue metabolism are already detectable in tissues and cells obtained from newborn animals (Jimenez et al. 1984, 1986a).

Immunologic Alterations

Although morphologic studies of affected organs from TSK mice have failed to show the mononuclear cell inflammatory infiltrates characteristic of human scleroderma (except for the neutrophilic cellular infiltrates found in the lungs as described above) some subtle immunologic abnormalities have been noted. The presence of nuclear-specific antibodies in TSK/+ mice was first observed by Osborn et al. (personal communication), but more detailed studies will be necessary to characterize their nature and possible pathogenetic role.

Other immunologic studies were performed by DeLustro et al. (1983), who examined the development of humoral and delayed-type hypersensitivity (DTH) to homologous connective tissue antigens in the TSK/+ mutant. TSK/+ mice did not display significant DTH responses when challenged with type I or IV collagens. In contrast, positive DTH responses to elastase-solubilized lung peptides were detected. These appeared at 10 weeks of age and increased in intensity until 22 weeks and could be adoptively transferred to normal and C57BL/6 mice with spleen cells from 30-week-old TSK/+ mice. Treatment with T-cell-specific antibodies plus complement significantly reduced DTH reactivity transfer by these TSK cells, suggesting abnormalities in T-cell function in the mutants. The significance of these abnormalities, however, requires further investigation.

Recent attention has been given to the possible role of mast cells in the pathogenesis of the proliferative and fibrotic lesions observed in rheumatoid arthritis and scleroderma, and it has been suggested that these cells may be important initiators of cutaneous fibrosis in PSS (Hawkins et al. 1985). In a detailed study of mast cells in TSK/+ mice, LeRoy and collaborators reported a more than twofold increase in the number of mast cells present in affected tissues of TSK/+ mice up to 6 months of age. At 11 months, however, the proportion decreased, and at 15 months the number of skin mast cells was similar in both groups of mice and significantly reduced from the number found in younger mice (Walker et al. 1985). In the same study, increased mast cell degranulation was found in TSK/+ mice skin. In 5-month-old animals the majority of mast cells degranulated. Increased mast cell degranulation persisted at 15 months, even though the total mast cell number per unit area was nearly equivalent in TSK/+ and normal mice. These results suggested a possible role of mast cells in the progressive connective tissue accumulation observed in the mutants. Further studies by the same investigators showed that administration of a specific inhibitor of mast cell degranulation to TSK/+ mice resulted in a marked decrease in the thickness of their skin (Walker et al. 1987).

Biochemical Alterations

Extensive biochemical studies have been performed to further characterize the connective tissue alterations in TSK mice and to attempt to determine the mechanisms responsible. These studies are reviewed below.

Analysis of Skin Collagen and Glycosaminoglycans.

The gross morphological and histological appearance of increased collagen deposition in TSK mice skin was quantitatively confirmed by performing direct measurements of the amounts of collagen present in the tissues by Jimenez et al. (1984) and Osborn et al. (1983). In our studies, constant diameter discs of normal and TSK/+ skin were removed from the interscapular region from mice of various ages. The specimens were homogenized and measured aliquots were used to determine their total protein, collagen, and DNA content. The results obtained utilizing skin samples from 6-month-old TSK/+ and normal mice are shown in Table 11. The average total collagen content per disc was about 2.5-fold greater in TSK/+ mice than in controls. The DNA content of the constant diameter discs was not different between TSK/+ and normal mice. Therefore, when the collagen content was expressed on a per DNA basis, a marked increase in the collagen per DNA ratio was observed. This finding supports the notion that the excessive accumulation of collagen in the skin of these animals is probably not due to increased fibroblast proliferation but most likely represents either increased collagen production or decreased collagen degradation.

The other major connective tissue component in skin besides collagen is represented by the glycosaminoglycans (GAG). Histologic studies suggested an increase in ground substance (which is mainly comprised of GAG) in TSK/+ mice. The content of dermal GAG was examined by Ross et al. (1983) utilizing large skin biopsy specimens after hydrolysis. These studies showed that there was no difference in the concentrations of hexosamine and uronic acid between TSK/+ and normal mouse skin when expressed on a wet weight basis. However, a significant increase in total hexosamine and total uronic acid per constant surface area of skin was found in 1-month-

Table 11. Collagen and DNA content of 4-mm diameter skin biopsies from 6-month-old TSK/+ and normal mice

Sample	TSK			Normal		
	Collagen (mg)	DNA (μg)	Collagen/DNA (μg/μg)	Collagen (mg)	DNA (μg)	Collagen/DNA (μg/μg)
1	1.58	48.4	32.6	0.95	45.9	20.7
2	1.60	30.4	52.7	0.67	21.2	31.8
3	1.53	49.5	30.9	0.32	40.9	7.7
4	1.31	45.6	28.8	0.64	42.5	15.0
5	1.14	27.9	41.0	0.28	52.1	5.4
$\bar{x}$	1.44 ± 0.1*	40.4 ± 10.4	37.2 ± 9.2**	0.57 ± 0.28*	40.5 ± 11.6	16.1 ± 10.7**

* Statistically significant differences between skin of TSK/+ and normal mice ($P < 0.0002$).
** Statistically significant differences between skin of TSK/+ and normal mice ($P < 0.006$).
From Jimenez et al. (1984).

old TSK/+ mouse skin as compared with normal skin. In biopsies from the 6-month-old age groups the differences were more pronounced. When the GAG concentration was measured, there was a significant increase in total GAG content per surface area of skin in 6-month-old TSK/+ mice, compared with age-matched normal mice.

The biochemical studies described above demonstrate that there is an increase in the net amounts of collagen and GAG in the skin of TSK mutant mice. Although the concentration of these macromolecules per unit of wet weight was not altered, their total amount expressed per surface area of skin was markedly elevated. These findings are similar to those previously reported in sclerodermatous human skin by Rodnan et al. (1979) who found an increase in the total amount of collagen present per surface area of skin from scleroderma patients when compared with skin from control individuals.

Enzymes Involved in Collagen Production; Post-Ribosomal Modifications and Degradation. It has been previously demonstrated that elevated rates of collagen production are usually associated with concomitant increases in the levels of various enzymes involved in the posttranslational modifications of newly synthesized collagen. Increased activity of prolyl and lysyl hydroxylases (EC 1.14.11.2 and 1.14.11.4) have been found in tissues undergoing active collagen synthesis (Kuutti-Savolainen et al. 1979) as well as in sclerodermatous skin (Keiser et al. 1971). To investigate whether changes similar to those found in PSS skin regarding the activity of these enzymes were present in TSK/+ mice skin, Shikata et al. (1986) studied the levels of prolyl hydroxylase in homogenates of skin from 3-week-old TSK/+

and normal mice. They found that the prolyl hydroxylase activity is about 2.8 times higher in TSK/+ mice skin than in normal controls.

The possibility that decreased degradation of collagen plays a role in the excessive connective tissue accumulation found in TSK/+ mice, as suggested by Brady (1975) for PSS skin, was examined by Shikata et al. (1986), who measured the activity of various enzymes responsible for collagen degradation. These investigators found that collagenase activity in the skin of TSK/+ mice is about 1.5 times higher than in normal skin. Also, gelatinase activity tends to be higher in the TSK/+ mice.

Skin Collagen Types of Normal and TSK Mice. Since the demonstration of biochemical heterogeneity in the molecular composition and structure of collagen (Miller 1976) and the characterization of the various tissue-specific collagens (Bornstein and Sage 1980), increasing attention has been given to the possible role of changes in collagen phenotype in various diseases. We therefore examined the possibility that alterations in the relative proportions of the various collagen types synthesized in TSK/+ tissues may be responsible for the excessive accumulation of collagen. Our results (Millan and Jimenez, unpublished data) failed to demonstrate any significant qualitative difference in the relative proportion of the various skin collagens examined. These findings are similar to those that did not show a phenotypic alteration in the proportion of the various collagen types in established sclerodermatous skin lesions (Lovell et al. 1979).

Biosynthesis of Collagen in Organ Cultures of Normal and TSK Skin. The excessive accumulation of

Table 12. Incorporation of [^{14}C]proline and synthesis of [^{14}C]hydroxyproline by skin biopsies from 6-month-old TSK/+ and normal mice in organ cultures[a]

Sample	[^{14}C]proline				[^{14}C]hydroxyproline			
	dpm/disc $\times 10^{-3}$		dpm/µg DNA $\times 10^{-1}$		dpm/disc $\times 10^{-3}$		dpm/µg DNA $\times 10^{-1}$	
	TSK	Normal	TSK	Normal	TSK	Normal	TSK	Normal
1	690.8	448.0	81.3	37.4	9.5	4.0	111.3	33.4
2	489.9	366.6	57.0	30.6	8.2	3.8	95.9	31.7
3	460.4	357.1	54.2	29.8	5.5	3.2	64.7	26.9
4	395.8	329.8	46.6	27.6	5.3	3.1	62.4	26.1
5	357.6	306.7	42.1	25.6	5.0	–	58.5	–
x̄	478.9 ± 129.4	361.6 ± 53.7	56.4 ± 15.2	30.2 ± 4.5	6.7 ± 2.0	3.5 ± 0.4	78.6 ± 23.6	29.5 ± 35.8
P	< 0.05		< 0.01		< 0.014		< 0.01	

[a] Skin discs (8 mm in diameter) obtained from the dorsum of TSK/+ and normal mice were incubated with [^{14}C]proline, and total [^{14}C]proline incorporation and [^{14}C]hydroxyproline synthesis were determined. Each value represents an average of two experiments.
From Jimenez et al. (1984).

collagen in TSK mice tissues could be either due to increased production of this protein by TSK fibroblasts or to an impairment in its degradation. To elucidate the role of these two mechanisms, in vitro collagen biosynthetic studies were performed. The results of these studies (Table 12) demonstrated that TSK/+ skin organ cultures synthesize substantially greater amounts of collagen than normal skin. In addition, it was found that this newly synthesized collagen is significantly more soluble. These data are similar to those previously described for scleroderma skin organ cultures (Jimenez et al. 1977). Electrophoretic analysis of the newly synthesized proteins from TSK/+ and normal skin organ cultures confirmed the increased production of collagen by mutant skin. These studies also showed that there were no qualitative differences in the complement of products biosynthesized by normal or TSK/+ skin organ cultures.

Growth and Biochemical Characteristics of TSK Fibroblasts in Monolayer Cultures. The establishment of fibroblastic cell lines from human normal and PSS skin was previously shown to be a powerful tool to examine collagen metabolism and regulation since it was demonstrated that cell lines obtained from affected tissue maintained their altered phenotype through several passages in culture (LeRoy 1974). We and others therefore performed studies of collagen metabolism and its regulation employing fibroblastic cultures of normal and TSK/+ cells.
To explore the possibility that the excessive collagen deposited in TSK tissues is due at least in part to increased fibroblast proliferation in the

mutants, studies to examine the growth characteristics of normal and TSK dermal fibroblasts were conducted by Osborn and Bauer (1985) and by ourselves (unpublished data). In our studies we examined the rates of proliferation in six control and six TSK fibroblast cell lines of similar passage number. We found that the growth of dermal fibroblasts from TSK/+ mice was significantly slower than that of normal fibroblasts, and the TSK fibroblasts reached confluency at a much lower cell density than the control fibroblasts. The lower cell density of confluent TSK fibroblasts was independent of the substratum on which the cells were grown. The availability of established dermal fibroblast cell lines from normal and TSK/+ mice allowed us to study collagen biosynthesis and regulation employing monolayer cultures (Jimenez et al. 1986a). In these studies, it was found that the average total protein biosynthesis was more than twice normal in TSK fibroblast cultures (Table 13). This increment was entirely accounted for by newly synthesized proteins secreted into the culture media. Similar results were obtained when collagen synthesis was analyzed (Table 14). Greater than twofold more collagen was synthesized by the TSK cell lines. Similar to the findings with total [^{14}C]proline incorporation, the increased amount of collagen synthesized by TSK/+ cultures was entirely accounted for by the fraction secreted into the culture media. These findings are strikingly similar to the results of studies of collagen and protein biosynthesis in cultures from normal and PSS dermal fibroblasts (Bashey et al. 1977; Perlish et al. 1976; Buckingham et al. 1978).
To determine whether there were qualitative dif-

Table 13. [^{14}C]Proline incorporation by confluent cultures of normal and TSK/+ dermal fibroblasts[a]

| Cell line | Total [^{14}C] (dpm/µg DNA × 10^{-3}) | | | | | |
| | Media | | Cell layers | | Total | |
	Normal	TSK	Normal	TSK	Normal	TSK
1	7.6	40.8	6.7	8.3	14.3	49.1
2	15.4	22.5	11.2	7.2	26.6	29.7
3	7.5	22.0	4.0	4.0	11.5	26.0
4	18.3	41.6	12.0	7.4	30.3	49.0
5	12.2	31.1	2.5	5.3	14.7	33.8
x̄	12.2±4.8	31.1±9.6	7.3±4.2	6.5±1.8	19.5±8.4	37.5±6.8
P	<0.004		<0.69		<0.019	

[a] Confluent fibroblasts from normal and TSK/+ mice were incubated with [^{14}C]proline in 35-mm plastic culture plates for 72 h. Cells and media were separated and total [^{14}C]proline incorporation was determined in a scintillation counter. Each value shown represents a mean of three culture dishes.
From Jimenez et al. (1986a).

Table 14. [^{14}C]Hydroxyproline synthesis by confluent cultures of five cell lines of normal and TSK/+ dermal fibroblasts[a]

| Cell line | [^{14}C]hydroxyproline (dpm/µg DNA × 10^{-2}) | | | | | |
| | Media | | Cell layers | | Total | |
	Normal	TSK	Normal	TSK	Normal	TSK
1	27.4	131.2	7.2	4.6	34.6	136.1
2	57.8	88.7	10.5	2.5	68.3	91.2
3	31.5	87.4	1.3	6.5	32.8	93.9
4	73.8	153.3	9.7	3.8	83.5	157.1
5	46.5	107.8	3.0	3.8	49.5	111.6
x̄	47.4±19.1	113.7±29.4	6.3±4.1	4.2±1.5	53.7±21.9	118.0±28.3
P	<0.003		<0.326		<0.004	

[a] Experimental conditions were the same as in Table 13. The amount of [^{14}C]hydroxyproline in each fraction was determined after hydrolysis of dialyzed samples.
From Jimenez et al. (1986b)

ferences in the populations of newly synthesized proteins between control and TSK fibroblasts, the labeled proteins present in the media and cell layers from cultures were analyzed by polyacrylamide slab-gel electrophoresis. A significantly higher proportion of radioactivity migrating in the region of collagenous polypeptides was detected in the media from the TSK/+ cultures. However, there were no appreciable qualitative differences in the populations of labeled proteins synthesized by the two cells. The electrophoretograms also showed that the amounts of radioactivity migrating in the position of fibronectin were substantially greater in the cultures from TSK cells.

This observation bears resemblance to the increased amounts of fibronectin demonstrated in PSS skin by immunofluorescent studies (Cooper et al. 1979) and to our own observations of in-creased biosynthesis of this protein in PSS dermal fibroblast cultures (unpublished observations).

Expression of Collagen Genes in TSK/+ and Control Mice Fibroblasts. To examine at the molecular level the mechanisms responsible for the increased collagen production demonstrated in TSK/+ skin organ cultures and cultured dermal fibroblasts, we studied the expression of three collagen genes in TSK fibroblasts employing Northern and dot blot hybridization with type-specific cDNA probes for alpha 1 (I), alpha 2 (I), and alpha 1 (III) procollagen chains. We chose to use the human collagen clones because of the extensive cross-hybridization of the human collagen cDNA probes to mouse RNA and DNA even under conditions of high stringency.

Table 15. Densitometric analysis of amounts of polyadenylated RNA from control and TSK/+ fibroblasts hybridized to specific α1 (I), α2 (I), and α1 (III) cDNA probes[a]

Collagen probe	Control fibroblasts	TSK/+ fibroblasts	TSK/ +/ratio/ control
α1 (I)	4.7	22.4	4.8
α2 (I)	8.4	41.2	4.9
α1 (III)	5.4	30.1	5.6

[a] Areas under each peak were obtained by densitometric analysis of radioautograms and were quantitated employing a planimeter. Each value represents a average of results obtained for multiple exposures and are expressed in cm^2.
From Jimenez et al. (1986b).

The results of Northern blot hybridization and dot blot hybridization of control and TSK-fibroblast-polyadenylated RNA are shown in Table 15. TSK fibroblasts showed an approximately fivefold increase in type I and III collagen-specific RNA transcripts when compared with equal amounts of RNA from control fibroblasts. The increased levels of collagen mRNAs were not the result of a more generalized phenomenon, since the levels of beta-actin-hybridizing mRNA were found to be essentially equal, suggesting that the increased levels of mRNA in the TSK fibroblast were selective for collagen. These results are also similar to the recent findings of Jimenez et al. (1986b) that demonstrated a coordinate increase in specific types I and III procollagen mRNAs in PSS dermal fibroblasts.

Other Studies. Physiologic studies of TSK/+ mice lungs demonstrated emphysematous changes such as increased total lung capacity, compliance, and specific compliance. Because of the possible role of antiprotease deficiency in the development of naturally occurring emphysema, the levels of antiprotease activity in TSK/+ mice were also investigated. Normal antiprotease activity was found; therefore, the mechanisms responsible for the pulmonary alterations in TSK/+ mice cannot be well understood and require further study. Biochemical studies of collagen content and characterization of collagen types in hearts from 12-month-old TSK/+ mice were performed by Osborn et al. (1987); they found a significant increase in total collagen content and a severe elevation of type I collagen with a proportional decrease of types III and V collagens in TSK/+ hearts.

Table 16. Similarities and differences between various alterations present in TSK/+ mice and progressive systemic sclerosis (PSS) in humans

	TSK/+ mutant	Human PSS
Cutaneous involvement	+	+
Visceral involvement		
Gastrointestinal	−	+
Vascular	−	+
Pulmonary	Emphysema	Fibrosis
Renal	?	+
Cardiac	+	+
Peritoneal fibrosis	+	?
Arthritis/calcinosis	−	+
Immunologic changes		
Mononuclear cellular infiltrates	−	+
Antinuclear antibodies	+/?	+
Other	+/?	+
Histologic and ultrastructural changes	+	+
Biochemical changes		
Increased collagen/surface area	+	+
Increased solubility of collagen	+	+
Collagen phenotype changes	−	−
Increased biosynthesis in skin	+	+
Increased levels of posttranslational enzymes	+	+
Normal collagenolytic activity	+	+
Increased glycosaminoglycan content	+	+
Abnormal collagen regulation		
Increased synthesis in fibroblast cultures	+	+
Increased procollagen gene expression	+	+
Increased fibronectin	+	+

Comparison with Other Species

Several experimental models resembling scleroderma (PSS) have been previously described (Stastny et al. 1963; Stastny and Ziff 1967; Ishikawa et al. 1975, 1978; Finch et al. 1980; Gershwin et al. 1981; van de Water and Gershwin 1985). A review of the features of these models, however, indicates that none reproduces all the features of the human disease.

The studies reviewed above demonstrate the remarkable similarities between the connective tissue abnormalities present in TSK/+ mice and those characteristic of human progressive systemic sclerosis (PSS or scleroderma). These similarities are particularly apparent in skin and in fibroblasts dervied from this tissue. Although these abnormalities are sufficient to propose the TSK mutation as a valuable experimental model for human PSS, there are many PSS features that are not present in TSK/+ mice (Table 16). The most salient differences are the absence of inflammatory and immunological alterations in the TSK/+ mice as well as the lack of vascular, gastrointestinal, and articular involvement. Despite these, however, it is clearly apparent that TSK/+ mice reproduce one of the cardinal characteristics of PSS, namely, the increased accumulation of collagen and other connective tissue components in skin and some internal organs. The observation that a genetic mutation in TSK mice can result in connective tissue alterations that closely resemble those present in PSS will undoubtedly be of great value in understanding the mechanisms that are responsible for tissue fibrosis in PSS at a molecular level. In addition, they will be useful in dissecting the mechanisms of normal and pathologic regulation of collagen production.

Acknowledgements. This work was supported by grant AM-32564 from the National Institutes of Health and by a grant from the Scleroderma Research Foundation. We gratefully acknowledge the excellent technical assistance of M. Billman in preparation of the manuscript.

References

Bashey RI, Jimenez SA, Perlish JS (1977) Characterization of secreted collagen from normal and scleroderma fibroblasts in culture. J Mol Med 2: 153–161

Bornstein P, Sage H (1980) Structurally distinct collagen types. Annu Rev Biochem 48: 957–1003

Brady AH (1975) Collagenase in scleroderma. J Clin Invest 56: 1175–1180

Buckingham RB, Prince PK, Rodnan GP, Taylor F (1978) Increased collagen accumulation in dermal fibroblast cultures from patients with progressive systemic sclerosis (scleroderma). J Lab Clin Med 92: 5–21

Cooper SM, Keyser AJ, Beaulieu AD, Ruoslahti E, Nimni ME, Quismorio FP Jr (1979) Increase in fibronectin in the deep dermis of involved skin in progressive systemic sclerosis. Arthritis Rheum 22: 983–987

DeLustro FA, Mackel AM, LeRoy EC (1983) Delayed-type hypersensitivity to elastase-soluble lung peptides in the tight-skin (Tsk) mouse. Cell Immunol 81: 175–179

Finch WR, Rodnan GP, Buckingham RB, Prince RK, Winkelstein A (1980) Bleomycin induced scleroderma. J Rheumatol 7: 651–659

Gershwin ME, Abplanalp HA, Castles JJ, Ikeda RM, van der Water J, Eklund J, Haynes D (1981) Characterization of a spontaneous disease of white leghorn chickens resembling progressive systemic sclerosis (scleroderma). J Exp Med 153: 1640–1659

Green MC, Sweet HO, Bunker LE (1976) Tight-skin, a new mutation of the mouse causing excessive growth of connective tissue and skeleton. Am J Pathol 82: 493–512

Hawkins RA, Claman HN, Clark RAF, Steigerwald JC (1985) Increased dermal mast cell populations in progressive systemic sclerosis: a link in chronic fibrosis? Ann Intern Med 102: 182–186

Ishikawa H, Saito Y, Yamakage A, Kitabatake M (1978) Sclerodermainducing glycosaminoglycan in the urine of patients with systemic scleroderma. Dermatologica 156: 193–204

Ishikawa H, Suzuki S, Horiuchi R, Sato H (1975) An approach to experimental scleroderma, using urinary glycosaminoglycans from patients with systemic scleroderma. Acta Derm Venereol (Stockh) 55: 97–107

Jimenez SA, Millan A, Bashey RI (1984) Scleroderma-like alterations in collagen metabolism occurring in the TSK (tight-skin) mouse. Arthritis Rheum 27: 180–185

Jimenez SA, Yankowski RI, Frontino PM (1977) Biosynthetic heterogeneity of sclerodermatous skin in organ cultures. J Mol Med 2: 423–430

Jimenez SA, Williams CJ, Myers JC, Bashey RI (1986a) Increased collagen biosynthesis and increased expression of type I and type III procollagen genes in tight-skin (TSK) mouse fibroblasts. J Biol Chem 261: 657–662

Jimenez SA, Feldman G, Bashey RI, Bienkowski R, Rosenbloom J (1986b) Co-ordinate increase in the expression of type I and type III collagen genes in progressive systemic sclerosis fibroblasts. Biochem J 237: 837–843

Keiser HR, Stein HD, Sjoerdsma A (1971) Increased protocollagen proline hydroxylase activity in sclerodermatous skin. Arch Dermatol 104: 57–60

Kuutti-Savolainen ER, Risteli J, Miettinen TA, Kivirikko KI (1979) Collagen biosynthesis enzymes in serum and hepatic tissue in liver disease. I. Prolyl hydroxylase. Eur J Clin Invest 9: 89–95

LeRoy EC (1974) Increased collagen synthesis by scleroderma skin fibroblasts in vitro: a possible defect in the regulation or activation of the scleroderma fibroblast. J Clin Invest 54: 880–889

Lovell CR, Nicholls AC, Duance VC, Bailey AJ (1979) Characterization of dermal collagen in systemic sclerosis. Br J Dermatol 100: 359–369

Menton DN, Hess RA (1980) The ultrastructure of collagen in the dermis of tight-skin (TSK) mutant mice. J Invest Dermatol 74: 139–147

Menton DN, Hess RA, Lichtenstein JR, Eisen AZ (1980) The structure and tensile properties of the skin of tight-skin (TSK) mutant mice. J Invest Dermatol 70: 4–10

Miller EJ (1976) Biochemical characteristics and biological significance of the genetically distinct collagens. Mol Cell Biochem 13: 165–192

Osborn TG, Bauer NE (1984) Physical and biochemical manifestations of a cardiomyopathy in the tight-skin mouse. Arthritis Rheumatol 27: S75A

Osborn TG, Bauer NE (1985) Growth assessment of dermal fibroblasts from tight-skinned mice. Arthritis Rheum 28: W81 (abstr)

Osborn TG, Bauer NE, Ross SC, Moore TL, Zuckner J (1983) The tight-skin mouse: physical and biochemical properties of the skin. J Rheumatol 10: 793-996

Osborn TG, Bashey RI, Moore TL, Fischer VW (1987) Collagenous abnormalities in the heart of the tight skin mouse. J Mol Cell Cardiol 19: 581-587

Perlish JS, Bashey RI, Stephens RE, Fleischmajer R (1976) Connective tissue synthesis by cultured scleroderma fibroblasts. I. In vitro collagen synthesis by normal and scleroderma dermal fibroblasts. Arthritis Rheum 19: 891-901

Rodnan GP, Lipinski E, Luksick J (1979) Skin thickness and collagen content in progressive systemic sclerosis and localized scleroderma. Arthritis Rheum 22: 130-140

Rosenberg GT, Ross SC, Osborn TG (1984) Glycosaminoglycan content in the lung of the tight-skin mouse. J Rheumatol 11: 318-320

Ross SC, Osborn TG, Dorner RW, Zuckner J (1983) Glycosaminoglycan content in skin of the tight-skin mouse. Arthritis Rheum 26: 653-657

Rossi GA, Hunninghake GW, Gadek JE, Szapiel SV, Kawanami O, Ferrans VJ, Crystal RG (1984) Hereditary emphysema in the tight skin mouse. Evaluation of pathogenesis. Am Rev Respir Dis 129: 850-855

Shikata H, Hiramatsu M, Kashimata M, Noguchi M, Masumizu T, Fugimoto D, Utsumi N (1986) Enzyme activities involved in connective tissue metabolism in the skin of tight-skin (TSK) mice. Arch Dermatol Res 278: 510-512

Stastny P, Ziff M (1967) Immunologically induced experimental models of human "connective tissue diseases." Rheumatology 1: 189-241

Stastny P, Stembridge VA, Ziff M (1963) Homologous disease in the adult rat, a model for autoimmune disease. I. General features and cutaneous lesions. J Exp Med 118: 635-648

Szapiel SV, Fulmer JD, Hunninghake GW, Elson NA, Kawanami O, Ferrans VJ, Crystal RG (1981) Hereditary emphysema in the tight-skin (TSK/+) mouse. Am Rev Respir Dis 123: 680-685

Van de Water J, Gerschwin ME (1985) Annual model of human disease. Avian scleroderma: an inherited fibrotic disease of white Leghorn chickens resembling progressive systemic sclerosis. Am J Pathol 120: 478-482

Walker M, Harley R, Maize J, DeLustro F, LeRoy EC (1985) Mast cells and their degranulation in the Tsk mouse model of scleroderma. Proc Soc Exp Biol Med 180: 323-328

Walker MA, Harley RA, LeRoy EC (1987) Inhibition of fibrosis in TSK mice by blocking mast cell degranulation. J Rheumatol 14: 299-301

Asebia, a Mutation Affecting Sebaceous Glands, Mouse

John G. Compton, Robert W. Dunstan, and John P. Sundberg

Gross Appearance

Homozygous mice carrying the asebia mutation *ab* or *ab^J* are characterized by defective sebaceous glands and other cutaneous abnormalities (*ab:* Gates and Karasek 1965; Josefowicz and Hardy 1978a; *ab^J*: Pennycuik et al. 1986). At 7 days of age, homozygous asebic mice display impaired hair growth. Alopecia increases in severity with successive hair cycles, and eventually only scattered hairs are present. The fine epidermal scaling is generally mild but tends to become more severe with aging. Asebic mice are light sensitive and have pruritus of the eyelids, and a sticky exudate typically encrusts the eyes (Fig. 280). They have a distinctive odor of undetermined origin. The severity of these phenotypic features varies, either due to genetic background or to allelic differences between the two known independent mutations, *ab* or *ab^J* (Pennycuik et al. 1986).

Microscopic Features

A significant feature of asebic skin is the lack of normal sebaceous glands (Gates and Karasek 1965; Josefowicz and Hardy 1978c). The sebaceous glands of asebic mice lack the orderly maturation of peripheral reserve cells into vacuolated cells that rupture and secrete their contents into the sebaceous duct (Fig. 281). Asebic glands appear disorganized with reserve cells interspersed among sebaceous cells that are in various stages of differentiation (Figs. 282 and 283).

Differentiated cells have fewer (<10%) and less uniform lipid droplets than those found in normal cells and stain more darkly with eosin. Mature mutant sebaceous cells may fail to rupture, and some have a "webbed" appearance (Josefowicz and Hardy 1978c). Acidophilic material observed within the follicular openings is probably undispersed sebum secreted from the asebic glands. The hypoplastic sebaceous glands appear

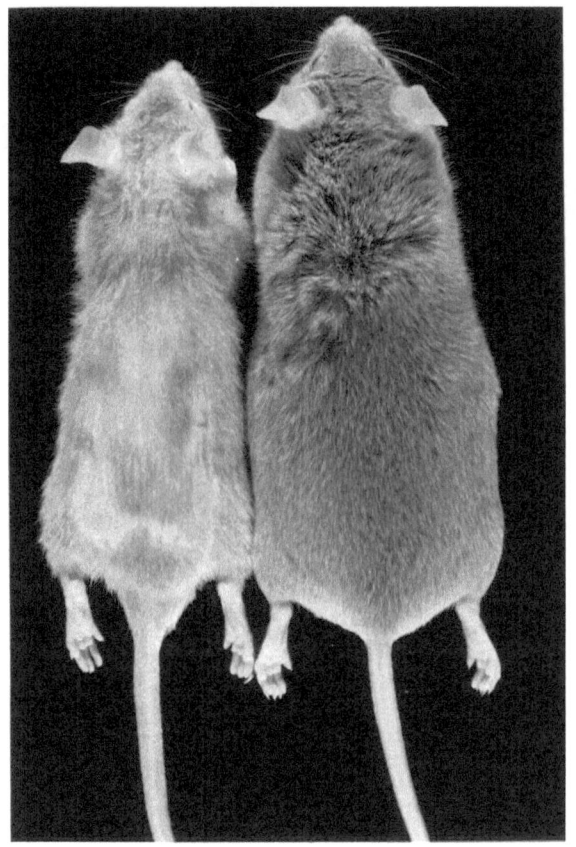

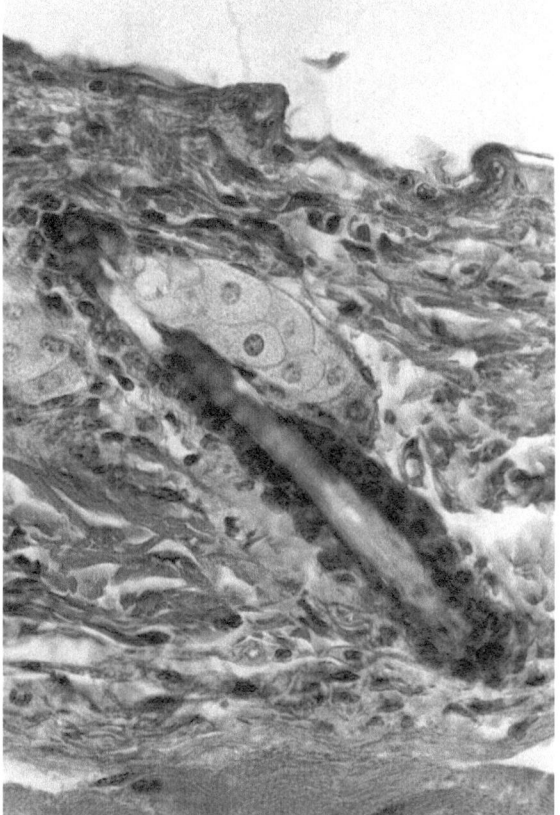

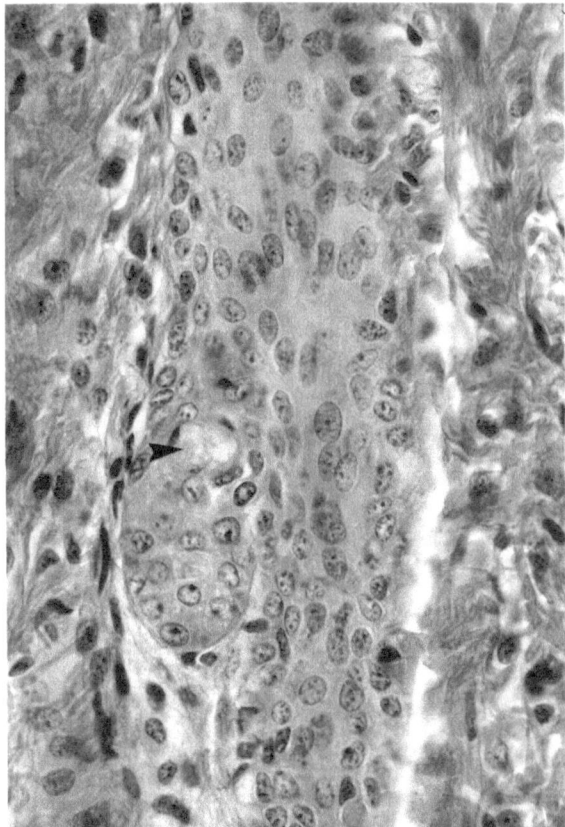

Fig. 280 *(upper left).* Nine-month-old ab^J/ab^J *(left)* and $ab^J/+$ *(right)* mice. Note encrustations over eye

Fig. 281 *(upper right).* Normal pilosebaceous unit of $ab^J/+$ mouse. H and E, ×300

Fig. 282 *(lower right).* Small, abnormal, sebaceous gland of ab^J/ab^J mouse (4 weeks old) with few differentiating cells *(arrowhead).* H and E, ×400

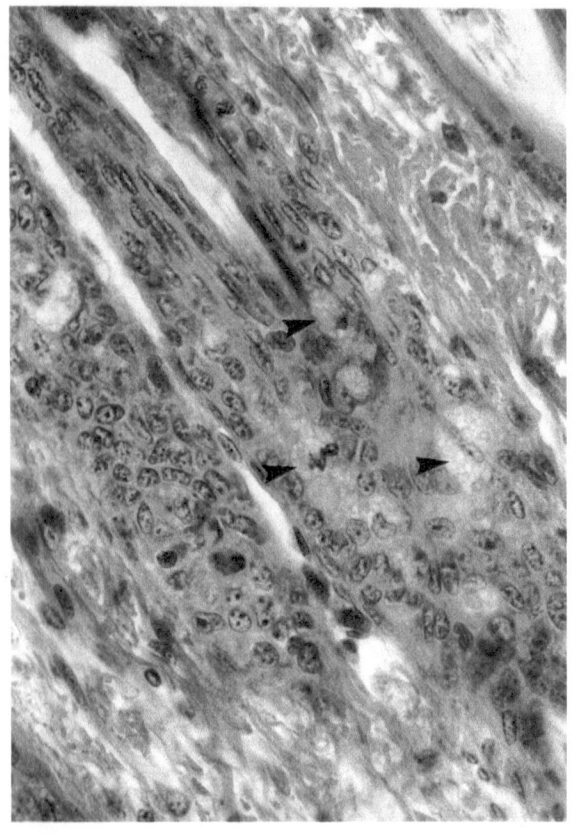

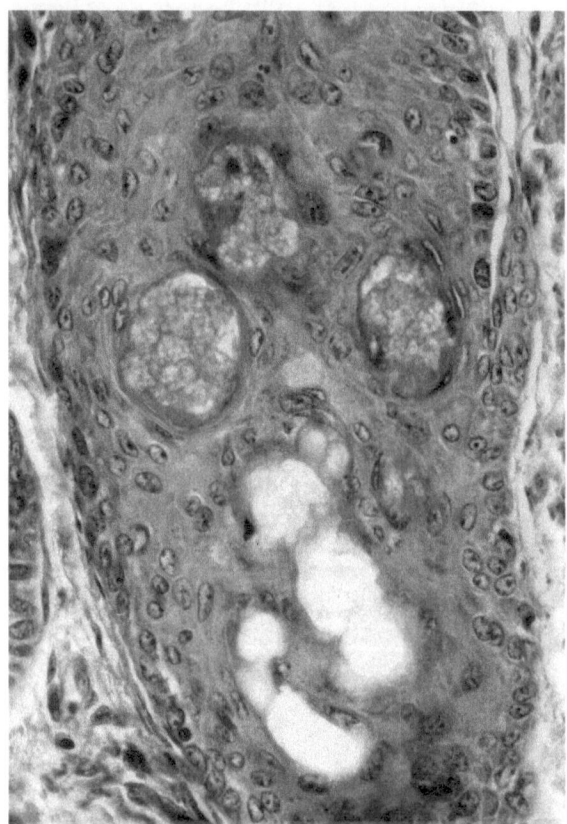

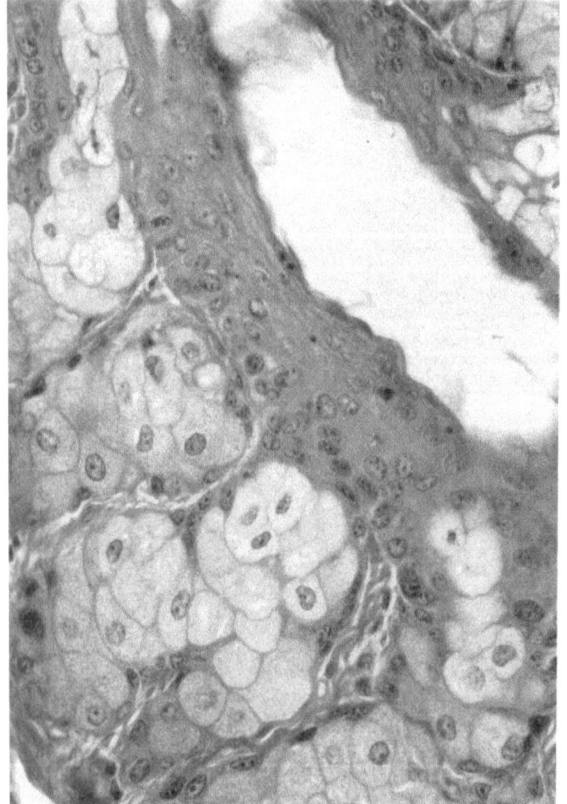

Fig. 283 *(upper left).* Sebaceous cells in various stages of differentiation *(arrowheads)* in *ab^J^/ab^J^* mouse. H and E, × 400

Fig. 284 *(lower left).* Meibomian gland from a normal mouse (4 weeks old). H and E, × 400

Fig. 285 *(upper right).* Disorganized, abnormally differentiated meibomian gland of an *ab^J^/ab^J^* mouse (4 weeks old). H and E, × 400

to bud from a site lower on the outer root sheath of the hair follicle than do normal glands. They develop initially as pairs of single lobes that extend abnormally deep into the dermis and mature into irregular, multilobed glands. Comparable defects are observed in asebic meibomian glands, namely, reduced size, irregular structure, and fewer, fully differentiated, deeply acidophilic cells (Figs. 284 and 285). In contrast, male preputial glands, female clitoral glands, and the anal glands of both sexes do not appear to be affected (Josefowicz and Hardy 1978c).

In addition to abnormal sebaceous glands, asebic mice display alterations in their epidermis (Gates and Karasek 1965; Josefowicz and Hardy 1978a), dermis (Josefowicz and Hardy 1978a), and hair follicles (Josefowicz and Hardy 1978b). Hyperplasia and orthokeratosis characterize the epidermis (Josefowicz and Hardy 1978a; Pennycuik et al. 1986). In asebic mice less than 4 months old, the stratum malpighii is twice normal thickness, and the stratum corneum is 2–10 times thicker than normal. The hyperplasia and orthokeratosis become more pronounced between 11 and 22 months, where the stratum malpighii and stratum corneum, respectively, are 4 and 6–20 times thicker than normal. In contrast, normal adult epidermis thins at this age to only a few cell layers. The epidermis of asebic mice is vaguely papillated and foci of spongiosis are occasionally present.

The dermis of mutant mice is about twice as thick and more vascular than normal siblings (Josefowicz and Hardy 1978a; Pennycuik et al. 1986). Suppurative inflammation is present in the dermis and in regions of degenerating follicles. Areas of mutant dermis contain cellular debris, indicative of extensive cytolysis. Spindle-shaped cells with abnormal morphologic features develop postnatally.

In the first hair cycle, late anagen asebic hair follicles are largely normal except for their excessive length (twice normal) and accompanying deep penetration into the hypodermis. In later hair cycles, the parallel alignment of follicles is replaced by a more random arrangement (Josefowicz and Hardy 1978b; Pennycuik et al. 1986). Abnormally twisted follicles and hyperplastic branched follicles develop. The inner root sheath is abnormal at the transition region near the sebaceous glands, lacking the typical PAS-positive transversely "corrugated" appearance of normal inner root sheath cells which interdigitate with outer root sheath cells. Rather than being short and round, the outer root sheath cells in this re-gion are elongated and have flattened nuclei. In later hair cycles, the inner root sheath cells at this level are partially degraded and adhere to the hair shaft, or are associated with keratinized plugs in the hair canals. The base of many hair follicles appear degenerated, with pyknotic nuclei and leukocytic infiltration.

Ultrastructure

Numerous spindle-shaped cells in asebic dermis contain a variety of abnormal organelles, including irregular lysosomes, tubelike inclusions, flocculent vacuoles, abnormal mitochondria, and dilated rough endoplasmic reticular cisternae (Josefowicz and Hardy 1978a). Extracellular matrix components are also affected. Collagen fiber periodicity is normal, but the fibers are smaller in diameter and less dense. Elastin fibers sheathing the hair follicles are sparse, and masses of the amorphous elastin component, lacking microfilaments, are distributed in the dermis.

Normal sebaceous gland cells have a system of smooth endoplasmic reticulum that becomes more prominent as the cells differentiate (Josefowicz and Hardy 1978c). Tubules of smooth endoplasmic reticulum appear to open into the lipid droplets. As cells differentiate and the smooth endoplasmic reticulum increases in complexity, there is a decrease in mitochondria, which degenerate into amorphous cytoplasmic structures. Asebic sebaceous gland cells also contain smooth endoplasmic reticulum of tubules, but these are less extensive and dilated, and, though associated with lipid droplets, they do not appear to interconnect them. This may account for the irregular sizes of the lipid vacuoles. The "webbed" appearing differentiated cells contain mostly disrupted tubules and droplets. Their mitochondria appear to resist degeneration, as intact mitochondria are present in addition to the amorphous structures.

Biologic Features

Two, independent, apparently allelic, asebia mutations exist, the original spontaneous mutant, *ab,* which occurred on BALB/cCrglGa-albino (Gates and Karasek 1965), and the *ab^J* mutation that arose on BALB/cJ at the Jackson Laboratory (maintained as the stock ABJ/Le-*ab^J*). The asebia allele *ab^J* has been shown to be autosomal recessive and fully penetrant, and it maps to the distal end of mouse chromosome 19 (Sweet and Lane 1977). No distinguishing features have been discerned between $+/+$ and $ab/+$ or $ab^J/+$ mice (Josefowicz and Hardy 1978a; Pennycuik et al. 1986).

The earliest gross identification of the homozygous asebia phenotype is 6–7 days, but the earliest abnormality described is increased dermal cellularity at 16 days gestation (Josefowicz and Hardy 1978a). At 18 days gestation, abnormal spindle-shaped cells appear, and epidermal hyperkeratosis develops. Progressive dermal and epidermal thickening, and increasing hyperkeratosis are characteristic postnatally. Defective differentiation of normal 18-day sebaceous gland rudiments leads to disorganized patterns of cellular maturation and incomplete terminal differentiation of many sebaceous cells. Asebic epidermis also has an abnormal lipid composition (a deficiency of esterified sterols, wax esters, and wax diesters; Wilkinson and Karasek 1966). Alopecia in asebia is associated with the production of increasing numbers of misshapened, elongated, and disoriented follicles, and failure of many hair shafts to emerge through the follicular ostia. Prolonged anagen stages and abnormal catagen is accompanied by failure of dermal papillae to form contiguously with the downwardly growing follicular matrix cells. Defective outer root sheath cells appear to contribute to the follicular abnormalities.

While the cellular function of the gene affected by the asebia mutation is unknown, the site of expression of asebia has been investigated. Normal epidermal development and function are subject to dermal influences. It has been postulated that the asebia mutation could cause the observed hyperplasias by altering the dermal environment since the sebaceous glands, interfollicular epidermis, and outer root sheath of hair follicles all arise from the same embryonic cell layer (Josefowicz and Hardy 1978c). The involvement of a systemic factor in hair cycle timing has been suggested from observations that the prolonged asebic hair cycle became apparently normal in skin grafted onto nude mice hosts (Pennycuik et al. 1986). However, embryonic dermal-epidermal recombination grafts demonstrated that sebaceous, epidermal, and follicular abnormalities occurred only in grafts containing mutant epidermis (Pennycuik et al. 1986). This is consistent with primary action of the asebia gene function in the epidermal cell lineage.

Comparison with Other Species

To our knowledge an analogous condition to that of asebia has not been identified in humans. Recently, a condition was described in standard poodles in which the absence of sebaceous glands was associated with hyperkeratosis (Rosser et al. 1987). However, the loss of sebaceous glands was secondary to granulomatous sebaceous adenitis.

References

Gates AH, Karasek M (1965) Hereditary absence of sebaceous glands in the mouse. Science 148: 1471–1473

Josefowicz WJ, Hardy MH (1978a) The expression of the gene asebia in the laboratory mouse. 1. Epidermis, dermis. Genet Res 31: 53–65

Josefowicz WJ, Hardy MH (1978b) The expression of the gene asebia in the laboratory mouse. 2. Hair follicles. Genet Res 31: 145–155

Josefowicz WJ, Hardy MH (1978c) The expression of the gene asebia in the laboratory mouse. 3. Sebaceous glands. Genet Res 31: 157–166

Pennycuik PR, Raphael KA, Chapman RE, Hardy MH (1986) The site of action of the asebia locus *(ab)* in the skin of the mouse. Genet Res 48: 179–185

Rosser ER, Dunstan RW, Breen PT, Johnson GR (1987) Sebaceous adenitis with hyperkeratosis in the Standard Poodle: a discussion of 10 cases. J Am Anim Hosp Assoc 23: 341–345

Sweet HO, Lane PL (1977) Asebia-J on chromosome 19. Mouse News Lett 57: 20

Wilkinson DI, Karasek MA (1966) Skin lipids of a normal and a mutant (asebic) mouse strain. J Invest Dermatol 47: 449–455

Ichthyosis, Inherited, Skin, Mouse *(ic/ic)*

Karen A. Holbrook

Gross Appearance

Homozygous ichthyotic *(ic/ic)* animals are easily distinguished from heterozygous littermates by their smaller size, short, sparse coat, scaliness of "bare" skin (paws, ears, tail), short vibrissae, and accumulation of scale superimposed upon segmental rings of the tail (Fig. 286). Expression of the *ic/ic* phenotype varies considerably, even among affected littermates (Carter and Phillips 1950; Jensen and Esterly 1977). Severely affected animals have thick, confluent, rigid, cutaneous plates that crack and are gradually shed. The hair is usually diminished in quantity, and animals can be nearly bald. Mildly affected animals have small scales surrounding the orifices of hair follicles confined to the feet, tail, and ears (Jensen and Esterly 1971) (Fig. 287).

Microscopic Features

The morphology of the epidermis may vary with the genetic background of the animals carrying the trait, but it is invariably altered from normal. Spearman (1960) investigated the ichthyotic offspring produced by *ic/ic* males [obtained from the original *ic/ic* mice of Carter and Phillips (1950)] outcrossed to normal CBA females. The stock was maintained by backcrossing +/*ic* females to *ic/ic* males. He described thickened tail epidermis in the *ic/ic* animals (the viable cell layers were nearly twofold greater in thickness than normal tail epidermis) with a patchy granular layer, thickened, flaky, orthokeratotic stratum corneum, and enlarged keratinocytes. Nuclei in these cells displayed "more active nucleoli" than normal keratinocytes.

The hairs of all affected animals are disarrayed (Fig. 288) fine, short, sparse (Fig. 289), uneven in thickness, curled or kinked, and may lack a cuticle (Fig. 290). Guard hairs are typically absent from the dorsal surface (Carter and Phillips 1950). The density and structure of the follicles, however, appears to be normal (Spearman 1960). Even though follicles of vibrissae are present, some adult *ic/ic* mice lack vibrissae, and the follicles are plugged with keratinous debris (Holbrook and Sybert 1985) (Fig. 291); in other animals, vibrissae are present but short (Carter and Phillips 1950).

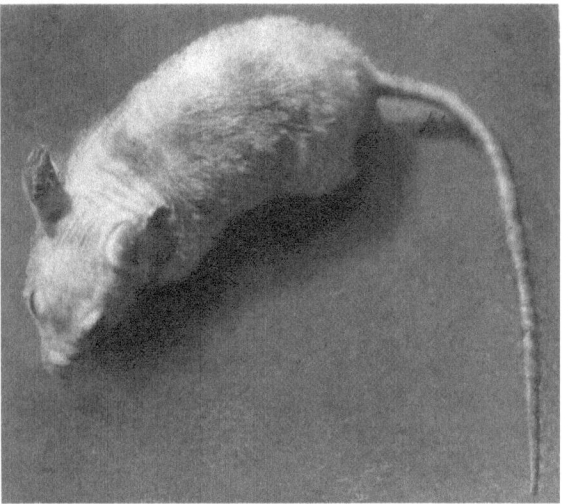

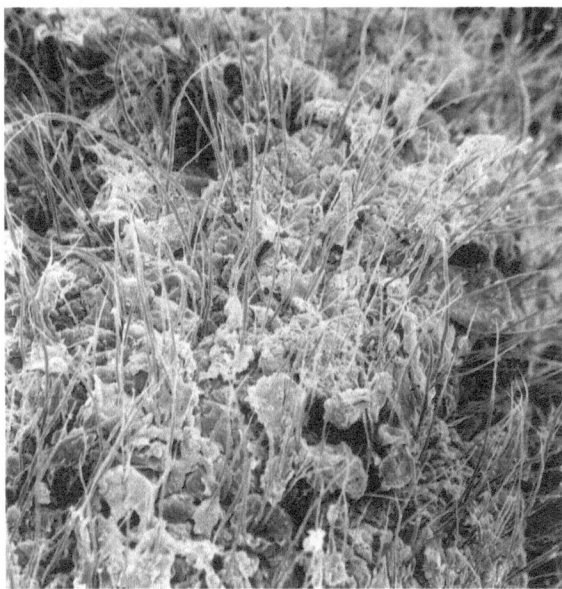

Fig. 286 *(above).* Adult *ic/ic* mouse. Note the bristly coat, lack of vibrissae, scaly ears, and segmental appearance of the tail

Fig. 287 *(below).* Skin, body of an adult *ic/ic* mouse. Note the loose scale accumulated on the surface, particularly at the orifices of hair follicles. This is a mild scaling compared to more severely affected animals. SEM, × 50

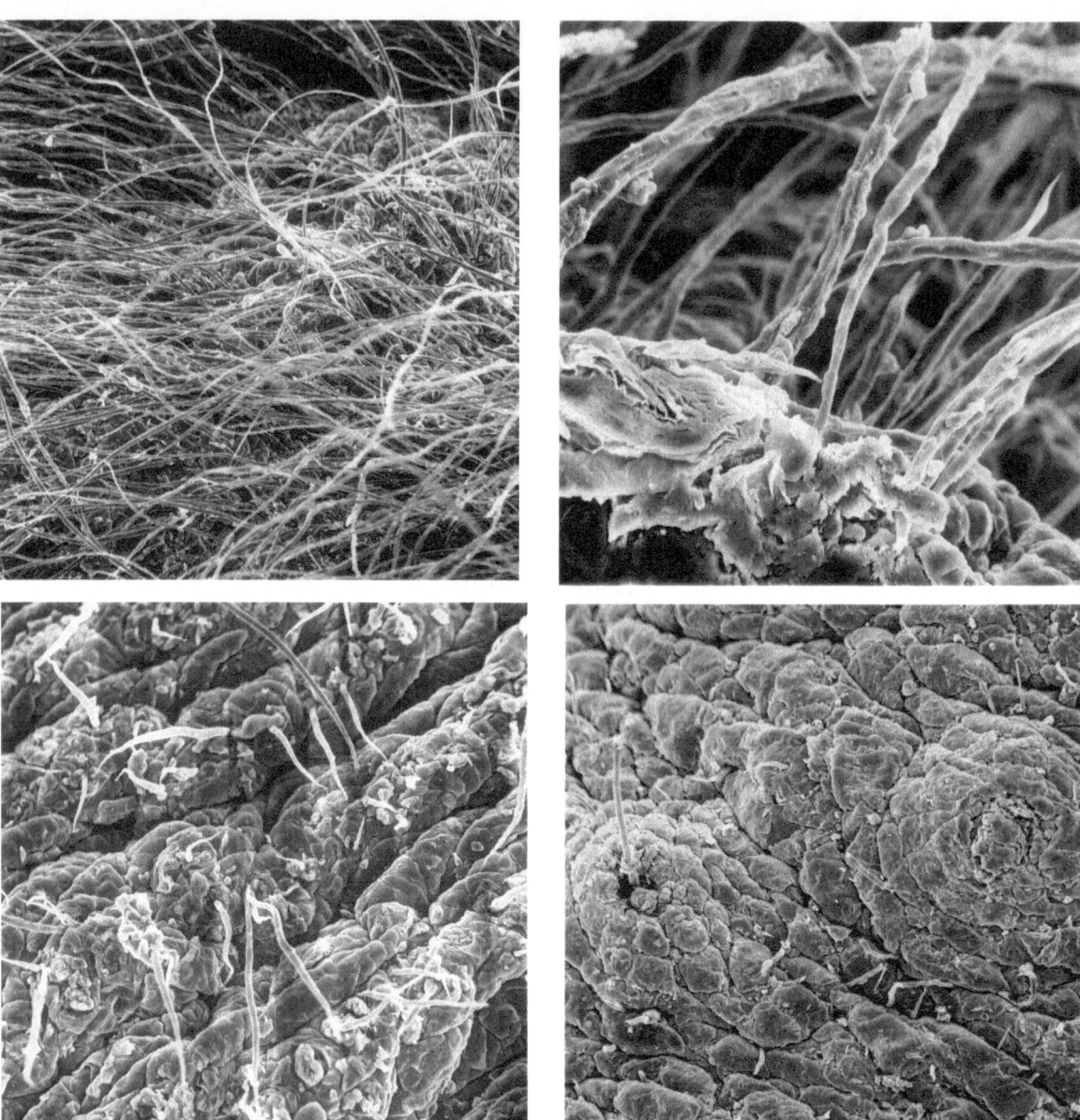

Fig. 288 *(upper left)*. Hair, adult *ic/ic* mouse. The hairs of the dorsum are nonparallel and disarrayed. SEM, × 50

Fig. 289 *(lower left)*. Hair, adult *ic/ic* mouse. Short, sparse hairs are present on the ears. SEM, × 100

Fig. 290 *(upper right)*. A higher magnification of body hairs from Fig. 289 reveals the absence of a cuticle and the variable diameter and structure of the hair. SEM, × 250

Fig. 291 *(lower right)*. Skin of snout of an adult *ic/ic* mouse showing the surface of two vibrissal follicles, one containing a small vibrissa and the other lacking a vibrissa. SEM, × 55

The rough appearance of the tail of the icythyotic mouse (Figs. 286 and 292) appears to be a consequence of thickened keratotic rings separated by exaggerated constrictions. Each of the rings is composed of keratinized plaques. Short and/or broken hairs emerge between the segments of the tail (Figs. 292 and 293). It has been shown that the constrictions are the consequence of atrophic regions of the dermis that become poorly vascularized and necrotic (Spearman 1960). Sections of the tail subsequently detach at these sites (Fig. 294). The surface morphology of the tail suggests also that the exaggerated segmental appearance of the tail also may be a consequence

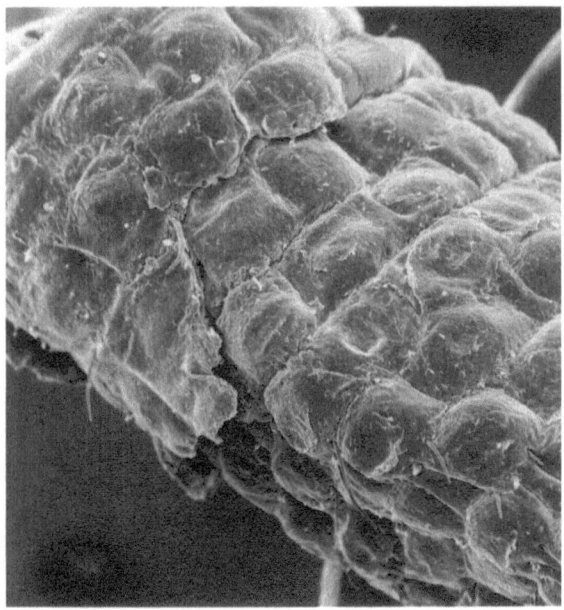

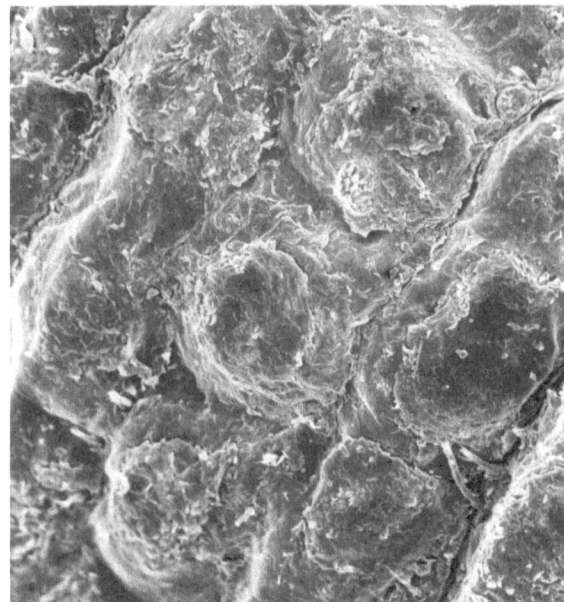

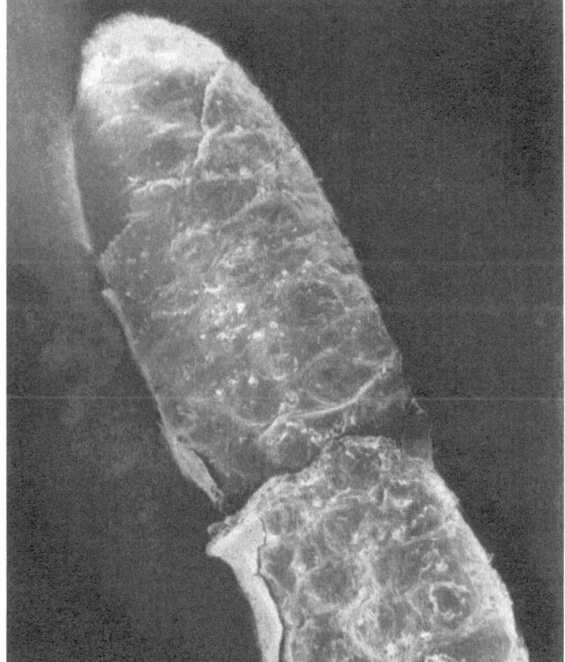

Fig. 292 *(upper left)*. Tail, adult *ic/ic* mouse. Note the segmental ring organization around the tail circumferentially and the individual plaques of each segment. Note also the apparent deep segmentation at one site. SEM, × 30

Fig. 293 *(upper right)*. Tail, adult *ic/ic* mouse. The plaque-like accumulations of scale and the broken hairs of the tail are seen at higher magnification. SEM, × 55

Fig. 294 *(lower right)*. Tail, adult *ic/ic* mouse. A deep constriction near the tip of the tail might foreshadow separation of the distal portion. SEM, × 25

of excessive layers of keratinized cells (Figs. 292 and 293).

Jensen and Esterly (1977) compared the histology, epidermal histochemistry, and ultrastructure of *ic/ic* and +/*ic* mice (obtained from an inbred ichthyotic line maintained by brother-sister matings at the Jackson Laboratory) with the same features in skin from normal Swiss S mice. They reported that the spinous, granular, and cornified layers of the dorsal epidermis of *ic/ic* mice were thickened and that abnormalities in this region

were not as marked as they were in the tail, where the stratum corneum was excessively thickened. Basal epidermal cells appeared normal, but the rete ridges were exaggerated.

The histology of the *ic/ic* epidermis of the same stock was also investigated by Holbrook and Sybert (1985). They observed less conspicuous alterations in the thickness of the trunk epidermis but marked alterations in the hair follicles of the body and vibrissae. The infundibular portions of the hair follicles on the body were thin-walled,

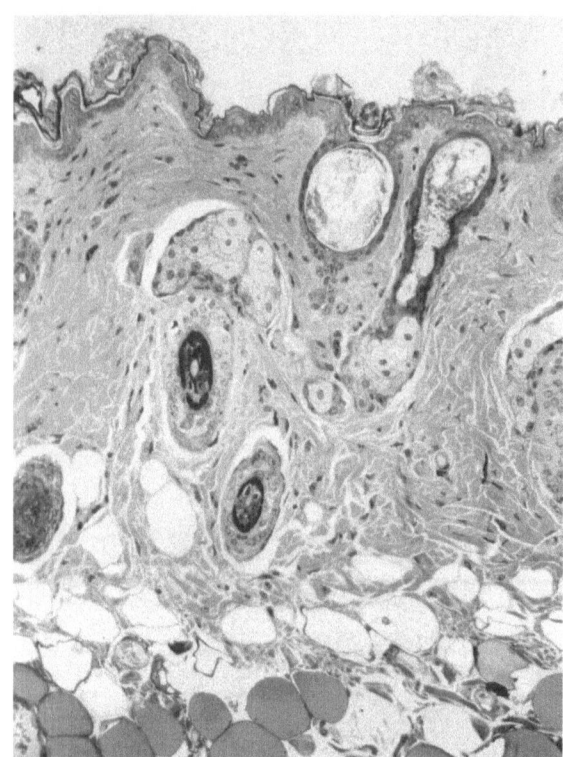

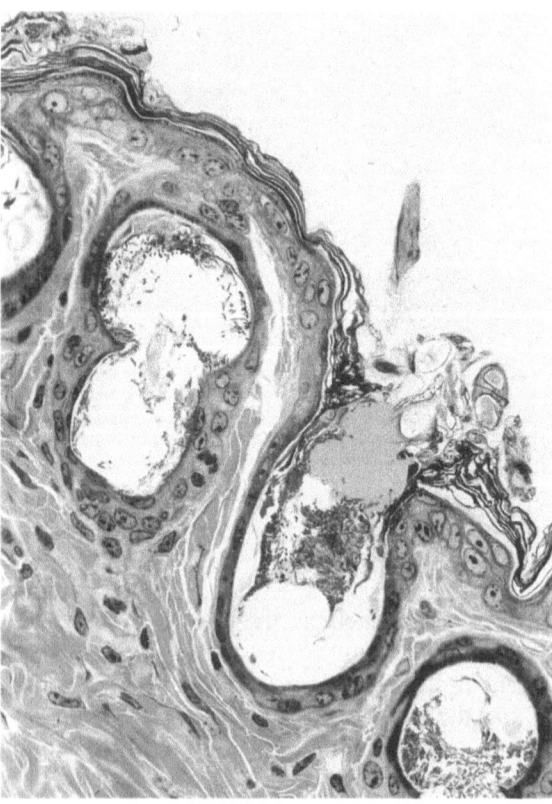

◀ **Fig. 295** *(above)*. Dorsal skin, adult *ic/ic* mouse. Full-thickness skin with a reasonably normal thickness epidermis, some accumulation of scale at the orifice of a follicle, and the cystlike infundibulum of each hair follicle. Toluidine blue, × 100

Fig. 296 *(below)*. Dorsal skin, adult *ic/ic* mouse. Bacteria, sebum, and scale accumulate at the orifices of the infundibulum. Note the relatively thin epidermis and lining of the infundibulum. Toluidine blue, × 420

cystlike structures lined with a few, thin, cornified cells (Figs. 295 and 296). A hair may or may not be present, and the cyst was often filled with bacteria. These structures opened broadly to the surface, where keratogenous debris and sebum accumulated (Fig. 296). Sebaceous glands were evident.

Autoradiographic studies using [³H]thymidine to investigate the mitotic rate of epidermal cells revealed no evidence of increased mitotic rate or epidermal transit time in either *ic/ic* or +/*ic* mice (Jensen and Esterly 1977).

Histochemical studies of the tail (Spearman 1960) and body epidermis (Jensen and Esterly 1977) have been reported. Increased levels of enzymes that signify elevated rates of epidermal metabolism (nonspecific esterases, acid phosphatase, oxidative enzymes) were observed (Jensen and Esterly 1971). High levels of cytoplasmic RNA were revealed by thioflavine T subsequent to DNAse digestion of DNA. Large nucleoli within the nuclei of epidermal cells suggested to Spearman (1960) that protein synthesis was increased. Tail epidermis oxidized in peracetic acid and then stained with thioflavine T fluoresced a bright yellow; this reaction indicates a high cystine content of the keratin proteins. Sections of mutant skin treated to reveal protein-bound sulfhydryl groups displayed a uniform strong positive reaction in both the tail and perifollicular epidermis (Spearman 1960). Elevated quantities of phospholipids were inferred from acid hematin staining of thickened scale and follicular epithelium from the ichthyotic mice (Spearman 1960).

Ultrastructure

Basal and lower spinous layers of the epidermis in the *ic/ic* mice are separated by greater intercellular distances than typical. Cells of the thickened granular and spinous layers (Fig. 297) contain aggregated keratin filaments, increased cyto-

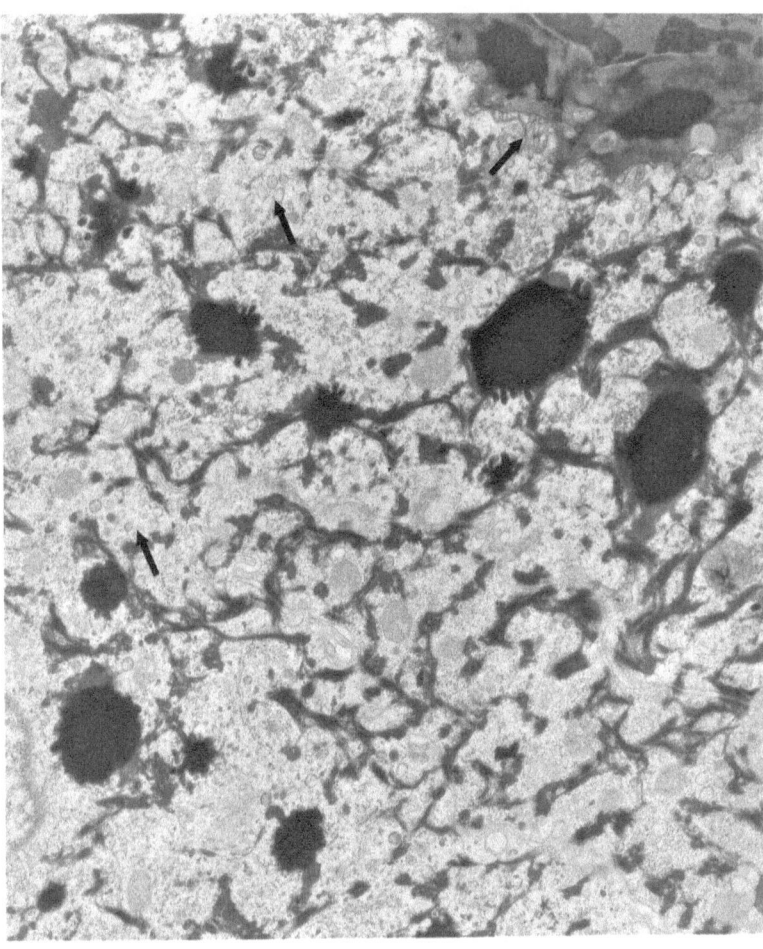

Fig. 297. Dorsal epidermis, adult *ic/ic* mouse. Note the high density of ribosomes, clumping of keratin filaments, abundance of lamellar granules *(arrows)*, and the abberrant structure of the keratohyaline granules. TEM, × 12 300

plasmic ribosomes and mitochondria, and abundant lamellar granules, both within cells and in the intercellular space. The keratohyaline granules of granular cells vary in number and morphology, although typically they were more numerous and prominent than in normal mice (Jensen and Esterly 1977). In some of the animals obtained from the Jackson Laboratory stock, the keratohyaline granules had irregular margins modified by fingerlike projections and blebs (new data, see Fig. 297). Normal-appearing, glubular, keratohyaline granules were the exception rather than the rule. Remnants of cellular organelles were retained in the cornified cells.

Animals with the ichthyotic genotype carry structural markers in the nuclei of leukocytes, plasma cells of the lymph node, intestinal epithelial cells, erythroblasts (Green et al. 1975), and certain populations of neurons (Goldowitz and Mullen 1982). They are evident, to a lesser extent, in the nuclei of these cells in +/*ic* heterozygotes. The nuclei of lymphocytes present in sections of lymph nodes, spleen, Peyer's patches, and thymus have two to three large clumps of heterochromatin that are not typically associated with the nuclear envelope. The heterochromatin in the normal mouse nucleus is dispersed in several, small clumps associated with the nuclear envelope and in a single centrally positioned clump. The markers are more variable in morphology in lymphocytes found in smears of peripheral blood and bone marrow and may not be distinguishable from normal (Green et al. 1975). In contrast, the markers are prominent in *ic/ic* eosinophils and neutrophils in smears of peripheral blood and bone marrow but are not seen as clearly in the same cells in tissue sections. In marrow smears, the nuclei of *ic/ic* neutrophils are round or oval instead of the normal polymorphic shape; the chromatin is located centrally within the nucleus with spokelike extensions radiating outward to the nuclear membrane. Eosinophils in the bone marrow of heterozygotes occasionally have nuclei similar to neutrophils. The nuclear markers in white cells of ic/ic animals are reminiscent of nuclear markers in neutrophils of humans and rabbits with the Pelger-Huet anomaly (Nachtsheim 1950); however, there are no skin or hair abnormalities in these animals.

The marker is also present in small-sized microneurons of the brain, granular cells of the cerebellum, external and internal granular layers of the olfactory bulb, and cochlear nucleus of affected mice. In these cells it is recognized as a single central accumulation of heterochromatin (Goldowitz and Mullen 1982). The nuclei in these cells in normal animals have an indistinct nucleolus and heterochromatin organized along the nuclear envelope. Granular cells of the dentate gyrus nucleus and cortical stellate cells of layer 2 display the marker only in early postnatal life. As with the leukocytes, the expression of the marker in heterozygous animals is intermediate between normal and mutant mice (Goldowitz and Mullen 1982).

Donor ic/ic cells transplanted to congenic mice retain the marker, suggesting that this feature is a property of the cell type rather than induced by the cell environment of the mutant animal (Green et al. 1975).

Biologic Features

Natural History. The ichthyotic mouse was first identified in 1950 in Edinburgh, Scotland, where it appeared in two parallel sublines of the common house mouse, *Mus musculus* (Carter and Phillips 1950). The mutation was considered to have arisen spontaneously in both lines from a common progenitor (Table 17).

The gene for ic/ic is located on chromosome 1 and is part of linkage group VIII (Altman and Katz 1979). Transplantation studies have shown that the abnormal gene is expressed in the epidermis (Green et al. 1974). Tissue recombinants prepared from 14-day ic/ic and +/+ mouse embryos grafted to the testis of a histocompatible adult mouse developed hair that was characteristic for the epidermal genotype. The genotype of the dermis appeared to have no influence on the phenotypic outcome of the recombinant explant (Green et al. 1974).

The abnormal gene appears to be responsible for alterations beyond those demonstrated in the

Table 17. Natural history of expression of the ic/ic phenotype described in the original mutant stock[a]

Postnatal age	Phenotypic characteristics of the skin
Days 2–3	short vibrissae; originally straight, then interlace and curl
Day 6	dorsal guard hairs barely visible; rough papillate, creased skin
Week 2	thin, short coat; low density of curled body hairs; short and curled vibrissae
Weeks 3–4	major period of expression of features of the ic/ic phenotype; hard, scaly, cracked skin that sloughs; severity is variable; scaly rings on tail; period of compromised viability
Older adults	thin, curly coat, small size

[a] Summary of data from Carter and Phillips 1950.

skin and its appendages. Some of these may be secondary to the skin changes (e.g., ectropion, eclabium, and restricted respiration are likely a consequence of the thickened epidermis), while others appear to bear no relationship. Growth is diminished, some of the animals are mute, and certain exocrine glands (Harderian glands) may be absent (Grüneberg 1954). Females are usually sterile because of aberrations in vaginal structure. Those which are fertile have short breeding lives and usually produce no more than two litters (Carter and Phillips 1950). Some of the more severely affected males lack a scrotum and may have a penis that is deflected forward, but those with descended testes are fertile (Carter and Phillips 1950). Viability of animals is in proportion to the severity of the disease.

Etiology. The disorder is caused by a simple recessive gene that arose as a spontaneous mutation (Carter and Phillips 1950). Carter and Phillips (1950) noted that matings between normal mice and either ic/ic males or females produced only normal offspring, indicating that the inheritance was neither X-linked nor autosomal dominant; however, the numbers of affected animals that resulted from matings between F2 and backcross generations were also lower than expected from single gene, autosomal recessive inheritance. This implied that there is high, early postnatal, selective mortality of homozygous mutant animals (Carter and Phillips 1950).

The trait is usually maintained by matings between ic/ic males and ic/+ females. Ichthyotic mice are available from the Jackson Laboratory and are maintained in other laboratories on various hybrid backgrounds (e.g., Goldowitz and Mullen 1982; Spearman 1960).

Comparison with Other Species

Ichthyosis is a group of diseases expressed in humans and in a number of domestic animals (Selmanowitz 1979; Goldsmith 1985; Holbrook and Sybert 1985). Several forms of inherited ichthyosis are well documented for humans (Feinstein et al. 1970; Frost et al. 1966). The disorder in mice has been linkened to ichthyosis vulgaris (Spearman 1960), lamellar ichthyosis (Jensen and Esterly 1977), and psoriasis (Spearman 1960) on the basis of the pattern of inheritance and the phenotypic expression of the disorder. Table 18 lists abnormal characteristics of the skin and biology of the *ic/ic* mouse and compares these features with expression of ichthyosis or scaly epidermis in different human disorders. Examination of the data in Table 18 suggests that the ichthyotic mouse does not appear to be an accurate model for any one of the human forms of ichthyosis.

Other features of the disorder may have a counterpart in human disease; the constricted rings of the tail, for example, have been likened to an inherited trait in humans called ainhum or pseudoainhum (Spearman 1960; Selmanowitz 1979), in which depressed rings about the digits lead to eventual amputation. Although the consequence in the two conditions is similar, the causes appear to be different; in the mouse it results from atrophy of dermal connective tissue, whereas in humans, it occurs because of constrictive fibrous bands in the dermis.

Irrespective of the precision with which the ichthyotic mouse fits as a model for human disease, studies of this mouse mutant will provide insight into the mechanism of abnormal keratinization and normal and pathologic processes in the epidermis.

Table 18. A comparison of the features of ichthyosis in the *ic/ic* mouse with human forms of ichthyosis

Mouse characteristics	Ichthyosis vulgaris	Psoriasis	Lamellar ichthyosis
Accelerated epidermal metabolism		×	
Parakeratotic stratum corneum		×	
Thickened orthokeratotic stratum corneum	×		×
Poorly developed granular layer	×		
Thickened stratum granulosum	×	×	×
Acanthosis of spinous layer		×	×
Increased lamellar granules			×
Expression of the disease typically begins postnatally	×		
Normal epidermal kinetics	×		
Altered hair structure			
Inheritance as an autosomal recessive trait			×

References

Altman PL, Katz DD (eds) (1979) Inbred and genetically defined strains of laboratory animals. Federation of American Societies for Experimental Biology, Bethesda, p 32 (Biological handbooks III)

Carter TC, Phillips RS (1950) Ichthyosis, a new recessive mutant in the house mouse. J Hered 41: 297–300

Feinstein A, Ackerman B, Ziprlowski L (1970) Histology of autosomal dominant ichthyosis vulgaris and x-linked ichthyosis. Arch Dermatol 101: 524–527

Frost P, Weinstein GD, van Scott EJ (1966) The ichthyosiform dermatoses. II. Autoradiographic studies of epidermal proliferation. J Invest Dermatol 47: 561–567

Goldowitz D, Mullen RJ (1982) Nuclear morphology of ichthyosis mutant mice as a cell marker in chimeric brain. Dev Biol 89: 261–267

Goldsmith LA (1985) Genetic models for ichthyosis. In: Maibach HI, Lowe N (eds) Models in dermatology, vol I. Karger, Basel, pp 127–131

Green MC, Alpert BN, Mayer TC (1974) The site of action of the ichthyosis locus (ic) in the mouse, as determined by dermal-epidermal recombinations. J Embryol Exp Morphol 32: 715–721

Green MC, Shultz LD, Nedzi LA (1975) Abnormal nuclear morphology of leukocytes in the mouse mutant ichthyosis. A possible transplantation marker. Transplantation 20: 172–175

Grüneberg H (1954) Exocrine glands and the Chievitz organ of some mouse mutants. J Embryol Exp Morphol 25: 247–261

Holbrook KA, Sybert VP (1985) Animal models of inherited ichthyoses and other forms of aberrant epidermal differentiation. In: Maibach HI, Lowe N (eds) Models in dermatology, vol 1. Karger, Basel, pp 132–158

Jensen JE, Esterly NB (1977) The ichthyosis mouse: histologic, histochemical, ultrastructural and autoradiographic studies of interfollicular epidermis. J Invest Dermatol 68: 23–31

Nachtsheim H (1950) The Pelger-anomaly in man and rabbit. A mendelian character of the nuclei of the leucocytes. J Hered 41: 131–137

Selmanowitz VJ (1979) Ectodermal dysplasias including epitheliogenesis imperfecta, ichthyoses and follicular/glandular anomalies. In: Andrews EJ, Ward BC, Altman NH (eds) Spontaneous animal models of human disease, vol II. Academic, New York, pp 3–10

Spearman RI (1960) The skin abnormality of ichthyosis, a mutant of the house mouse. J Embryol Exp Morphol 8: 387–395

The Mammary Gland

Morphology and Development of the Rat Mammary Gland

Irma H. Russo, Muneesh Tewari, and Jose Russo

Introduction

The mammary gland is an organ whose description in either morphology, physiology, or biochemistry requires one to specify the species, sex, age, reproductive history, and physiologic condition of the host before any definitive conclusion can be drawn. These variables pose a great burden on researchers in the field, since the massive literature available in some species might not apply to others, and extrapolations become necessary, though speculative and subject to further corroboration.

The mammary gland of mice and rats has been extensively studied in its intrauterine development, both in vivo (Balinsky 1950; Turner and Gomez 1933; Sakakura et al. 1979) and in vitro (Ceriani 1970; Hardy 1950) and in its postnatal development in both virgin and pregnant animals (Astwood et al. 1937; Bassleer 1970; Cowie and Folley 1961; Raynaud 1961; Russo IH and Russo J 1978, 1986; Russo J and Russo IH 1978, 1987; Russo J et al. 1979, 1982).

The development of this ectodermal derivative is so unique that its study requires a multidisciplinary approach in order to understand the role that genetic, environmental, end endogenous influences play in this system's final morphology and function.

The fact that the mammary glands are markedly underdeveloped at birth (Hardy 1950; Raynaud 1961), that inductive interactions between epithelium and mesenchyme are essential for normal morphogenesis (Sakakura et al. 1979), and that complete development and differentiation are reached only in adulthood and only after full-term pregnancy and lactation (Ast-wood et al. 1937; Russo J et al. 1982) emphasize the importance of taking into consideration a series of nonmammary factors for fully understanding this organ's morphology, development, and function (Astwood et al. 1937; Cowie and Folley 1961; Raynaud 1961; 1971).

The observation that the development and differentiation of the mammary gland influence its susceptibility to carcinogenesis (Russo IH and Russo J 1978, 1986; Russo J and Russo IH 1987, 1980, 1978; Russo J et al. 1977, 1979, 1982, 1983a, b; Van Zwieten 1984) has awakened the need to further understand these influences. In addition, the discovery that the parenchyma in the various pairs of mammary glands does not respond as a unit to systemic hormonal influences, but exhibits variations in the rate of development which seem to be modulated by the location of the gland in the body as well as by the topographic location of specific ductal structures within the mammary gland tree (Russo J and Russo IH 1987) further stress the need to understand this complex picture which requires the development of schemes for unifying different experimental protocols and for facilitating comparisons among investigators using different experimental models.

Mammary Development

Prenatal Development

Descriptive work on the morphogenesis and histogenesis of the rat mammary gland dates back to the excellent publication of Myers (1917), in which he makes reference to the works of Bonnet, Brouha, Bresslau, and Schil, authors who published their observations in 1897, 1905, 1910, and 1912, respectively.

In his publication, Myers (1917) reviewed more extensively the work of Henneberg published in 1900. An extensive bibliography on the morphogenesis and the physiology of the rodent mammary apparatus has accumulated over the years (Anderson 1978; Astwood et al. 1937; Balinsky 1950; Cowie and Folley 1961; Raynaud 1961, 1971), including the effect of hormones on the developing gland (Ceriani 1970; Jean 1968; Heuberger et al. 1982; Knight and Peaker 1982; Kratochwil 1977; Raynaud 1961, 1971).

The embryonal and fetal development of the albino rat mammary gland have been divided into anatomically distinct stages:

1. The mammary band or streak stage, observed in the 6-10-mm crown-rump length embryo, at the 11th day of pregnancy (Anderson 1978; Myers 1917). The anlage of the mammary streak is composed of a single layer of cuboidal cells appearing unilaterally in the region of the dorsal limiting furrow (Myers 1917). By the 12th day of pregnancy the streak becomes bilateral, with the cephalic and caudal ends blending with the cubical epithelium of the limb anlages. By the 12th day and 13 h of intrauterine life the cells of the mammary streak are larger; a second layer of cells starts to condense beneath the mammary streak. By the 13th day and 1 h of pregnancy the mammary streak is composed of two distinct cell layers, a stratum corneum and a stratum mucosum, which is separated from the underlying mesenchyme by a basement membrane.

2. The next stage is the mammary line stage, which is observed in the 6-14-mm crown-rump length embryo between the 11th and 13th day of pregnancy, according to Anderson (1978). According to Myers (1917), the mammary line consists of a thickening of parts of the mammary streak due either to cell enlargement or to the appearance of a third layer of round cells between the stratum corneum and the stratum mucosum. Mammary gland development progresses in a cephalo-caudal sequence and even in these early stages it is observed that in the thoracic region the mammary line is distinct, whereas in the inguinal region it is indistinguishable, being possible to identify it only with special techniques (Myers 1917).

3. The hillock follows the mammary line stage. It is observed on day 13 (Anderson 1978) or 14 (Myers 1917) of intrauterine life in the crown-rump length 17-18-mm fetus. This stage is characterized by the formation of the biconvex lens-shaped structure on the cephalic end of the mammary line. This represents the first pectoral mammary hillock. The second and third pectoral and the abdominal hillocks begin to appear, and at the same time the portions of the mammary line remaining between the hillocks start to atrophy (Myers 1917). The mammary hillocks persist through the 16th day, then they become less evident, although they apparently occupy the position of the future nipples.

4. The "mammary point" stage is described by Myers (1917) in the 15-day-old fetus. In it, the thoracic mammary gland anlages are no longer elevated above the surface but are pressed into the mesenchyme in what represents the mammary point stage, whereas the inguinal mammary glands still remain in a more immature form. In 15 day and 14 h embryos the six pairs of mammary glands occupy their definitive positions (Myers 1917).

5. The mammary bud stage is observed in the fetus with a crown-rump length of 18-19 mm. On the surface of the skin at this stage is a small eminence over each developing gland. A spheroidal mass of epithelial cells surrounded by the basement membrane forms the gland anlage. The stratum germinativum of the epidermis is in continuity with the circular mass of cells and forms the basal layer of the mass, although the basal cells appear much more elongated than those in the stratum germinativum of the adjacent epidermis. The cells occupying the center are irregular in shape and closely packed (Myers 1917). Superficially the gland anlage projects somewhat, producing the eminence visible from the surface. The mesenchymal cells around the developing mammary gland are somewhat elongated and arranged in two or three concentric and regular layers containing occasional small blood vessels.

6. The stage of teat formation is described by Anderson (1978) in the 15-day fetus. This is the stage that Myers (1917) described in fetuses of 16 days and 12 h, in which the mammary eminences still appear on the surface of the skin as slightly elevated areas. In some places the epidermis is slightly thickened to form hair anlages and the mesenchymal cells become more condensed than in the previous stage, thus forming a definitive layer; the mesenchyme becomes less cellular and with no regular arrangement in the deeper layers. Mitotic figures are very common in the mesenchyme immediately surrounding the gland.

At 17 days and 2 h the eminences described in the previous stage have disappeared. The gland areas instead appear as slight depressions or pits on the surface of the skin, which represent the point of ingrowth of the epithelium. Fetuses of 18 days and 9 h show a defined mammary pit on the surface of the epidermis over each feature nipple area. The stratum germinativum is depressed, forming a shallow, funnel-shaped outline, the mouth of which is directed toward the surface and is partly filled with epithelial cells showing cornification and desquamation. The outlet of the funnel extends into the corium and becomes continuous with the anlage of the primary mammary duct. The gland anlage increases in length and its deeper portion becomes the anlage of the primary duct, while its superficial portion undergoes vacuolization, cornification, and desquamation.

7. Primary sprout stage. In this stage, the anlage elongates, penetrating more deeply into the condensed mesenchyme, which completely surrounds it (Myers 1917). The "primary sprout" stage was described by Anderson (1978) in the fetus having a crown-rump length of 18–32 mm. The primary duct starts to branch into two secondary ducts representing the "secondary sprout" stage that Anderson (1978) describes in the 19-day-old or 40-mm fetus.

The primary duct of most of the glands possesses a basal layer of cuboidal cells with large oval nuclei resting on a somewhat indistinct basement membrane, while the opposite ends are directed toward the center of the duct. The center of the duct is filled with cells of irregular shape which show a tendency towards separation from each other, thus producing small cavities or lacunae, the first appearance of a definitive lumen.

By the 19th day of intrauterine life, the primary mammary duct has made rapid growth and has sprouted into secondary and tertiary ducts in most glands. The formation of lumina in the two inguinal glands lags behind their formation in the thoracic and abdominal mammary glands. Many of the cells near the developing lumina are undergoing mitotic divisions. There is no pyknosis or other evidence of cell degeneration (Myers 1917).

At 20 days 6 h there are well-defined mammary pits in the epidermis; at the bottom of each pit there is a rounded, elevated portion of the epidermis, the anlage of the nipple. The depression or funnel described in the preceding stage becomes partly filled with cells that become cornified and are cast out, deepening the mammary pit. The anlage of the nipple protrudes from the bottom of the mammary pit toward the surface, leaving a surrounded furrow or sulcus. The superficial part of the epidermis over the nipple anlage now appears no thicker than that in the adjacent regions. From the surface of the nipple anlage, the primary duct courses through the corium to the subcutaneous tissue, where it divides into secondary and tertiary ducts, which begin to branch into quaternary ducts. The terminal ducts end in small knoblike enlargements or end buds. Lobules have not yet formed in the mammary gland (Myers 1917).

In newborn rats the lumina extend through the primary ducts into the secondary ducts, reaching the end buds. No lumen, however, is observed through the intraepidermal portion. In the primary ducts the lumina are small, irregular, slitlike spaces which become continuous with the more regular, rounded lumina of the distal ducts. The process of lumen formation that began in the 18–20-day fetus continues until the time of birth, but still their formation is incomplete. The mechanism of lumen formation is considerably controversial. Although it has been postulated that in humans lumina are formed as a result of degeneration of the central cells of the solid epithelial ducts anlage, in the rat lumen formation appears to be more a process of cell rearrangement rather than cell degeneration (Myers 1917).

Effect of Hormones on the Morphogenesis of the Fetal Mammary Gland

The effect of sex hormones on the morphogenesis of the fetal mouse mammary has been extensively studied (Hardy 1950; Heuberger et al. 1982; Kratochwil 1977; Raynaud 1961, 1971; Wasner et al. 1983). The knowledge of these hormonal influences on the developing rat mammary gland is considerably less developed and fragmentary. In the mouse it has been observed that mammary buds are identical in both intact or gonadectomized males and females (Raynaud 1961, 1971); however, in the male, at the 12th day of intrauterine life under the influence of testosterone, the epithelial buds become surrounded by condensed mesenchyme and subsequently are destroyed by testosterone-activated mesenchymal cells (Heuberger et al. 1982; Raynaud 1971). This phenomenon occurs about 36–84 h after morphological differentiation of the testes. The androgen responsiveness of the mammary rudiment lasts approximately 36 h and gradually disappears (Kratochwil 1977). As a result of this process, the mammary glands are reduced in the male fetus, and those that persist lack connection with the ectoderm (Raynaud 1971). The loss of androgen responsiveness is of importance for the survival of the mammary glands in female embryos, since their high sensitivity to testosterone would cause their destruction when ovaries produce these hormones in later fetal and postnatal life (Kratochwil 1977). Sex-related differences are not so well-established in the rat. It has been observed, however, that estrogens injected into rats on the 14th day of pregnancy produce a dose-dependent enlargement of the nipple in all six pairs of glands except the second thoracic pair, in which this treatment has an inhibitory effect, producing also a partial or total inhibition of mammary development (Jean 1968). Estrogenic hormones injected into the pregnant mouse or directly into the embryo produce premature development of the nipples in the embryos of the two sexes and arrests the development of the mammary anlage (Raynaud 1971). Estrogenic hormones are toxic to the mammary anlage of the 17-day-old rat fetus grown in vitro (Ceriani 1970).

Postnatal Development

From Birth to Puberty

Anatomy. The rat's mammary glands are distributed in pairs along the milk line, with one pair located in the cervical, two in the thoracic, one in the abdominal, and two in the inguinal regions (Astwood et al. 1937; Van Zwieten 1984). The nipples are medially located, and from there the mammary ductal system extends subcutaneously into the mammary fat pad, progressing dorsolaterally (Young and Hallowes 1973; Russo IH and Russo J 1978; Van Zwieten 1984).

Subgross Anatomy. At birth the six pairs of mammary glands consist of one or two main lactiferous ducts arising from the nipple. The mammary gland of newborn female Fisher rats, as shown by Ceriani (1970), is composed of a main lactiferous duct branching into at least four or five secondary ducts, and these further branch dichotomously into a third generation of ducts. The male mammary gland does not differ greatly from that of newborn females (Ceriani 1970). In the mouse, however, the male mammary anlage detaches from the epidermis and undergoes inhibition of growth (Heuberger et al. 1982; Raynaud 1961, 1971; Wasner et al. 1983).

Since the basic structure of the gland follows a uniform pattern during development, the nomenclature utilized and the criteria developed for evaluating mammary gland growth, development, and differentiation will be defined in general terms applicable to all glands, as shown in Fig. 298. Essentially during the 1st week of life, the mammary gland of the female rat consists of one to three main lactiferous ducts opening into the nipple. These ducts, considered to be the first generation of ducts, are straight and broad; in young animals they are free of lateral branches until they bifurcate dichotomously into two similar branches, forming the second generation of ducts, or sympodially, emitting lateral branches which are also called second generation. In the newborn, as well as in the 5-day-old rat, successive branching up to a fourth or fifth generation of ducts is observed (Fig. 298). The main branches of the mammary tree are straight with only occasional small buds sprouting laterally in a sympodial manner; these are called lateral buds (Fig. 298). In the 5-day-old rat the mammary parenchyma occupies an area ranging from 0.89 mm^2 for the first pair of glands to 7.9 mm^2 for the fourth or abdominal mammary gland, which is the largest. The average area for each of the glands in 4.80 mm^2. By 21 days of age the mammary glands have expanded to occupy an average area of 26.50 mm^2 (Fig. 299).

In order to quantitate the number of structures present in areas representing different stages of development, the mammary gland parenchyma is divided into thirds along the longitudinal axis. The third closest to the nipple, called zone A (Fig. 301), is composed of the main lactiferous ducts; the intermediate area, called zone B (Figs. 298, 300, 301, 303, 304), contains more abundant lateral buds; in this area most of the secondary ducts arise. The distal third of the gland, or zone C, contains the terminal ductal structures ending in bulbous clubs terminal end buds (TEBs) (Figs. 298, 300, 302, 303, 305).

Although each of the mammary glands is basically composed of the three zones described above, there are differences in glandular area, as well as in number and size of individual structures, which depend upon the location of the gland (cervical, thoracic, abdominal, or inguinal region). Thoracic glands, mainly the third pair, are composed of more numerous and larger TEBs, especially those located in zone C, which measure an average of $25 \times 10^3 \pm 12 \times 10^3$ μm^2 (Figs. 300 and 302) (Table 19) whereas TEBs located in abdominal mammary glands (Figs. 303 and 305) are slightly smaller (Table 19). Gland development progresses with age by successive dichotomous or sympodial branching of new

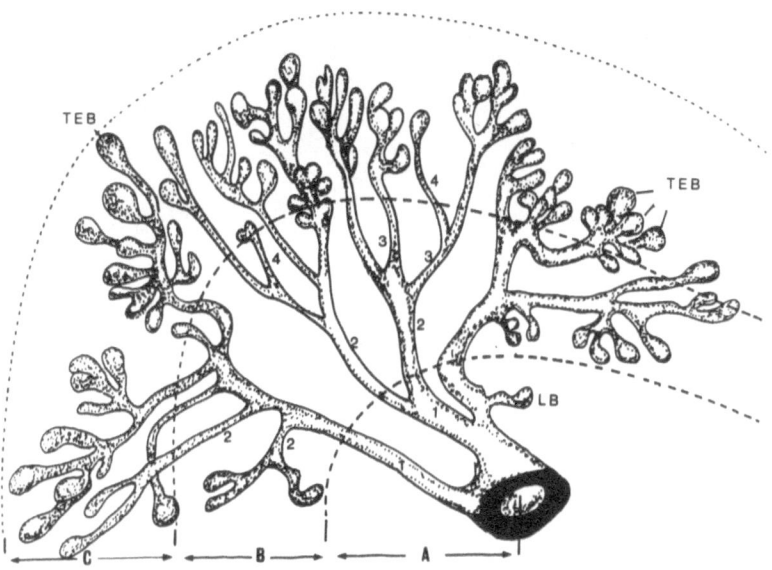

Fig. 298. Schematic representation of the third (thoracic) mammary gland of a 21-day-old female rat, based on the whole mount of the gland shown in Fig. 300. The gland was divided into three zones: *A*, proximal to the nipple; *B*, medial; *C*, distal to the nipple. Branching pattern is identified sequentially as 1st generation or primary ducts *(1)*, 2nd generation or secondary ducts *(2)*, 3rd generation or tertiary ducts *(3)*, fourth generation or quaternary ducts *(4)*, terminal end buds *(TEB)*, lateral buds *(LB)*

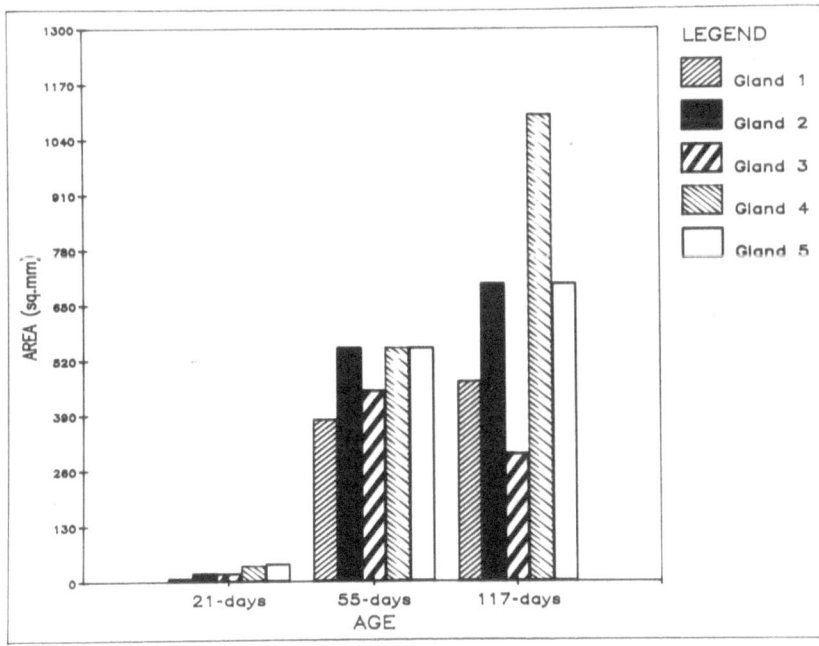

Fig. 299. Histogram of mammary gland area *(ordinate)* of the 1st, 2nd, 3rd, 4th, and 5th pairs of mammary glands at 21, 55, and 117 days of age *(abscissa)*. Mammary gland area was measured by tracing the gland with a stylus in the whole mount preparation projected on a digitizer tablet of a MOP-Videoplan Image Analysis System (Carl Zeiss, Oberkochen, FRG). The values shown represent the average of five animals per group

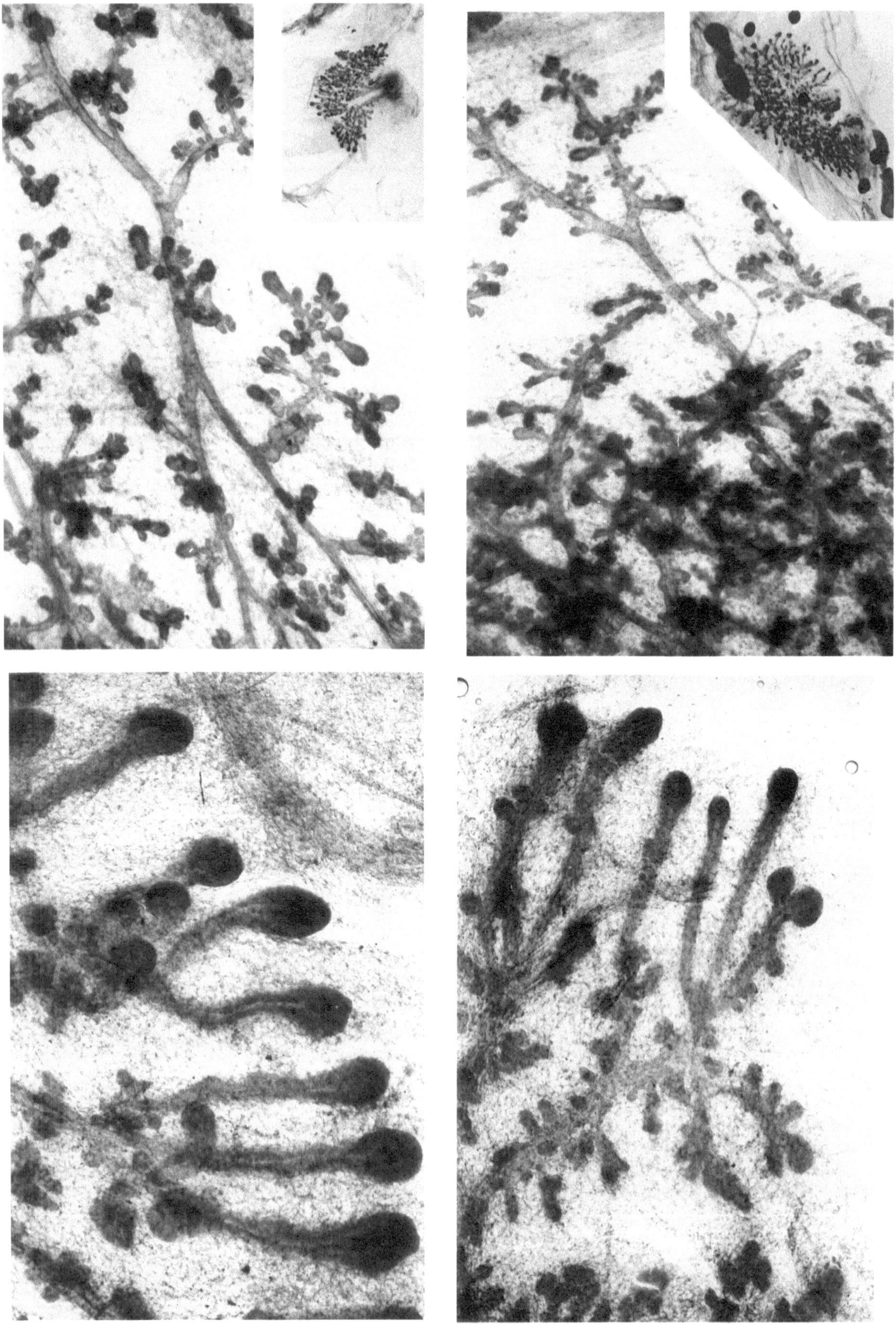

Figs. 300–320 *(pp. 238–243).* Whole mount preparations of mammary glands of animals ranging from 21 to 117 days of age. Mammary glands were removed attached to the skin pelt and fixed in 10% neutral buffered formalin for 24 h. Then the glands were dissected from the skin, dehydrated, and defatted in acetone for 2 days. Tissues were rehydrated in decreasing concentrations of ethanol, stored in distilled water overnight, and stained with 0.025% toluidine blue (Sigma Chemical, St. Louis) in McFloaine buffer at pH 4.0 for 2 h. The tissues were washed in 4% ammonium molybdate, differentiated in methanol for 30 min. Tissues were dehydrated, cleared in xylene, and mounted on glass slides

◄ **Fig. 300** *(inset of Fig. 301).* Third (thoracic) mammary gland of a 21-day-old female rat from which the diagram for Fig. 298 was taken. × 3

Fig. 301 *(upper left).* Zone B of the thoracic mammary gland shown in Fig. 300, which contains numerous lateral buds, occasional alveolar buds, and terminal ducts. × 55

Fig. 302 *(lower left).* Zone C of the gland shown in Fig. 300, which is almost exclusively composed of darkly stained, club-shaped terminal end buds. × 55

Fig. 303 *(inset of Fig. 304).* Abdominal (4th) mammary gland of a 21-day-old female rat in which the mammary ducts are reaching the vicinity of the lymph node. × 3

Fig. 304 *(upper right).* Zone B of the gland shown in Fig. 303 containing numerous lateral buds and occasional alveolar buds. Secondary branching is abundant. × 55

Fig. 305 *(lower right).* Zone C of the gland shown in Fig. 303. Although terminal end buds are bulbous and darkly stained, their average diameter is slightly smaller than those present in the thoracic gland shown in Fig. 300 and 302. The ducts also contain more lateral buds. × 55

Table 19. Size of terminal end buds (TEB) in the different zones of the rat mammary gland: variations with age and gland location

Age	Gland	Zone	TEB Area[a] ($\mu m^2 \times 10^3$)
21 days	Thoracic	A	24 ± 14
		B	19 ± 8
		C	25 ± 12
	Abdominal	A	16 ± 8
		B	17 ± 13
		C	18 ± 8
55 days	Thoracic	A	No TEB
		B	11 ± 2
		C	20 ± 15
	Abdominal	A	No TEB
		B	10 ± 6
		C	18 ± 12
117 days	Thoracic	A	No TEB
		B	21 ± 11
		C	28 ± 11
	Abdominal	A	No TEB
		B	16 ± 5
		C	10 ± 3

[a] Mean of TEBs measured in five animals per group, ± standard deviation.

ducts, sprouting of lateral buds, elongation of existing ducts, and cleavage of TEBs or lateral buds into two or more small ductules or alveoli, called at this stage alveolar buds (ABs) (Figs. 308–310), which are more numerous in the 1st and 5th pair of glands, although they are universally present.

Postpubertal Development

Subgross Anatomy. The estrous cycle in Sprague-Dawley rats fed a regular diet (Alvarez Sanz et al. 1986; Huang et al. 1982) begins at 35 ± 2 days of age. From 21 to 55 days of age, the mammary gland undergoes rapid growth which may be prevented by ovariectomy on the 22nd day (Cowie and Folley 1961). This growth is characterized by lengthening of existing ducts and dichotomous and sympodial branching of major ducts. The

portion of the gland proximal to the nipple (zone A) and the intermediate portion (zone B) (Fig. 298) exhibit abundant sprouting of lateral buds, which are always small in size and tend to cleave into two smaller ductules or alveoli (Figs. 308–310) or form small primitive lobular structures (Fig. 311), whereas the distal third of the gland (zone C) still contains long ducts ending in prominent TEBs and exhibiting scanty lateral branching (Fig. 307). Though lobular density increases progressively after the female animals reach the age of 42 days, the formation of lobules is infrequent, and it soon reaches a plateau that remains constant as long as the animal is virgin (Russo J and Russo IH 1980). Mammary gland development is a progressive, though uneven process. Although numerous TEBs progress to ABs (Figs. 308–310) and these to lobules (Fig. 311), a large number of TEBs in the virgin rat never differentiate. They become progressively smaller and finger-shaped; the diameter, that in the TEB is 103.0 ± 16.7 µm, reduces to 69.6 ± 1 µm; at this stage, these former TEBs are called terminal ducts (TD) (Figs. 316–320). TDs appear palely stained in whole mount preparations due to thinning of the walls and widening of the lumen. TDs do not undergo further morphologic changes as long as the animals remain virgin.

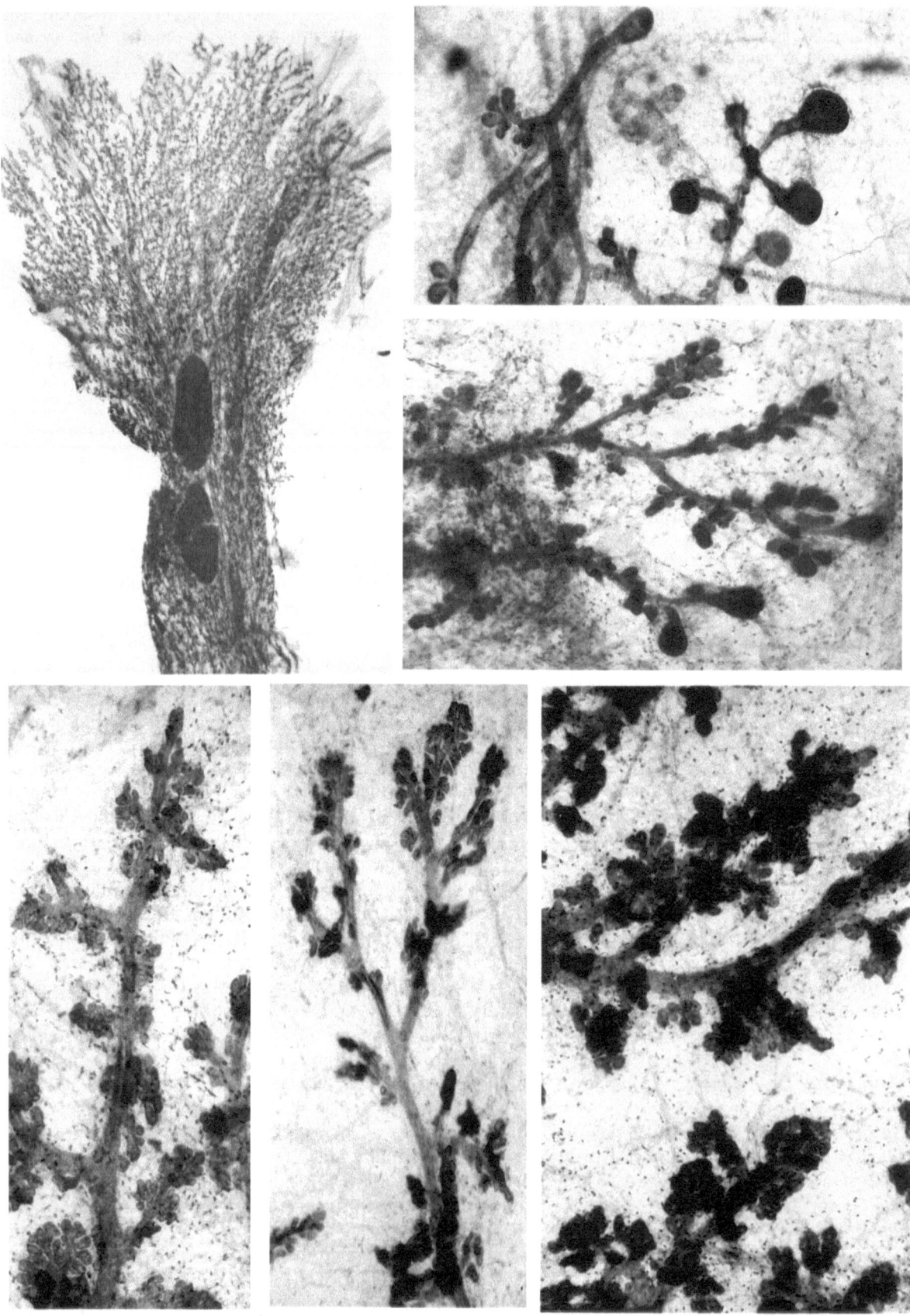

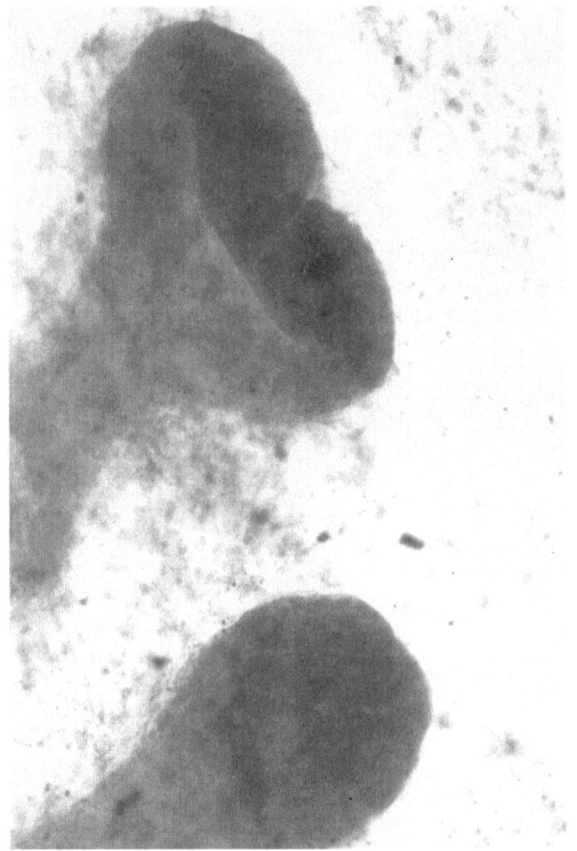 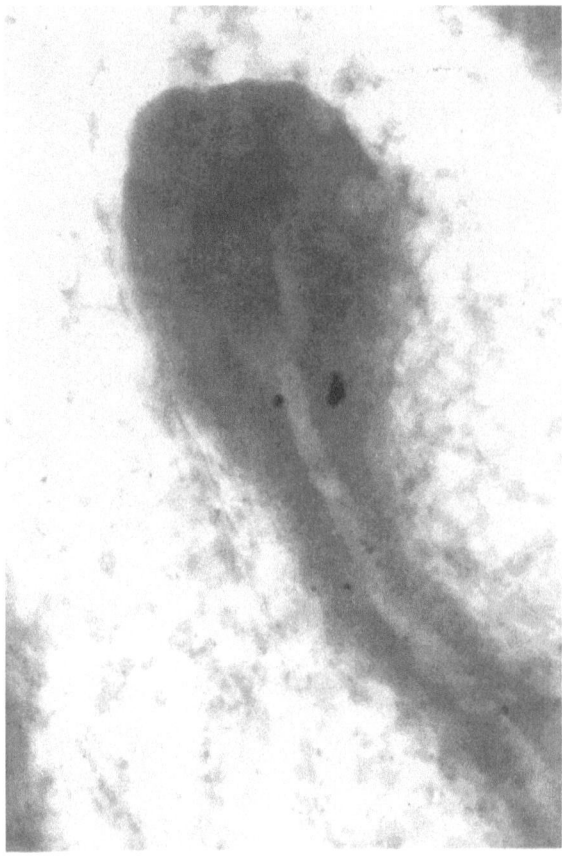

Fig. 312. Two terminal end buds in zone C of the thoracic mammary gland of a 21-day-old rat. They are club-shaped, solid in appearance, and the one in the *upper left corner* has undergone early cleavage. × 100

Fig. 313. Terminal end bud in zone C of the abdominal mammary gland of a 21-day-old rat. The TEB is solid at the tip, although a centrally located patent lumen may be identified. × 100

◄ **Fig. 306** *(upper left)*. Abdominal mammary gland of a 55-day-old virgin female rat with profuse branching and extension of the mammary parenchyma beyond the lymph nodes. × 3

Fig. 307 *(upper right first from top)*. Terminal end buds present in zone C of the thoracic mammary gland of a 55-day-old virgin female rat. × 55

Fig. 308 *(upper right second from top)*. Zone C of the abdominal mammary gland of a 55-day-old female rat. This zone is composed of more lateral buds and alveolar buds. There are two terminal end buds which are smaller in size than those seen in the thoracic gland. × 55

Fig. 309 *(lower left)*. Another area in the zone C of the 4th (abdominal) gland of a 55-day-old virgin female rat contains almost exclusively alveolar buds and lateral buds. × 55

Fig. 310 *(lower middle)*. Zone C of the inguinal mammary gland of a 55-day-old virgin female rat, almost exclusively composed of alveolar buds and lateral buds. × 55

Fig. 311 *(lower right)*. Zone B of the mammary gland of a 55-day-old virgin female rat contains primitive lobules. × 55

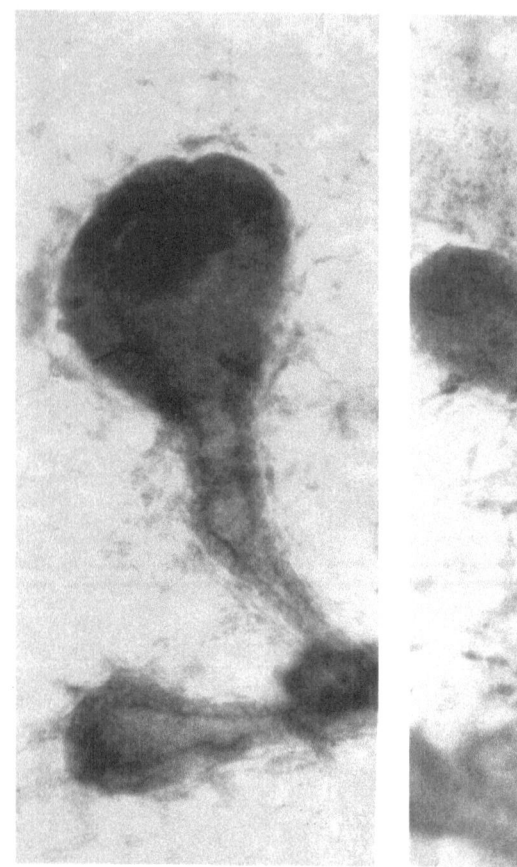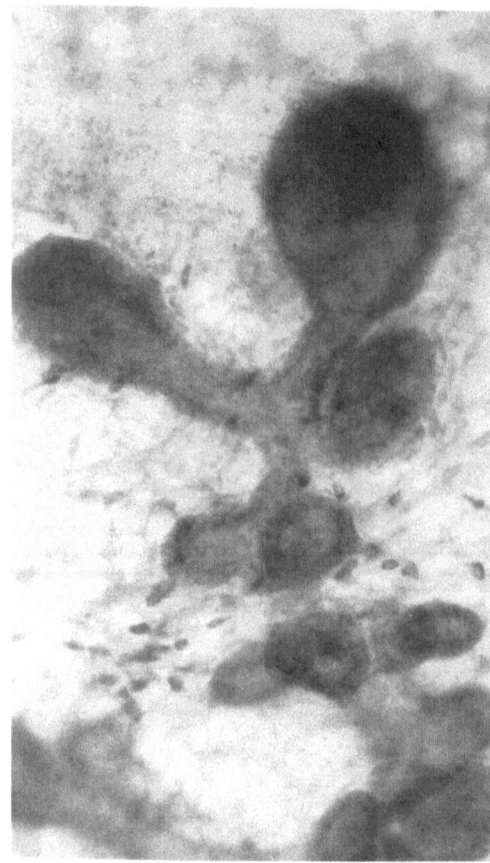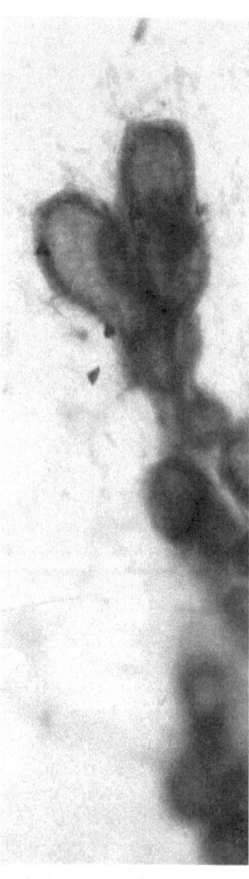

Fig. 314 *(left)*. Terminal end bud and terminal duct in zone C of the thoracic mammary, gland of a 55-day-old virgin female rat. × 100

Fig. 315 *(middle)*. Terminal end bud, terminal duct, and numerous lateral buds in zone C of the abdominal gland of the animal shown in Fig. 314. × 100

Fig. 316 *(right)*. Cluster of terminal end buds and terminal ducts present in zone B of the abdominal gland of the animal shown in Fig. 314. × 100

Fig. 317 *(upper left)*. Terminal end buds and terminal ▶ ducts present in zone C of the thoracic mammary gland of a 117-day-old virgin female rat. × 100

Fig. 318 *(lower left)*. Terminal ducts and lateral buds present in zone C of the abdominal mammary gland of the animal shown in Fig. 317. × 100

Fig. 319 *(upper right)*. Terminal ducts and alveolar buds present in zone B of the abdominal gland of a 117-day-old virgin rat. × 100

Fig. 320 *(lower right)*. Primitive lobules present in zone B of the abdominal gland of a 117-day-old virgin rat. × 100

Between the ages of 35 and 55 days, as a consequence of progressive branching, the mammary gland occupies larger areas of the mesenchyma or mammary fat pad. By 55 days of age the total mammary gland area has increased to an average of 553.15 mm² (Figs. 299 and 306). The number of TEBs decreases markedly in zones A and B in all glands (Figs. 308-311) but not in zone C (Figs. 307 and 308). Lateral buds, ABs, and small lobules, each composed of more than 10 ductules, become more abundant, mainly in zones A and B (Fig. 311).

The reduction in number of TEBs in zones A and B is also accompanied by a reduction in size of individual structures (Table 19; Fig. 302, 307, 312, 314). During this period, except for differences in the total area occupied by individual glands (Fig. 299), all the pairs of glands appear similar in architecture. However, mammary glands located in the thoracic region, namely the third pair, contain an area apparently derived from a single branch that grows into the layer of subcutaneous muscle and is composed of straight ducts ending in club shaped TEBs mea-

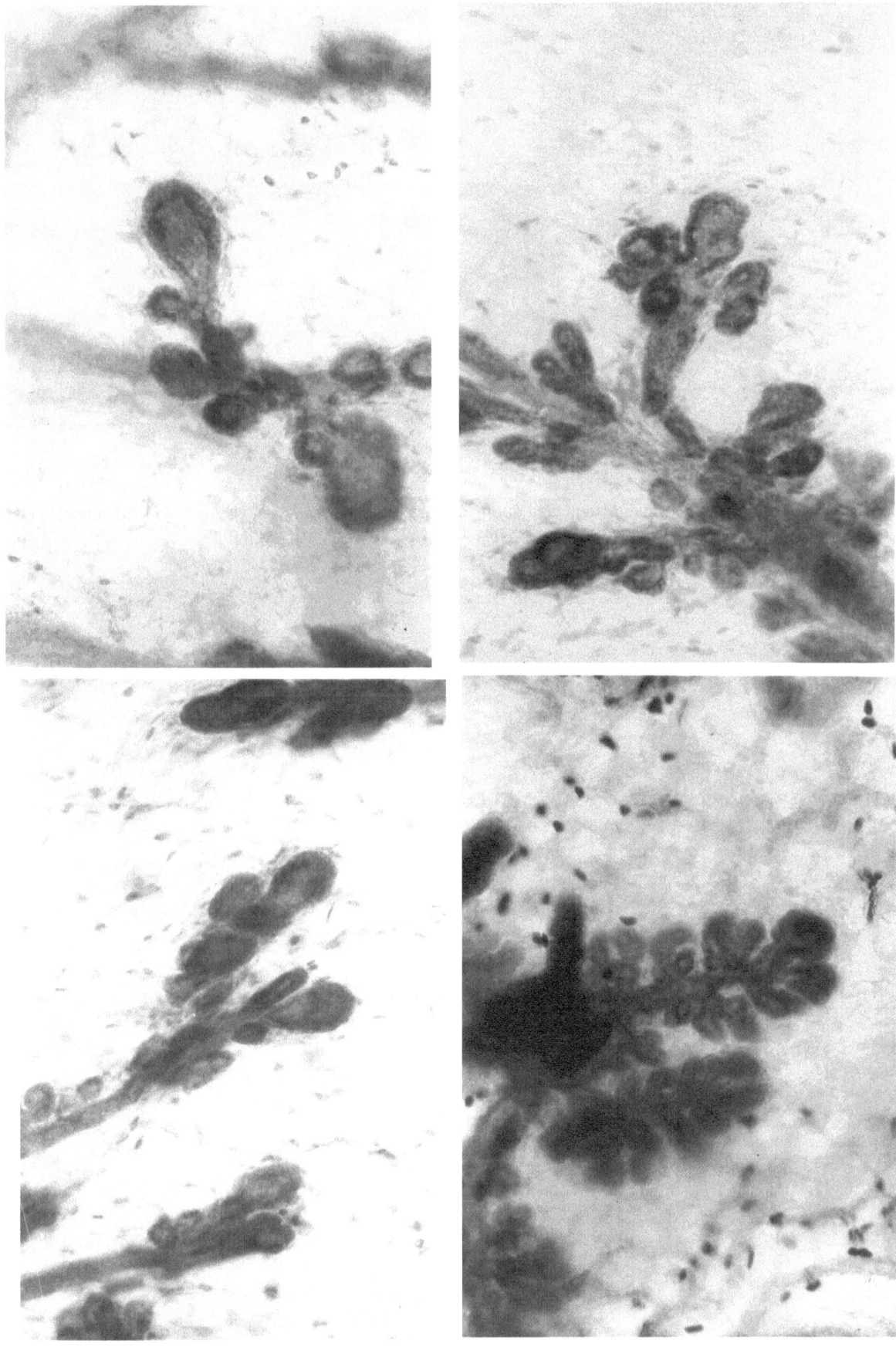

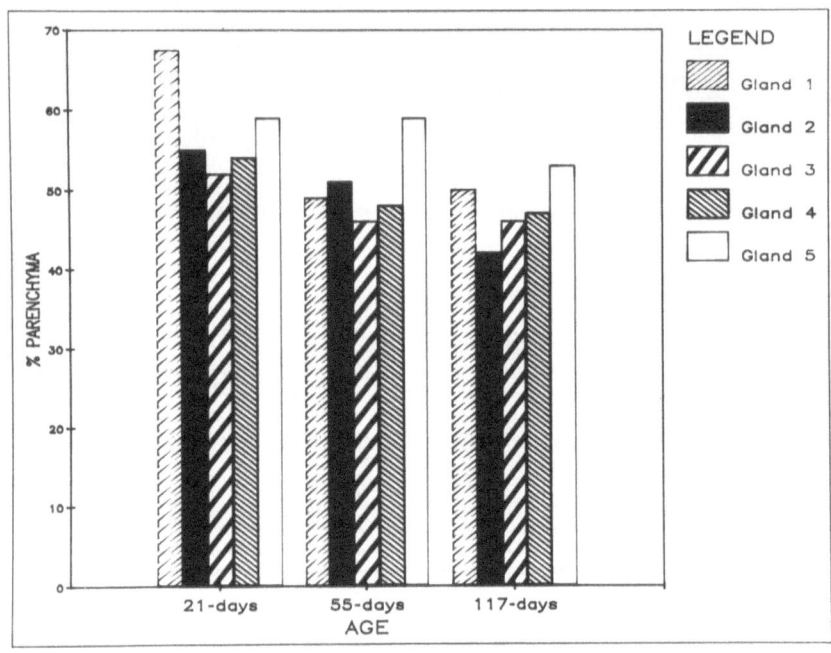

Fig. 321. Percentage of parenchyma per total area of the mammary gland *(ordinate)* in glands 1–5 in virgin female rats aged 21, 55, and 117 days *(abscissa)*. Each *bar* represents the mean of five animals per group

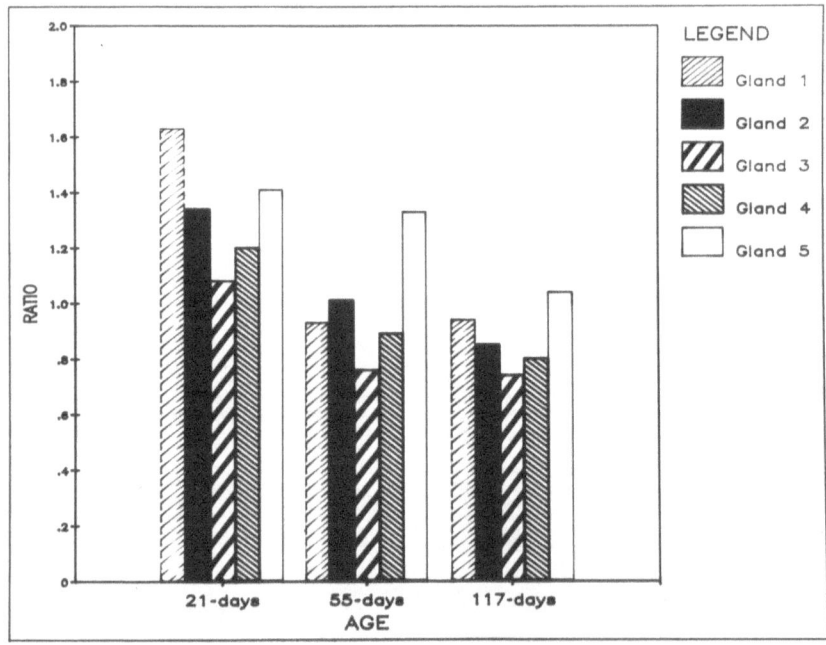

Fig. 322. The parenchyma-stroma ratio *(ordinate)* in glands 1–5 of virgin female rats aged 21, 55, and 117 days *(abscissa)*. Each *bar* represents the mean of five animals per group

suring an average of approximately 20×10^3 μm^2 (Table 19; Figs. 307, 313, 314, 315). This area that lags behind in development suggests that the mammary gland parenchyma responds unevenly to systemic hormonal stimuli.

With aging, the reduction of TEBs becomes more evident. TEBs disappear from zone A of both thoracic and abdominal glands by 55 days of age (Table 19). Between 55 and 117 days of age (Figs. 316–320) there are no great variations in the total area of the glands, except for a significant increase in area of the fourth gland in older animals (Fig. 299), but the thinner branches of the older animals's mammary gland result in a lower percentage in the amount of parenchyma (Fig. 321) and in a lower parenchyma-stroma ratio (Fig. 322). There is a little variation in the number of ABs and lobules and in the size of lobule development in older animals in comparison with the 55-day-old ones, as long as the animals remain virgin.

Histology. The mammary gland of prepubertal female rats is composed of occasional large ducts lined by a single or double layer of epithelial cells, which becomes multilayered at the TEB (Fig. 323). Individual epithelial cells are cuboidal and have scanty acidophilic cytoplasm. The nuclei are medium-sized or large, round or oval. The heterochromatin is finely granular, and nucleoli are inconspicuous. The nucleocytoplasmic ratio is high (Fig. 323). The epithelium rests on a discontinuous layer of elongated myoepithelial cells. The supporting connective tissue consists of a few bundles of collagen fibers containing some interspersed fibroblasts, a few capillaries, and lymphatic vessels. External to this, adipose cells, with laterally displaced nuclei, constitute the bulk of the stroma (Fig. 323), although in young animals there are focal areas in which the stroma has a myxomatous appearance.

With progressive branching, the diameter of the ducts becomes narrower; however, at their terminal end, most ducts retain a broad lumen ending in the club-shaped TEBs which are lined by a thick epithelium composed of 5–10 layers of cells. The mammary gland of mature or old virgin animals (Figs. 324–328) varies little in its histology from that of prepubertal animals, except for the more abundant branching, narrower ducts, and more numerous ABs and lobules (Figs. 327 and 328).

ABs appear as clusters of 3–5 tubules, each one having a centrally located lumen surrounded by a layer of cuboidal epithelial cells (Fig. 327). The diameter of each AB, as determined in both histologic section and whole mount preparation, is 31.9 ± 4.5 μm. ABs are composed of an almost constant number of cells which, in transverse section, is 13.9 ± 2.2 μm. With each successive estrous cycle ABs burst into smaller alveoli, whose number increases progressively, forming lobules, which are composed of clusters of alveoli of small diameter, with a small but patent lumen lined by a single layer of low cuboidal epithelial cells (Fig. 328).

Ultrastructure. The treelike structure that composes the parenchyma of the young virgin rat mammary gland is lined by two main cell types: an external layer of myoepithelium and an internal layer of epithelial cells. In hematoxylin and eosin stained sections very little variation in individual cell morphology is seen in the epithelia lining the main lactiferous ducts, TEBs, ABs, or lobules of young prepubertal, sexually mature, or old virgin rats. On the other hand, 1-μm sections of plastic embedded material and electron micrographs reveal that slight variations in cell size, shape, or nucleocytoplasmic ratio observed by light microscopy are associated with ultrastructural differences in nuclear shape and nuclear and cytoplasmic electron densities. When ultrastructural criteria such as cell and nuclear size, nucleocytoplasmic ratio, amount and distribution of chromatin, electron density of nucleus and cytoplasm, and number and distribution of organelles are analyzed in combination with histochemical criteria, namely detection of Mg^{2+}- and Na^+/K^+-dependent ATPases, three subtypes of mammary epithelial cells emerge: dark cells, intermediate cells, and light cells (Russo J et al. 1983a). In sections of plastic-embedded tissue, dark cells (DCs) appear as the smallest of all epithelial cells with darkly stained cytoplasm and an oval, small, convoluted nucleus (Figs. 329 and 330); under the electron microscope they are characterized by their small, irregular nucleus that contains coarsely clumped and electron-dense heterochromatin (Figs. 331, 334, 335). The cytoplasm is electron dense and contains a moderate number of mitochondria and few stacks of rough endoplasmic reticulum. Ribosomes are numerous, and Golgi complexes are well-developed. This is the type of cell in which numerous lipid droplets and secretory vacuoles are more frequently seen (Figs. 331, 334, 336). Although fat distribution within the cell seems to be random, with either subnuclear, paranuclear, or supranuclear localization, the number and size of fat

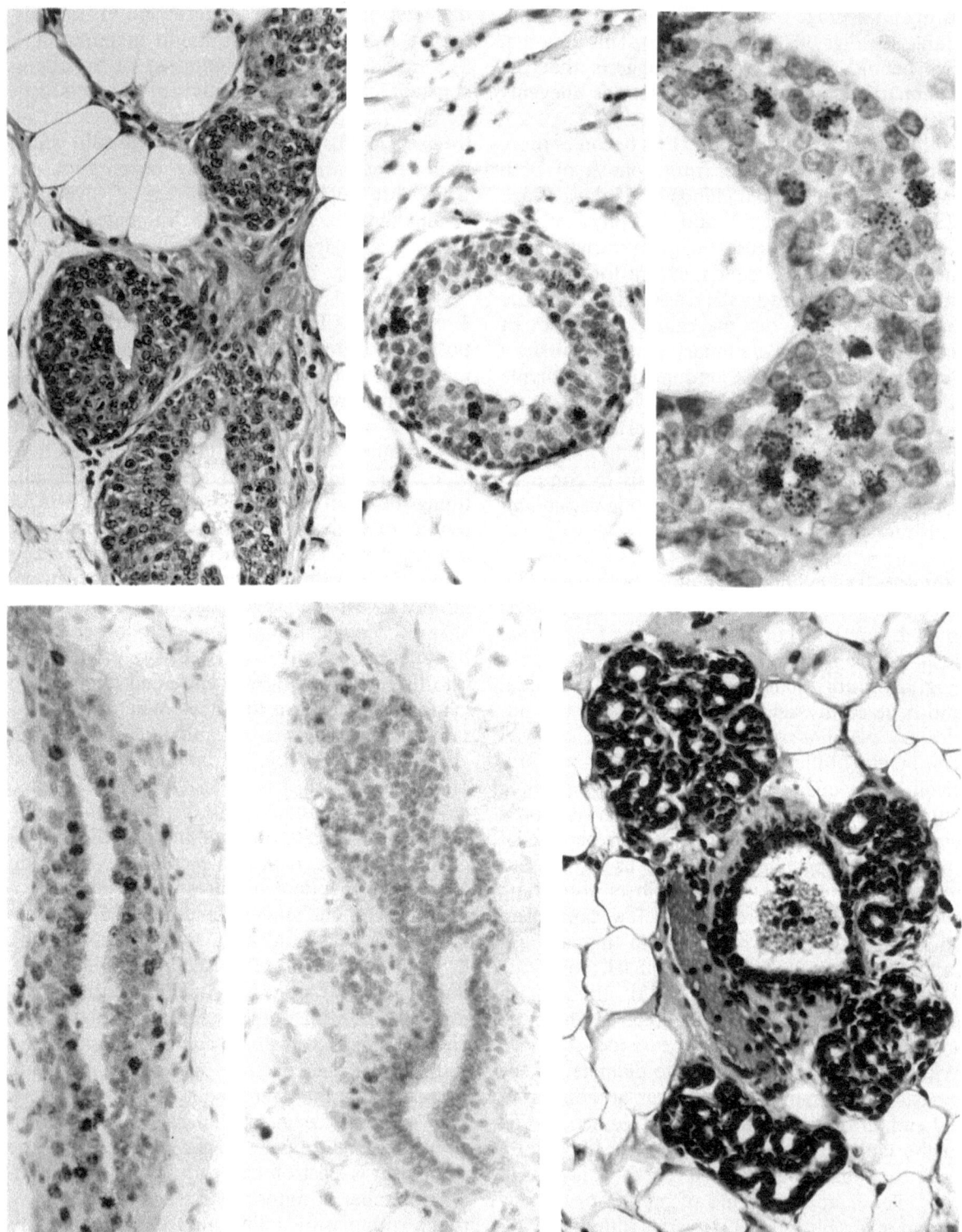

Fig. 323 *(upper left).* Thoracic mammary gland, 21-day-old female rat, containing one duct and two terminal end buds surrounded by fibrous and adipose tissue. H and E, ×65

Fig. 324 *(upper middle).* Terminal end bud (TEB) in the thoracic mammary gland of a 55-day-old virgin female rat is composed of fewer epithelial layers than the TEB in the 21-day-old animal shown in Fig. 323. There is incorporation of [³H]-thymidine in the lining epithelium. H and E, ×65

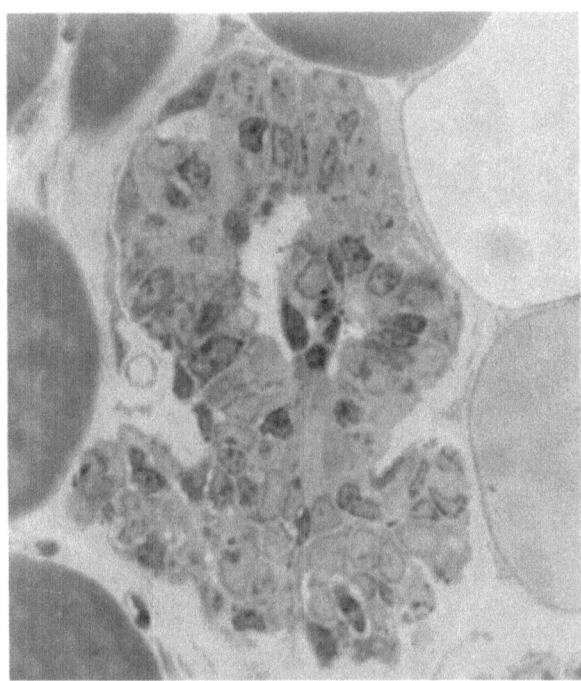

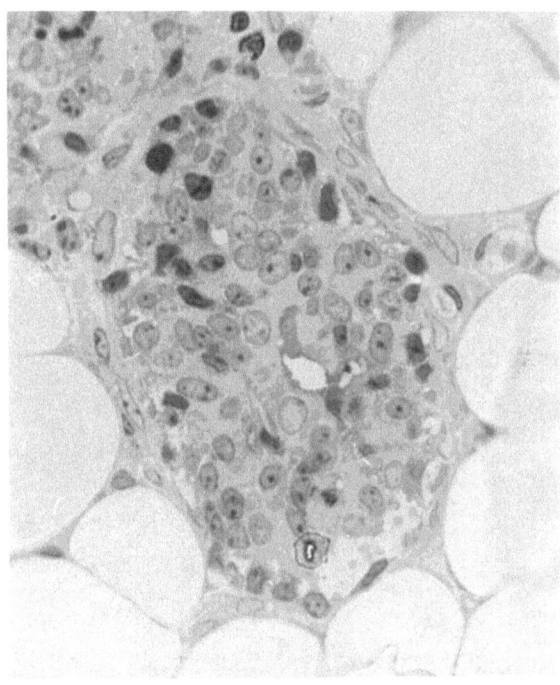

Fig. 329. Ductal structure with budding alveolar buds in the thoracic mammary gland of a 55-day-old virgin female rat. There is a layer of elongated myoepithelial cells between the stroma and the epithelium. Dark and intermediate cells are seen in the lining epithelium. Toluidine blue, × 450

Fig. 330. Terminal end bud in the thoracic mammary gland of a 55-day-old virgin female rat. The lining epithelium is composed of several layers of dark and intermediate cells surrounding a narrow lumen. Toluidine blue, × 450

◀ **Figs. 324–327.** Autoradiograms of virgin rat mammary glands. DNA synthesis was studied in animals injected intraperitoneally with 2.5 µCi methyl-[³H]-thymidine per body weight (specific activity 25 Ci/mM; Amersham Searle, Arlington Heights). The animals were killed by decapitation 1 h after injection. The skin with the attached mammary glands was removed, stretched on a corkboard, and fixed for 24 h in 10% neutral buffered formalin. The mammary tissue was dissected, dehydrated, embedded in paraffin, and sectioned at a thickness of 5 µm. Deparaffinized sections were coated with Kodak NTB-2 photographic emulsion (Eastman Kodak, Rochester, stored in light-proof boxes at 4 °C for 1–2 weeks, developed with microdol-X (Eastman, Kodak, Rochester), fixed, and counterstained with hematoxylin and eosin. The DNA labeling index was determined by a count of the number of labeled nuclei per total number of cells composing the epithelium of terminal end buds, terminal ducts, alveolar buds, ducts, and lobules and expressed as a percentage

Fig. 325 *(upper right).* Higher magnification of the terminal end bud shown in Fig. 324 to demonstrate the incorporation of [³H]-thymidine in the lining epithelium and in occasional myoepithelial cells. H and E, × 100

Fig. 326 *(lower left).* Autoradiograph with [³H]-thymidine incorporation into the lining epithelium and the surrounding stroma in a mammary duct contained in zone B of the abdominal mammary gland of a 55-day-old virgin female rat. H and E, × 65

Fig. 327 *(lower middle).* Duct and alveolar buds present in the mammary gland of a 117-day-old virgin female rat containing only occasional epithelial cells incorporating [³H]-thymidine. H and E, × 65

Fig. 328 *(lower right).* Abdominal mammary gland, 117-day-old virgin female rat, containing a main lactiferous duct surrounded by primitive lobules. H and E, × 65

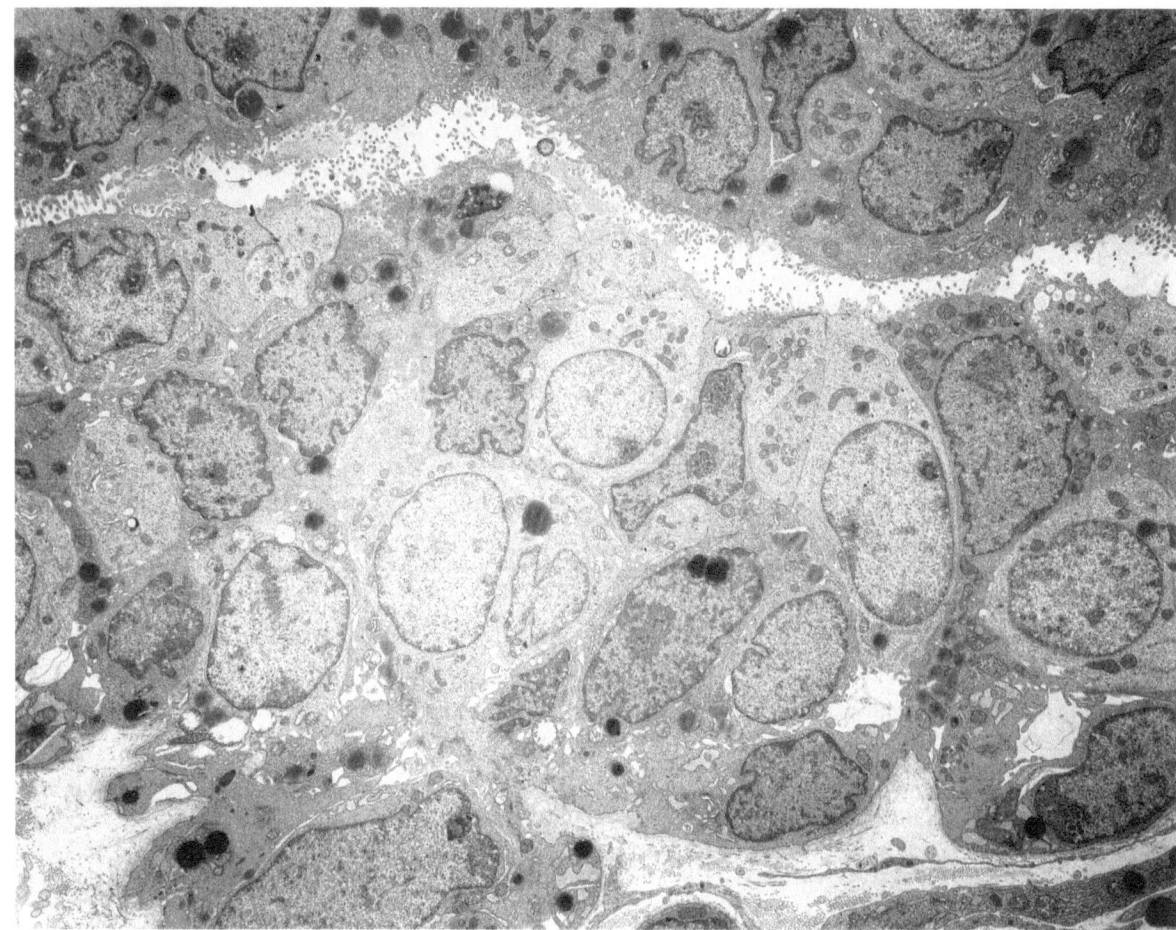

Fig. 331. Higher magnification of terminal end bud shown in Fig. 330. Myoepithelial, dark, and intermediate cells are seen lining the structure. Dark cells contain a few lipid droplets. Uranyl acetate-lead citrate, TEM, × 2500

droplets varies, primarily with the physiological condition of the animal and secondarily with the location of the DCs within the mammary gland tree. DCs located in TEBs (Fig. 331) and TDs (Fig. 334) of virgin animals have 3–4, small- to medium-sized droplets of lipids, whereas those located in alveoli of pregnant or hormonally treated animals contain numerous, large droplets occupying most of the cytoplasm of the cell (Figs. 335 and 336). These cells also contain in the apical portion numerous, electron-dense, condensed areas of fibrillar material surrounded by a clear halo, enclosed by a membrane that represents protein. DCs react positively for Mg^{2+}-dependent ATPase and negatively for Na^+/K^+-dependent ATPase (Russo J et al. 1983b).

Intermediate cells (ICs) have round to oval nuclei with a smooth or only slightly indented nuclear membrane containing finely dispersed heterochromatin (Figs. 331 and 334). The cyto-

Fig. 332 *(upper left first from top)*. Ductal structures in the ▶ mammary gland of a 117-day-old virgin female rat. Toluidine blue, × 450

Fig. 333 *(upper left second from top)*. Alveolar structure in the mammary gland of a virgin female rat treated with chorionic gonadotropin for 21 days. The lining epithelium has secretory activity. Toluidine blue, × 450

Fig. 334 *(upper right)*. Ductal structure shown in Fig. 332, which is lined by a layer of dark and intermediate cells. Uranyl acetate-lead citrate, TEM, × 2500

Fig. 335 *(lower left)*. The lining epithelium of the alveolus shown in Fig. 333; note the presence of lipid droplets and proteins in the cytoplasm of dark cells, adjacent to a light cell. Uranyl acetate-lead citrate, TEM, × 4000

Fig. 336 *(lower right)*. The alveolar lumen of the hormonally treated animal shown in Fig. 333 is lined by a single layer of cuboidal dark cells containing lipid droplets in the cytoplasm. The lumen contains secretory material. Uranyl acetate-lead citrate, TEM, × 4000

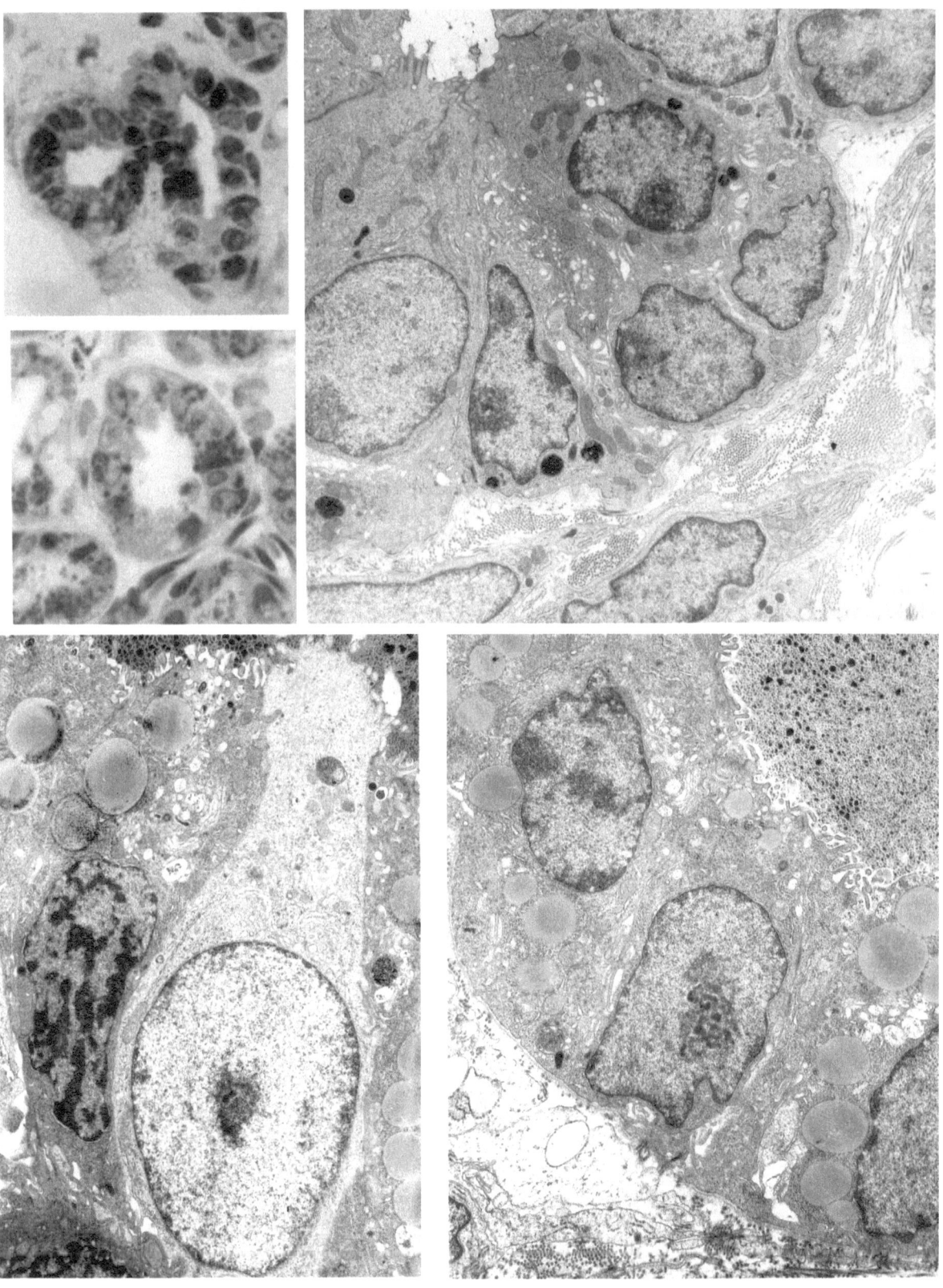

plasm is of moderate electron density, and organelles are more numerous than in DCs, particularly mitochondria (Figs. 331 and 334). Cytoplasmic lipids are absent regardless of the location of the cell, although occasional ICs contain a single lipid vacuole. ICs are in general seen occupying the full thickness of the epithelium; more frequently, the basal portion is in contact with myoepithelial cells, although occasionally they are in direct contact with the basement membrane (Figs. 335 and 336). The Mg^{2+}-dependent ATPase reaction is positive in these cells, whereas the Na^+/K^+-dependent ATPase reaction is negative (Russo J et al. 1983b).

Light cells (LCs) are large, with a round nucleus that contains scanty but finely clumped heterochromatin and an electron-lucent cytoplasm; they contain a moderate number of a small mitochondria and Golgi complexes (Fig. 335). Lipids are conspicuous absent. LCs, like DCs and ICs, show a positive reaction for Mg^{2+}-dependent ATPase but are negative for Na^+/K^+-dependent ATPase.

At the light microscopic level, myoepithelial cells (MCs) appear similar to DCs, but they are readily identifiable by their location adjacent to and interior to the basal lamina (Figs. 329, 330, 332). Ultrastructurally, MCs are characterized by a moderately electron-dense cytoplasm containing thick bundles of tonofilaments, the presence of numerous pinocytotic vesicles along the plasma membrane, and hemidesmosomes joining the cell membrane to the basal lamina (Figs. 331 and 334). Myoepithelial cells differ from all the epithelial cell types in their positive reaction with both Mg^{2+}- and Na^+/K^+-dependent ATPases (Russo J et al. 1983b).

TEBs (Figs. 330 and 331) are composed of five to eight layers of cells, 77% of which are DCs, 11% ICs, and 12% MCs. TDs are lined by a single layer of cells, 76% of which are DCs, 12% ICs, and 12% MCs (Figs. 332, 334). ABs that appear as clusters of ductules are lined by a double layer of cells consisting of 62% DCs, 21% ICs, and 17% MCs. The fraction of DCs is slightly lower, while that of ICs and MCs is slightly higher in ABs than in TEBs or TDs, but the differences are not statistically significant (Russo J et al. 1983b).

Cell Kinetics. The mammary gland of young virgin female rats exhibits a profuse mitotic and DNA synthetic activity which is highest in TEBs (Figs. 324 and 325) and lower in ducts (Fig. 326) and ABs (Fig. 327) (Russo J et al. 1979). Stromal cells are occasionally labeled (Fig. 326). Although

the number of TEBs reduces progressively with aging, as long as these structures are present in the mammary gland they retain a higher proliferative activity than other terminal ductal or lobular structures. In both old and young virgin rat mammary glands 100% of TEBs are labeled, although the number of labeled cells per TEB is markedly lower in older than in young virgin animals. Aging also reduces the percentage of labeled TDs and ABs, and their DNA-labeling indices (Russo J et al. 1979). Lobular structures in the resting virginal gland rarely incorporate DNA precursor into their epithelial cells, and myoepithelial cells are only occasionally labeled.

Further Considerations on Mammary Development

The development of the mammary gland is deeply influenced by genetically determined factors, by systemic influences during growth and development, and by focal factors. The most important factor for final morphology and function is genetically determined, and it is sex. The presence of an X or Y chromosome determines the formation of an ovary or testis, and these in turn manifest their influence on mammary development early in fetal life. The response of this organ to both endogenous and exogenous hormones depends upon the presence in both the mammary mesenchyme and parenchyma of specific receptors (Kratochwil 1977). Although it is known that mammary gland development is influenced from prenatal life in adulthood by various circulating endogenous and exogenous hormones (Ciocca et al. 1982; Raynaud 1961, 1971), very little is known about local regulatory factors or topographically determined variations in the response of the mammary gland to circulating hormonal levels, which might be modulating the final gland structure.

Even though there is a greater understanding of the role of circulating natural or synthetic hormones on mammary gland structure (Russo IH and Russo J 1986; Russo J and Russo IH 1987), much less is known on the local control of gland development. The influence of local factors in the response of the fetal mammary gland to hormones was observed by Raynaud (1961, 1971) and Jean (1968), and the importance of the mesenchyme as an inductor of morphogenesis has been highlighted by Sakakura et al. (1979) and Kratochwil (1977). However, these authors did not identify what substances were modulating that growth, and only recently the direct effect of a growth factor on mammary gland development has been demonstrated in the mouse (Silberstein and Daniel 1987).

The identification of local growth regulatory factors is a novel, developing field that will deeply modify our traditional concepts on the effect of hormones on endocrine responsive organs. The observation of topographic differences in mammary gland development in a single animal (Russo J and Russo IH 1987) suggests that local regulatory factors play an equal or even more important role than circulating hormonal levels (Ciocca et al. 1982). It is possible to postulate that the asynchronous development of thoracic and abdominal mammary glands is due to variations in the steroid hormone receptor content of the mammary epithelium. These hormones, which act via their specific receptors, may act as mitogens, in part inducing endocrine and/or autocrine mediators that serve as necessary intermediates, or they may produce specific gene products that induce eventually terminal differentiation of the cell (Danielpour and Sirbasku 1984). It is not known whether they affect thoracic and abdominal mammary glands differently, either as a consequence of variations in receptor content, which may be genetically determined (Jean 1968; Raynaud 1961, 1971), or secondary to local circulatory or stromal factors (Ciocca et al. 1982; Kratochwil 1977; Sakakura et al. 1979). It is also possible to postulate that it is the presence of stimulatory growth factors or their receptors that modulates the rate of cell proliferation in the different compartments of the mammary gland, or influences their ability to differentiate, by acting on specific cell types, epithelial, myoepithelial, or stromal cells, thus influencing the ability of the mammary gland to undergo normal differentiation. Whether all these factors play a role either independently or interrelatedly requires further investigation.

References

Alvarez Sanz MC, Liu JM, Huang HH, Hawrylewicz EJ (1986) Effect of dietary protein on morphologic development of rat mammary gland. JNCI 77: 477–487

Anderson RR (1978) Embryonic and fetal development of the mammary apparatus. In: Larson BL (ed) Lactation: a comprehensive treatise. Academic, New York, pp 3–40

Astwood EB, Geschickter CF, Rausch EO (1937) Development of the mammary gland of the rat. Am J Anat 61: 373–405

Balinsky BI (1950) On the prenatal growth of the mammary gland rudiment in the mouse. J Anat 84: 227–235

Bassleer R (1970) The morphology of hormone-induced structural changes in the female breast. In: Altman HW (ed) Current topics in pathology, vol 53. Springer, Berlin Heidelberg New York, pp 1–89

Ceriani RL (1970) Fetal mammary gland differentiation in vitro in response to hormones. I. Morphological findings. Dev Biol 21: 506–529

Ciocca DR, Parente A, Russo J (1982) Endocrinologic milieu and susceptibility of the rat mammary gland to carcinogenesis. Am J Pathol 109: 47–56

Cowie AT, Folley SJ (1961) The mammary gland and lactation. In: Young WC (ed) Sex and internal secretion, vol I, 3rd edn. Williams and Wilkins, Baltimore, pp 590–641

Danielpour D, Sirbasku DA (1984) New perspectives in hormone-dependent (responsive) and autonomous mammary tumor growth: role of autosimulatory growth factors. In Vitro 20: 975–980

Hardy MH (1950) The development in vitro of the mammary glands of the mouse. J Anat 84: 388–393

Heuberger B, Fitzka I, Wasner G, Kratochwil K (1982) Induction of androgen receptor formation by epithelium-mesenchyme interaction in embryonic mouse mammary gland. Proc Natl Acad Aci USA 79: 2957–2961

Huang HH, Hawrylewicz EJ, Kissane JQ, Drab EA (1982) Effects of protein diet on release of prolactin and ovarian steroids in female rats. Nutr Rep Int 26: 807–820

Jean C (1968) Nature et frequence des malformations mammaires du rat noveau-ne en fonction de la dose d'oestradiol injectee a la mere gravide. CR Soc Biol (Paris) 162: 1144–1149

Knight CH, Peaker M (1982) Development of the mammary gland. J Reprod Fertil 65: 521–536

Kratochwil K (1977) Development and loss of androgen responsiveness in the embryonic rudiment of the mouse mammary gland. Dev Biol 61: 358–365

Myers JA (1917) Studies on the mammary gland. II. The Fetal development of the mammary gland in the female albino rat. Am J Anat 22: 195–223

Raynaud A (1961) Morphogenesis of the mammary gland. In: Konan SK, Cowie AT (eds) Milk: the mammary gland and its secretions, vol 1. Academic, New York, pp 3–45

Raynaud A (1971) Fetal development of the mammary gland and hormonal effects on its morphogenesis. In: Falconer IR (ed) Lactation. Pennsylvania State University Press, University Park and London, pp 1–29

Russo IH, Russo J (1978) Developmental stage of the rat mammary gland as determinant of its susceptibility to 7,12-dimethylbenz(a)anthracene. JNCI 61: 1439–1449

Russo IH, Russo J (1986) From pathogenesis to hormone prevention of mammary carcinogenesis. Cancer Surv 5: 649–670

Russo J, Russo IH (1978) DNA labeling index and structure of the rat mammary gland as determinants of its susceptibility to carcinogenesis. JNCI 61: 1451–1459

Russo J, Russo III (1980) Susceptibility of the mammary gland to carcinogenesis II. Pregnancy interruption as a risk factor in tumor incidence. Am J Pathol 100: 497–512

Russo J, Russo IH (1987) Biological and molecular bases of mammary carcinogenesis. Lab Invest 57: 112-137

Russo J, Saby J, Isenberg WM, Russo IH (1977) Pathogenesis of mammary carcinomas induced in rats by 7,12-dimethylbenz(a)anthracene. JNCI 59: 435-455

Russo J, Wilgus G, Russo IH (1979) Susceptibility of the mammary gland to carcinogenesis. I. Differentiation of the mammary gland as determinant of tumor incidence and type of lesion. Am J Pathol 96: 721-736

Russo J, Tay LK, Russo IH (1982) Differentiation of the mammary gland and susceptibility to carcinogenesis. Breast Cancer Res 2: 5-73

Russo J, Tait L, Russo IH (1983a) Susceptibility of the mammary gland to carcinogenesis. III. The cell of origin of rat mammary carcinoma. Am J Pathol 113: 50-66

Russo J, Tay LK, Ciocca DR, Russo IH (1983b) Molecular and cellular basis of the mammary gland susceptibility to carcinogenesis. Environ Health Perspect 49: 185-199

Sakakura T, Nishizuka Y, Dawe CJ (1979) Capacity of mammary fat pads of adult C3H/HeMs mice to interact morphogenetically with fetal mammary epithelium. JNCI 63: 733-736

Silberstein GB, Daniel CW (1987) Reversible inhibition of the mammary gland growth by transforming growth factor-beta. Science 237: 291-293

Turner CW, Gomez ET (1933) The normal development of the mammary gland of the male and female albino mouse. Bull Mo Agric Exp Sta Res 182: 3-43

Young S, Hallowes RC (1973) Tumours of the mammary gland. In: Turusov VS (ed) Pathology of tumors in laboratory animals, vol 1. Tumours of the rat, pt 1. IARC, Lyon, pp 31-73

Wasner G, Hennermann I, Kratochwil K (1983) Ontogeny of mesenchymal androgen receptors in the embryonic mouse mammary gland. Endocrinology 113: 1771-1780

Van Zwieten MJ (1984) Normal anatomy and pathology of the rat mammary gland. In: The rat as animal model in breast cancer research. Martinus Nijhoff, Kluwer, Hingham MA, pp 53-134

Endocrine Influences on the Mammary Gland

Irma H. Russo, Josephine Medado, and Jose Russo

Introduction

The mammary gland is an organ whose morphology and physiology are constantly during the life span of an animal. Therefore, the study of the mammary gland has to be done taking into consideration the four major phases of its development: (a) prenatal; (b) postnatal, divided into pre- and postpubertal phases; (c) pregnancy-mediated, encompassing pseudopregnancy, pregnancy, lactation, and postlactational involution; and (d) age-related involution (Cowie and Folley 1961; Munford 1963).

All these phases of mammary gland development are strongly influenced by the hormones produced by the pituitary, ovaries, adrenal glands, and placenta (Knight and Peaker 1982). These hormones permanently affect mammary gland morphology and development; therefore, the assessment of this organ's condition requires the knowledge of present and past hormonal influences (Russo IH and Russo J 1986; Russo IH et al. 1985a, b, 1986; Russo J et al. 1977, 1979, 1982, 1983).

Endocrine Influences on Mammary Development

A number of interacting mechanisms are involved in the control of mammary growth. Maternal hormones influence fetal gland development. Fetal hormones in turn, produced by the testis, ovary, adrenal glands, or placenta, influence both the fetal and the maternal mammary gland.

Development in the fetus is controlled largely by local factors of mesenchymal origin, although the gland rudiments are capable of responding to hormonal stimulation before birth (Heuberger et al. 1982; Kratochwil 1969, 1977; Wasner et al. 1983). Development of the duct system during postnatal life is stimulated by mammatrophic hormones of the anterior pituitary, ovaries, and adrenals, but local factors are once again important in determining the actual configuration of the growing mammary tree (Russo IH et al. 1986; Russo J and Russo IH 1978, 1987a; Sakakura et al. 1979).

Pregnancy represents the summation of hormonal influences leading the mammary gland to its peak of development, which culminates in the maximal expression of differentiation that is milk secretion (Russo J and Russo IH 1987b). The maternal endocrine mechanisms that stimulate mammogenesis and lactogenesis are intimately concerned in the maintenance of pregnancy, development of the fetuses, and initiation of parturition. The developing fetuses are instrumental in producing other strongly mammotropic hormones (placental lactogens and estrogens), and thereby directly influence the degree of mammary development. After parturition, although the suckling young are no longer capable of having a direct endocrine effect on the gland, they do have an indirect one, via their influence on maternal hormone secretion. Also, the degree of frequency of suckling and gland emptying may affect the way in which local factors within the gland control further development (Forsyth 1986; Knight and Peaker 1982).

The mammotropic functions of prolactin, growth hormone, progesterone, estrogens, and corticosteroids were established initially by gland extirpation and hormone replacement experiments in immature rats (Lyons 1958). The same hormones also promote mammary development in intact, virgin animals (Meites 1961) and stimulate DNA synthesis and cell proliferation in mammary tissue in vitro (Forsyth and Jones 1976). In vitro and in vivo experiments established the following points: prolactin and/or growth hormone are essential for normal mammary development in the young animal and if given in high enough quantities will promote some growth even if the absence of steroids (Russo J and Russo IH (1987a). If in addition to prolactin, estrogens are also present, duct growth (only) will be stimulated, and if progesterone is then added, development will proceed to the lobulo-alveolar tissue stage (Russo IH and Russo J 1986). However, showing that the circulating concentration of a particular hormone is high at the time that mammary growth is stimulated is not necessarily evidence of cause and effect. Hormone concentrations can be misleading, partly because the most commonly used technique, radioimmunoassay, measures the immunoreactive properties of the hormone rather than its biological activity and partly because several factors other than concentration affect the activity of the hormone. First, specific receptor sites must be present on the cell membrane or within the cytosol of the target cells. Receptors for estrogens, progesterone, corticosteroids, prolactin, and growth hormone have been detected in mammary tissue, and it has been shown that their numbers vary with different stages of the reproductive cycle (Muldoon 1986). Prolactin is bound relatively poorly by

pregnant rat mammary tissue but well by lactating tissue (Hayden et al. 1979a). Progesterone receptors on the other hand are present in pregnant, but not lactating mouse tissue (Haslam and Shyamala 1979), although they are found in lactating goat tissue (Markland and Hutchens 1977). Since receptor levels are themselves under endocrine control, positive and negative feedback loops may be set up. Although some authors consider that estrogen receptors are generally estrogen independent (Knight and Peaker 1982), others suggest that two forms of estrogen receptor exist, one in immature and another in mature rats, this latter one being sensitive to bromocriptine (Muldoon 1986). Estrogen receptors are induced by prolactin and are inhibited by progesterone. Estrogens increase the binding of both progesterone and prolactin, and self-regulation of prolactin receptors by prolactin has also been demonstrated (Knight and Peaker 1982). This introduces a very important aspect of endocrine control, namely the interactions that occur between different hormones. The importance of the combination of peptide and steroid hormones has already been stressed; a more specific example is found in the action of estrogens, which not only stimulate the release of prolactin from the pituitary (Meites and Clemens 1972) but also have localized effects on mammary tissue, sensitizing it to the action of prolactin, possibly by inducing prolactin receptors (Butcher et al. 1974; Nagasawa and Yanai 1971a).

Two other hormones, thyroxine and relaxin, have been implicated in the control of mammary growth, which is inhibited and accelerated in young hypo- and hyperthyroid rats, respectively (Vonderhaar and Greco 1979). This is most probably a result of the action of thyroxine on general metabolism, rather than a direct effect on the gland. Relaxin synergizes with pituitary and ovarian hormones to stimulate growth in young ovariectomized-hypophysectomized rats (Harness and Anderson 1977) but inhibits steroid-induced mammary development in virgin goats (Cowie et al. 1965); hence its role may vary from species to species.

Feto-Maternal Interactions in the Control of Mammogenesis

There is considerable evidence that the placenta is the prime source of mammotrophic hormones, secreting a considerable amount of a peptide hormone similar to prolactin, called placental lactogen, and a chorionic gonadotropin (CG) composed of an alpha and a beta subunit structurally similar to human CG (Wide et al. 1980). The pituitary seems to be relatively unimportant, since in those species in which pregnancy is maintained after hypophysectomy, mammogenesis is either totally unaffected (Anderson 1975a) or only partly inhibited (Buttle et al. 1979; Denamur and Martinet 1961). Ovariectomy or fetectomy of pregnant rats has no significant effect on mammogenesis, provided that the placentae remain intact; if the placentae are removed then mammogenesis ceases (Desjardins et al. 1968). Placental extracts also stimulate mammary growth in hypophysectomized, ovariectomized, virgin rats when given together with steroids (Ray et al. 1955), and in vitro, growth of mammary explants is promoted by co-culture with placental fragments (Forsyth and Jones 1976). Placental lactogen cannot be detected during the first third of gestation, but from then on its concentration rises and is maintained at a high level until just before parturition (Kelly et al. 1976). Mammary growth seems to be correlated with placental lactogen secretion, since both are maximal during the last two-thirds of gestation. Mammary growth is initiated between days 4 and 6 of pregnancy in rats, and cell proliferation is at its highest on day 12. The earliest that rat placental lactogen has been detected is day 6, and the peak values occur at midpregnancy, i.e., around day 12 (Kelly et al. 1976). A positive correlation between mean placental lactogen concentration during the second half of gestation and milk yield in the succeeding lactation has been demonstrated by Hayden et al. (1979b). The influence of CG on gland development during pregnancy has not been assessed, although it has been observed that administration of CG to virgin animals produces a profuse lobulo-alveolar development (Russo J and Russo IH 1987a). Several factors other than concentration may be important in regulating the action of placental hormones. The same lactogenic hormone receptors that bind prolactin also bind placental lactogen, therefore the number of these receptors will be important, as will the affinity of placental lactogen for the receptor and the amount of competitive binding by nonbiologically active compounds (Knight and Peaker 1982). There is evidence that fetuses are able to influence mammogenesis in most species since a correlation has been demonstrated between fetal number and maternal gland development. Experiments in mice have demonstrated that fetal number and mammary growth are correlated up to a maximum of eight feto-placental units; thereafter, either placental lactogen secretion is not enhanced or the gland is unable to respond further to the hormone (Nagasawa and Yanai 1971b).

Rats need a minimum of only three feto-placental units to ensure maximum mammary development (Anderson 1975a; Hayden et al. 1979b). However, prolactin secretion may be enhanced in pregnant rats by self-licking of nipples, a phenomenon which is apparently necessary for normal mammogenesis, since its prevention results in reduction of mammary growth (Roth and Rosenblatt 1968). In guinea pigs, mammary gland weight and milk yield at peak lactation are both correlated with the number of young born, rather than the number suckled (Davis et al. 1979), which is once again indicative of fetal effect on mammogenesis. In conclusion, it is well-established that a peptide mammotrophic hormone is essential for normal mammogenesis in all species.

Mammary Gland Development During Pregnancy

The study of the development of the mammary gland in rats during their first pregnancy reveals that the gland structure changes progressively, and these changes affect total gland area (Fig. 337), parenchymal area (Fig. 338), and the parenchyma-stroma ratio (Fig. 339).

Measurements of the percentage increase in both wet weight and defatted dry weight of the six pairs of glands of rats during pregnancy vary from 50% to 120%, whereas the equivalent figures for DNA range from 200% to 300%. Since the latter reflects cell numbers and hence the size of the functional portion of the gland, it is obvious that weight determinations alone seriously underestimate the increase in secretory potential. The data of Munford (1963) demonstrated a roughly linear increase of log DNA with time throughout pregnancy and for the first 5 days of lactation. A similar relationship exists in mice from day 12 of pregnancy to day 5 of lactation (Knight and Peaker 1982). It would appear, therefore, that mammary cell number increases in an exponential fashion during gestation in these two species. The mouse has a cell population doubling time at 6 days; in the rat it is somewhat longer. Grahame and Bertalanffy (1972) indicated that in the rat the proportion of dividing cells declines during the second half of pregnan-

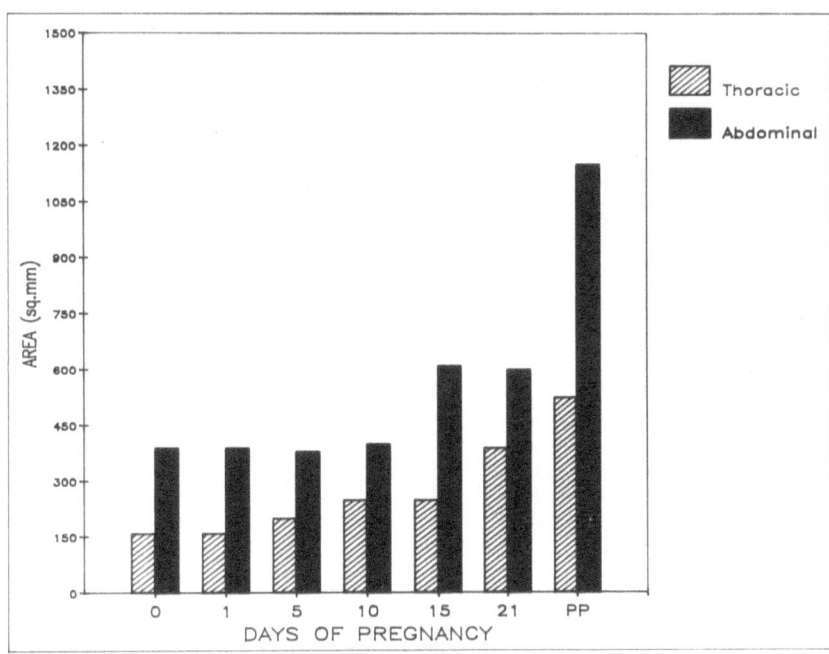

Fig. 337. Rat mammary gland area *(ordinate)* in thoracic and abdominal glands at 0, 1, 5, 10, 15, and 21 days of pregnancy and 1 day postpartum *(pp) (abscissa)*

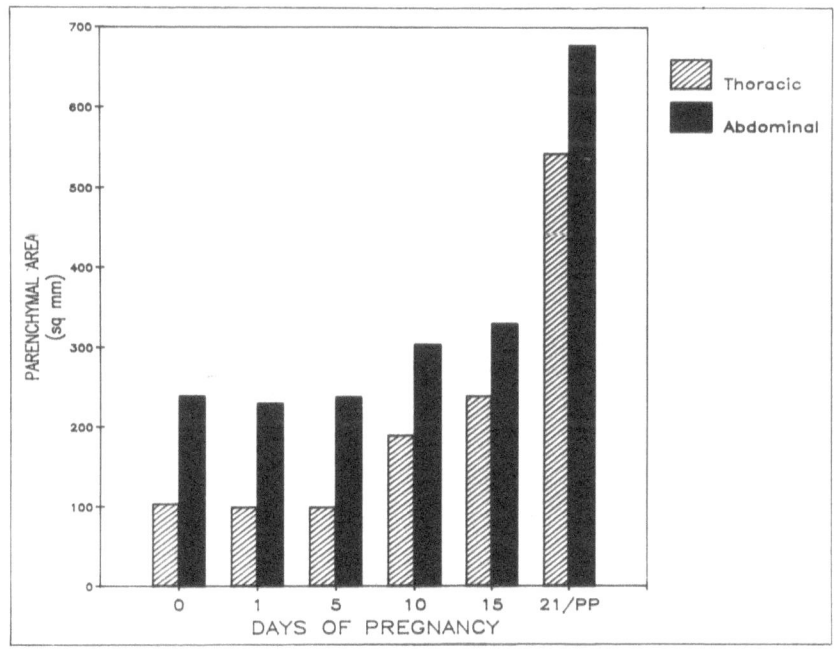

Fig. 338. Mammary parenchymal area *(ordinate)* of thoracic and abdominal glands of rats at 0, 1, 5, 10, and 15 days of pregnancy. Values obtained at the 21st day of pregnancy were combined with those obtained at 1 day postpartum *(pp)* and expressed as an average

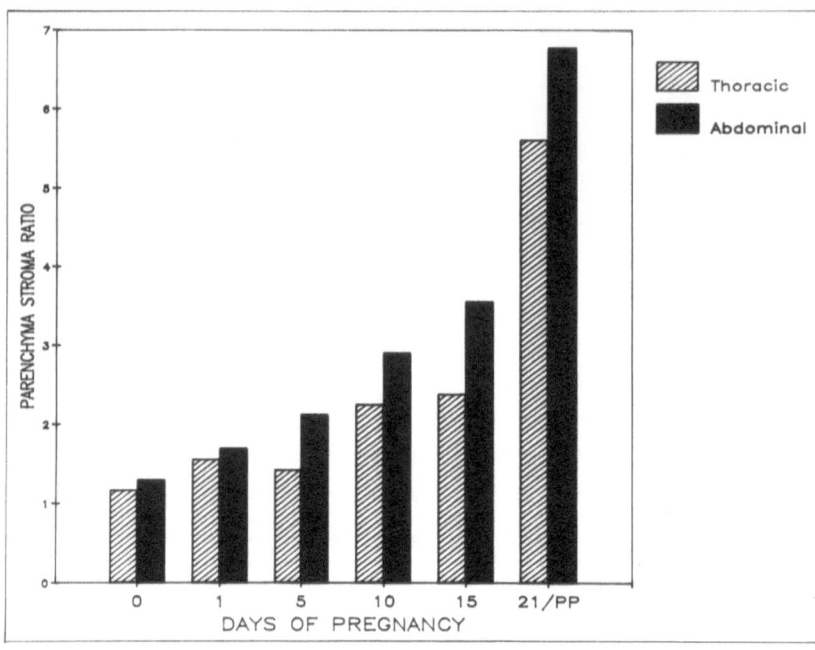

Fig. 339. Mammary parenchyma-stroma ratio *(ordinate)* in thoracic and abdominal glands of rats shown in Figs. 337 and 338; postpartum

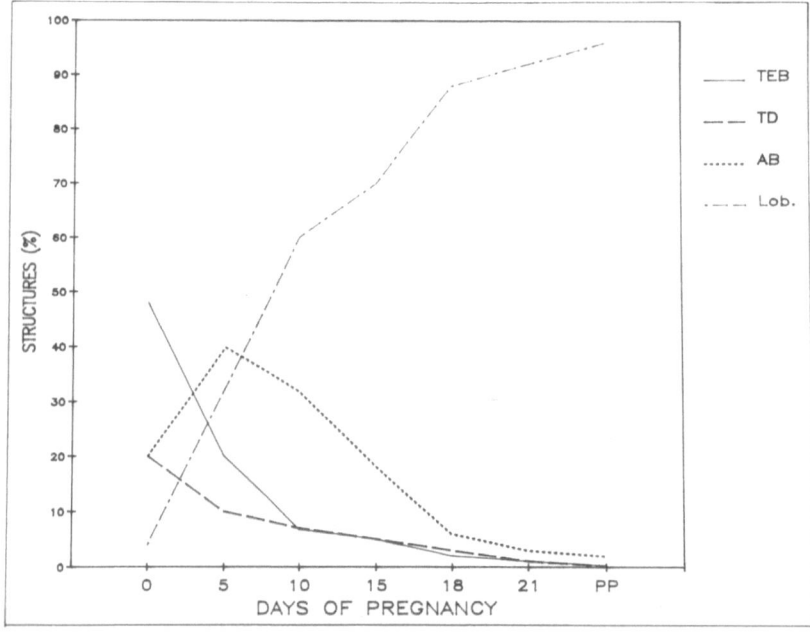

Fig. 340. Mammary gland, rat. Percentage of terminal ductal structures *(ordinate)* at 0, 5, 10, 15, 18, and 21 days of pregnancy and 1 day postpartum *(pp) (abscissa)*. *TEB*, terminal end bud; *TD*, terminal duct; *AB*, alveolar bud; *Lob*, lobules

cy. Thus, in order to maintain exponential growth the time taken for each cell to divide must decrease, as is known to occur under the influence of ovarian steroids (Bresciani 1971).

The morphological bases of these changes consist predominantly in profuse lobular development, whose proportion start increasing from the time of conception (Fig. 340). Histological studies have shown that during gestation the duct system increases in size and complexity, and epithelial cells proliferate, displacing adipose tissue and forming the first true lobulo-alveloar tissue. However, the comprehension of the process requires one to examine all the pairs of glands, as well as all topographic areas of each gland (Russo IH et al. 1986; Russo J and Russo IH 1987a). It has been observed that mammary glands located in the thoracic region differ in degree of development from those located in the abdominal region (Russo J and Russo IH 1987a), even though both of them are under systemic hormonal stimulation. These differences consist in varia-

tion in the degree of development of terminal ductal structures located in specific topographic areas of the mammary gland, which persist during the full length of pregnancy and even during lactation. The various terminal ductal structures that have been identified in the virgin rat mammary gland are terminal end buds (TEBs), terminal ducts (TDs), alveolar buds (ABs), and lobules (Russo IH and Russo J 1986; Russo IH et al. 1985a, b; Russo J and Russo IH 1987a; Russo J et al. 1982).

The mammary glands of virgin female rats as well as that of rats recently mated contain a large proportion of TEBs (Figs. 340–342), TDs and ABs (Figs. 340, 343, 344), and few lobules (Figs. 340 and 345). During the first 10 days of pregnancy, TEBs decrease not only in percentage number but also in size (Figs. 340, 346, 347, 348), due to their differentiation to ABs, and the further differentiation of ABs to lobules, the percentage of which reaches a maximum after the second half of pregnancy (Figs. 340, 350, 351).

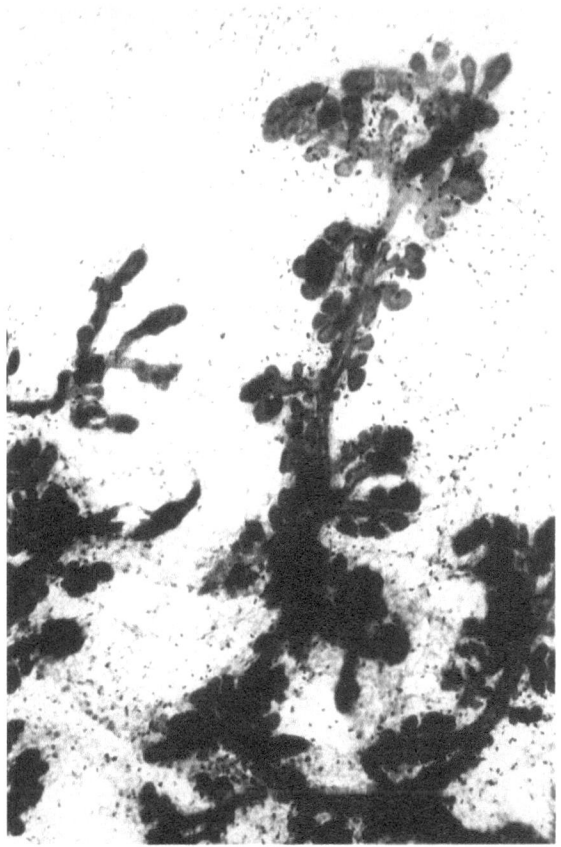

Fig. 341. Abdominal mammary gland, 55-day-old female rat on the first day of pregnancy. Whole mount, toluidine blue, × 55

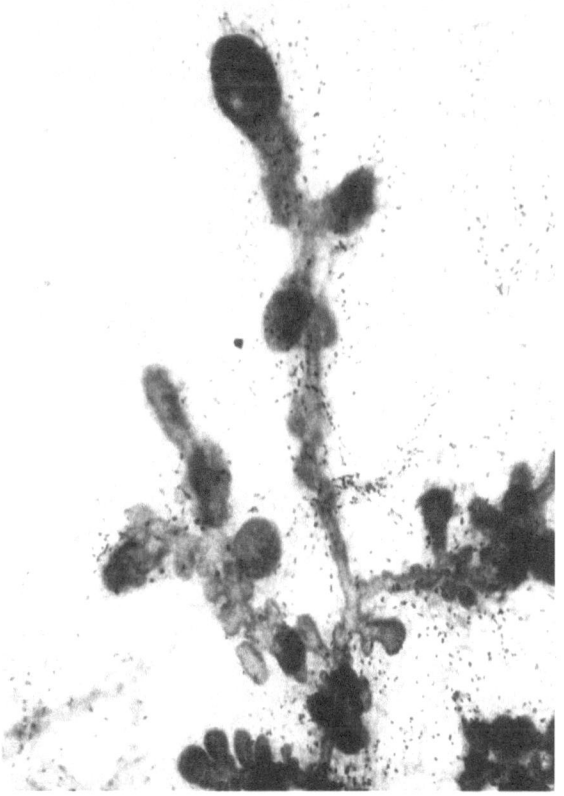

Fig. 342. Thoracic mammary gland, 55-day-old rat on the first day of pregnancy. Whole mount, toluidine blue, × 55

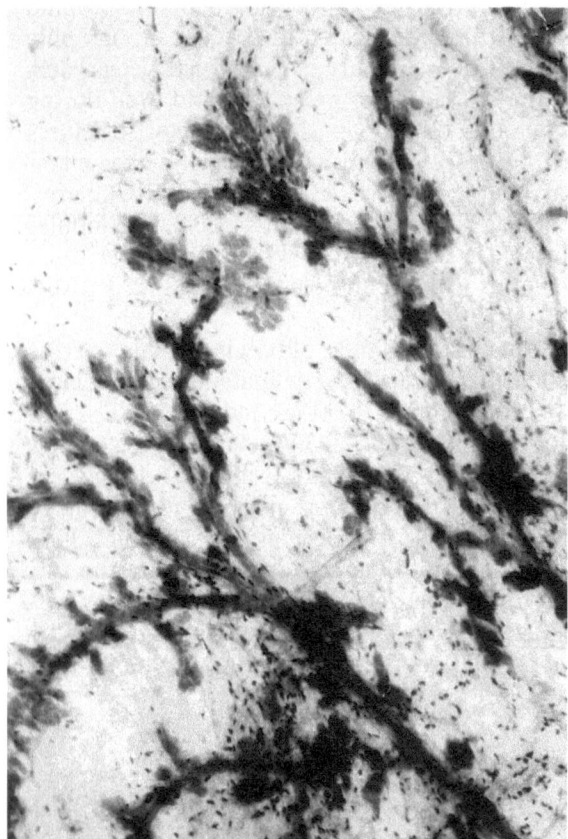

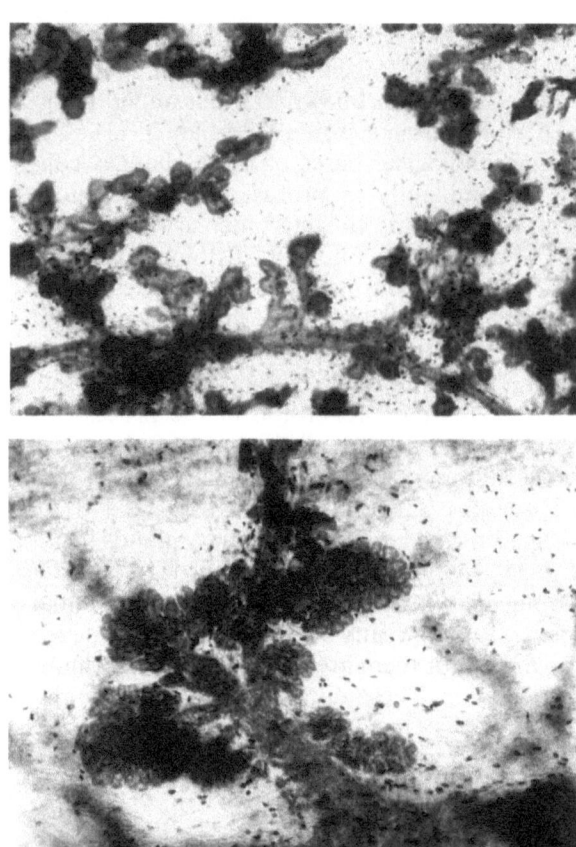

Figs. 343 *(left)* and **344** *(upper right)*. Terminal ducts and alveolar buds are more abundant in abdominal mammary gland, rat, on the first day of pregnancy. Whole mount, toluidine blue, × 55

Fig. 345 *(lower right)*. Early lobular formation, inguinal mammary gland, 1-day pregnant rat. Whole mount, toluidine blue, × 55

Fig. 346 *(upper left)*. Mammary gland, rat. At the fifth day of pregnancy terminal end buds are smaller, being rapidly replaced by alveolar buds and lobules. Whole mount, toluidine blue, × 55

Fig. 347 *(top)*. Mammary gland, rat. Cleavage of a terminal end bud into two terminal ducts *(center)*. Whole mount, toluidine blue, × 55

Fig. 348 *(upper right)*. Distal portion of the abdominal gland, rat. Note abundance of alveolar buds and lateral buds at the 10th day of pregnancy. × 65

Fig. 349 *(lower left)*. Profuse lobular development, abdom- ▶ inal mammary gland, 18-day pregnant rat. Whole mount, toluidine blue, × 55

Fig. 350 *(middle right)*. Higher magnification of lobular structures shown in Fig. 349. × 100

Fig. 351 *(lower right)*. Mammary gland, rat. Cystic terminal end bud present in a thoracic mammary gland at the end of pregnancy. Whole mount, toluidine blue, × 55

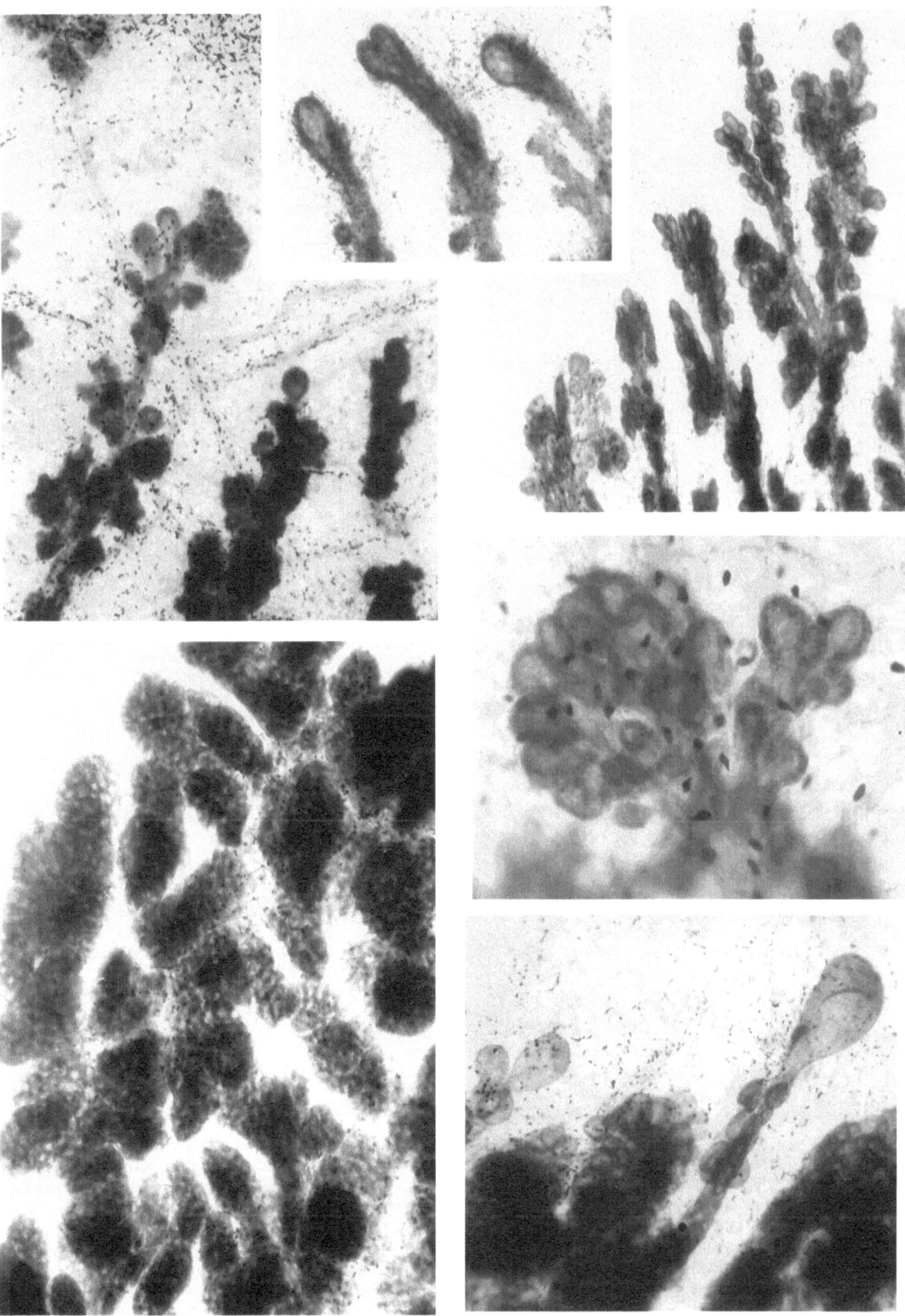

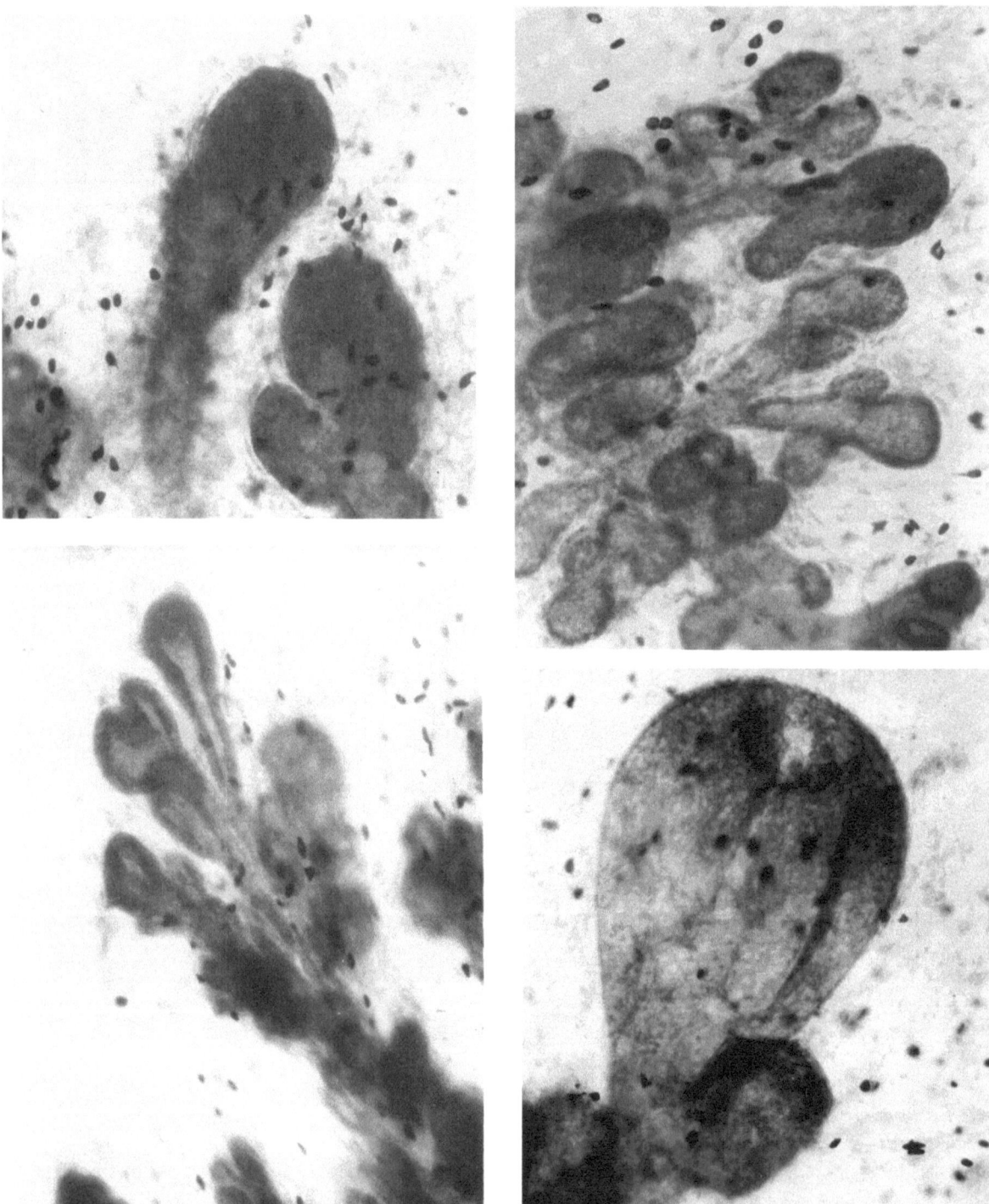

Fig. 352 *(upper left)*. Solid terminal end buds, thoracic mammary gland, rat, on the 1st day of pregnancy. Whole mount, toluidine blue, × 100

Fig. 353 *(lower left)*. Mammary gland rat. By the 10th day of pregnancy, terminal end buds become smaller with thinning of the walls and a more widely patent lumen. Whole mount, toluidine blue, × 100

Fig. 354 *(upper right)*. Mammary gland, rat. At the end of pregnancy, most terminal ductal structures and lateral buds are lined by a single layer of epithelial cells, and the lumen has become distended. Whole mount, toluidine blue, × 100

Fig. 355 *(lower right)*. Mammary gland, rat. Cystic terminal end bud, thoracic gland, at the 1st day of lactation. Whole mount, toluidine blue, × 100

At the end of pregnancy, the mammary gland is almost totally composed of lobular structures, although occasional glands contain isolated cystically dilated TEBs (Figs. 351 and 355).

The hallmark of mammary gland differentiation during pregnancy is the disappearance of TEBs, and a progressive modification of its cytoarchitecture. At the beginning of pregnancy, TEBs are numerous with a solid appearance in whole mount preparations (Fig. 352), whereas at the middle of pregnancy they decrease in number (Fig. 340), and the number of cell layers decreases, with subsequent cleavages to ABs (Fig. 353). At the end of pregnancy only a few TEBs with a cystic appearance are present (Figs. 350, 354, 355). The other important change observed during pregnancy, in addition to the disappearance of TEBs and ABs, is the formation of lobules, which exhibit a six-fold increase by the end of pregnancy (Figs. 340, 349). The lobules are formed by an increase in number of individual alveoli (Figs. 356–360). At the end of pregnancy, the alveoli exhibiting secretory activity are called acini; they are lined by cuboidal epithelium with secretory material in the apical portion. Myoepithelial cells are compressed against the basement membrane (Fig. 360). These differences are better observed ultrastructurally in comparison with the resting gland (Figs. 361 and 362).

Mammary Gland During Lactation

Milk yield is a function of the number of secreting cells and the activity of each cell. The number of secretory cells increases dramatically during gestation, although this is not a terminal event since in some species a transient surge of cell proliferation occurs 2 or 3 days postpartum, e.g., mouse (Traurig 1967; Knight and Peaker 1982) and rat (Greenbaum and Slater 1957). DNA continues to increase in a logarithmic fashion for at least the first 5 days of lactation in these species. Milk yield increases gradually for the first 7 days of lactation.

In the guinea pig there is relatively little change in DNA during gestation, but there is a large increase within 2 days after parturition (Nelson et al. 1962). This may result from a wave of mitosis prepartum rather than from proliferation during lactation. The glands of rabbits apparently increase in size and DNA content late in lactation (Lu and Anderson 1973), although studies of the [3H]-thymidine labeling index have failed to detect any increase in cell proliferation at this time. DNA concentration remains relatively unchanged during early lactation in sheep (Anderson 1975b), goats (Anderson et al. 1981; Fleet et al. 1975), and cows (Baldwin 1966), although possible variations in the size of the glands and retained milk content of the tissue mean that this observation alone is not indicative of a lack of growth. When lactation is extended in rodents by litter replacement, a gradual decline in milk yield is accompanied by a fall in DNA and by a larger decrease in total content of ribonucleic acid (RNA), which suggests that decreased secretion relates more to reduced cellular activity than to loss of cells (Nagasawa and Yanai 1976).

Cessation of lactation may be brought about by increased intramammary pressure due to nonremoval of secretion, as in goats (Peaker 1980), or to removal of the hormonal galactopoietic stimulus after suckling ceases, as in rats (Hanwell and Linzell 1972). RNA starts to fall within 12 h of weaning in rats; the fall in DNA (loss of cells) starts 24–36 h later and lasts for up to 20 days (Ota 1964). A period of involution is an essential prerequisite for successful redevelopment and subsequent lactation (cows milked continuously until parturition yield considerable less milk than normal in the next lactation) (Wheelock and Dodd 1969). This indicates that secretory epithelial cells have a limited life span and must eventually be replaced. Apart from certain exceptions, mentioned above very little cell division occurs in lactating tissue; hence involution must take place before extensive cell replacement can occur. There is some disagreement as to whether with involution the gland reverts to its mature, virgin state completely or incompletely, in that some cells are carried over into the next lactation. By labeling mammary epithelial cells of rats with [3H]-thymidine during one lactation and counting the number of labeled cells during the next lactation, Pitkow et al. (1972) estimated that carryover might be as high as 50%. This suggests that a substantial number of epithelial cells may remain in the gland after involution. Thus mammary development is likely to be incremental in successive gestations, which could explain why milk yield of cattle is more closely related to parity than to age (Wada and Turner 1959).

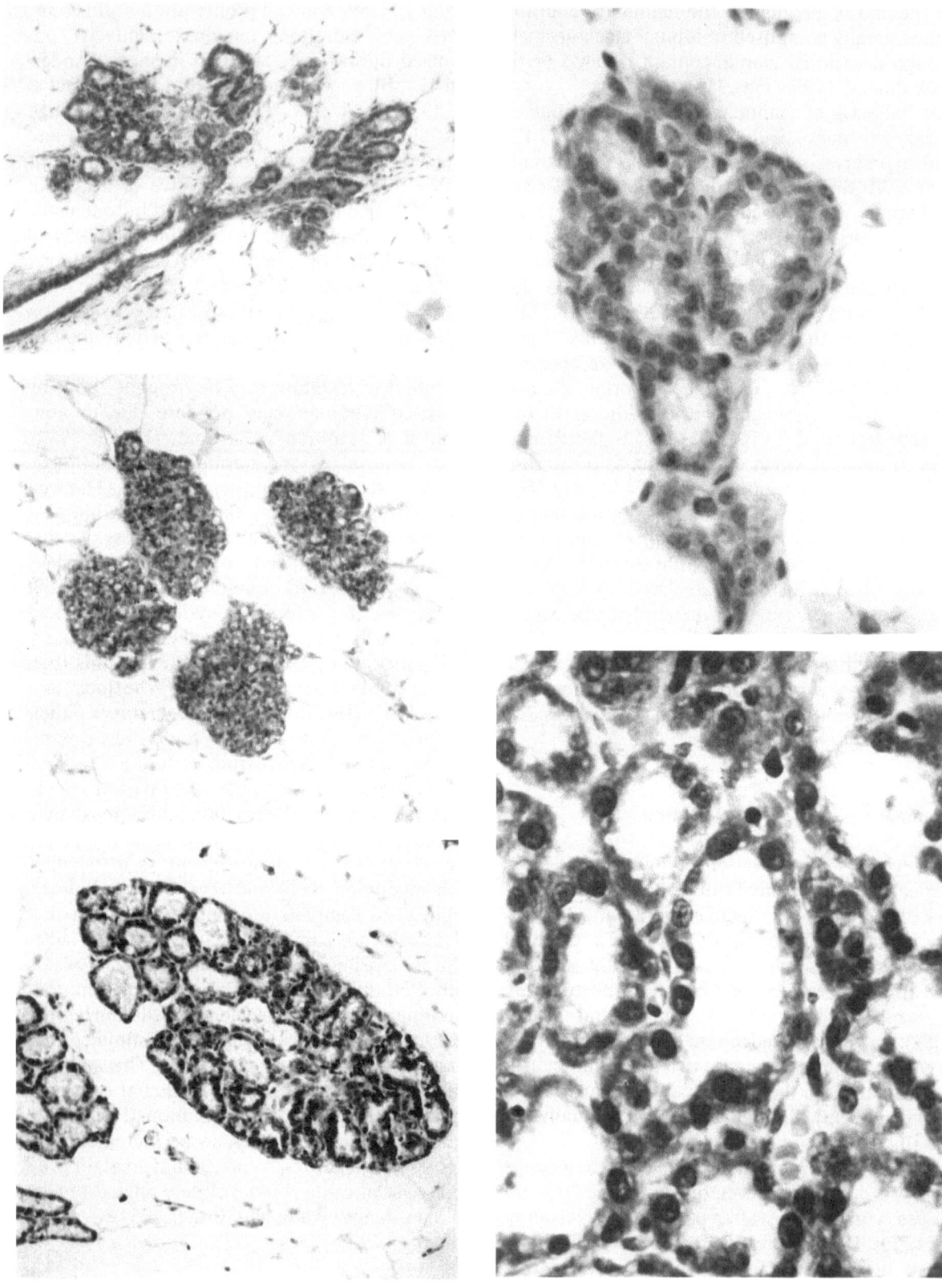

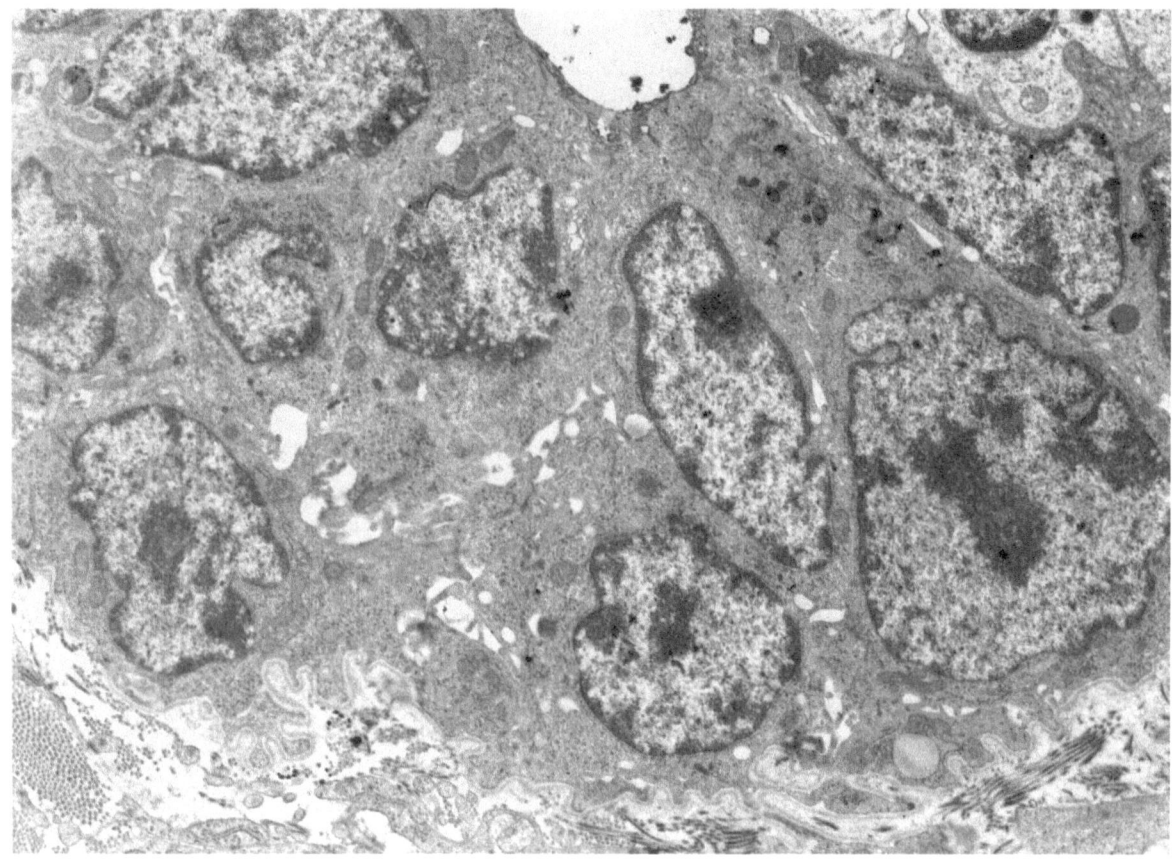

Fig. 361. Resting mammary gland alveolus, rat, lined by a single layer of epithelium and an external layer of myoepithelial cells lying on a convoluted basement membrane. Uranyl acetate-lead citrate, TEM, × 4000

◀ **Fig. 356** *(upper left).* Mammary gland, rat, during the 1st day of pregnancy; alveoli and primitive lobular structures composed of alveolar buds. H and E, × 100

Fig. 357 *(upper right).* Higher magnification of the lobular structures shown in Fig. 356. H and E, × 450

Fig. 358 *(middle left).* Mammary gland, rat. Lobules at the 15th day of pregnancy are composed of more numerous

alveolar structures per lobule than those shown in Fig. 356. H and E, × 100

Fig. 359 *(lower left).* Mammary gland, rat. At the end of pregnancy, the lobules enlarge due to distention of the lumen by secretion. H and E, × 100

Fig. 360 *(lower right).* Higher magnification of Fig. 359. H and E, × 450

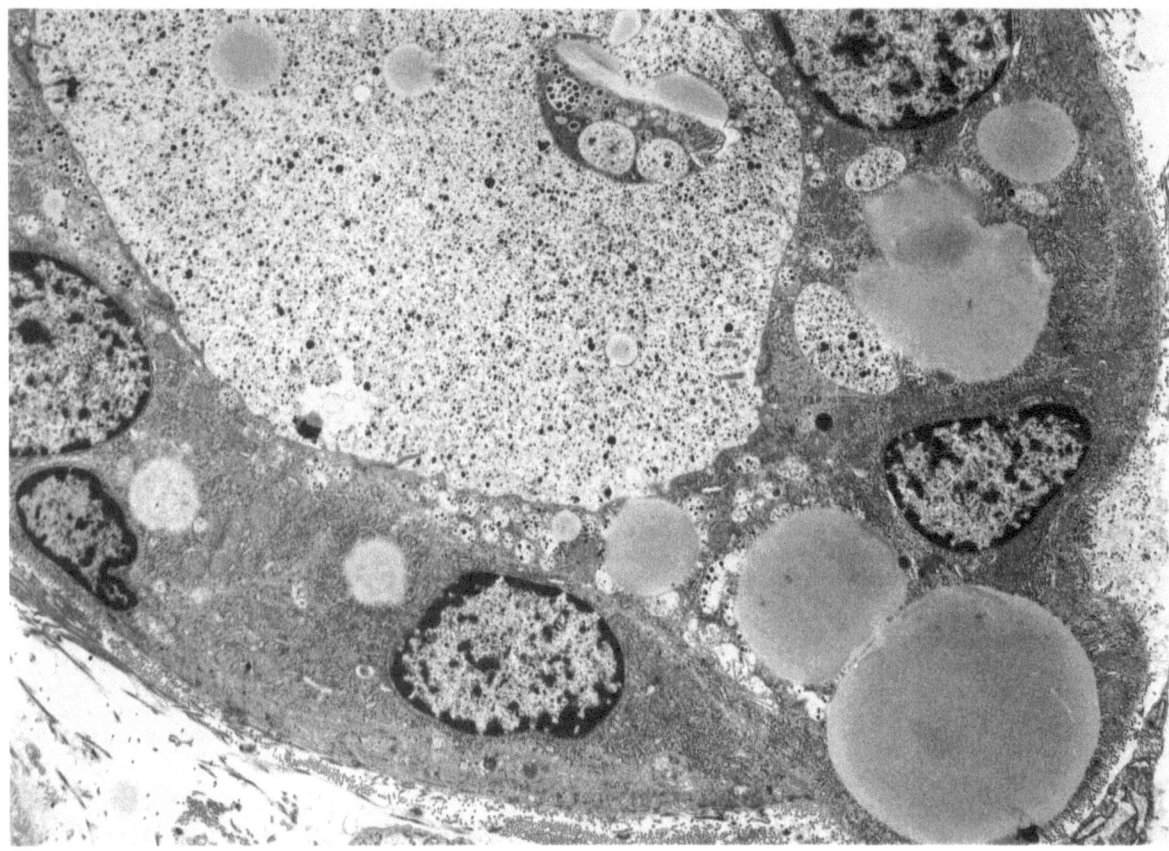

Fig. 362. Acinus of a lactating gland, mammary gland, rat. The epithelial cells contain large confluent lipid droplets and proteinaceous secretion which also fill the lumen. Uranyl acetate-lead citrate, TEM, × 4000

References

Anderson RR (1975a) Mammary gland growth in the hypophysectomized pregnant rat. Proc Soc Exp Biol Med 148: 283-287

Anderson RR (1975b) Mammary gland growth in sheep. J Anim Sci 41: 118-123

Anderson RR, Harness JR, Snead AF, Salah MS (1981) Mammary growth pattern in goats during pregnancy and lactation. J Dairy Sci 64: 427-432

Baldwin RL (1966) Enzymatic activities in mammary glands of several species. J Dairy Sci 49: 1533-1542

Bresciani F (1971) Ovarian steroid control of cell proliferation in the mammary gland and cancer. In: Hubinont PO, Leroy F, Galand P (eds) Basic actions of sex steroids on target organs. Karger, Basel, pp 130-159

Butcher RL, Collins WE, Fugo NW (1974) Plasma concentration of LH, FSH, prolactin, progesterone and estradiol-17 beta throughout the 4-day estrous cycle of the rat. Endocrinology 94: 1704-1708

Buttle HL, Cowie AT, Jones EA, Turvey A (1979) Mammary growth during pregnancy in hypophysectomized or bromocriptine-treated goats. J Endocrinol 80: 343-351

Cowie AT, Folley SJ (1961) The mammary gland and lactation. In: Young WC (ed) Sex and internal secretions, vol 1. Williams and Wilkins, Baltimore, pp 590-642

Cowie AT, Cox CP, Folley SJ, Hoskins ZD, Naito M, Tindal JS (1965) The effects of the duration of treatments with oestrogen and progesterone on the hormonal induction of mammary growth and lactation in the goat. J Endocrinol 32: 129-139

Davis SR, Mepham TB, Lock KJ (1979) Relative importance of prepartum and postpartum factors in the control of milk yield in the guinea-pig. J Dairy Res 46: 613-621

Denamur R, Martinet J (1961) Effects del l'hypophysectomie et de la section de la tige pituitaire sur la gestation de la brebis. Ann Endocrinol (Paris) 22: 755-759

Desjardins C, Paape MJ, Tucker HA (1968) Contribution of pregnancy, fetuses, fetal placentas and deciduomas to mammary gland and uterine development. Endocrinology 83: 907-910

Fleet IR, Goode JA, Hamon MH, Laurie MS, Linzell JL, Peaker M (1975) Secretory activity of goat mammary glands during pregnancy and the onset of lactation. J Physiol (Lond) 251: 763-773

Forsyth IA (1986) Variation among species in the endocrine control of mammary growth and function: the roles of prolactin, growth hormone, and placental lactogen. J Dairy Sci 69: 886-903

Forsyth IA, Jones EA (1976) Organ culture of mammary gland and placenta in the study of hormone action and placental lactogen secretion. In: Balls M, Monnickendam MA (eds) Organ culture in biomedical research. Cambridge University Press, pp 201-221

Grahame RE, Bertalanffy FD (1972) Cell division in normal and neoplastic mammary gland tissue in the rat. Anat Rec 174: 1-7

Greenbaum AL, Slater TF (1957) Studies of the particulate components of rat mammary gland. 2 Changes in the levels of the nucleic acid of the mammary glands of rats during pregnancy, lactation and mammary involution. Biochem J 66: 155-161

Hanwell A, Linzell JL (1972) A simple technique for measuring the rate of milk secretion in the rat. Comp Biochem Physiol [A] 43: 259-270

Harness JR, Anderson RR (1977) Effect of relaxin and somatotrophin in combination with ovarian steroids on mammary glands in rats. Biol Reprod 17: 599-603

Haslam SZ, Shyamala G (1979) Progesterone receptors in normal mammary glands in mice: characterization and relationship to stage of development. Endocrinology 105: 786-795

Hayden TJ, Bonney RC, Forsyth IA (1979a) Ontogeny and control of prolactin receptors in the mammary gland and liver of virgin, pregnant and lactating rats. J Endocrinol 80: 259-269

Hayden TJ, Thomas CR, Forsyth IA (1979b) Effect of number of young born (litter size) on milk yield of goats: role for placental lactogen. J Dairy Sci 62: 53-63

Heuberger B, Fitzka I, Wasner G, Kratochwil K (1982) Induction of androgen receptor formation by epithelium-mesenchyme interaction in embryonic mouse mammary gland. Proc Natl Acad Sci USA 79: 2957-2961

Kelly PA, Tsushima T, Shiu RPC, Friesen HG (1976) Lactogenic and growth hormone-like activities in pregnancy determined by radioreceptor assays. Endocrinology 99: 765-774

Knight CH, Peaker M (1982) Development of mammary gland. J Reprod Fertil 65: 521-536

Kratochwil K (1969) Organ specificity in mesenchymal induction demonstrated in the embryonic development of the mammary gland of the mouse. Dev Biol 20: 46-71

Kratochwil K (1977) Development and loss of androgen responsiveness in the embryonic rudiment of the mouse mammary gland. Dev Biol 61: 358-365

Lu MH, Anderson RR (1973) Growth of the mammary gland during pregnancy and lactation in the rabbit. Biol Reprod 9: 538-543

Lyons WR (1958) Hormonal synergism in mammary growth. Proc R Soc Biol 149: 303-325

Markland FS Jr, Hutchens TW (1977) Characterization of the progestin receptor from lactating mammary glands of the goat. In: McGuire WL et al. (eds) Progesterone receptors in normal and neoplastic tissues. Raven, New York, pp 23-28

Meites J (1961) Farm animals: hormonal induction of lactation and galactopoiesis. In: Kon SK, Cowie AT (eds) Milk: the mammary gland and its secretion, vol 1. Academic, New York, pp 321-367

Meites J, Clemens JA (1972) Hypothalmic control of prolactin secretion. Vitam Horm 30: 165-221

Muldoon TG (1986) Steroid hormone receptor regulation by various hormonal factors during mammary development and growth in the normal mouse. Ann NY Acad Sci 464: 17-36

Munford RE (1963) Changes in the mammary glands of rats and mice during pregnancy, lactation and involution (2) Levels of deoxyribonucleic acid, and alkaline and acid phosphatase. J Endocrinol 28: 17-34

Nagasawa H, Yanai R (1971a) Increased mammary gland response to pituitary mammotrophic hormones by estrogen in rats. Endocrinol Jpn 17: 53-56

Nagasawa H, Yanai R (1971b) Quantitative participation of placental mammotrophic hormones in mammary development during pregnancy of mice. Endocrinol Jpn 18: 507-510

Nagasawa H, Yanai R (1976) Mammary nucleic acids and pituitary prolactin secretion during prolonged lactation in mice. J Endocrinol 70: 389-395

Nelson WL, Heytler PG, Ciaccio EI (1962) Guinea-pig mammary gland growth changes in weight, nitrogen and nucleic acids. Proc Soc Exp Biol Med 109: 373-375

Ota K (1964) Mammary involution and engorgement after arrest of suckling in lactating rats indicated by the contents of nucleic acids and milk protein of the gland. Endocrinol Jpn 11: 146-152

Peaker M (1980) The effect of raised intramammary pressure on mammary function in the goat in relation to the cessation of lactation. J Physiol (Lond) 301: 415-428

Pitkow HS, Reece RP, Waszilycsak GL (1972) The integrity of mammary alveolar cells in two consecutive lactations. Proc Soc Exp Biol Med 139: 845-850

Ray EW, Averill SC, Lyons WR, Johnson RE (1955) Rat placental hormonal activities corresponding to those of pituitary mammotrophin. Endocrinology 56: 359-373

Roth LL, Rosenblatt JS (1968) Self-licking and mammary development during pregnancy in the rat. J Endocrinol 42: 363-378

Russo IH, Russo J (1986) From pathogenesis to hormone prevention of mammary carcinogenesis. Cancer Surv 5: 649-670

Russo IH, Al-Rayess M, Sabharwal S (1985a) Effect of contraceptive agents on mammary gland structure and susceptibility to carcinogenesis. Proc Am Assoc Cancer Res 26: 460a

Russo IH, Al-Rayess M, Russo J (1985b) Role of contraceptive agents in breast cancer prevention. Biennial Int Breast Cancer Res Conf, London, March 24-28, p 87

Russo IH, Pokorzynski T, Russo J (1986) Contraceptives as hormone-preventive agents in mammary carcinogenesis. Proc Am Assoc Cancer Res 27: 912a

Russo J, Russo IH (1978) DNA-labeling index and structure of the rat mammary gland as determinants of its susceptibility to carcinogenesis. JNCI 61: 1451-1459

Russo J, Russo IH (1987a) Biological and molecular bases of mammary carcinogenesis. Lab Invest 57: 112-137

Russo J, Russo IH (1987b) Development of the human mammary gland. In: Neville MC, Daniel CW (eds) The mammary gland. Plenum, New York, pp 67-93

Russo J, Russo IH, Ireland M, Saby J (1977) Increased resistance of multiparous rat mammary gland to neoplastic transformation by 7,12-dimethylbenz(a)-anthracene. Proc Am Assoc Cancer Res 18: 149a

Russo J, Wilgus G, Russo IH (1979) Susceptibility of the mammary gland to carcinogenesis. I. Differentiation of the mammary gland as determinant of tumor incidence and type of lesion. Am J Pathol 96: 721-736

Russo J, Tay LK, Russo IH (1982) Differentiation of the mammary gland and susceptibility to carcinogenesis. Breast Cancer Res Treat 2: 5–73

Russo J, Tait L, Russo IH (1983) Susceptibility of the mammary gland to carcinogenesis. III. The cell of origin of rat mammary carcinoma. Am J Pathol 113: 50–66

Sakakura T, Nishizuka Y, Dawe CJ (1979) Capacity of mammary fat pads of adult C3H/HeMs mice to interact morphogenetically with fetal mammary epithelium. JNCI 63: 733–736

Traurig HH (1967) A radioautographic study of cell proliferation in the mammary gland of the pregnant mouse. Anat Rec 159: 239–247

Vonderhaar BK, Greco AE (1979) Lobulo-alveolar development of mouse mammary glands is regulated by thyroid hormones. Endocrinology 104: 409–418

Wada H, Turner CW (1959) Effect of recurring pregnancy on mammary gland growth in mice. J Dairy Sci 42: 1198–1202

Wasner G, Hennermann I, Kratochwil K (1983) Ontogeny of mesenchymal androgen receptors in the embryonic mouse mammary gland. Endocrinology 113: 1771–1780

Wheelock JV, Dodd FH (1969) Non-nutritional factors affecting milk yield in dairy cattle. J Dairy Res 36: 479–493

Wide L, Hobson B, Wide M (1980) Chorionic gonadotropin in rodents. In: Segal SJ (ed) Chorionic gonadotropin. Plenum, New York, pp 37–51

Histologic/Immunocytochemical Markers, Mammary Gland, Rat

Barry A. Gusterson, Michael J. Warburton, and Paul Monaghan

Introduction

Recent ultrastructural and immunocytochemical evidence indicates that within the normal female rat breast the epithelial component consists of two distinctive cell types – a luminal epithelial cell and an outer layer of myoepithelial (basal) cells. During development there are, in addition, intermediary forms identifiable in the terminal end bud structures (Williams and Daniel 1983). In the breast there is an intimate structural and functional interaction between these epithelial cells and the surrounding stroma. Much effort has therefore been put into producing markers for the cell types in the breast and the identification of the distribution of the components of the extracellular matrix. On the basis of a better understanding of the structure of the normal breast it is then possible to characterize the tumors that arise from the epithelial component and to identify the cell types involved in the early stages of carcinogenesis. This section considers some of the recent developments in immunocytochemical markers that are of value in the normal rat breast and lays the foundation for the paper following on p. 314 in which the application of these reagents to chemical carcinogen-induced rat mammary tumors is considered.

Histology of the Rat Mammary Gland

In the resting state the mammary epithelium, composed of luminal epithelial cells and an outer myoepithelial layer, is separated from the surrounding mesenchymal cells and connective tissue by the basement membrane. Early studies relied upon the use of enzyme histochemical techniques or nonspecific staining methods to identify the major cellular and matrix components (Dempsey et al. 1947; Hamperl 1970). The most useful markers of myoepithelial cells were alkaline phosphatase and Coomassie blue, the latter identifying the myofilaments present within the cytoplasm. Adenosine triphosphatase (ATPase) activity is present in the breast in two forms. Mg^{2+}-dependent ATPase is found in both luminal epithelial and myoepithelial cells, whereas Na^+/K^+-dependent ATPase is generally confined to myoepithelial cells (Russo and Wells 1977). The periodic acid-Schiff (PAS) technique delineates the basement membrane.

Biochemical analyses of the cellular components of the breast and of the extracellular matrix have recently identified a number of components of these structures, and well-characterized antibodies that recognize these components are now permitting a more defined assessment at the immunohistochemical level.

Luminal Epithelial Cells

A number of markers are available for the luminal epithelial cells of the breast which react with either membrane or cytoplasmic components. Peanut lectin is a useful reagent in this context as are antisera to the milk fat globule membrane (MFGM) both of which specifically stain the luminal surface of the epithelial cells (Fig. 363). In the lactating gland, both the membrane and the cytoplasm of the secretory cells are stained using MFGM-specific antiserum, whereas in the involuting gland, the staining is confined to the luminal surface and the lumen contents (Fig. 369). Antisera which recognize the enzyme thioesterase II have been shown to be useful cytoplasmic markers for epithelial cells in the rat breast (Pasco et al. 1983).

Recently, it has become clear that the protein constituents of the cytoskeleton of cells can be used as cellular markers, and much effort has been directed towards producing specific antibodies against these components. These reagents can then be used to define individual cell populations.

Originally, five classes of intermediate filaments (cytoskeletal elements) were described (Lazarides 1980), but more recently on the basis of cDNA and protein analysis (Steinert and Parry 1985) these filaments have been divided into four major groups (see Table 20), which define the major cell types within tissues. The keratins, which are encompassed in the intermediate filament groups type I and type II, have been further categorized by Moll et al. (1982) who have classified keratins 1–19 based on their size and charge. Using this nomenclature, keratins 1–8 are within the type II group and keratins 9–19 are in type I. In epithelial cells, where keratins are the cytoskeletal element, the typical 10-nm filaments are formed only when a keratin polypeptide from both type I and type II are co-expressed in the same cell. Individual epithelia express a re-

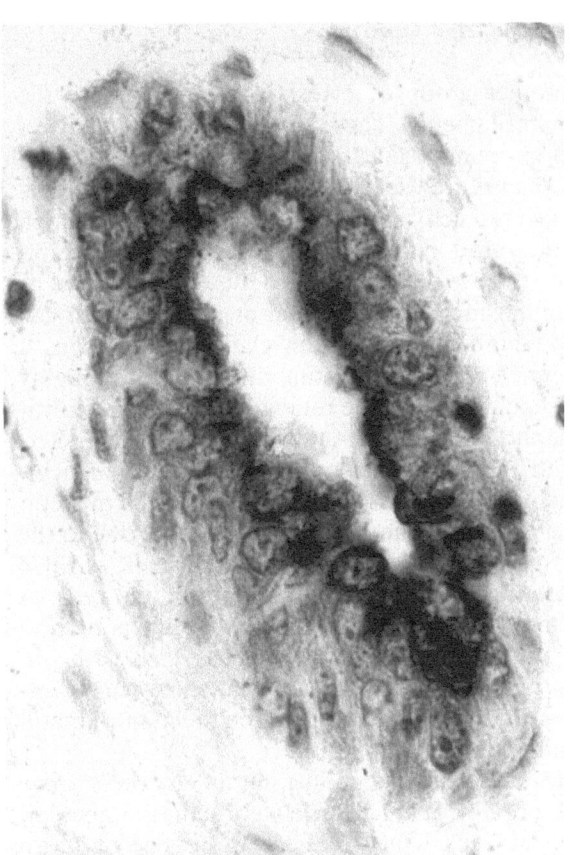

Fig. 363. Resting rat mammary gland stained with milk fat globule membrane-specific antibodies. The luminal membrane of the epithelial cells is intensely stained. × 1200

stricted pattern of these keratin polypeptides, thus enabling a classification of epithelial cells based upon their cytokeratin content. It is also of interest that, with minor variations, the keratins are highly conserved across species. Thus, the keratins present in the human breast find close parallels in the rodent, although differences in physiology and development may be reflected in differential cytokeratin expression. It is now becoming clear that certain keratin polypeptides can be identified as being characteristic of different cell types. Two antibodies, LE61 and LE65, which react with keratin 18, have been shown to stain selectively luminal cells in the rat and mouse breast (Lane 1982; Lane and Klymkowsky 1982), while other antibodies described later can be used to define the myoepithelial layer. Allen et al. (1984), using markers for basal (myoepithelial) cells (1A10) and for luminal cells (24B42), have demonstrated the use of the luminal marker to define the cells in the epidermis which are the "precursors" of the developing mammary gland.

Table 20. Classification of intermediate filaments

Group	Filament	Cells
Type I	Keratin (9–19)	Epithelium
Type II	Keratin (1–8)	Epithelium
Type III	Vimentin	Mesen-
	Desmin	chyme
	Glial fibrillary acidic protein	Muscle
		Astrocytes
Type IV	Neurofilaments	Neurones

Myoepithelial Cells

Another group of cytoskeletal proteins are the microfilaments. These are 4–6 nm in diameter and contain actin and myosin. Although microfilaments are widely distributed among epithelial and mesenchymal cells, they are found in high concentration in myoepithelial cells, thus permitting the use of antibodies to these components as cellular markers. The basal or myoepithelial cell population in the human gland also contains a defined set of cytokeratins, and this will probably be equally true in the rodent (Taylor-Papadimitriou and Lane 1987). Antibody LP34, which reacts with both luminal epithelial cells and myoepithelial cells in the human, is restricted to myoepithelial cells in the rat. This is probably due to the absence of keratin 18 in rat luminal cells, as LP34 identifies this keratin in human luminal cells. A polyclonal antibody produced by our laboratory is also a very good marker of basal cells in the rat breast, presumably because it reacts with keratins 5 or 14 which appear to be the major keratin pair in this situation.

More recently some membrane markers have been defined which selectively stain the myoepithelial cells. One of these is pokeweed lectin which also reacts with vascular endothelium (Leatham et al. 1983). The common acute lymphoblastic leukemia antigen (CALLA) is also expressed on myoepithelial cells in both humans and rats (Gusterson et al. 1986).

Using such reagents, the processes of myoepithelial cells appear to be continuous around both ducts and alveolar buds in the resting gland (Fig. 364). During pregnancy the myoepithelial cell processes, as visualized by staining with the appropriate keratin-specific or myosin-specific serum, are prominent in the main ducts but appear attenuated and discontinuous in the alveoli. In lactating glands, the myoepithelial cells are even more attenuated, with large gaps between the cells, whereas in the involuting gland the myoepithelial cells are distorted around the collapsed alveoli and gaps between adjacent cells can be clearly seen (Fig. 370).

Basement Membrane and Stroma

The basement membrane can be seen at the ultrastructural level as an electron-lucent layer, the lamina lucida, directly adjacent to the epithelial and myoepithelial cells, and an electron-dense layer, the lamina densa, located between the lamina lucida and the connective tissue. In the rat mammary gland, laminin and type IV collagen are constituents of the basement membrane at all stages of development, whereas fibronectin and type V collagen are present only in the alveolar basement membrane region during lactation (Warburton et al. 1982). Entactin, a sulphated glycoprotein, is present in the basement membrane of the secretory alveoli in the lactating mammary gland but is absent from this structure in the resting gland (Warburton et al. 1984). Some of these basement membrane and basal surface-associated proteins are also found within the stroma; for example, fibronectin and type V collagen are both constituents of vascular basement membranes and the interstitial connective tissue throughout all developmental phases in the rat. Similarly, entactin is found associated with interstitial collagen.

The best basement membrane markers are laminin and type IV collagen which can be immunocytochemically localized to the basement membrane surrounding the ductal system and the blood vessels. The basement membrane, as visualized by these two markers, appears to be continuous around both ducts and alveoli, and in some cases can be clearly seen to interdigitate between the myoepithelial cells (Figs. 365 and 366). In mature virgin rats there is no cytoplasmic staining for type IV collagen or laminin, but in the terminal end buds of the developing gland cytoplasmic staining can be seen for both of these proteins, probably indicating local synthesis at this stage of development (Ormerod and Rudland 1984). Both fibronectin and type I collagen can be identified in tissue sections using the appropriate antibodies. Fibronectin is localized throughout the stroma, while type I collagen appears to be concentrated beneath the basement membrane.

During pregnancy the basement membrane, as visualized with laminin-specific or type IV collagen-specific antibodies, remains continuous around the ducts and acini (Fig. 367). During lactation there is little change in the distribution of these constituents (Fig. 368); however, fibronectin now appears to be distributed in a similar pattern to type IV collagen in addition to being a component of the connective tissue. In the involuting gland the basement membrane appears to be thickened, and there is diffuse staining of the distorted cellular clusters with basement membrane antibodies (Figs. 371 and 372).

Although the staining of the basal lamina with antisera to type IV collagen and laminin appears

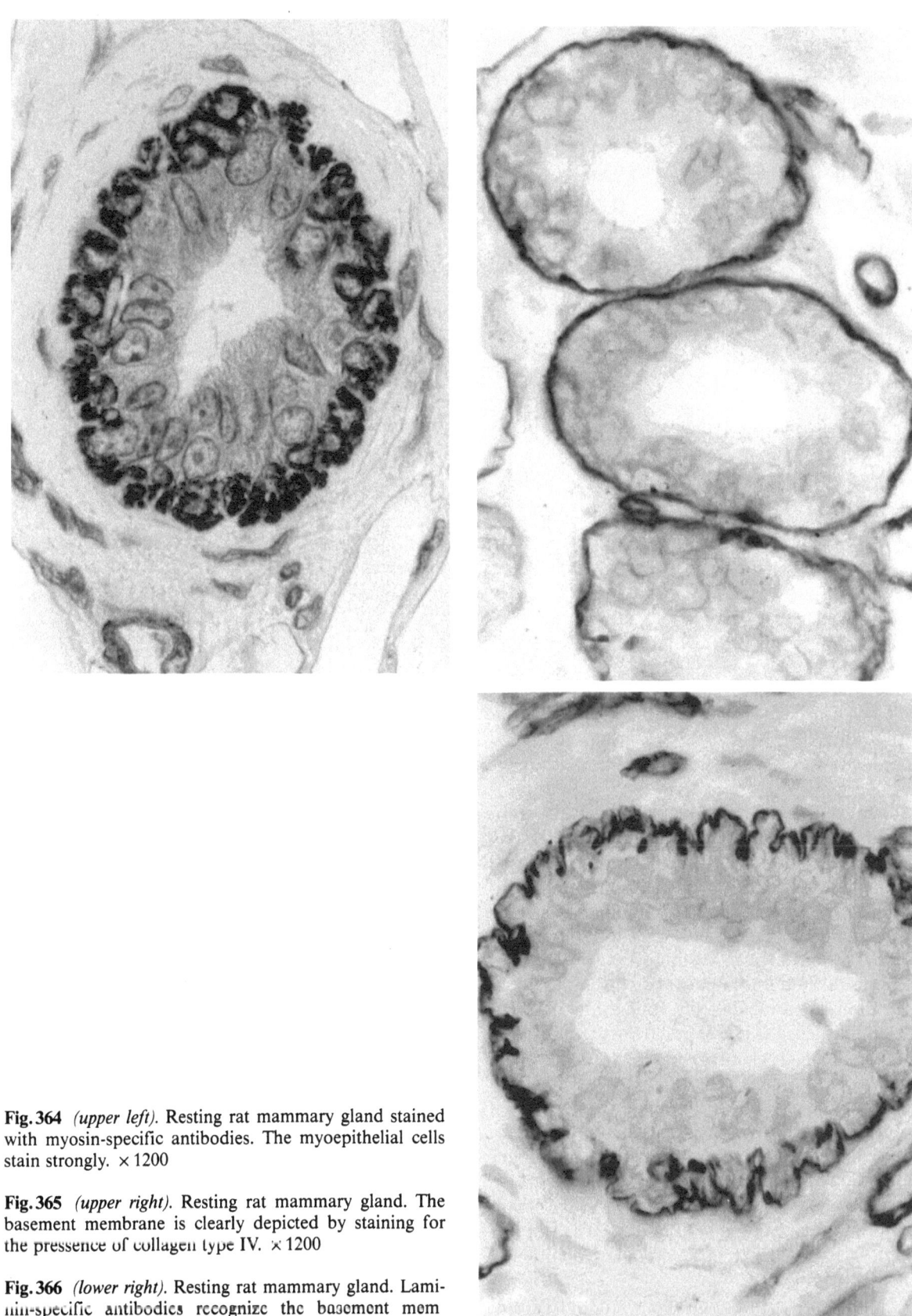

Fig. 364 *(upper left).* Resting rat mammary gland stained with myosin-specific antibodies. The myoepithelial cells stain strongly. × 1200

Fig. 365 *(upper right).* Resting rat mammary gland. The basement membrane is clearly depicted by staining for the presence of collagen type IV. × 1200

Fig. 366 *(lower right).* Resting rat mammary gland. Laminin-specific antibodies recognize the basement membrane, giving a similar pattern to collagen type IV-specific antibodies (Fig. 365). × 1000

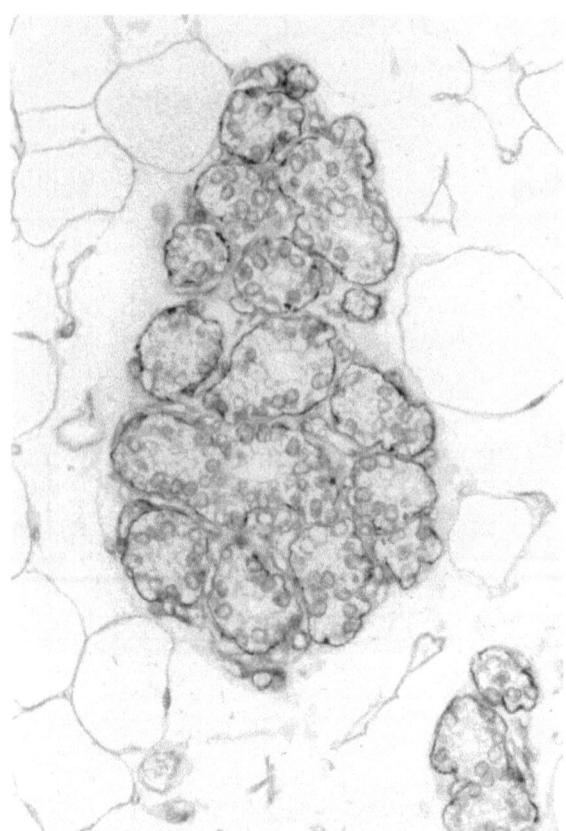

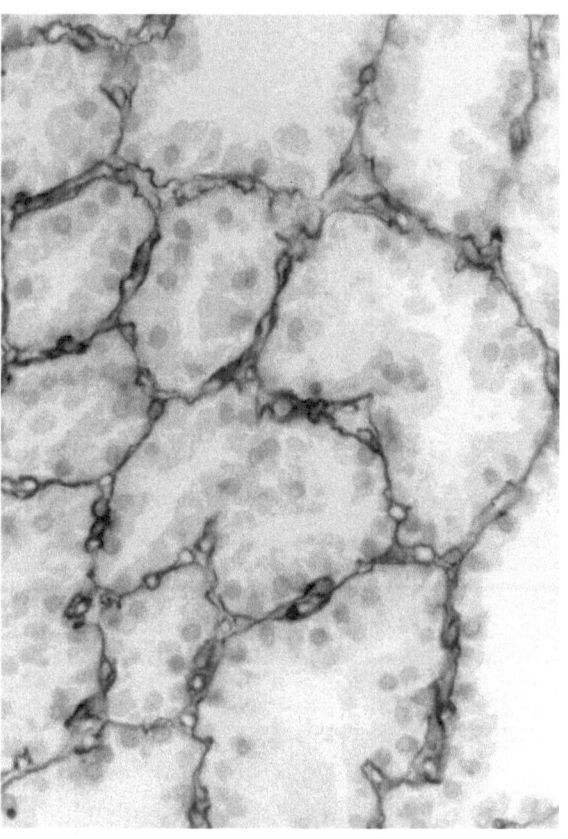

Fig. 367. Pregnant rat mammary gland. The basement membrane remains intact as shown by staining with laminin-specific antibodies. × 300

Fig. 368. Lactating rat mammary gland. Collagen type IV-specific antibody stain. × 400

uniform at the light microscope level, its complexity of organization is revealed by observing the staining patterns at the ultrastructural level (Monaghan et al. 1983). Thus, although the lamina densa in the rat lactating mammary gland is stained uniformly with antibodies to laminin and type IV collagen, both of these constituents are also present in the semiperiodic clusters that traverse the lamina lucida from the basal surface to the lamina densa (Fig. 373). Ultrastructural localization of entactin demonstrates it on the basal surface of epithelial cells and also within both the lamina densa and the lamina lucida (Warburton et al. 1984). Type V collagen is predominantly a matrix protein, but in the rat mammary gland it has been described on the basal surface of epithelial cells where they abut the basement membrane (Warburton et al. 1983). It is not apparent on the basal surface of myoepithelial cells.

The contribution of immunohistochemistry and ultrastructural techniques has also enabled identification of a dendritic cell within the breast epi-

Fig. 369 *(upper left)*. Lactating rat mammary gland. Milk ▶ fat globule membrane-specific antibodies depict the epithelial cell luminal membranes and lumen contents. × 500

Fig. 370 *(lower left)*. Involuting rat mammary gland. The disorganized myoepithelial cells are clearly seen stained with myosin-specific antibodies. × 600

Fig. 371 *(upper right)*. Involuting rat mammary gland. The basement membrane is distorted with focal thickening. Collagen type IV-specific antibodies. × 400

Fig. 372 *(lower right)*. Involuting rat mammary gland. The irregularities in the basement membrane are also seen with laminin-specific antibodies. × 1000

thelium of the rat (Fig. 374) bearing a close similarity to Langerhans' cells in the skin (Joshi et al. 1985). The extensive processes of these dendritic cells are only readily detected by the immunocytochemical localization of the cell membrane using Ia-specific antibodies.

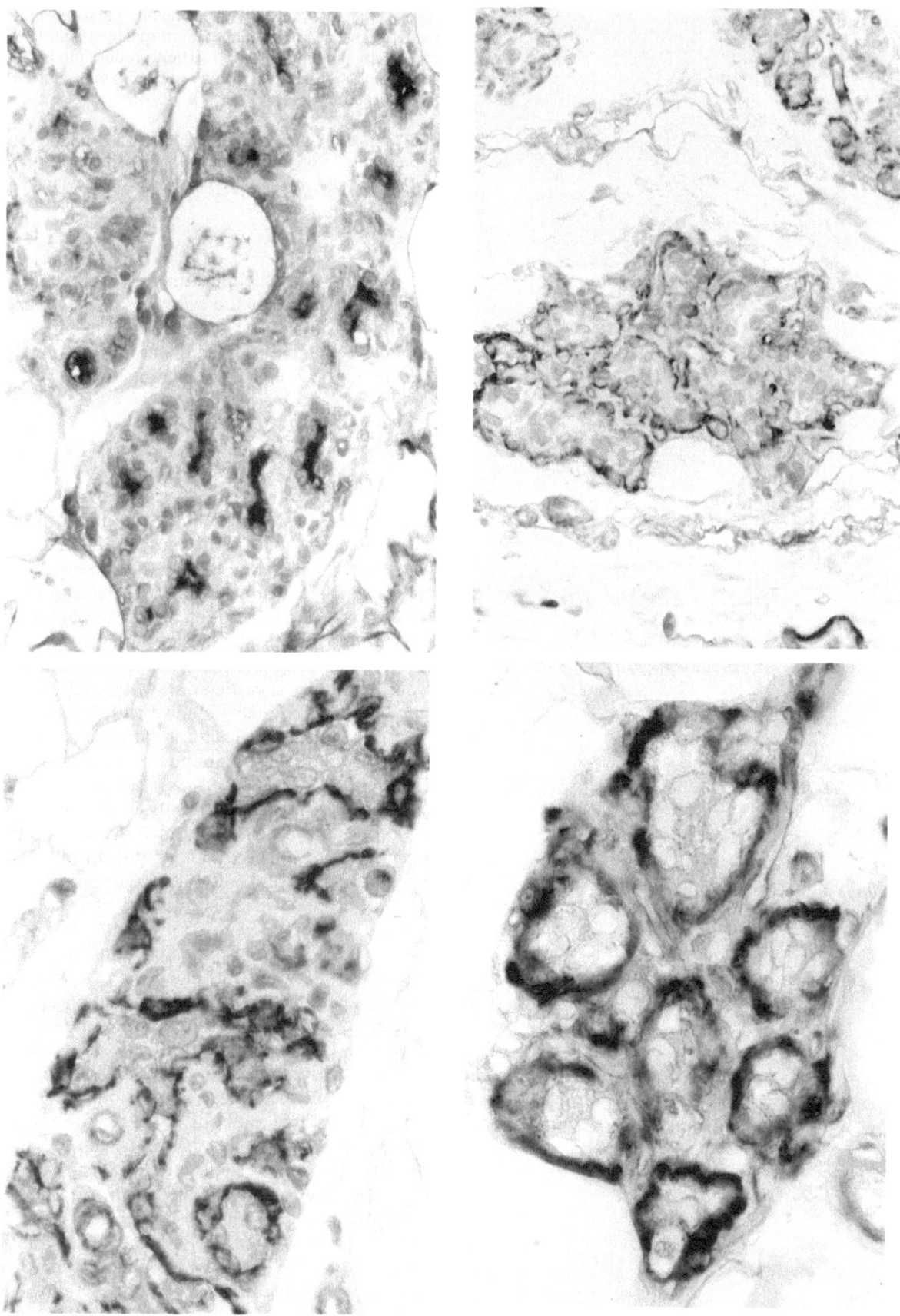

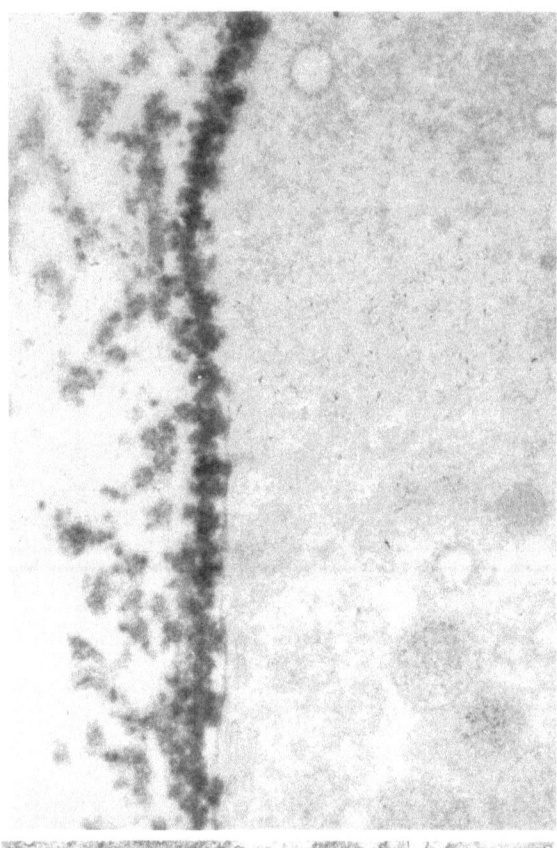

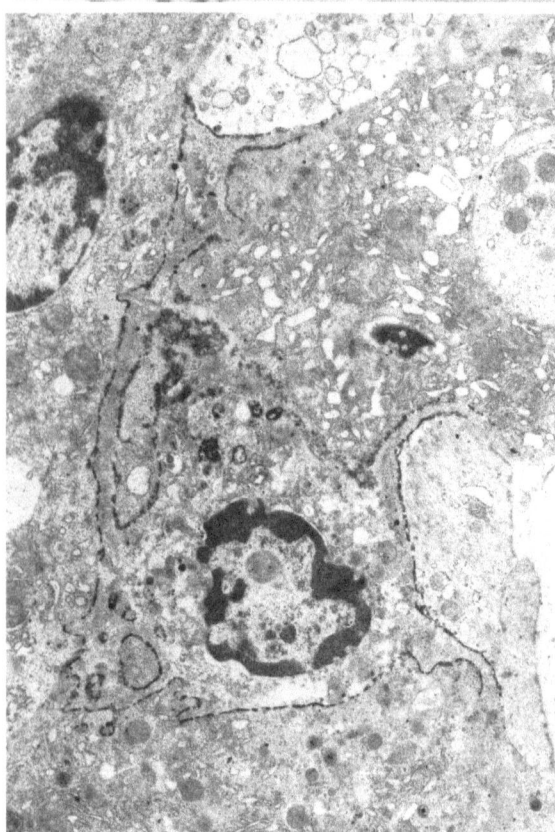

◀ **Fig. 373** *(above)*. Lactating rat mammary gland. Electron micrograph showing staining pattern obtained with laminin-specific antibodies, with reaction product present in the lamina densa and focally in the lamina lucida. × 45 000

Fig. 374 *(below)*. Electron micrograph of a dendritic cell in pregnant rat breast. The immunoperoxidase reaction product clearly outlines the dendritic cell membranes. × 8000

These immunocytochemical markers can be used to define more clearly the cell types in the breast and the constituents of the basement membrane and connective tissue in both the normal gland and the tumors which arise from it.

Immunocytochemical Techniques Used

Light Microscopy. It is our experience that methacarn fixation (60% methanol, 30% chloroform, and 10% acetic acid) is the most useful fixative for tissues which are subsequently to be studied immunocytochemically. Tissues are cut into thin slices (1 mm thick) and fixed at 4 °C for 24 h prior to undergoing a standard processing procedure and embedding in paraffin wax. All staining in our laboratory is carried out by the indirect alkaline phosphatase technique which is simple to use and produces sufficient amplification of the signal for the relatively abundant antigens to be identified.

For staining using antibodies to cytokeratins, fibronectin, and the basement membrane components type IV collagen and laminin, prior pronase treatment is often advisable. Our protocol is to incubate the dewaxed sections with phosphate buffered saline (PBS) at 37 °C for 15 min followed by a further 15-min incubation at 37 °C with trypsin (0.05 mg/ml) or collagenase (Sigma type VI, 0.1 mg/ml) for fibronectin staining. This is followed by rinsing in running tap water.

All sections are then treated with 15% acetic acid for 5 min to inhibit endogenous alkaline phosphatase. After washing in PBS, sections are incubated with the first antibody at the required dilution in PBS for 1½ h at room temperature. Sections are then washed with PBS containing 0.01% Tween 80 and incubated with the appropriate alkaline phosphatase-conjugated second antibody [diluted with 0.5% bovine serum albumin (BSA) in PBS] at room temperature for 1 h. Sections are then rewashed with PBS followed by water and then incubated with naphthol AS

B1 phosphate (0.5 mg/ml) and fast red TR (0.5 mg/ml) in veronal buffer, ph 9.2 at room temperature for 1 h. After further rinsing in running water, sections are counterstained with Mayer's hemalum and mounted in buffered glycerin jelly. To accentuate the staining for black and white photomicrography it is advisable to use a green filter.

Ultrastructural Immunocytochemistry. Many antigens that are studied in the breast do not survive aldehyde fixation. For membrane and extracellular antigens, satisfactory results can be obtained using a pre-embedding staining procedure. Lobulo-alveolar units are dissected from the surrounding stroma and incubated with the required antibody at room temperature for 2 h, washed for 15 min in PBS, and then incubated with an appropriately screened antibody conjugated to horseradish peroxidase for 2 h at room temperature. For pre-embedding staining in this tissue, colloidal gold conjugates appear to have less ability to penetrate the tissue and give markedly reduced antigen localization. The tissue is then rinsed with PBS and incubated for 5 min with 0.05% diaminobenzidine and 0.06% hydrogen peroxide in PBS. At this stage tissue can be fixed in 2% glutaraldehyde and postfixed in 1% osmium tetroxide for 16 h at 4°C. Tissues are then processed for electron microscopy using the method previously described (Monaghan et al. 1984).

Other ultrastructural techniques that are suitable for immunolocalization have been described in detail elsewhere (Polak and Van Noorden 1986).

Controls

1. No staining should be present if the staining schedule is followed with the first antibody omitted. This excludes staining due to the second antibody and endogenous alkaline phosphatase or peroxidase activity (depending upon the system used).
2. Staining should be totally extinguished by prior incubation of the antisera with the appropriate antigen (1 mg/ml) at 37°C for 3 h.

References

Allen R, Dulbecco R, Syka P, Bowman M, Armstrong B (1984) Developmental regulation of cytokeratins in cells of the rat mammary gland studied with monoclonal antibodies. Proc Natl Acad Sci USA 81: 1203–1207

Dempsey EW, Bunting H, Wislocki GB (1947) Observations on the chemical cytology of the mammary gland. Am J Anat 81: 309–341

Gusterson BA, Monaghan P, Mahendran R, Ellis J, O'Hare MJ (1986) Identification of myoepithelial cells in human and rat breasts by anti-common acute lymphoblastic leukemia antigen antibody A12. JNCI 77: 343–349

Hamperl H (1970) The myothelia (myoepithelial cells): Normal state; regressive changes; hyperplasia; tumors. Curr Top Pathol 53: 161–220

Joshi K, Monaghan P, Neville AM (1985) Ultrastructural identification of Ia positive dendritic cells in the lactating rat mammary gland. Virchows Arch [A] 406: 17–25

Lane EB (1982) Monoclonal antibodies provide specific intramolecular markers for the study of epithelial tonofilament organization. J Cell Biol 92: 665–673

Lane EB, Klymkowsky MW (1982) Epithelial tonofilaments: investigating their form and function using monoclonal antibodies. Cold Spring Harbor Symp Quant Biol 46: 387–402

Lazarides E (1980) Intermediate filaments as mechanical integrators of cellular space. Nature 283: 249–256

Leatham A, Dokal I, Atkins N (1983) Lectin binding to normal and malignant breast tissue. Diagn Histopathol 6: 171–180

Moll R, Franke WW, Schiller DL, Geiger B, Krepler R (1982) The catalog of human cytokeratins: patterns of expression in normal epithelia, tumors and cultured cells. Cell 31: 11–24

Monaghan P, Warburton MJ, Perusinghe N, Rudland PS (1983) Topographical arrangement of basement membrane proteins in lactating rat mammary gland: comparison of the distribution of type IV collagen, laminin, fibronectin, and Thy.1 at the ultrastructural level. Proc Natl Acad Sci USA 80: 3344–3348

Monaghan P, Sappino AP, Roberts JDB, Knight MA, Ellis J, Nakajima T (1984) Monoclonal antibody LICR-LON-E36 recognizes gonadotrophs in female rat pituitaries. J Histochem Cytochem 32: 1048–1054

Ormerod EJ, Rudland PS (1984) Cellular composition and organization of ductal buds in developing rat mammary glands: Evidence for morphological intermediates between epithelial and myoepithelial cells. Am J Anat 170: 631–652

Pasco D, Smith S, Quan A, Richards J, Nandi S (1983) The use of thioesterase II as a rat mammary epithelial cell-specific marker. Cell Tissue Res 234: 57–70

Polak JM, Van Noorden S (1986) Immunocytochemistry – modern methods and applications, 2nd edn. PSG, Littleton MA

Russo J, Wells P (1977) Ultrastructural localizations of adenosine triphosphatase activity in resting mammary gland. J Histochem Cytochem 25 (2): 135–148

Steinert PM, Parry DAD (1985) Intermediate filaments: conformity and diversity of expression and structure. Ann Rev Cell Biol 1: 41–65

Taylor-Papadimitriou J, Lane EB (1987) Keratin expression in the mammary gland. In: Neville MC, Daniel CW (eds) The mammary gland: development, regulation and function. Plenum, New York, pp 181–215

Warburton MJ, Mitchell D, Ormerod EJ, Rudland PS (1982) Distribution of myoepithelial cells and basement membrane proteins in the resting, pregnant, lactating, and involuting rat mammary gland. J Histochem Cytochem 30 (7): 667-676

Warburton MJ, Monaghan P, Ferns SA, Hughes CM, Rudland PS (1983) Distribution and synthesis of type V collagen in the rat mammary gland. J Histochem Cytochem 31: 1265-1273

Warburton MJ, Monaghan P, Ferns SA, Rudland PS, Perusinghe N, Chung AE (1984) Distribution of entactin in the basement membrane of the rat mammary gland. Exp Cell Res 152: 240-254

Williams JM, Daniel CW (1983) Mammary ductal elongation: differentiation of myoepithelial and basal lamina during branching morphogenesis. Dev Biol 97: 274-290

Classification of Neoplastic and Nonneoplastic Lesions of the Rat Mammary Gland

Jose Russo, Irma H. Russo, Mathew J. van Zwieten, Adrianne E. Rogers, and Barry A. Gusterson

Introduction

The rat mammary gland is one of the most widely studied and useful models of mammary carcinogenesis (Dao 1962, 1964; Gullino et al. 1975; Huggins et al. 1959; Huggins and Yang 1962; Ito 1981; Russo IH and Russo J 1978; Russo J and Russo IH 1978, 1980; Russo J et al. 1982; Shirai et al. 1981; Van Zwieten 1984; Young and Hallowes 1973). Many strains of rats develop spontaneous tumors and respond to a variety of chemical carcinogens and radiation with the development of hormone-dependent mammary tumors. The classification presented attempts to provide a working framework for diagnosing the type of lesions found in the mammary glands of rats treated with chemical carcinogens or radiation, and to clarify criteria for establishing two basic characteristics of tumors: (a) whether they are epithelial or stromal in origin, and (b) whether they are benign or malignant.

This classification (Table 21) is based upon a pathogenetic concept. It may be too broad for the histopathologist or too detailed for those that need to evaluate tumorigenic response in carcinogenic testing. However, this classification should begin to fill the need for definitive parameters for establishing tumor type and malignancy. One important message that we try to convey is that, whatever the final use or need that researchers have for classifying mammary tumors in the rat, histological study is mandatory.

In those situations in which it is necessary to simplify or combine related categories – for instance, in order to utilize statistical data – a working classification scheme is proposed (Table 22). The definitive histological criteria used in the scheme are the same as in Table 21, but many of the detailed and descriptive categories are not used.

Table 21. Classification of rat mammary gland tumors

I. *Epithelial neoplasms*
 A. Benign lesions
  1. Intraductal papilloma
  2. Papillary cystadenoma
  3. Adenoma
   (a) Tubular
   (b) Lactating
 B. Malignant lesions
  1. Noninvasive carcinoma
   (a) Ductal papillary
   (b) Ductal cribriform
   (c) Ductal comedo
  2. Invasive carcinoma
   (a) Papillary
   (b) Cribriform
   (c) Comedo
   (d) Tubular

II. *Stromal neoplasms*
 A. Benign: Fibroma
 B. Malignant: Fibrosarcoma

III. *Epithelial-stromal neoplasms*
 A. Benign: Fibroadenoma
 B. Malignant: Carcinosarcoma

IV. *Nonneoplastic lesions*
  Cystic changes
  (a) Ductal
  (b) Lobular

Table 22. Consolidated classification of rat mammary tumors

I. Epithelial neoplasms
 A. Benign (papilloma, adenoma)
 B. Malignant (carcinoma)

II. Stromal neoplasms
 A. Benign (fibroma)
 B. Malignant (fibrosarcoma)

III. Epithelial-stromal neoplasms
 A. Benign (fibroadenoma)
 B. Malignant (carcinosarcoma)

IV. Nonneoplastic lesions

Histological Classification of Mammary Gland Tumors

Rat mammary tumors may be composed of a single histologic type or of combinations of several patterns. In Table 21 are depicted the main histological types of mammary tumors found in the rat.

Epithelial Neoplasms

Benign Lesions

Intraductal Papilloma. Lesions that are circumscribed by a fibrous stromal reaction and are characterized by papillary projections which protrude into the dilated ductal lumens are intraductal papillomas. The papillae are composed of a fibrous core lined by a single layer of cuboidal or low cylindrical epithelial cells that in some areas appear pseudostratified. In Fig. 406 one can see a typical benign intraductal papilloma. Some intraductal papillomas appear to be composed of interconnecting bridges of connective tissue, with the free surfaces lined by a single layer of tall columnar cells, and occasinally myoepithelial cells are also seen. The epithelial cells are homogeneous in size and shape; they have leptochromatic nuclei, and the nucleolus is either absent or small and inconspicuous. The cells of these papillary lesions (Fig. 407 and 409) are less pleomorphic than those observed in the papillary carcinoma, shown in Figs. 410–413. Some cellular atypia and mitoses may be present. These lesions may evolve from the classical intraductal papilloma shown in Fig. 406.

Papillary Cystadenoma. Well-circumscribed lesions that are composed of papillary projections protruding into cystic spaces are papillary cystadenomas (Fig. 375). The papillae are lined by a single, double, or pseudostratified layer of low columnar epithelial cells; the lining cells may have small projections or "snouts" that give the epithelium an apocrine appearance (Fig. 377). The basal layer is low cuboidal. Cells with small, hyperchromatic nuclei may be desquamated into the lumen or the markedly edematous core (Fig. 376).

Adenomas. Rat mammary gland adenomas are benign epithelial neoplasms that form glandular patterns of two types: tubular and lactating. Tubular ones are characterized by proliferation of

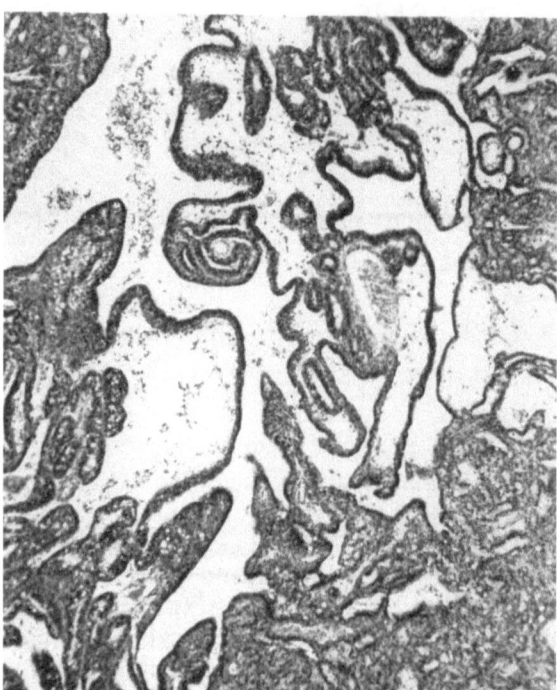

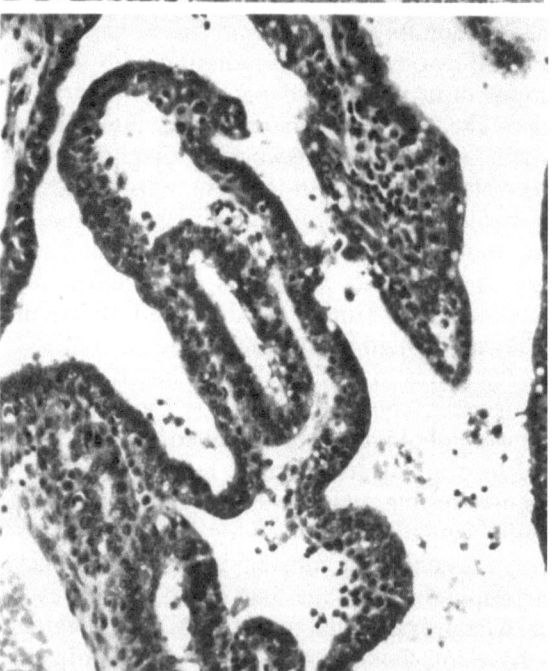

Fig. 375 *(above).* Papillary cystadenoma of the mammary gland. Papillae lined by epithelial cells project toward a cystic cavity. The fibroconnective tissue in the papillary core is edematous. H and E, × 60

Fig. 376 *(below).* Detail of a papilla in a cystadenoma. The edematous core of the papillae is infiltrated by lymphocytes and contains cell detritus, which is also seen in the cystic lumen. H and E, × 150

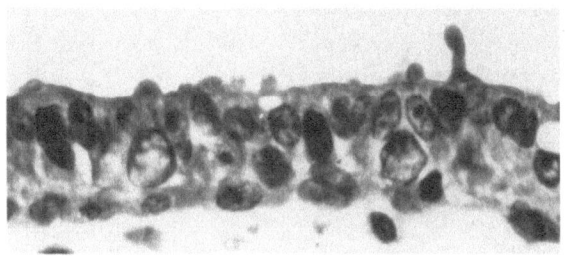

Fig. 377. Epithelium lining the papillae of the tumor shown in Figs. 375 and 376. The cells are tall, columnar, with round to oval nuclei. There are cytoplasmic projections at the luminal surface. The basal layer is composed of smaller cells. H and E, × 400

tubular or alveolar structures arranged in clusters and separated by scanty connective tissue (Figs. 378–380). The lesions consist of an increase in the number of individual alveoli, giving an appearance suggestive of a larger lobule with more alveoli than usual. Individual alveoli are lined by low cuboidal epithelial cells arranged in a single layer and may have a secretion-filled lumen. Epithelial cells have small nuclei with one, small, inconspicuous nucleolus (Fig. 383). In some tubular adenomas of older animals, mainly those located in inguinal mammary glands, a more atypical appearance of the cells lining the alveoli is observed; this phenomenon could represent an early transition to adenocarcinoma (Fig. 380). In Fig. 384 can be seen the larger nuclei with coarser chromatin and prominent nucleoli that characterize the adenocarcinoma, in contrast to the appearance of ductal cells (Fig. 382) and tubular adenoma (Fig. 383). The lumen of the alveoli composing a tubular adenoma is round and smooth, while the lactating adenoma (Fig. 381) has a serrated lumen due to cell decapitation or supranuclear vacuolization. Lactating adenomas

vary from small ones measuring less than 1 mm in diameter (Fig. 385), that are indistinguishable from hyperplastic lobules, to ones greater than 2 cm. The secretion-filled alveoli are lined by a single layer of low cuboidal epithelium with basal nuclei and vacuolated cytoplasm (Figs. 386–389). Each individual alveolus is surrounded by a thin layer of connective tissue, whose amount progressively increases from the adenoma to the fibroadenoma. Lactating adenomas exhibit marked variation in the size of individual alveoli, some of which acquire large dimensions due to accumulations of secretion fluid, eventually forming cysts, with flattening of the lining epithelium (Figs. 388–390).

Malignant Lesions

Noninvasive Carcinomas. The earliest change observed in the mammary parenchym after carcinogen treatment of virgin rats is the dilatation of terminal ductal structures and multilayering of the epithelial lining, which may be up to six layers thick (Fig. 391). The cells have a large, round nucleus, prominent nucleoli, and coarse chromatin along the inner leaflet of the nuclear membrane (Figs. 396 and 397). These early lesions, intraductal proliferations (IDPs) (Russo J et al. 1977), represent the transition between the normal terminal and bud (TEB) (Russo J et al. 1977, 1979) and carcinoma in situ; the criteria for identifying these three types of structures are outlined in Table 23. IDPs appear to evolve into carcinoma in situ through the development of: (a) micropapillae, which might be the only pattern present (Figs. 392–395) or combined with cribriform pattern (Fig. 394); (b) pseudolumina, forming a cribriform pattern (Figs. 398–401); or (c) a comedo pattern (Fig. 402–405; Table 23).

Table 23. Differential diagnosis of terminal end bud (TEB), intraductal proliferation (IDP), and carcinoma in situ (CIS)

Components	TEB	IDP	CIS
Basement membrane	Present	Present	Present
Surrounding stroma	Normal	Moderate desmoplastic reaction	Marked desmoplastic reaction
Inflammatory reaction	Absent	Moderate	Marked
Luminal border	Smooth	Serrated	Irregular
Secondary lumina	Absent	Absent	Present in cribriform pattern
Micropapillae	Absent	Some	May be prominent
Epithelium	Heterogeneous three cell types	Predominance of one cell type	Predominance of one cell type
Mitoses	Numerous	Numerous	Numerous

Data adapted from Russo IH and Russo J (1978); Russo IH et al. (1976); Russo J and Russo IH (1978, 1980, 1987); Russo J et al. (1977, 1979, 1982, 1983).

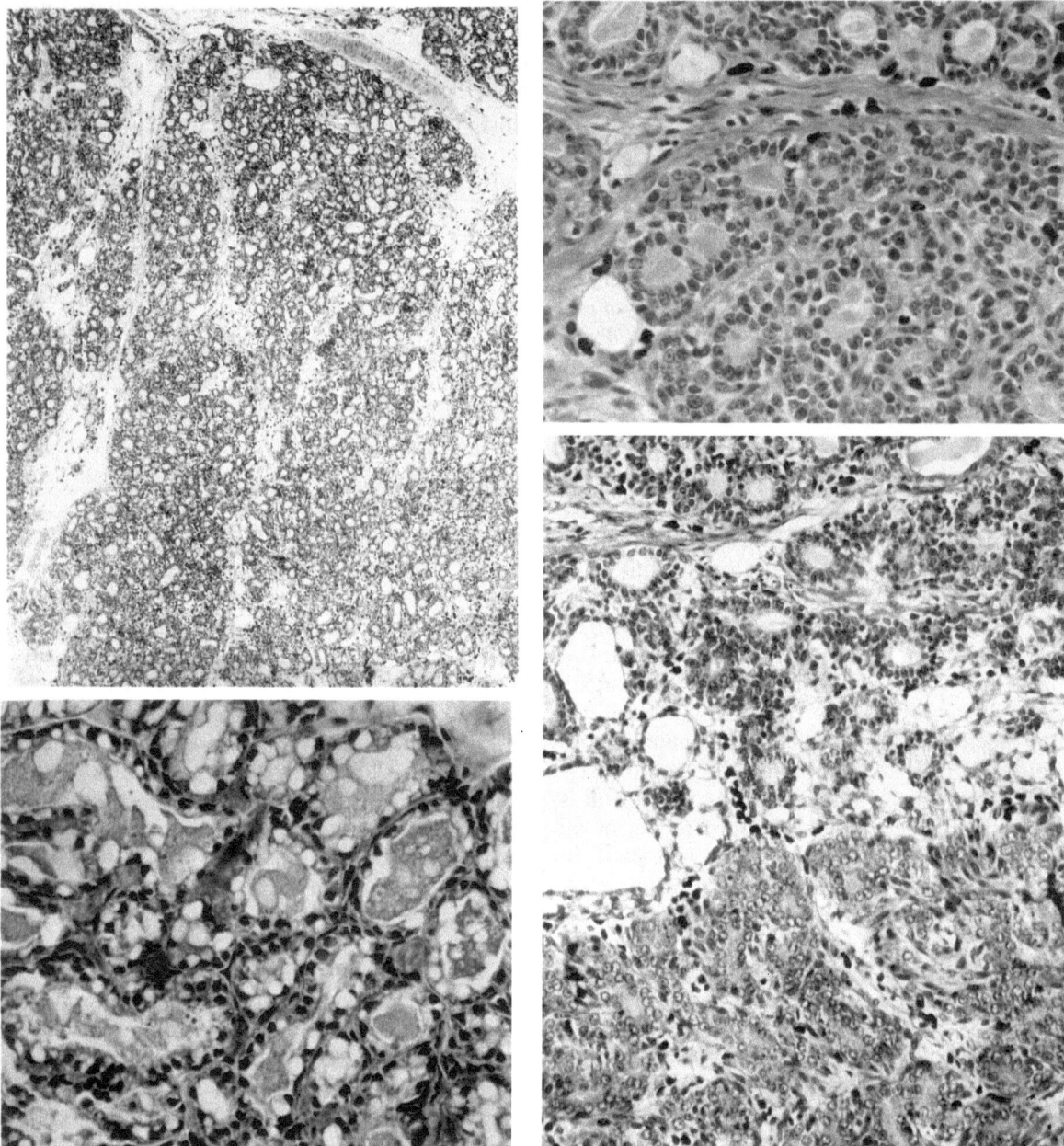

Fig. 378 *(upper left)*. Tubular adenoma. Closely apposed alveolar or tubular structures are separated by a small amount of connective tissue. H and E, ×60

Fig. 379 *(upper right)*. Tubular adenoma in which the tubular structures exhibit a regular contour. Individual alveoli are surrounded by a small amount of connective tissue. H and E, ×160

Fig. 380 *(lower right)*. Transition between tubular adenoma *(upper half)* and adenocarcinoma *(lower half)*. H and E, ×100

Fig. 381 *(lower left)*. Lactating adenoma. H and E, ×150

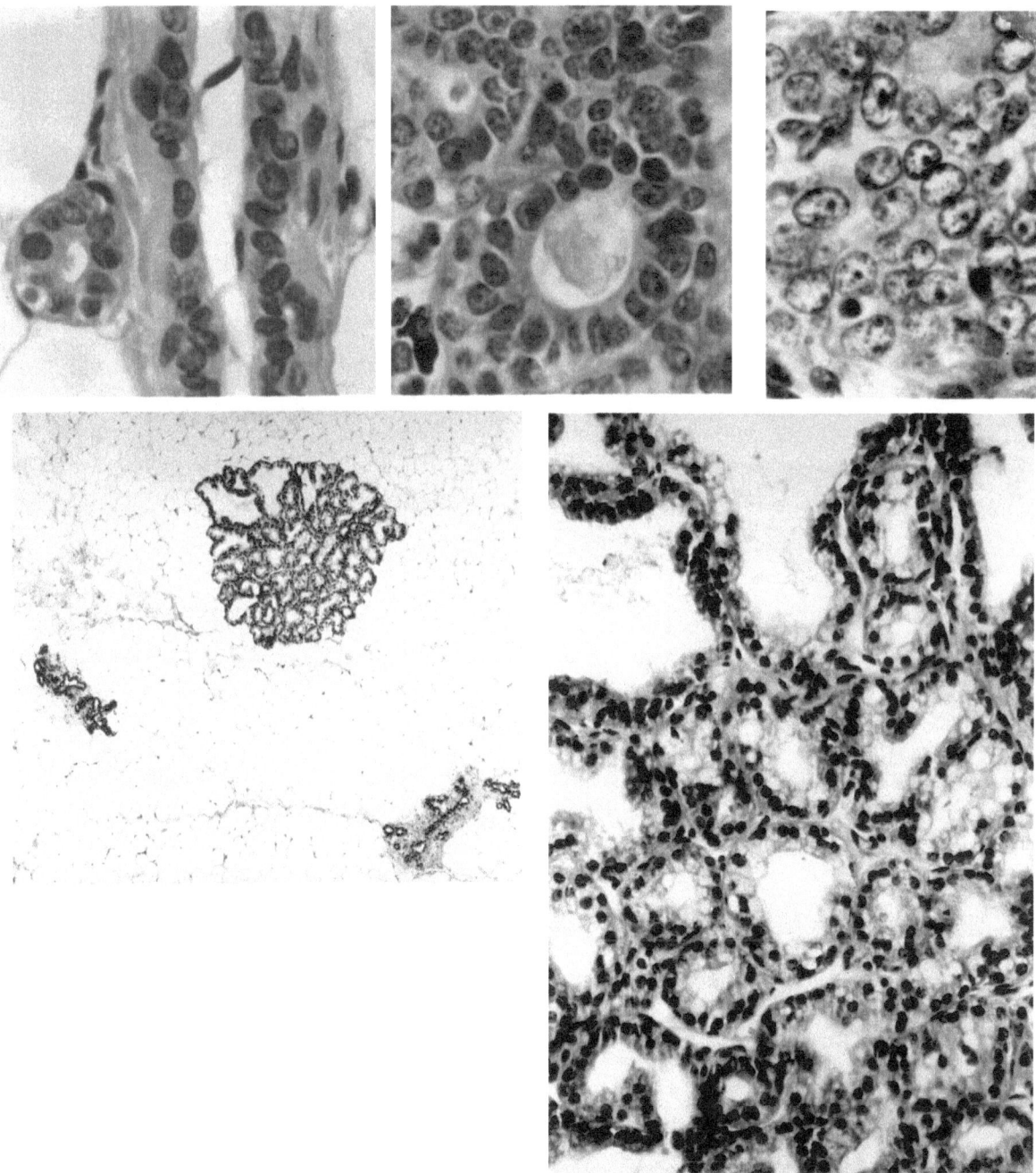

Fig. 382 *(upper left).* Ductal structure and alveolar bud of the normal mammary gland. H and E, ×400

Fig. 383 *(upper middle).* Alveolar or tubular structure from a tubular adenoma. H and E, ×400

Fig. 384 *(upper right).* Higher magnification of the adeno-carcinoma shown in Fig. 380. H and E, ×400

Fig. 385 *(lower left).* Hyperplastic alveolar nodule of the rat mammary gland. Compare with the normal ductal and primitive alveolar structures in the *lower right* and *left corners.* H and E, ×60

Fig. 386 *(lower right).* Detail of the alveolar components of the lesion shown in Fig. 385. H and E, ×150

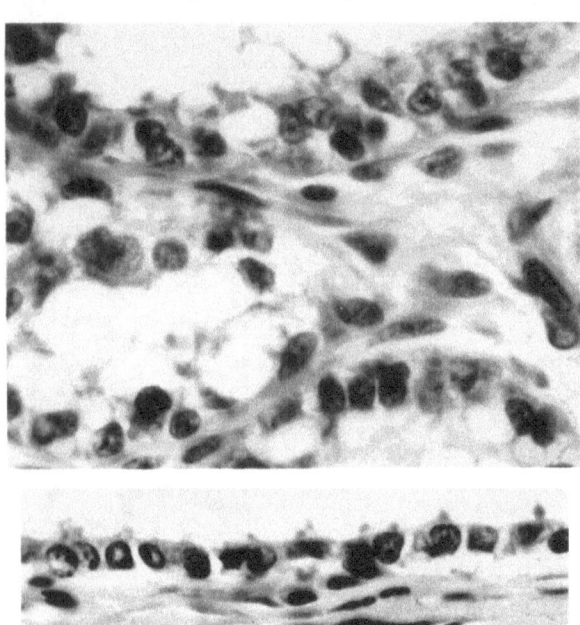

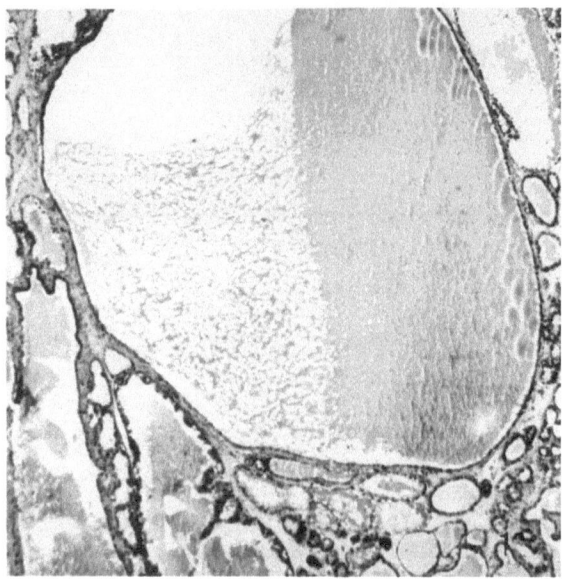

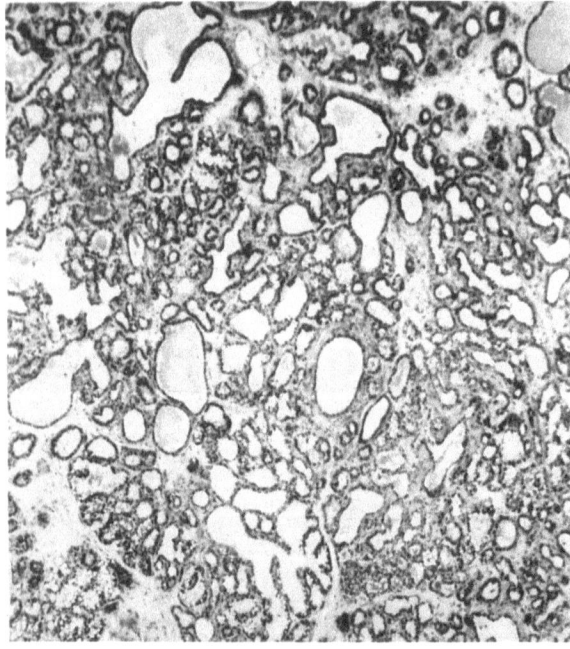

Fig. 387 *(upper left).* Higher magnification of the epithelium of a lactating adenoma showing the accumulation of secretory material in the lumen as well as in the supranuclear portion of the cells. H and E, ×400

Fig. 388 *(middle left).* Lining epithelium of the cystic structure shown in Fig. 390. H and E, ×400

Fig. 389 *(lower left).* Cystic changes in a lactating adenoma. H and E, ×60

Fig. 390 *(upper right).* Cystic structure originated from a lactating adenoma. H and E, ×60

Fig. 391 *(upper left).* Intraductal proliferation (IDP) in the rat mammary gland. This lesion is observed 21–41 days postcarcinogen (DMBA) administration. The proliferation starts in the terminal end buds and expands to the ductal structures. A very small desmoplastic reaction is observed in the stroma. The lumen in IDP is smooth. H and E, ×60

Fig. 392 *(middle left).* Intraductal carcinoma, papillary and cribriform patterns, exhibiting stromal desmoplastic reaction. H and E, ×60

Fig. 393 *(upper right).* Papillary carcinoma in situ. H and ▶ E, ×100

Fig. 394 *(lower left).* Multiple areas of carcinoma in situ showing early papillary and cribriform patterns and intense desmoplastic reaction in the stroma. H and E, ×60

Fig. 395 *(lower right).* Higher magnification of a papillary structure in the intraductal carcinoma described in Fig. 393. H and E, ×400

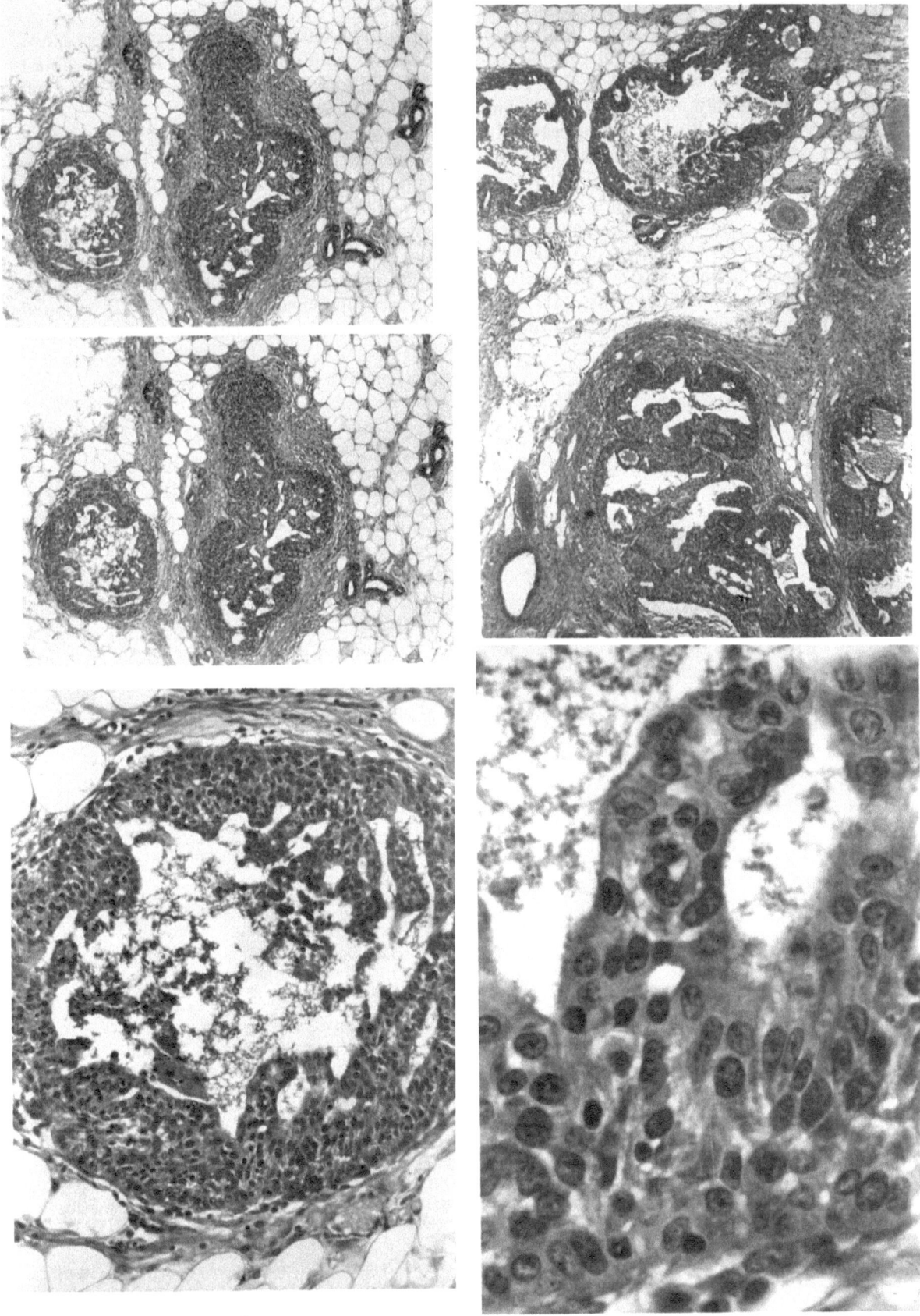

1. Ductal Papillary Carcinoma. The ductal structures are dilated, and the lining epithelium grows inward, forming epithelial papillae devoid of fibrovascular core. Most of the epithelial cell population is uniform in size and shape. Russo J et al. (1982, 1983) described the lesion as consisting of predominantly of a single cell type, the intermediate cell. Intermediate cells are characterized by an increased nucleocytoplasmic ratio and a prominent nucleolus. Mitotic figures are often found. The luminal cells stain for a mixture of acid and neutral mucopolysaccharides (Russo IH et al. 1976). The stroma, which is separated from the epithelium by a well-defined basement membrane, exhibits a slight to marked desmoplastic reaction, with replacement of fat by fibroblasts and infiltration by lymphocytes and mast cells (Figs. 392–394).

2. Ductal Cribriform Carcinoma. This tumor type is the result of epithelial cell proliferation in a solid pattern with formation of secondary lumina (Figs. 398–401). This type of tumor is cytologically similar to papillary carcinomas and like them elicits a sromal reaction and lymphocytic infiltration (Figs. 399 and 400). The secondary lumina stain intensely for acidic mucopolysaccharides that contrast with the neutral

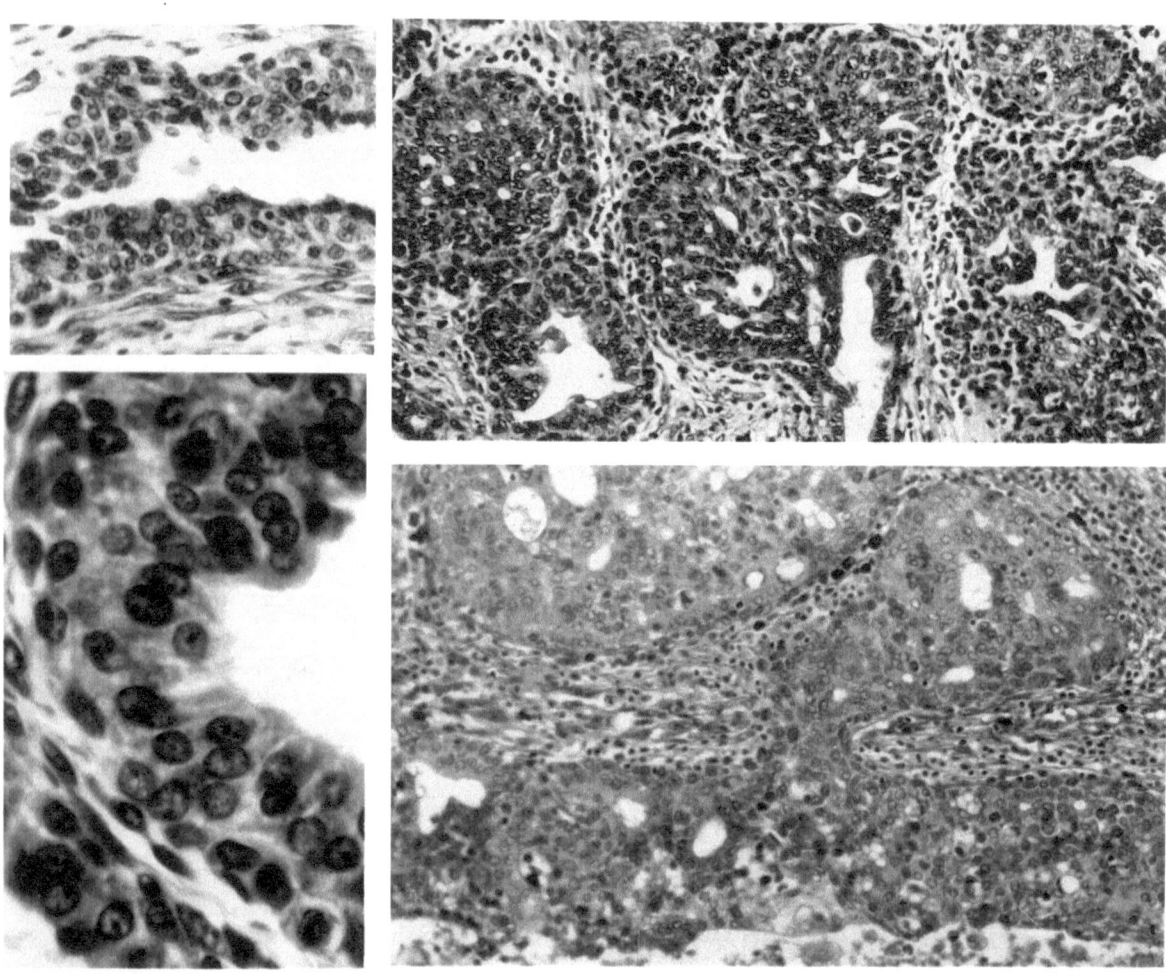

Fig. 396 *(upper left).* Intraductal proliferation in which there are clearly five to six layers of cells. H and E, × 100

Fig. 397 *(lower left).* Higher magnification of Fig. 396 in which large nuclei and prominent nucleoli are seen. The luminal border is smooth, and there is no secretory material or detritus in the lumen. H and E, × 400

Fig. 398 *(upper right).* Intraductal carcinoma, cribriform pattern. The terminal end buds have been affected by the carcinogen, and epithelial proliferation is seen extending towards the ducts. H and E, × 100

Fig. 399 *(lower right).* Intraductal carcinoma, cribriform pattern; epithelial clusters are surrounded by intense desmoplastic reaction and lymphocytic infiltration. H and E, × 160

mucopolysaccharides of the basement membrane. In early lesions, such as those shown in Fig. 398, the origin from the TEB and the extension to the ducts is quite evident.

3. *Ductal Comedocarcinoma.* This lesion is characterized by intraductal growth of epithelium and accumulation of necrotic cellular debris in the lumen (Fig. 402–405). The surrounding stroma may exhibit a marked desmoplastic reaction. The cytological pattern of the lesion is similar to that of the other intraductal carcinomas. The comedo and the cribriform patterns may occur in the same tumor, such as shown in Fig. 403; less frequently, a papillary component is present as well.

The differentiation of noninvasive from invasive carcinoma (Table 21) is based upon the unequivocal growth of the invasive carcinoma into adjacent tissues. This is clear evidence of the malignant potential of the tumor. The usual decision to consider a rat mammary tumor malignant despite the absence of invasion or metastasis is based upon the many similarities in histologic and cytologic features between the invasive and noninvasive varieties. The similar features seen in

Table 24. Differential diagnosis between papillary carcinoma grades I and II

Components	Grade I	Grade II
Fibrovascular core	Prominent	Sparse
Epithelium	3 layers thick	5–10 layers thick
Micropapillae	Present	Present
Luminal border	Smooth	Serrated
Cytological characteristics	Moderate pleomorphism	Marked pleomorphism
Nucleolus mitoses	Inconspicuous, scarce	Prominent

mammary tumors which have metastasized is another item of evidence of potential malignancy of the "noninvasive carcinoma" (Van Zwieten 1984). Additional studies are urgently needed on the long-term behavior of rat mammary tumors to provide the data necessary for a better understanding of the biological behavior of these neoplasms.

Invasive Ductal Carcinomas. The presence of invasion can be difficult to judge because the mammary glands spread diffusely in the fat pad and

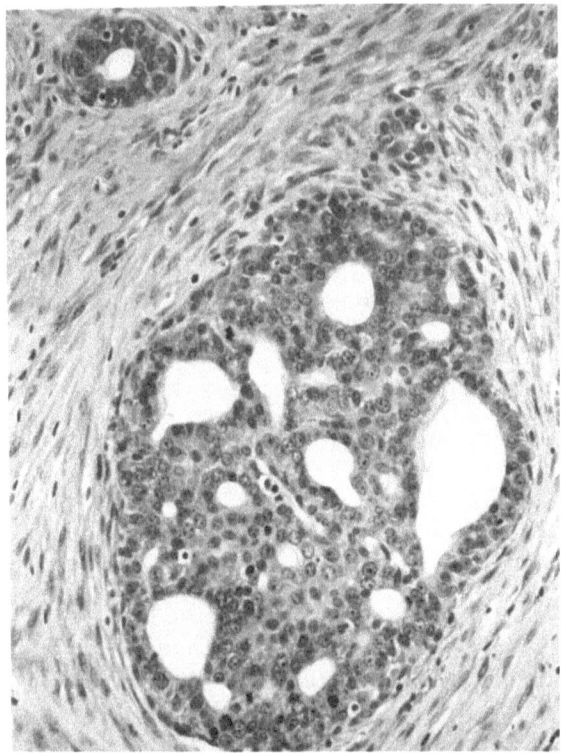

Fig. 400. Intraductal carcinoma, cribriform pattern. H and E, × 160

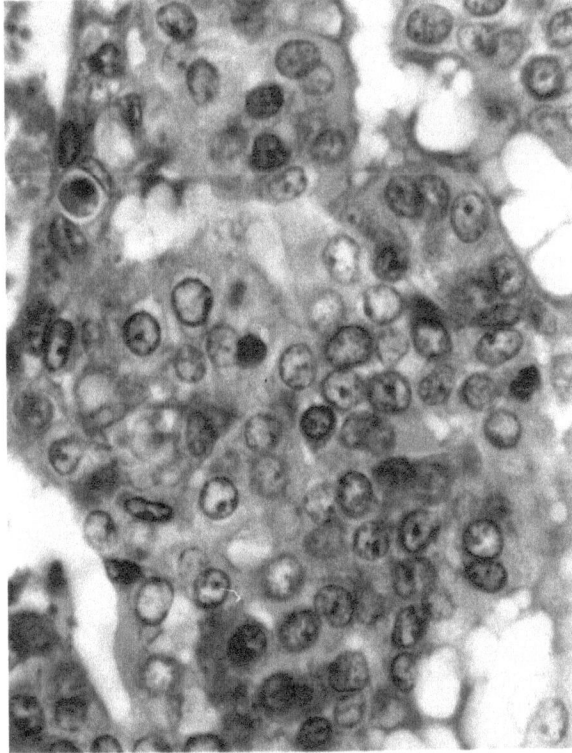

Fig. 401. Higher magnification of the lesion shown in Fig. 399, in which large cells with prominent nucleoli are present. H and E, × 400

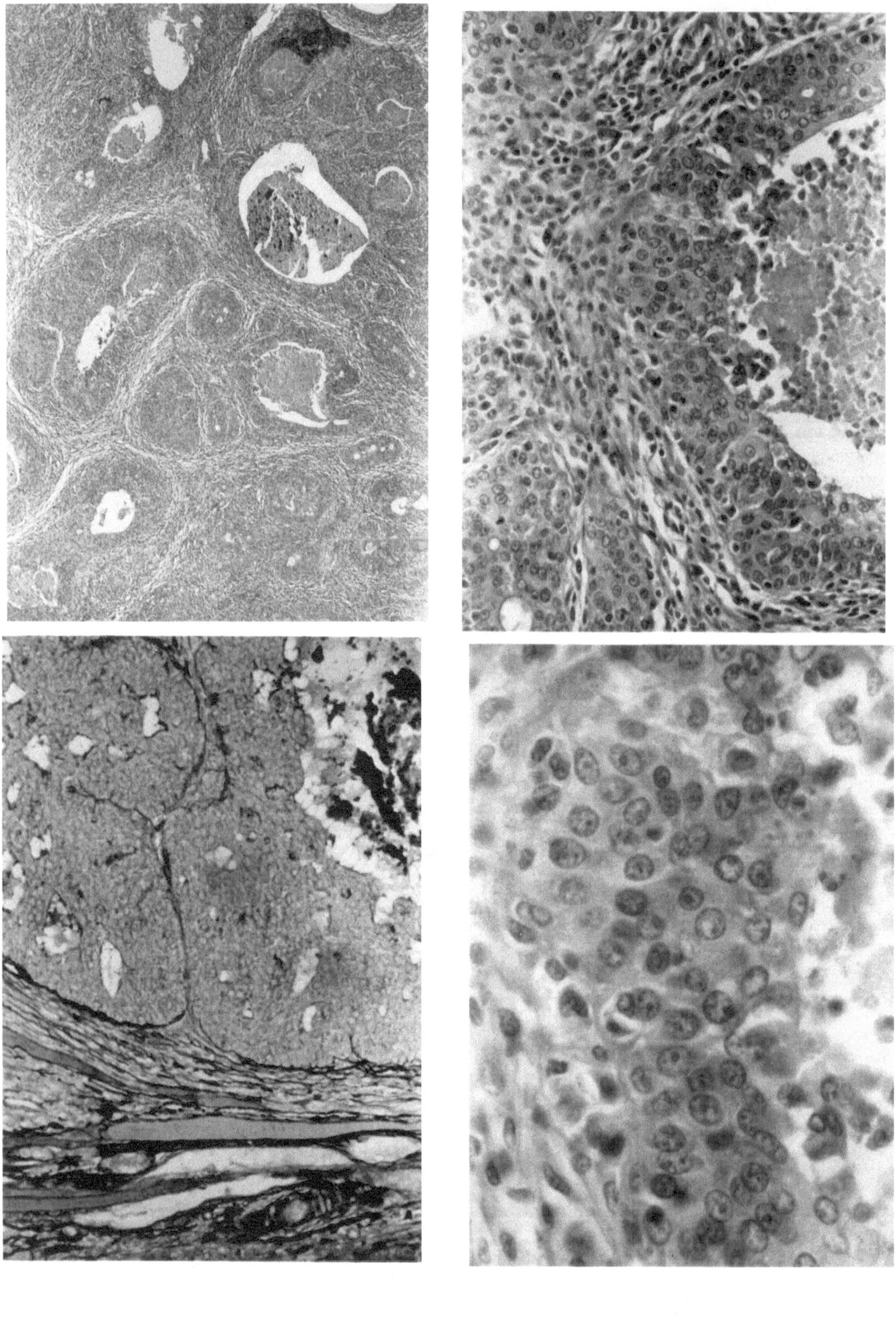

◀ **Fig.402** *(upper left).* Intraductal carcinoma, comedo type. Observe that individual ductal structures have been dilated by epithelial proliferation. There is necrotic material in the center of the tumor masses and an intense desmoplastic reaction in the stroma. H and E, × 60

Fig.403 *(lower left).* Combination of a cribriform carcinoma with a comedo component. Observe the basement membrane delimiting the individual components. Reticulum stain, × 100

Fig.404 *(upper right).* Observe the homogeneous appearance of the cells in comedo carcinoma with accumulation of cell detritus and necrosis in the lumen. H and E, × 160

Fig.405 *(lower right).* Higher magnification of the epithelium of the comedo carcinoma shown in Fig.404. H and E × 400

adjacent muscle. Intraductal lesions may appear invasive (Fig.429).

1. Papillary Carcinomas. The most typical and frequent of the 7,12-dimethylbenz[*a*]anthracene (DMBA)- and *N*-methyl-*N*-nitrosourea (NMU)-induced tumors are papillary carcinomas (Gullino et al. 1975, Russo J et al. 1977, 1979; Van Zwieten 1984; Young and Hallowes 1973). Most of them are detectable by palpation; they efface the normal architecture of the gland, invading surrounding structures; when they invade the skin, they ulcerate and undergo local necrosis. They contain delicate fibrovascular cores, often heavily infiltrated by lymphocytes and mast cells (Fig.408). The fibrovascular cores are considerably thinner than those seen in intraductal papillomas (Figs.406 and 407). On top of the fibrovascular core grows the epithelium, which depending upon its thickness and cytologic characteristics allows one to classify these lesions into two grades, I and II Table 24). Papillary carcinomas grade I are composed of 1–2 layers of epithelial cells, which in turn emit short epithelial papillae devoid of fibrovascular core.

The nuclei of most of these cells are less pleomorphic than those described in the intraductal carcinoma (Figs.380 and 411), but they are significantly different from those lining the intraductal papilloma (Fig.409). Nucleoli tend to be inconspicuous. Some papillae are lined by a single layer of columnar epithelium that is continuous with a multilayered, pleomorphic epithelium. The papillary carcinoma grade II is also characterized by papillary projections; however, the core of connective tissue is more sparse than that observed in the papillary carcinoma grade I, and the secondary projections (papillae) of epithelium are solid clusters of cells. The luminal borders of these cell projections are serrated (Figs.412 and 413), whereas those in papillary carcinoma grade I are smooth (Figs.410 and 411). Epithelial cells in this tumor type are more pleomorphic than those of the papillary carcinoma grade I (Fig.413). In Table 24 are depicted the basic histological and cytological differences between these tumor subtypes. Occasionally, in papillary carcinomas grade II, the luminal spaces may become dilated or cystic; these lesions are called cystic papillary carcinomas (Figs.414–417). They may well represent a further evolution of a papillary or cribriform type.

2. Cribriform Carcinoma. The invasive cribriform carcinoma exhibits the same cellular arrangement as the in situ lesion, in which the solid sheets of neoplastic epithelial cells are interrupted by round or irregularly shaped secondary lumina of variable size. Invasion is characterized by penetration of haphazardly arranged, fingerlike projections of epithelium into the surrounding stroma (Figs.418–423). Even small clusters of cells infiltrating the dermis (Fig.426), skeletal muscle, and connective tissue (Figs.427 and 428) still exhibit a cribriform pattern. The cribriform pattern may be maintained in metastatic lesions (Figs. 431–435). Individual neoplastic cells are moderately to markedly pleomorphic (Figs.420, 421, 430), the degree of pleomorphism varying from tumor to tumor (Figs.419–431) and even in different areas of the same tumor (Figs.426–430). Interstingly enough, even in the most pleomorphic areas (Figs.420 and 421) the glandular pattern is still present, with secretory material within the newly formed lumina. Occasional areas of squamous metaplasia may be found (Figs.422 and 423).

The infiltrating neoplastic cells are in general surrounded by a connective tissue exhibiting a marked desmoplastic reaction and heavy lymphocytic and mast cell infiltrations. These tumors may metastasize after several months postinitiation (Van Zwieten 1984). The cribriform type of tumor appears in general as a uniform pattern, but it may be associated with papillary- or comedo-type patterns in the same tumor.

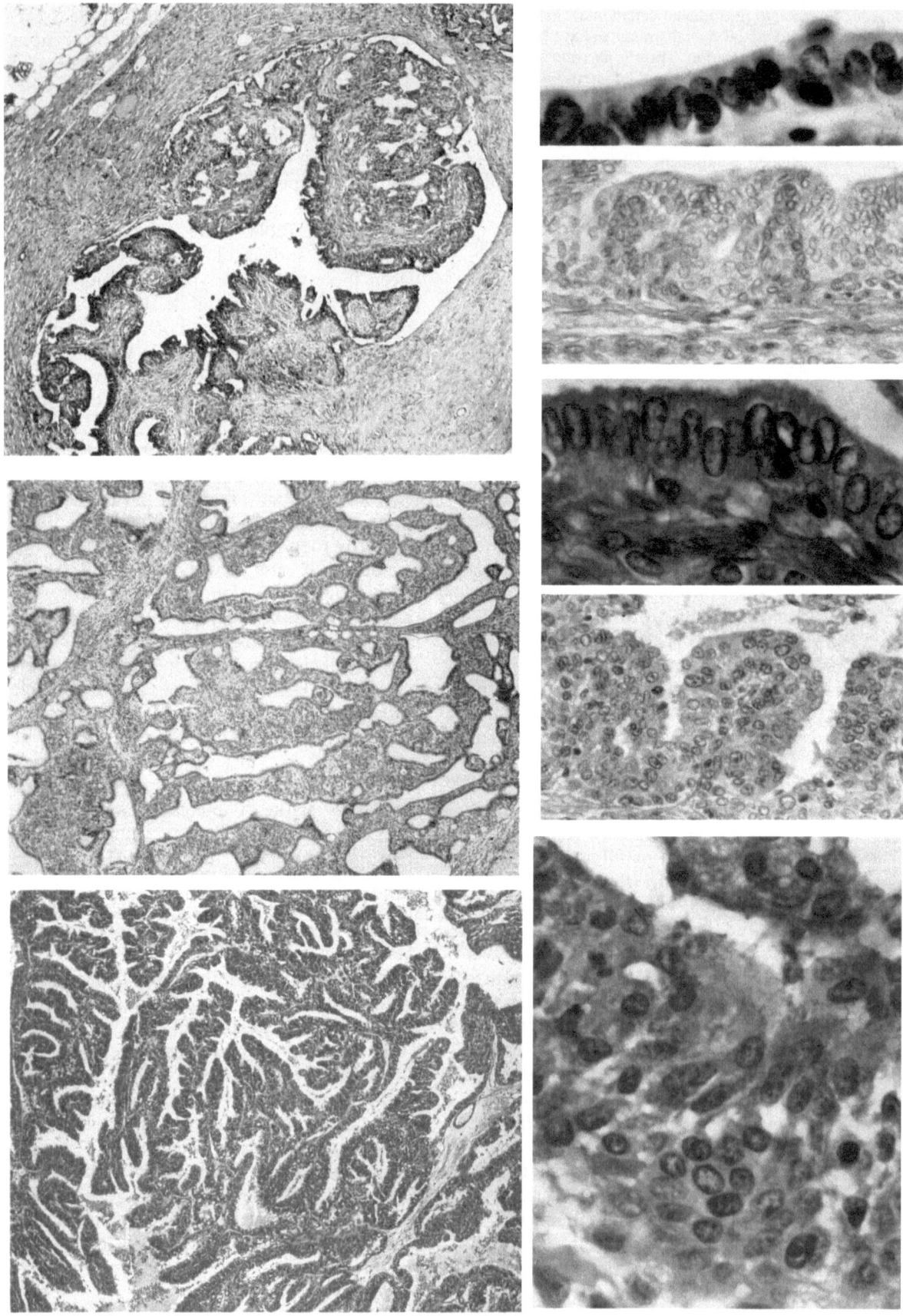

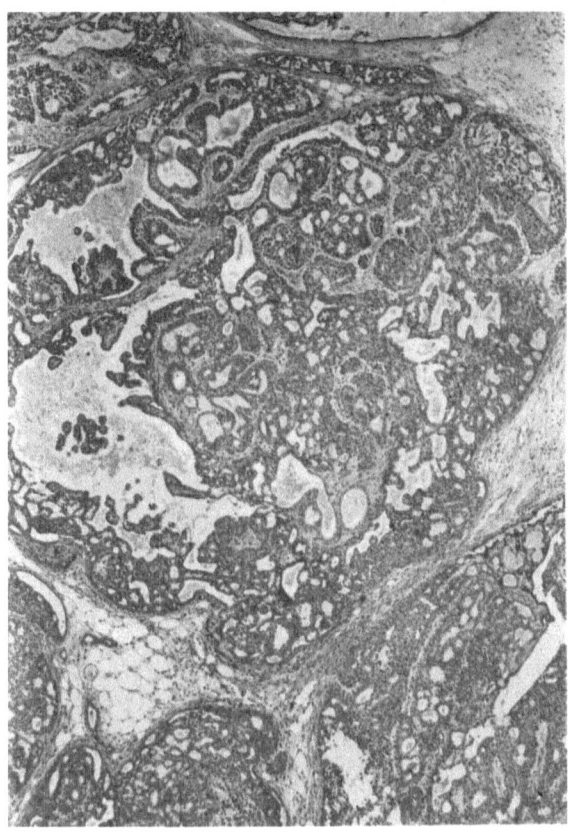

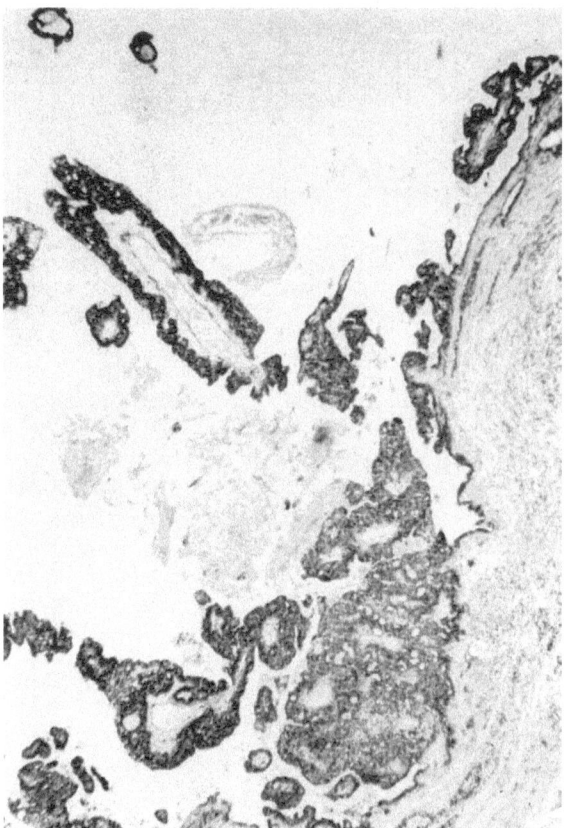

Fig. 414. Papillary carcinoma with cystic components. H and E, × 60

Fig. 415. Detail of the papillary carcinoma shown in Fig. 414. H and E, × 100

◄ **Fig. 406** *(upper left)*. Intraductal papilloma. H and E, × 60

Fig. 407 *(middle left)*. A variety of intraductal papilloma in which most of the epithelium has been flattened, and the stroma contains an abundant amount of connective tissue. H and E, × 60

Fig. 408 *(lower left)*. Papillary carcinoma, grade II. Observe the numerous papillary projections sustained by very small, thin, connective tissue cores. H and E, × 60

Fig. 409 *(right top)*. Epithelium lining the intraductal papilloma shown in Fig. 407. H and E, × 400

Fig. 410 *(right second from top)*. Epithelial lining found in a papillary carcinoma, grade I. Observe the smooth appearance of the cell border. H and E, × 160

Fig. 411 *(right third from top)*. Tall columnar cells lining the papillae of a papillary carcinoma, grade 1. H and E, × 400

Fig. 412 *(right fourth from top)*. Papillary projection in a papillary carcinoma, grade II, in which the number of cells per layer is higher, and the degree of pleomorphism is quite evident. The luminal border has an irregular appearance. H and E, × 160

Fig. 413 *(right bottom)*. Higher magnification of the epithelium lining the papillary carcinoma, grade II. Observe the homogeneous appearance of the cells with large nuclei and prominent nucleoli. H and E, × 400

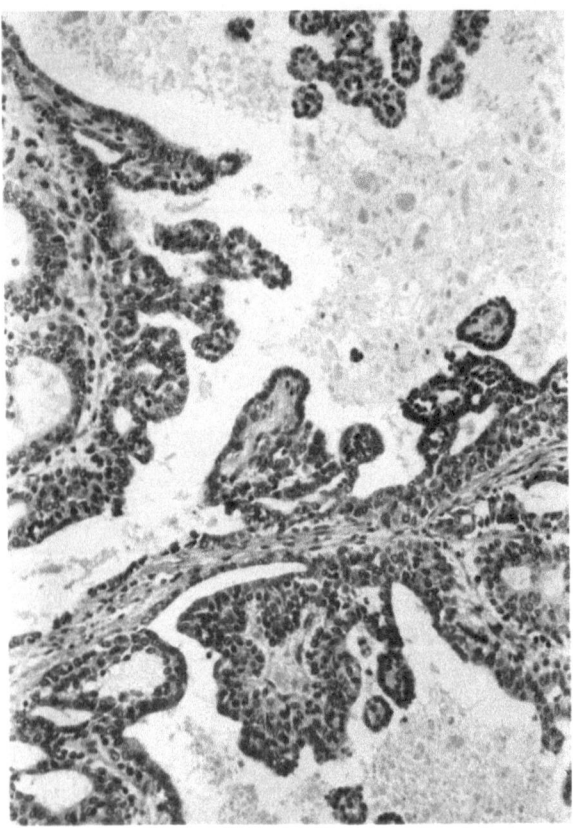

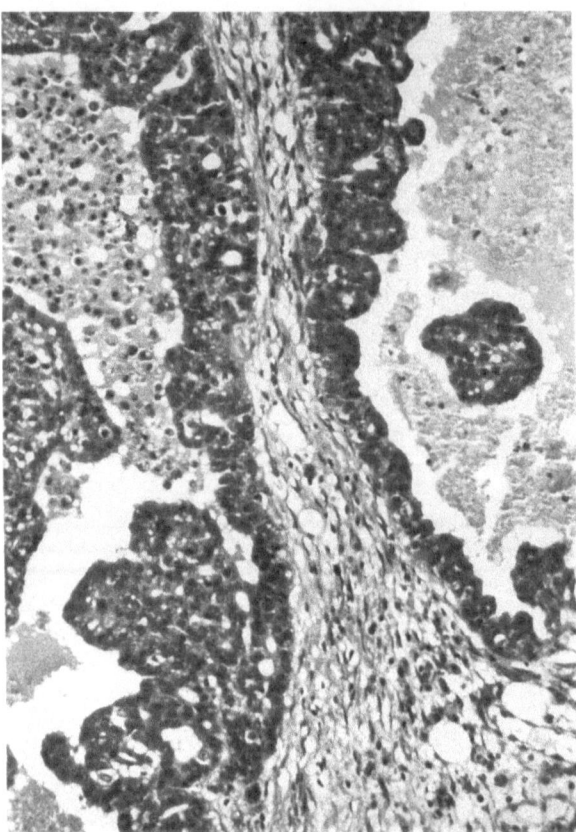

Fig.416. Detail of the papillary structures protruding toward the cystic lumen. H and E, ×160

Fig.417. The epithelial lining of the papillae in the papillary carcinoma shown in Fig.414 emits solid projections of cells. Papillary and cribriform pattern are seen in the same papillae. H and E, ×150

Fig.418 *(upper left).* Infiltrating cribriform carcinoma. H and E, ×60

Fig.419 *(lower left).* Detail of the cribriform pattern showing secondary lumina. Epithelial clusters are surrounded by lymphocytes and marked desmoplastic reaction. H and E, ×160

Fig.420 *(upper right).* Detail of glandular formations ▶ found in a cribriform carcinoma containing abundant secretion in the secondary lumina. H and E, ×160

Fig.421 *(lower right).* Detail of the cribriform carcinoma infiltrating type, in which the marked nuclear pleomorphism is clear, but the cells are still found around lumina containing secretory material. H and E, ×400

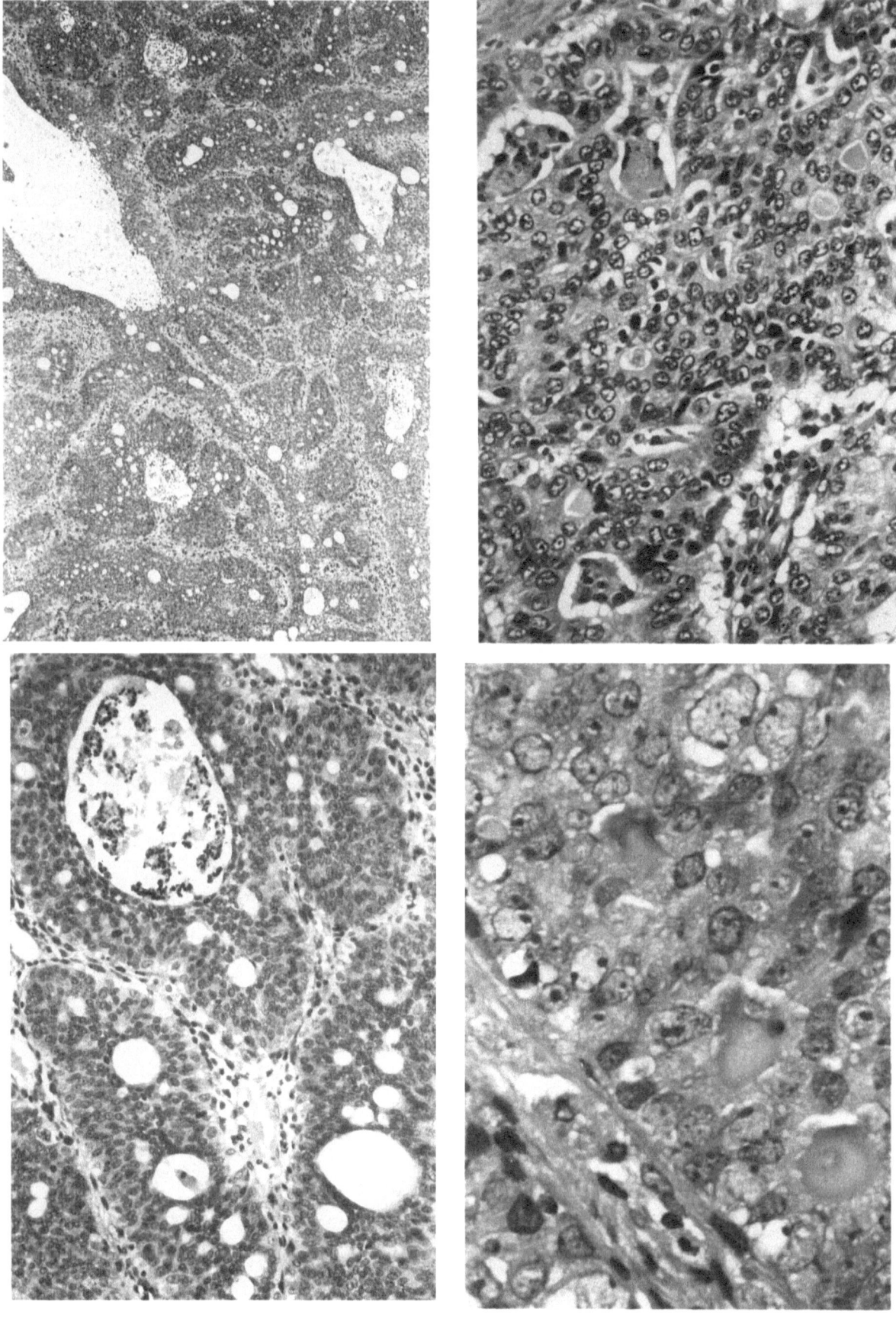

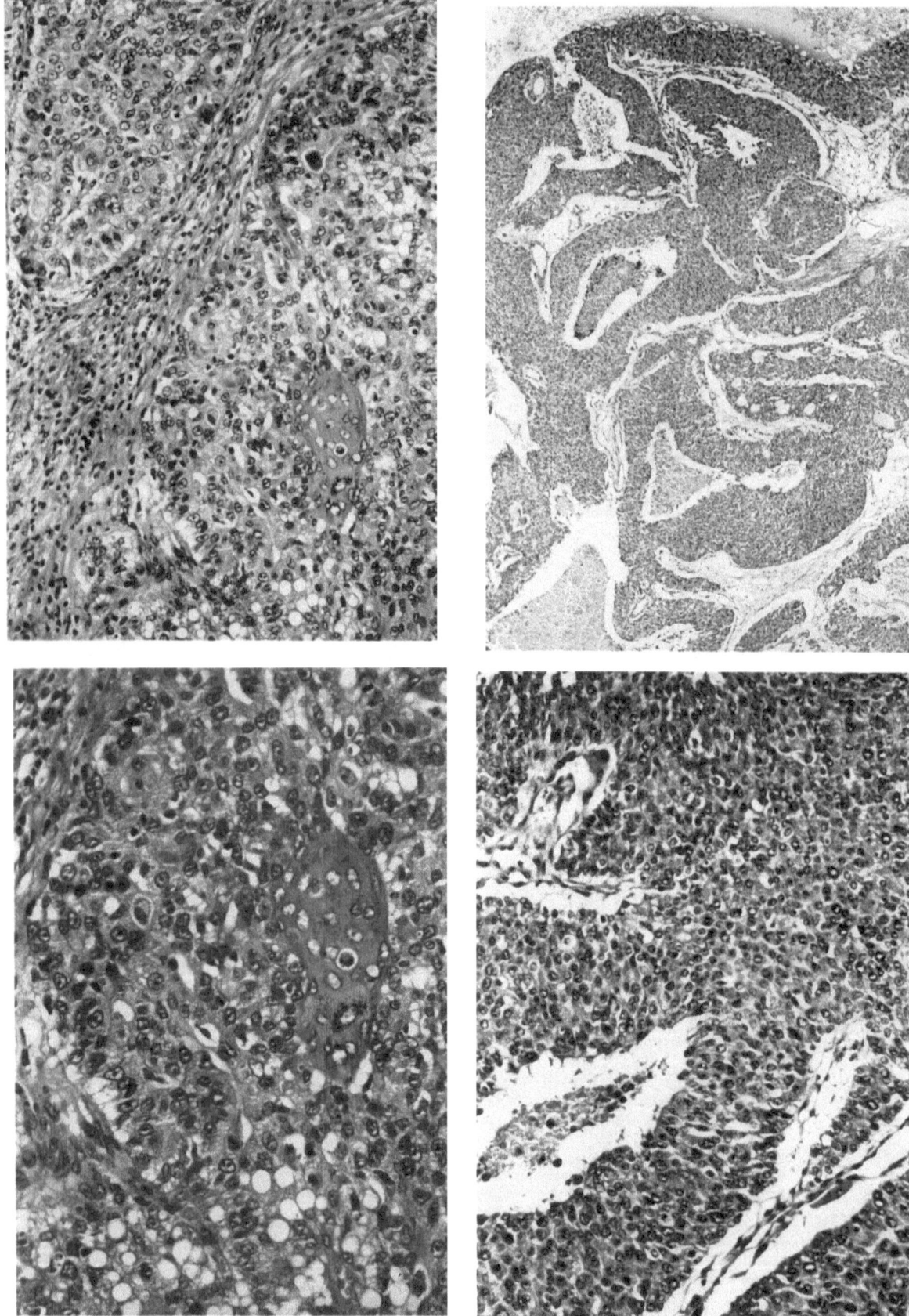

◀ **Fig. 422** *(upper left)*. A cribriform carcinoma containing an area of squamous metaplasia. H and E, × 100

Fig. 423 *(lower left)*. A cribriform carcinoma containing an area of squamous metaplasia. H and E, × 160

Fig. 424 *(upper right)*. Infiltrating carcinoma, comedo type. H and E, × 60

Fig. 425 *(lower right)*. Detail of infiltrating carcinoma, comedo type. The cells are not separated from the stroma by a basement membrane. H and E, × 100

Table 25. Differential diagnosis between tubular adenomas and adenocarcinomas

Components	Adenoma	Tubular carcinoma
Tubular structure	Present	Present
Lumen	Prominent	Present or absent
Secretion in lumen	Present	Present; in some cases prominent
Epithelium	Three cell types	Almost always one cell type
Cell morphology	Cuboidal polarity preserved	Pleomorphic, loss of polarity
Nuclear features	Round	Oval, enlarged, and with prominent nucleolus
Stroma	Scanty	Scanty or absent

3. Comedo Carcinoma. The tumor type found quite frequently in animals that have been treated at younger ages is comedo carcinoma. The lesions appear as distended ductal structures lined by a multilayered epithelium surrounding necrotic debris. Invasion occurs as an extension of ductlike structures or sheets of epithelial cells arranged in a serpiginous pattern into a stroma in which desmoplastic reaction and inflammatory cell infiltration may occur. Individual neoplastic cells are moderately pleomorphic (Figs. 424 and 425). These tumors resemble the comedo carcinoma of the human breast (Fisher et al. 1975).

4. Tubular Carcinoma. Under the category of tubular carcinoma are classified those tumors that are composed of well-defined tubular or alveolar structures; it is postulated that this type originates from alveolar buds or from alveolar bud-derived adenomas, whereas all the other types of carcinomas described above are ductal in origin. Several transitional steps between adenomas and fully manifest carcinomas are found, which in some cases makes it difficult to differentiate one from the other. Tubular carcinomas, however, differ cytologically enough from tubular adenomas to allow identification. In Figure 380 one can see a tumor composed of a portion of tubular adenoma and another of carcinoma. The epithelial cells composing the tubular carcinoma have increased nuclear size, and the nuclei contain prominent nucleoli; tubular adenomas, on the other hand, have cells with smaller nuclei, and nucleoli are absent or inconspicuous. In Fig. 453, the differences in nuclear area in normal ductal structures (Fig. 382), tubular adenoma (Fig. 383), and adenocarcinoma (Fig. 384)

are shown. Whereas the nuclei of epithelial cells in both normal ducts and tubular adenomas have similar surface areas, the nuclei in adenocarcinomas have larger areas, increased nucleocytoplasmic ratios, and a greater degree of nuclear pleomorphism; they are similar to those of IDPs, intraductal carcinomas, and infiltrating carcinomas. Table 25 depicts the basic features used for differentiating adenomas from adenocarcinomas.

Two variants of tubular carcinoma may be found in some irradiated animals (Van Zwieten 1984). One of the variants is composed of tubular structures in which the lumens are empty, narrow, and lined by a single layer of low cuboidal dark cells, with an underlying 6–8-layer thick epithelium (Figs. 436, 437, 439). These cells are large, with abundant, finely granular, acidophilic, and often vacuolated cytoplasm and round or oval, centrally located nuclei, an appearance that is consistent with the intermediate cell type observed in DMBA-induced tumors (Russo J et al. 1983) (Figs. 437 and 439); mitotic figures are frequent. Cell disposition in this tumor variant is quite different from that observed in tumors induced by chemical carcinogens such as DMBA or NMU in which the intermediate cells surround the lumen and the dark cells are peripheral. The second variant of tubular carcinoma consists of a tumor in which the tubular elements are lined by a single layer of epithelial cells, and the lumen is wide and irregular, containing abundant secretory material (Figs. 438 and 440).

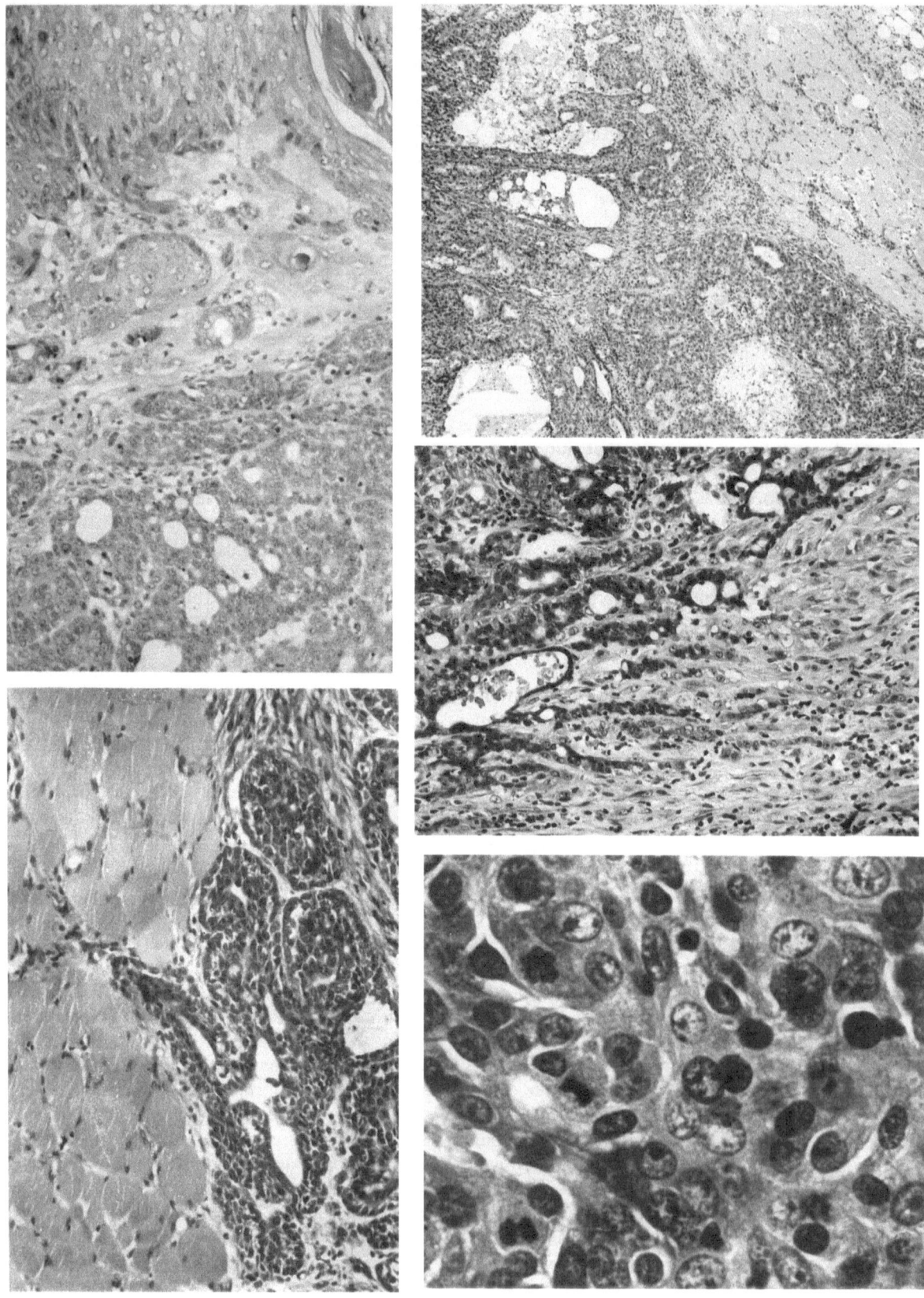

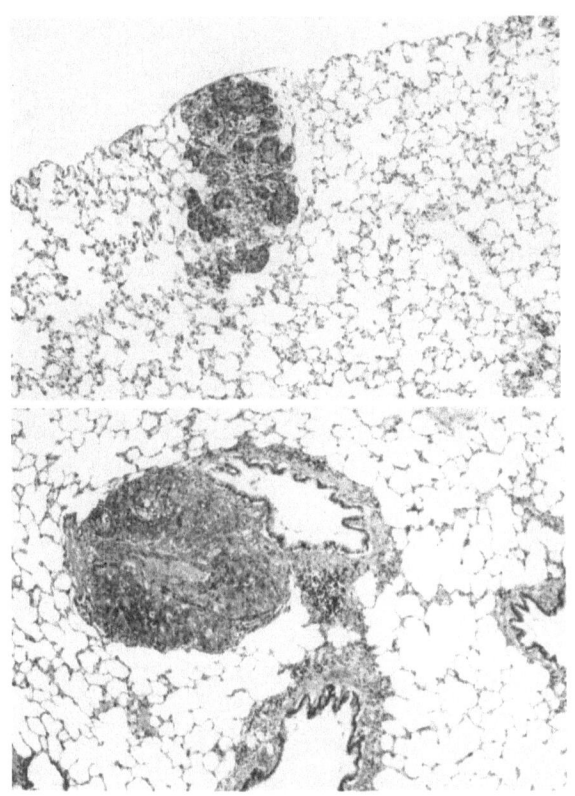

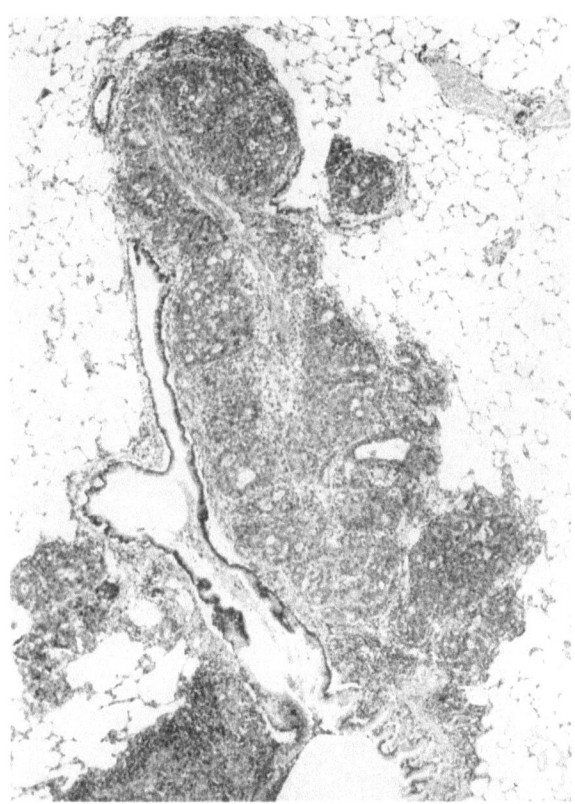

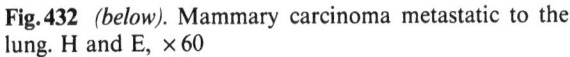

Fig. 431 *(above).* Mammary carcinoma metastatic to the lung. H and E, ×60

Fig. 432 *(below).* Mammary carcinoma metastatic to the lung. H and E, ×60

Fig. 433. Mammary carcinoma metastatic to the lung. H and E, ×60

◄ **Fig. 426** *(upper left).* Invasive ductal carcinoma, cribriform type involving the dermis. H and E, ×100

Fig. 427 *(upper right).* Invasive cribriform carcinoma in which penetration to skeletal muscle is evident. H and E, ×60

Fig. 428 *(middle right).* Invasive cribriform carcinoma. H and E, ×100

Fig. 429 *(lower left).* Invasion of muscle by neoplastic cells of a cribriform carcinoma. H and E, ×100

Fig. 430 *(lower right).* Individual cells in an infiltrating cribriform carcinoma exhibit nuclear pleomorphism. H and E, ×4000

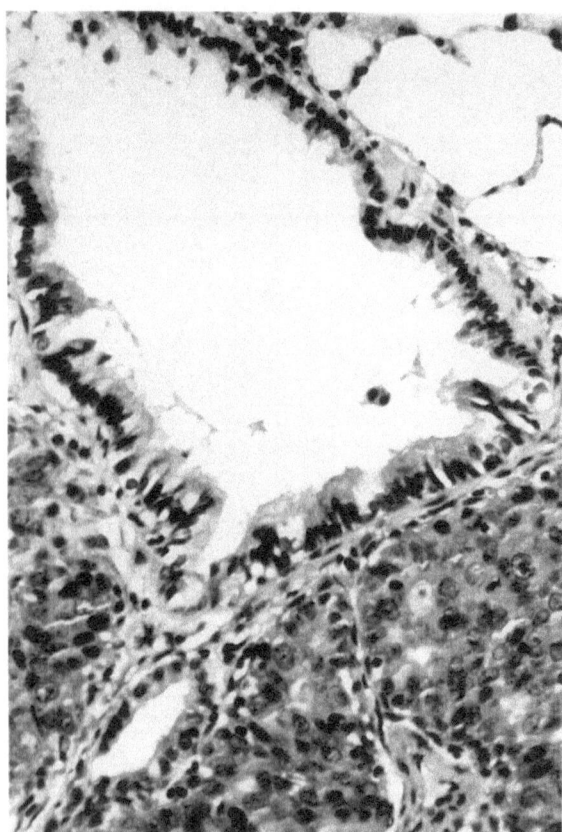

Fig. 434. Higher magnification shows a cribriform pattern in this metastatic lesion. H and E, × 160

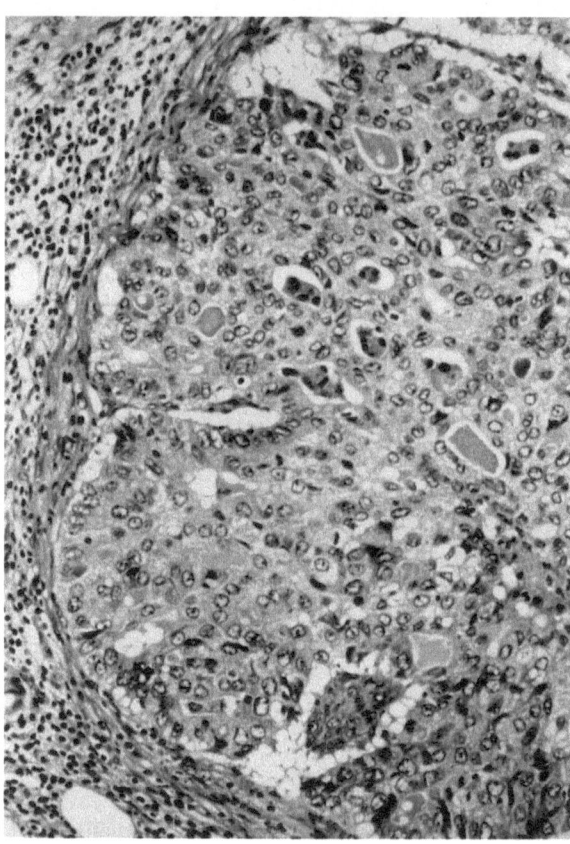

Fig. 435. Detail of an infiltrating carcinoma, cribriform pattern, metastatic to the lung. Observe the desmoplasia around the neoplastic cells and the lymphocytic infiltration. H and E, × 160

Fig. 436 *(upper left).* Tubular adenocarcinoma. Observe the narrow lumen and the thickening of the cellular lining. H and E, × 60

Fig. 437 *(upper right).* Same tubular adenocarcinoma as shown in Fig. 436; observe distribution of neoplastic cells around the lumen. H and E, × 400

Fig. 438 *(middle right).* Tubular adenocarcinoma, secretory type. H and E, × 60

Fig. 439 *(lower left).* Higher magnification of tubular adenocarcinoma showing nuclear details. H and E, × 400 ▶

Fig. 440 *(lower right).* Detail of Fig. 438 in which the monolayers of cells line tubular structures with serrated lumina containing secretory material. H and E, × 160

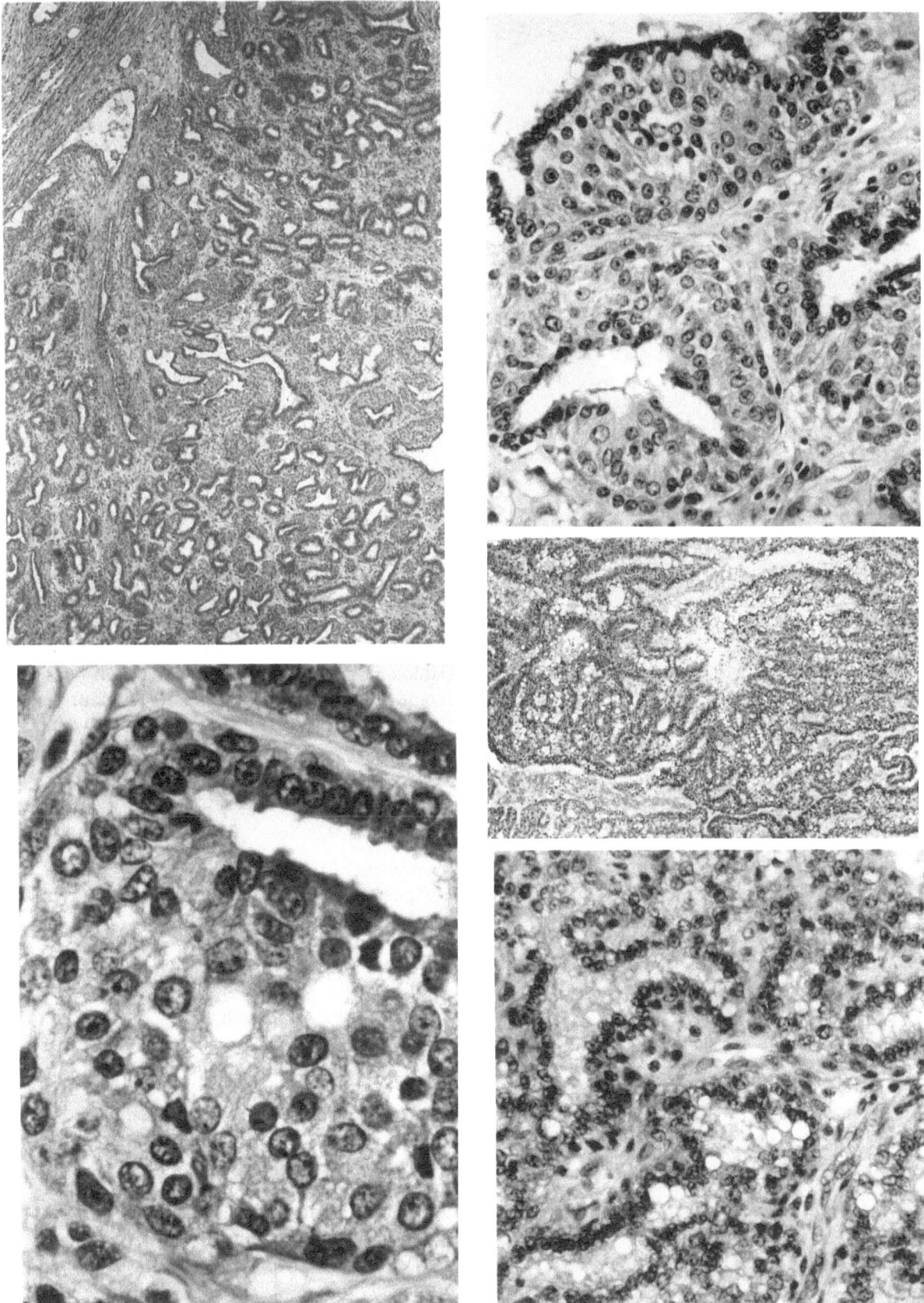

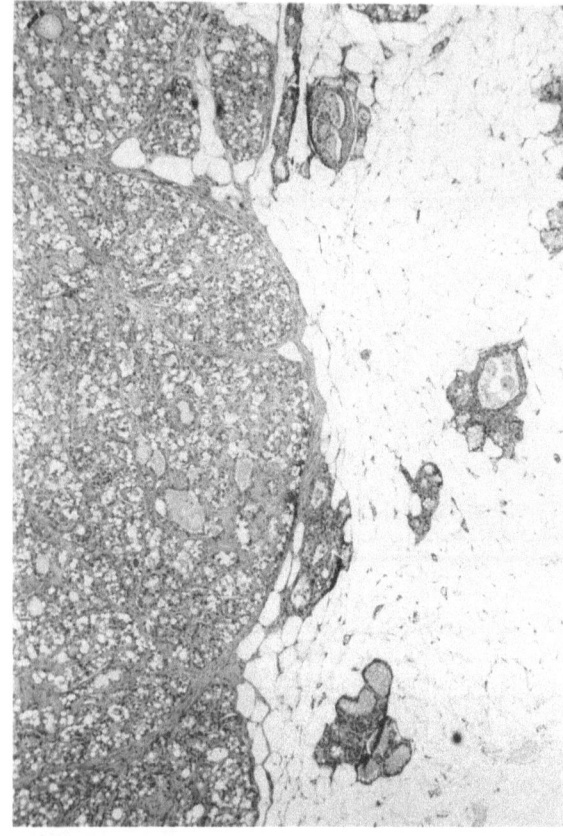

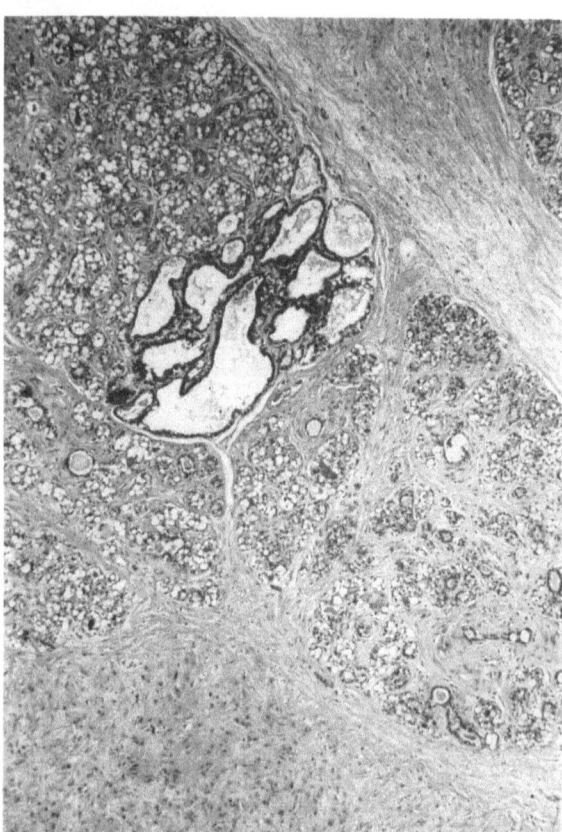

◀ **Fig. 441** *(above)*. Lactating adenoma with increased amount of connective tissue, probably going through the process of fibroadenoma formation. H and E, × 60

Fig. 442 *(below)*. Fibroadenoma with some remnants of lacting adenoma. Observe in the lower portion in increment in connective tissue that is obliterating the luminal spaces. H and E, × 60

Fig. 443 *(upper left)* and **444** *(lower left)*. Details of tubular ▶ elements in a lactating adenoma showing compression by connective tissue proliferation. H and E, × 160

Fig. 445 *(upper right)*. Fibroadenoma in which the desmoplastic reaction is compressing the tubular alveolar components. H and E, × 60

Fig. 446 *(lower right)*. Detail of the tubular elements composing the fibroadenoma shown in Fig. 445. H and E, × 400

Stromal Neoplasms

Benign Lesions

Fibroma. Well-circumscribed, nonencapsulated tumors composed of proliferating fibroblasts arranged in interlacing bundles and embedded in variable amounts of collagen fibers are fibromas. In some tumors there are isolated remnants of glandular epithelium (Figs. 447 and 448), which suggests that they originate from fibroadenomas.

Malignant Lesions

Fibrosarcoma. Malignant fibroblasts exhibiting the expected anaplastic characteristics and increased number of mitoses are the essential components of fibrosarcomas.

Epithelial-Stromal Neoplasms

Benign Lesions

Fibroadenoma. Benign tumors composed of mammary epithelium and connective tissue are fibroadenomas. The gross appearance of these tumors is soft, rubbery, paler, and less vascular than the carcinomas. Histologically, they exhibit variations with a transition from the mainly epithelial tumors which appear as adenomas (Figs. 441–444) to a more predominant proliferation of connective tissue, which determines the characteristic architecture of the fibroadenoma,

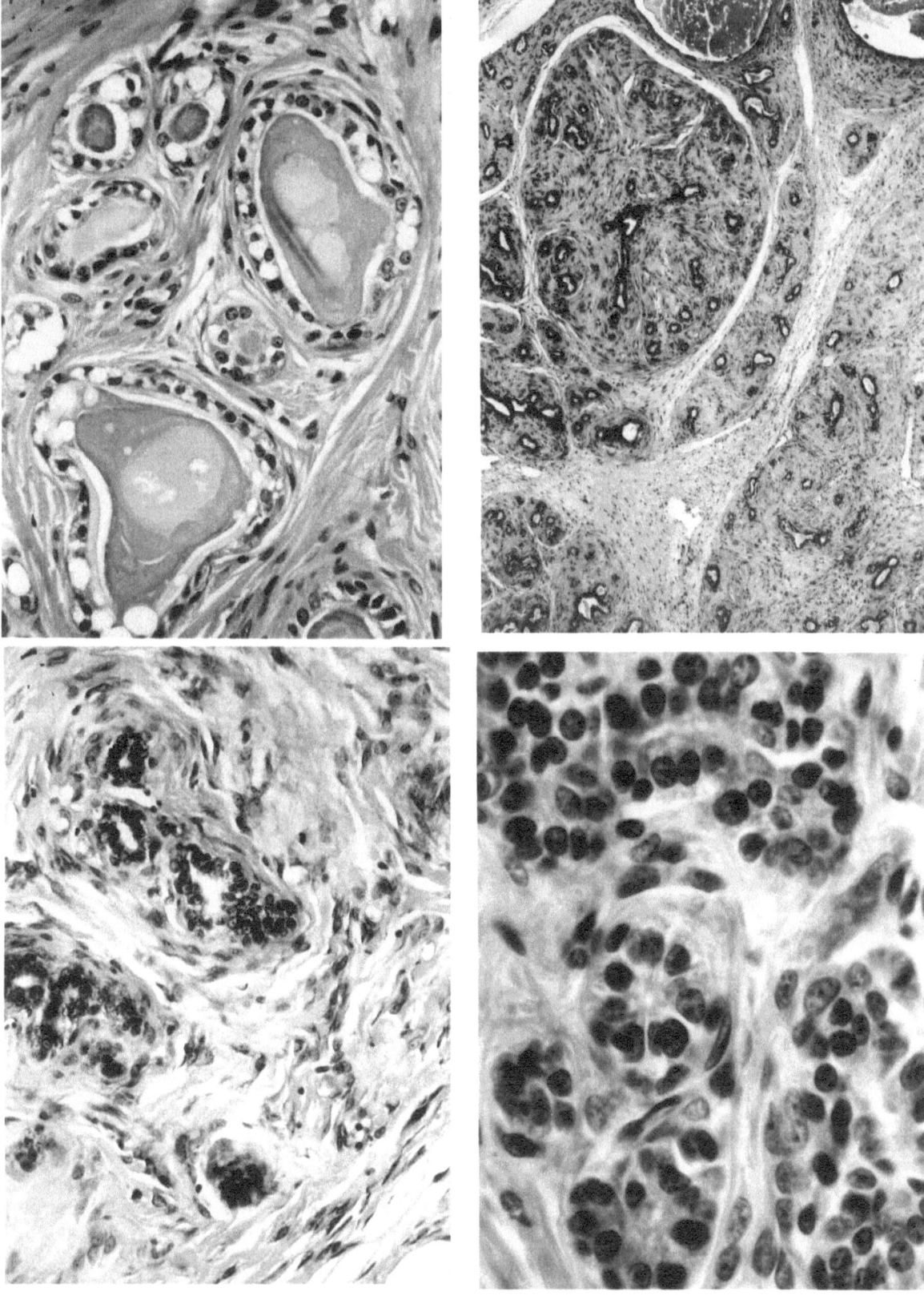

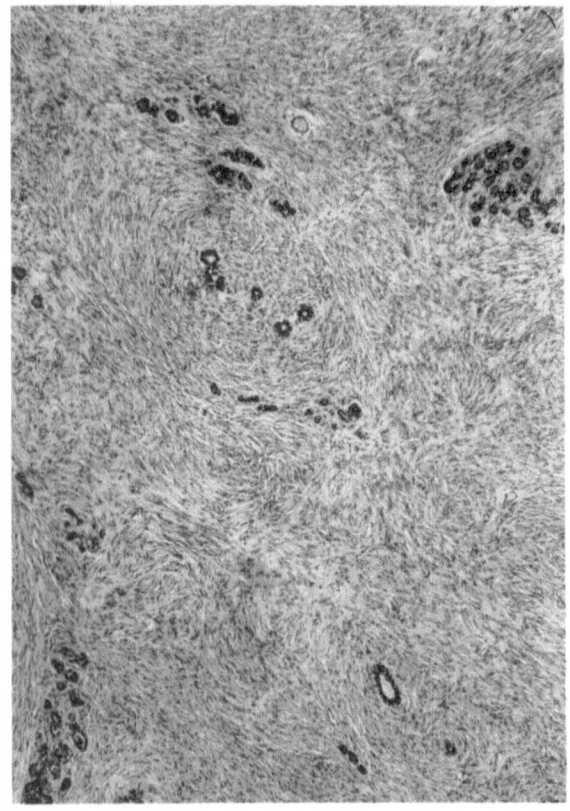

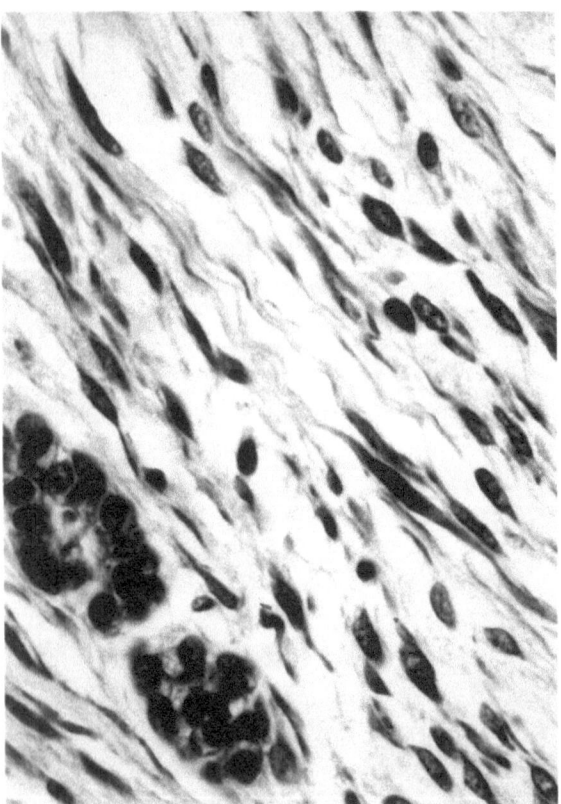

◀ **Fig. 447** *(above).* Fibroma in which small remnants of tubular epithelial elements are preserved. H and E, × 60

Fig. 448 *(below).* Detail of Fig. 447, in which the dense connective tissue contains fibroblastic proliferation. H and E, × 400

Fig. 449 *(upper left).* Carcinosarcoma of the breast. H and ▶ E, × 100

Fig. 450 *(lower left).* Detail of the tumor shown in Fig. 448 composed of stellated or elongated cells. H and E, × 400

Fig. 451 *(upper right).* Cells of the carcinosarcoma reacting positively for vimentin. Peroxidase-anitperoxidase (PAP), × 400

Fig. 452 *(lower right).* Cells from the carcinosarcoma shown in Fig. 449, in which clusters or rows of cells react positively against keratin. Peroxidase-antiperoxidase (PAP), × 400

pericanalicular type. Ductal and lobular structures are surrounded by layers of fibrous tissue (Figs. 443–446). The intracanalicular type of fibroadenoma that occurs in humans (Rosai 1981) is found only occasionally in the rat. In both types of tumors the secretory epithelium is usually one layer thick and maintains the same relation to the myoepithelium and basement membrane as does the normal mammary gland. When the fibrous tissue overgrows the epithelium to an extreme degree, ducts and alveoli become constricted, distorted, and widely separated by contracting bands of collagen (Fig. 444).

Malignant Lesions

Carcinosarcoma. A rare entity, the carcinosarcoma has frankly malignant characteristics in both the epithelium and the stroma. The epithelial component varies from well-differentiated, tubular structures to poorly demarcated and elongated cells which are difficult to differentiate from neoplastic stromal cells (Figs. 449–452). The specific markers keratin, myoglobin, desmin, and vimentin are useful for separating spindle-shaped epithelial cells from the stromal component. Nuclei vary in size and shape, and giant, multinucleated cells may be found. Mitoses are common in both the epithelium and the stroma.

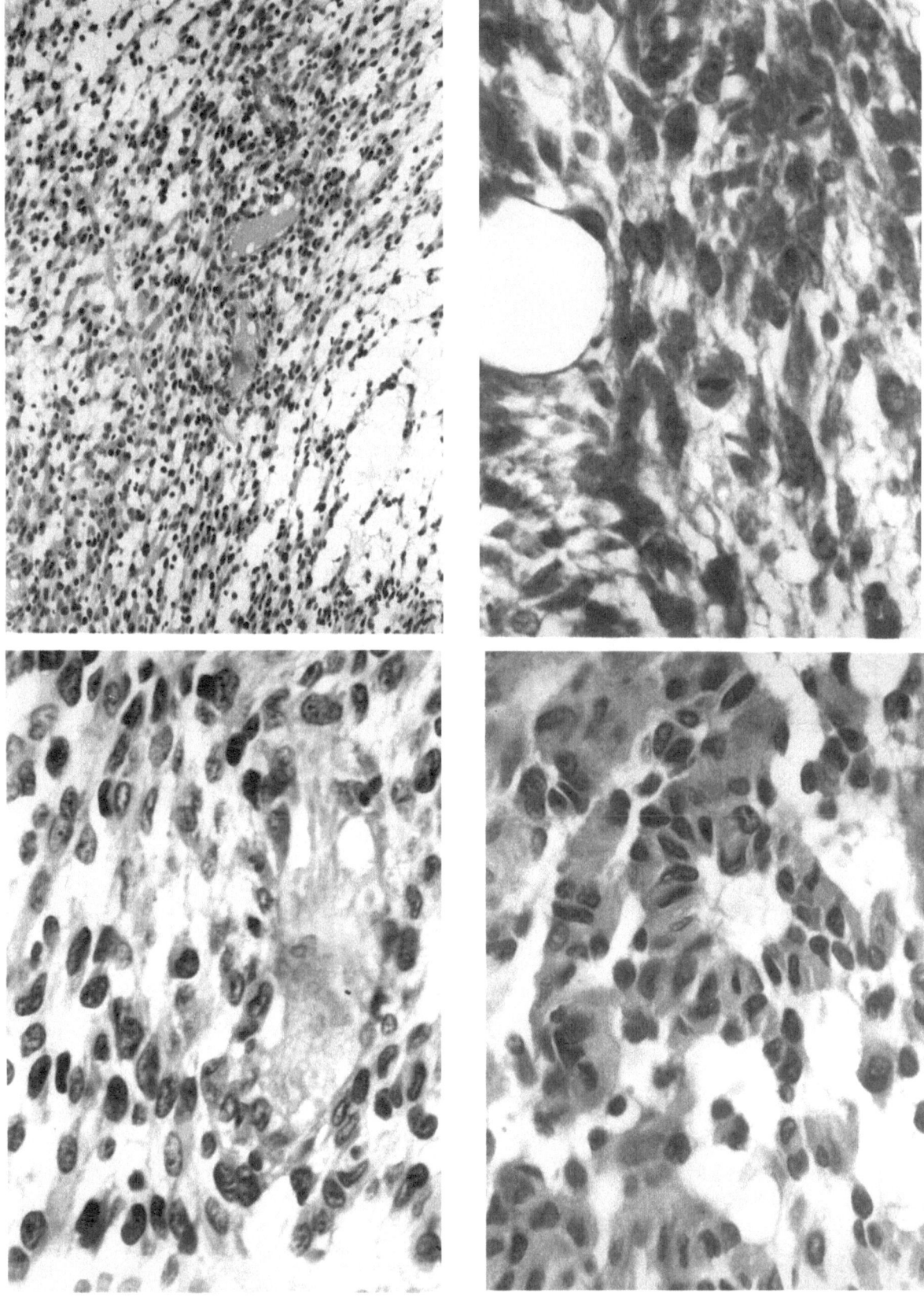

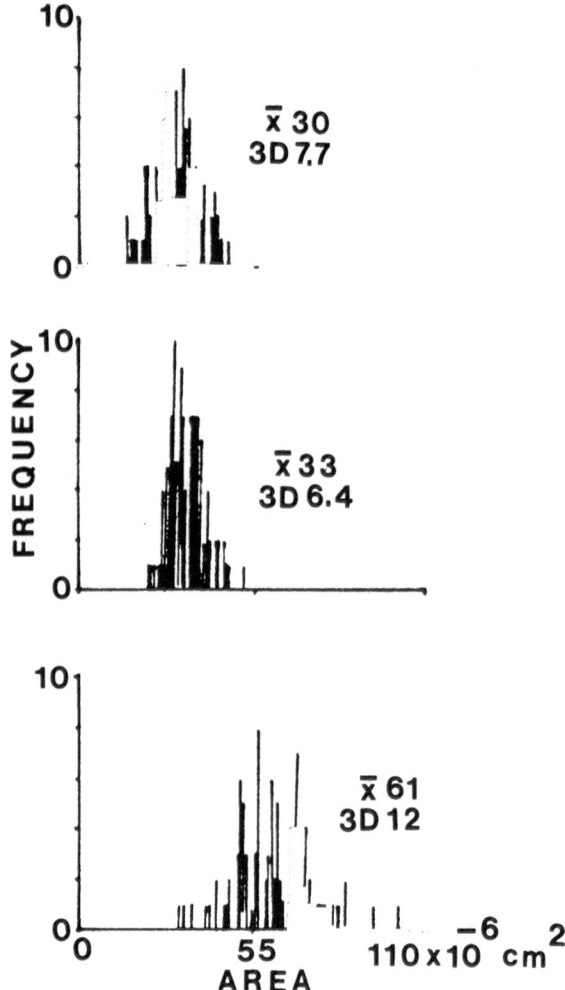

Nonneoplastic Lesions

Among the nonneoplastic lesions in the mammary gland, cystic changes are the ones most frequently found. They can originate from either ductal or lobular elements. Cysts derived from ducts range in size from 10 to 100 times the normal diameter, are lined by flat, cuboidal, epithelial cells, and have myoepithelial cells which are compressed against the basement membrane. In general, these ductal changes, that are also called duct ectasia or galactocele, are characterized by the accumulation within the lumen of eosinophilic granular material composed of lipids and protein secretion. Crystals similar to cholesterol and focal calcification are common. Lobular cysts are characterized by a grapelike configuration. The small cystic dilatations can be confluent, forming one large cyst (Fig. 390) lined by low cuboidal epithelial cells (Fig. 388), although some may contain cells with large vacuoles and decapitation of the apical portion of the cytoplasm. The nuclei are in general round or oval and are compressed against the basement membrane.

◀ **Fig. 453.** Frequency distribution of nuclear area of normal ducts *(upper)*; adenoma *(middle)*, and adenocarcinoma *(lower)*

▼ **Fig. 454.** Pathogenetic route of mammary carcinogenesis in the rat. *TEB*, terminal and bud; *TD*, terminal duct; *AB*, alveolar bud; *IDP*, intraductal proliferation

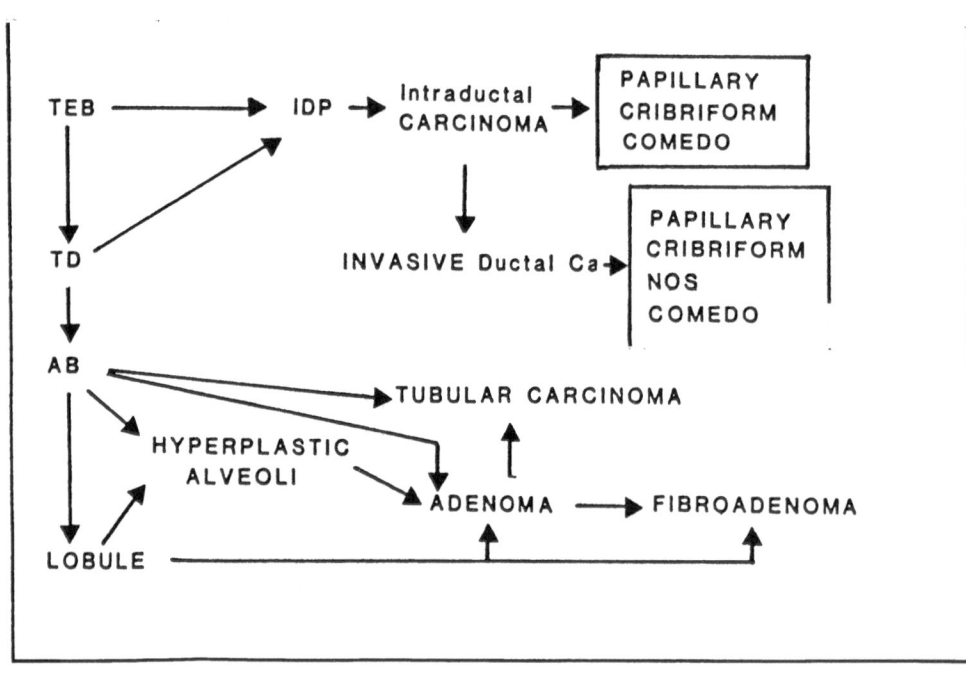

A ruptured galactocele (possibly by palpation) may evoke an intense inflammatory foreign body reaction which will require some time to be completely resolved.

Differential Diagnosis of Mammary Tumors

Although a common practice for evaluating the tumorigenic response of the rat mammary gland to carcinogens in the quantitation of palpable tumors, it is important to keep in mind that palpable lesions are lumps or swellings whose nature can be determined only through histologic examination. In Table 26 are listed normal organs, nonneoplastic lesions, and tumors of nonmammary origin that under gross examination can be confused with mammary tumors.

Physiological enlargement of the mammary gland during pregnancy and lactation generally is uniform and affects all glands; the gland regresses and involutes after weaning.

Salivary glands, particulary the parotid, are large and voluminous, extend well down into the neck, and become surrounded by the parenchyma of the first pair of mammary glands. When a biopsy is taken from mammary tumors of the first gland, it is easy to remove accidentally a piece of salivary gland as well. Two types of histology are found, depending upon whether the gland is of serous or mucinous type. The secreting acini of salivary glands are regular in appearance, and the ducts are lined by columnar epithelium. They should not be confused with mammary adenocarcinoma or with lactating gland.

The preputial gland (also referred to as the clitoral gland in the female) is a paired organ located in the ventral midline cranial to the urethra, between the inguinal mammary glands, and tends to develop hyperplasia, duct ectasia, and squamous metaplasia in carcinogen-treated animals. These enlarged glands are usually detected during tumor palpation, and under histologic examination they have been confused with mammary adenomas exhibiting squamous metaplasia.

Lymph nodes draining areas in which a tumor has formed or in which infections have occurred are prone to become enlarged and palpable. The sinuses are dilated and packed with mononuclear cells, and the characteristic lymph node structure is distorted due to sinus histiocytosis.

Abscess formation is not uncommon in animals repeatedly biopsied for mammary tumor examination. Such abscesses are well-encapsulated, tense, or fluctuant. On histologic section, the di-

Table 26. Differential diagnosis of tumors developing in mammary region

Structure or lesion	Main features
Lactating gland	Enlargement of the gland, uniformly affects all the pairs of glands
Salivary gland	Located in neck; serous or mucinous type, epithelium
Preputial gland (Clitoral gland)	Located in the inguinal region; uniformly large cells with round, leptochromatic nuclei arranged in acini
Lymph nodes	Normal or reactive, characteristic architecture
Abscesses	Encapsulated, tense, or fluctuant. Numerous polymorphonuclear leukocytes, macrophages, and necrotic material
Skin and adnexal tumors	Basal and squamous cell carcinomas, trichoepithelioma, tricholemmoma, sebaceous adenomas and carcinomas, fibromas, fibrosarcomas
Hibernomas	Typical architecture with numerous fat droplets of varying sizes

agnosis is obvious, with accumulation of polymorphonuclear leukocytes, macrophages, and cell detritus.

Epidermal inclusion cysts, lined by a maturing squamous epithelium and containing desquamated material within the lumen, can be mistaken during palpation for small mammary tumors.

Basal and squamous cell carcinomas, when they occur in the skin overlying the mammary glands, may be confused with tumors originating from this organ. Carcinogen-treated rats may develop trichoepitheliomas, which are small, firm tumors in the skin, not adherent to the underlying connective tissue. They ulcerate early, and some of them acquire a considerable size. Histologically they are composed of structures suggestive of hair follicle formation; in transverse sections the epithelial cells are arranged in concentric rings surrounding a characteristic keratinous core. Other adnexal tumors of the skin, such as tricholemmoma, sebaceous adenomas, and carcinomas, or fibromas and fibrosarcomas arising in the dermis can be found.

Hibernomas are tumors of the specialized brown fat that is located in the interscapular region of the rat. These benign tumors are made up of uniform eosinophilic fat cells with varying amounts of intracytoplasmic granules and uniformly small, round vacuoles resembling normal brown fat.

Table 27. Criteria of malignancy in mammary tumors

I. *Macroscopic criteria*
   a) Rapid growth and skin ulceration in short period of time.
   b) Soft, fleshy appearance with or without areas of necrosis and hemorrhage.

II. *Histopathologic criteria*
   a) Loss of normal architecture with varying pleomorphism and layering or formation of papillae.
   b) One cell type, basically intermediate cells, predominate over the dark or myoepithelial cells. Varying response of the host such as fibrosis or inflammatory response.
   c) Increased nucleocytoplasmic ratio, round to oval nuclei with smooth contour, leptochromatic appearance, and 1 or 2 nucleoli, numerous mitoses.
   d) Invasiveness: Neoplastic cells infiltrating surrounding structures such as muscle, dermis, and fat.

III. *Biologic criteria*
   a) Metastases to lymph nodes and lung. Occasionally found in older animals, rarely found in young animals.
   b) Transplantability, although it may not be a reliable criterion because benign fibroadenomas may be also transplantable.
   c) Angiogenic response in anterior chamber of the eye, found in malignant and premalignant lesions.

Criteria of Malignancy

Whether spontaneous or carcinogen-induced rat mammary tumors are benign or malignant can be determined by applying the following criteria: gross examination, histopathologic examination, and observation of the biologic behavior of the tumor (Table 27).

Macroscopic (Gross) Criteria. The two major criteria to be taken into consideration upon gross examination of a tumor are its rate of growth and gross appearance. Generally, malignant tumors tend to grow faster; however, some exceptions to this rule are observed. We have also found that tumors in the mammary glands located in the thoracic region grow faster than those arising in glands located in the abdominal region (Russo J and Russo IH 1987). The gross appearance of carcinomas is generally soft and fleshy, with areas of necrosis and hemorrhage. Some have cysts containing blood and necrotic material. Fibroadenomas, on the other hand, are white, with a rubbery and firm consistency, and they shell out from their capsule when they are sectioned. Carcinomas can be firm if they have elicited a desmoplastic response.

Histopathologic Criteria. Among the criteria of malignancy, the most important one is the loss of the tubulo-alevolar pattern of the normal mammary gland, a pattern maintained in the adenomas and fibroadenomas. Cytologically, malignant cells are larger than their normal counterparts and have an increased nucleocytoplasmic ratio. The enlarged nuclei contain coarse chromatin and more prominent nucleoli. The epithelial heterogeneity expressed by the normal gland, or even by benign lesions, in which at least myoepithelial, dark, and intermediate or clear cell types are identified, is rarely observed in malignant lesions (Russo J et al. 1983). The predominant cell in malignancy is the intermediate type, dark cells are rarely observed, and very few myoepithelial cells remain, especially in the invasive lesions. The number of mitoses is generally higher in malignant lesions than in benign ones.

Finally, invasion of the stroma and neighboring tissues, such as muscle and dermis, is a hallmark of malignant tumors. The stromal response to invasion, as demonstrated by fibrosis and inflammatory infiltration, is generally more prominent in the malignant lesions than in the noninvasive or benign ones.

Biologic Criteria. The most reliable criterion of malignancy is the ability of a tumor to metastasize to distant organs, such as lymph nodes or lungs. Very few authors report the finding of metastases from either spontaneous or experimentally induced rat mammary tumors. This lack of metastasizing ability of rat tumors could be attributed to the short period of time that treated animals have been followed in most studies, since only when the study is prolonged for 2 or 3 years, or essentially the whole life span of the animal, do metastases become evident. The histopathologic type of a tumor does not seem to affect its metastasizing ability, since it has been found that cribriform, comedo, or papillary carcinomas produce metastases with similar frequency (Van Zwieten 1984).

Transplantability (Young and Hallowes 1973) has not been considered a reliable criterion of malignancy in rats because fibroadenomas are transplantable. The ability of neoplastic lesions to elicit angiogenesis has been postulated to be a biological marker of malignancy but has not been extensively used (Brem et al. 1978; Maiorana and Gullino 1978).

Pathogenesis of Mammary Tumors

Induction of rat mammary carcinomas by administration of certain chemical carcinogens such as 7,12-dimethylbenz[a]anthracene (DMBA) requires the carcinogen to act on a specific compartment of the mammary gland, that is the TEB (Russo J et al. 1977, 1982; Tay and Russo 1981a, b, 1985). The rat mammary gland is composed of a branching parenchyma in which the terminal ductal structures end in TEBs which progressively differentiate into alveolar buds (ABs). ABs differentiate into lobules (Russo IH and Russo J 1978; Russo J 1983). This process does not occur simultaneously in all glands, but it differs depending upon the topographical location of each gland (Russo J and Russo IH 1987). Thoracic mammary glands, in general, contain significantly more abundant and prominent TEBs than abdominal glands. With aging, there is a proportional reduction in the number of TEBs in all mammary glands. This reduction is mostly due to the progression of TEBs to ABs and lobules (Russo J and Russo IH 1987). The administration of DMBA to virgin rats of different ages induces tumors with an incidence that is directly proportional to the number of highly proliferating TEBs. An incidence of carcinoma of 100% is obtained when DMBA is administered to rats 30–55 days of age, but the highest number of tumors per animal is observed when the carcinogen is given to animals when they are 40–46 days of age, a period in which TEBs are most actively differentiating to ABs. The sharp decrease in the number of TEBs observed in animals older than 55 days, and to a greater degree in abdominal than in thoracic mammary glands, is also accompanied by a lower incidence of tumors and a lower number of tumors per animal. The difference in degree of development observed between thoracic and abdominal glands explains the higher incidence of ductal carcinomas originating from the former. These results indicate that it is the presence of the TEBs which makes the mammary gland the target of the carcinogenic action of DMBA (Russo J et al. 1979, 1987).

The pathogenic pathway of rat mammary carcinogenesis has originated from the study of the DMBA-induced mammary carcinoma model (Fig. 454). However, data obtained from nonsequential observations of tumor types induced by other carcinogens and radiation (Van Zwieten 1984) seem to confirm that a common pathway exists for different etiologic agents.

References

Brem SS, Jensen HM, Gullino PM (1978) Angiogenesis as a marker of preneoplastic lesions of the human breast. Cancer 41: 239–244

Dao TL (1962) The role of ovarian hormones in initiating the induction of mammary cancer in rats by polynuclear hydrocarbons. Cancer Res 22: 973–981

Dao TL (1964) Carcinogenesis of mammary gland in rat. Prog Exp Tumor Res 5: 1547

Fisher ER, Gregorio RM, Fisher B (1975) The pathology of invasive breast cancer. A syllabus derived from findings of the National Surgical Adjuvant Breast Project (protocol no 4). Cancer 36: 1–85

Gullino PM, Pettigrew HM, Granthan FH (1975) N-Nitrosomethylurea as mammary gland carcinogen in rats. JNCI 64: 401–414

Huggins C, Yang NC (1962) Induction and extinction of mammary cancer. A striking effect of hydrocarbons permits analysis of mechanisms of causes and cure of breast cancer. Science 137: 257–262

Huggins C, Grand LC, Brillantes FP (1959) Critical significances of breast structure in the induction of mammary cancer in the rat. Proc Natl Acad Sci USA 45: 1294–1300

Ito N (1981) In vivo carcinogenesis of 4-Nitroquinoline 1-oxide and related compounds. In: Sugimura T (ed) The Nitroguinolines. Carcinogenesis, a comprehensive surgery, vol 6. Raven, New York, pp 117–153

Maiorana A, Gullino PM (1978) Acquisition of angiogenic capacity and neoplastic transformation in the rat mammary gland. Cancer Res 38: 4409–4414

Rosai J (1981) Ackerman's surgical pathology. Mosby, St Louis, pp 1087–1149

Russo IH, Russo J (1978) Developmental stage of the rat mammary gland as determinant of its susceptibility to 7,12-dimethylbenz(a)anthracene. JNCI 61: 1439–1449

Russo IH, Saby J, Isenberg W (1976) Early signs of malignant transformation in rat mammary carcinoma. Proc Am Assoc Cancer Res 17: 116

Russo J (1983) Basis of cellular autonomy in susceptibility to carcinogenesis. Toxicol Pathol 11: 149–166

Russo J, Russo IH (1978) DNA-labeling index and structure of the rat mammary gland as determinants of its susceptibility to carcinogenesis. JNCI 61: 1451–1459

Russo J, Russo IH (1980) Influence of differentiation and cell kinetics on the susceptibility of the rat mammary gland to carcinogenesis. Cancer Res 40: 2677–2687

Russo J, Russo IH (1987) Biology of disease. Biological and molecular bases of mammary carcinogenesis. Lab Invest 57: 112–137

Russo J, Saby J, Isenberg WM, Russo IH (1977) Pathogenesis of mammary carcinomas induced in rats by 7,12-dimethylbenz(a)anthracene. JNCI 59: 435–445

Russo J. Wilgus G, Russo IH (1979) Susceptibility of the mammary gland to carcinogenesis. I. Differentiation of the mammary gland as determinant of tumor incidence and type of lesion. Am J Pathol 96: 721–734

Russo J, Tait L, Russo IH (1983) Susceptibility of the rat mammary gland to carcinogenesis. III. The cell of origin of rat mammary carcinoma. Am J Pathol 113: 50–66

Russo J, Tay LK, Russo IH (1982) Differentiation of the mammary gland and susceptibility to carcinogenesis. Breast Cancer Res Treat 2: 5-73

Shirai T, Fysh JM, Lee MS, Vaught JB, King CM (1981) Relationship of metabolic activation on N-hydroxy-N-acylaryamines to biological response in the liver and mammary gland of the female CD rat. Cancer Res 41: 4346-4353

Tay LK, Russo J (1981a) 7,12-Dimethylbenz(a)anthracene-induced DNA binding and repair synthesis in susceptible and nonsusceptible mammary epithelial cells in culture. JNCI 67: 155-161

Tay LK, Russo J (1981b) Formation and removal of 7,12-dimethylbenz(a)anthracene nucleic acid adducts in rat mammary epithelial cells with different susceptibility to carcinogenesis. Carcinogenesis 2: 1327-1333

Tay LK, Russo J (1985) Effect of human chorionic gonadotropin or 7,12-dimethylbenz(a)anthracene-induced DNA bindung and repair synthesis by rat mammary epithelial cells. Chem Biol Interact 55: 13-21

Van Zwieten MJ (1984) The rat as an animal model in breast cancer research. Martinus Nijhoff, Boston

Young S, Hallowes RC (1973) Tumours of the mammary gland. In: Turusov VS (ed) Pathology of tumours in laboratory animals, vol 1. Tumours of the rat, pt 1. IARC, Lyon, pp 31-74

Factors That Modulate Chemical Carcinogenesis in the Mammary Gland of the Female Rat

Adrianne E. Rogers

Introduction

Susceptibility of the female rat mammary gland to chemical carcinogenesis is strongly influenced by age, reproductive, and endocrine status and can be further modulated by diet, hormones, and drugs. Estrous cycle status at the time of exposure to the carcinogen has a small effect. Unknown factors also influence tumorigenesis, which can vary between experiments performed under apparently identical conditions.

Examples of mammary tumorigenesis in the major rat models are given in Tables 28-31. A given carcinogen dose induces tumors within a range of latency periods of several weeks, and incidence varies in different experiments in the same or different laboratories. Route of administration of 7,12-dimethylbenz[a]anthracene (DMBA) appears not to have a major effect on tumor latency, incidence, or number of tumors per animals. DMBA is effective when administered orally or parenterally or when injected directly into the gland, a procedure useful in separating local from systemic effects of modulating factors. N-methyl-N-nitrosourea (MNU) must be given parenterally to induce mammary tumors and is reported to be equally effective by the intravenous and subcutaneous routes. Both carcinogens are effective in a single dose. Dose response of tumorigenesis to DMBA or MNU is generally, but not always, clear in experiments designed to detect it (Table 31) and may differ greatly between experiments.

Single-dose models have been used to develop theories of the carcinogenic process in the mammary gland and have produced data on the events and modulating factors in initiation, promotion, and progression of tumors. Tumorigenesis results are expressed as latency (time between carcinogen administration and detection of palpable tumor), cumulative or final incidence of tumors, and tumor burden (number, weight, or geometric mean diameter of tumors per rat or per group of rats). Data obtained at necropsy should include histologic diagnosis of tumors; the data should be recorded separately for benign and malignant tumors. All the different expressions of results are useful in detecting modulating factors, but changes in latency and incidence probably indicate the most powerful effects of modulators and are the most easily interpreted. However, subtle effects may be detectable only in examination of tumor burden or histology.

Table 28. Mammary tumors induced by DMBA[a] in female Sprague-Dawley rats fed natural ingredient diets

Dose of DMBA (mg/kg)	Mammary tumors			Reference	Comment
	Latency[b] (weeks)	% Incidence[c]	No./rat[d]		
20	12	91 (32)	5.4	McCormick et al. 1982	At 20 mg dose:
20	20	60 (28)	0.7	Minton et al. 1983	Threefold variation in latency and large differences in tumor incidence and number, not due to difference in necropsy time
20	7	85 (17)	2.6	Thompson et al. 1982	Large effect on latency between 20 and
15	16	89 (40)	1.0		15 mg doses
20	–	100 (11)	3.9	Welsch and Dehoog 1983	Little or no difference between 20 and
10	–	90 (12)	4.5		10 mg doses, large difference between them and 5 mg dose; latency not given
5	–	85 (26)	2.0		
15	–	75 (30)	1.6	Moon et al. 1976	Large differences between three doses;
5	–	46 (30)	0.6		latency not given
2.5	–	8 (30)	0.1		

[a] DMBA given by gastric gavage to rats at 50-60 days of age; DMBA, 7,12-dimethylbenz[a]anthracene.
[b] Determined from graphs if not stated in paper.
[c] At necropsy, weeks after DMBA exposure given in parentheses.
[d] Calculated from data given if not stated in paper.

Table 29. Mammary tumors induced by DMBA in female Sprague-Dawley rats fed purified diets, 3%-5% fat

DMBA[a] (mg/rat)	Mammary tumors		No./rat at risk[d]	Reference
	Latency[b] (weeks)	% Incidence[c]		
7.5	12	47 (19)	1.2	Sylvester et al. 1986a
	11	76 (22)	2.4	Ip 1986a
	12	84 (22)	2.8	
5	–	70 (17)	2.3	Hopkins and Carroll 1979
	11	77 (17)	2.3	Carroll and Khor 1971
	–	46 (20-22)	1.3	Ip and Ip 1981
	13	40 (22)	0.9	Ip and Sinha 1981
	17	44 (22)	1.0	Carter et al. 1983
2.5-3.5	22	83 (35)	1.7	Lee and Rogers 1983
	16	52 (32)	1.4	Rogers et al. 1985
	9	78 (11)	2.9	Rogers et al. 1986
	16	68 (35)	1.4	
	27	38 (26)	0.5	Clinton et al. 1984

[a] DMBA given by gavage to 50-55-day-old rats; in some experiments purified diets were fed after DMBA exposure only; DMBA, 7,12-dimethylbenz[a]anthracene.
[b] Determined from graphs if not stated in paper.
[c] At necropsy, weeks after DMBA exposure given in parentheses.
[d] Calculated from data given if not stated in paper.

Table 30. Mammary tumors induced by MNU given intravenously to Sprague-Dawley rats[a] fed natural ingredient diets

MNU (mg/kg)	Latency[b] (weeks)	Mammary tumors		Reference
		% Incidence[c]	No./rat at risk[d]	
50	15	70 (26)	3.3	Chan and Dao 1981
50	8	100 (32)	4.8	McCormick et al. 1982
50	11	90 (26)	4.5	Grubbs et al. 1983a
50	11[d]	80 (21)[d]	1.7[d]	Ratko and Beattie 1985
50	10	90 (26)	4.3	Thompson and Meeker 1983
50 × 2	15	41 (25)	1.1	Rose et al. 1980
50 × 2	9	94 (26)	6.8	Grubbs et al. 1983b
25 × 2	–	73 (31)	2.7	Welsch et al. 1980
12.5 × 2	–	27 (25)	0.5	

MNU, *N*-methyl-*N*-nitrosourea.
[a] Rats 50–60 days of age.
[b] Calculated from data given if not stated in paper.
[c] At necropsy, weeks after MNU exposure given in parentheses.
[d] Average for rats treated at different stages of estrous cycle.

Table 31. Mammary tumors induced by parenteral MNU in female Sprague-Dawley rats[a] fed purified diets, 3%–5% fat

MNU (mg/kg)	Mammary tumors		No./rat at risk[d]	Reference
	Latency[b] (weeks)	% Incidence[c]		
50 iv	14	88 (26)	6.4	Chan and Dao 1981
50 iv	11	91 (18)	2.4	Silverman et al. 1980
50 iv	14	50 (18)	1.0	Wei et al. 1985
	16	90 (28)	1.8	
50 sc	7	100 (26)	7.6	Thompson et al. 1984, 1985
35 sc	11	96 (26)	4.1	

MNU, *N*-methyl-*N*-nitrosourea; iv, intravenous; sc, subcutaneous.
[a] Rats 50–60 days of age.
[b] Determined from data given if not stated in paper.
[c] At necropsy, weeks after MNU exposure given on parentheses.
[d] Calculated from data given if not stated in paper.

Modulating Factors

Age

Rats are most sensitive to DMBA tumorigenesis between approximately 35 and 60 days of age. This is the period beginning shortly after opening of the vagina and ending after establishment of regular estrous cycles. The mammary gland of older rats is less susceptible to chemical carcinogenesis, and the proportion of benign tumors is increased (Russo and Russo 1987; Sinha et al. 1983). The epithelium in older rats is relatively resistant and has a low growth fraction and lengthened G_1 phase in the cell cycle (Russo and Russo 1987). Susceptibility to tumorigenesis by MNU also is decreased when older animals are used. Chan and Dao (1983) and Grubbs et al. (1983a) reported decreased tumor incidence and multiplicity with age in Sprague-Dawley or Fischer 344 rats given MNU at ages up to 200 days.

An effect of age can be detected on binding of DMBA to mammary gland DNA. In rats of different ages (35, 50, or 120 days), binding was directly related to final tumor incidence and, therefore, inversely related to age, but only in rats of the most sensitive age (50 days) was binding proportional to dose (Janss and Ben 1978). The effect of age on binding was demonstrated also in vitro; binding was proportional to dose at all ages studied (Tay and Russo 1981).

Reproductive and Endocrine Status

Induction, development, and continued growth of tumors are dependent upon a normal hormonal environment. Hormone dependence can be shown in about 80% of DMBA-induced tumors and 70%–90% of MNU-induced tumors. The hormone-dependent tumors regress if circulating estrogen and prolactin are reduced or if tissue hormone receptors are blocked. Only a small number of tumors is induced in rats treated at the time of DMBA administration with tamoxifen or bromocriptine to block estrogen effects and prolactin release, respectively. The tumors induced in the presence of blockers are much less likely to be hormone dependent than tumors induced in normal rats (Sylvester et al. 1983, 1986a).

Endocrine influences on mammary tumorigenesis have been reviewed recently (Welsch 1985, 1986, 1987) and can be summarized as follows. Prolactin, growth hormone, estrogen, progesterone, glucocorticoids, insulin, and thyroxine all influence tumorigenesis. Hyperprolactinemia after carcinogen treatment increases the development and growth of mammary tumors in intact or ovariectomized rats, but hyperprolactinemia induced before carcinogen exposure inhibits tumorigenesis.

Estrogens are required for the development and growth of DMBA-induced mammary tumors. Ovariectomy of rats before DMBA treatment blocks tumorigenesis; ovariectomy after DMBA treatment reduces tumor development and causes tumor regression. The effects of castration are reversed by administration of estrogen. In intact animals, the administration of estrogens after carcinogen exposure can enhance tumor growth. Estrogen given before MNU administration reduces tumor development (Grubbs et al. 1985). Enhancement by estrogen does not occur in hypophysectomized rats, indicating that estrogen acts, at least in part, by inducing prolactin secretion.

Progesterone is less important than prolactin or estrogen in mammary tumorigenesis in rats, but it can increase or inhibit tumor development under certain experimental conditions. Glucocorticoids inhibit chemical carcinogenesis and growth of transplanted rat mammary carcinomas (Hilf et al. 1971). Induced diabetes inhibits the development or induces regression of tumors, and insulin treatment causes increased tumor growth (Heuson and Legros 1972). Thyroid hormones may increase mammary tumorigenesis; however, the effects of the thyroid hormones, insulin, glucocorticoid, and other hormones have not been examined in studies that take account of total caloric consumption and weight gain. Since caloric supply is a major modulating factor in tumorigenesis, further studies are needed.

There is an influence on tumorigenesis of the stage of the estrous cycle at the time of carcinogen exposure. Tumorigenesis is greater in rats given MNU at proestrus or estrus than at diestrus (Lindsey et al. 1981; Ratko and Beattie 1985). Cycle stage at MNU exposure had no significant effect on percentage of tumors positive for cytosolic or nuclear estrogen receptors (71%–89%) or on results of flow cytometric analysis of tumors for DNA content and cell cycle stage. However, tumors induced in rats given MNU at diestrus or metestrus grew more rapidly and regressed more rapidly in response to ovariectomy than tumors in rats given MNU at estrus or proestrus (Braun et al. 1987).

Tumorigenesis is reduced by prior pregnancy and lactation (Grubbs et al. 1983b, 1986). Grubbs et al. (1986) have presented two hypotheses for mechanisms by which parity prevents mammary carcinogenesis: (a) Early pregnancy alters the mammary epithelial cells by hormonal influences, making them less susceptible to subsequent carcinogen exposure; (b) initiated cells present before pregnancy are destroyed or inhibited from progressing to tumor by endocrine changes of pregnancy. Evidence in favor of the first hypothesis has been reported in several studies (Russo and Russo 1987). Grubbs et al. (1986) studied the effect on tumorigenesis of pregnancy beginning 10–28 days after a single dose of DMBA or MNU. In all experiments, pregnancy and lactation reduced tumorigenesis. Prolactin treatment of parous rats after lactation did not decrease the latency or increase the incidence of cancers; the same prolactin treatment did decrease tumor latency and increase tumor incidence and number in carcinogen-treated virgin rats. These investigators concluded that the hormonal changes of pregnancy caused differentiation of pre-neoplastic cells to a secretory state that prevented progression to tumor.

Carcinogen Dose

Tumor latency is inversely related, and tumor incidence, burden, and malignancy are directly related to the dose of DMBA or MNU. Isaacs (1985) reported that the number and percentage of malignant tumors increased synergistically with 2, 3, or 4 repeated doses of DMBA; results were similar with MNU. Dose-response relationships for the induction of mammary tumors by a single i.v. injection of MNU were reported by McCormick et al. (1981) in 50-day-old, female, Sprague-Dawley rats given single doses of 10–50 mg MNU per kg body weight. Malignant and benign mammary tumors occurred in all groups. Incidence and number of tumors per animal increased, and the latent period for cancer decreased with increasing doses of MNU. Malignant tumors appeared earlier than benign tumors, and benign tumors, as percentage of total tumors, decreased with increasing dose.

Fat

Dietary fat content has significant, reproducible, and consistent effects on chemically induced, mammary gland tumorigenesis in female rats in both the DMBA and MNU models (Tables 32 and 33). The fats that are effective reduce tumor latency and increase tumor incidence and number. The enhancement of tumorigenesis by fat

Table 32. Mammary tumorigenesis by DMBA or MNU in rats fed different amounts of corn oil or fat blend in nutritionally balanced, complete diets and response of tumorigenesis to diet restriction

% Corn oil in diet		Restriction[a] (% of calories in an ad libitum diet)	Mammary tumors		Reference
Before carcinogen	After		% Incidence[b]	Latency (weeks)	
5	5	0	68	16	Wetsel et al. 1981
5	20	0	87	12	
20	20	0	83	14	
5	5	0	36	11	Chan and Dao 1983
25	25	0	79	8	
5	5	0	38[c]	27	Clinton et al. 1984
10	10	0	36	19	
25	25	0	65	17	
5	10	0	55[c]	20	Clinton et al. 1986
10	10	0	65	18	
25	10	0	76	16	
14	14	0	80	–	Kritchevsky and Klurfeld 1986
14	14	40	20	–	
5	5	10[d]	74[e]	–	
5	17.5	10[d]	69	–	
5	30	10[d]	82	–	
5	5	0	30	–	Cohen 1987
5	10	0	56	–	
5	20	0	67	–	
5	10	25	8	–	
5	20	25	3	–	
Natural product diet	10[f]	0	67	18	Beth et al. 1987a
	16	0	77	17	
	22	0	77	14	
	10	30	50	24	
	16	30	63	21	
	22	30	57	20	

DMBA, 7,12-dimethylbenz[a]anthracene; MNU, N-methyl-N-nitrosourea.
[a] After carcinogen exposure.
[b] Calculated from published data if not explicity stated in paper.
[c] Tumor incidence correlated with caloric intake across diet groups, but effect of fat not attributable to caloric intake.
[d] For 5 weeks, then ad libitum intake.
[e] Tumor incidence paralleled caloric intake irrespective of dietary fat content.
[f] Blend of fats similar to average West German diet.

can be reduced by addition of selenium to the diet, by treatment with indomethacin, and by hormonal manipulations. Fat is effective if it is fed throughout the rat's lifetime or if it is fed for restricted periods before or after carcinogen exposure (Rogers and Lee 1986; Rogers and Longnecker 1988).

The fat content of diets used in studies generally has been between 3%-5% (by weight) for control and 20%-25% for high-fat diets. Diets lower than 3% fat are often not fully supportive of growth, may be deficient in essential fatty acids (EFA), and may not permit normal hormone synthesis and secretion or growth and differentiation of the mammary gland (Knazek et al. 1980; Welsch et al. 1985).

Polyunsaturated (ω-6) fats from vegetable sources have the greatest effects on tumorigenesis; monounsaturated fats have variable effects; saturated or polyunsaturated ω-3 fats have little or no effect (Rogers and Lee 1986; Rogers and Longnecker 1988). The effect of a fat is partly due to its linoleic acid content (Ip et al. 1985); several fatty acids contribute to the effect (Chan et al. 1983). In DMBA-treated rats fed a high lard diet, tumor latency was decreased, and tumor number, incidence, and fraction of tumors that were malignant were increased compared with control rats. There was no effect of dietary fat content on the growth rate of tumors classified histologically as benign or malignant (Rogers et al. 1985, 1986). Lard is composed of a mixture of polyunsaturated, monounsaturated, and saturated fatty acids. Similar results in detailed studies of tumorigenesis in DMBA-treated rats fed a diet high in corn oil indicate that enhancement is related specifically to fat but also to calories consumed irrespective of dietary fat content (Clinton et al. 1984, 1986). It appears that the effective high-fat diets do not influence growth of a

Table 33. Mammary tumorigenesis by DMBA or MNU in rats fed high levels of different types of fat in nutritionally balanced diets

Dietary fat[a] type	%	Mammary tumors		Reference
		% Incidence	Latency (weeks)	
Corn oil	5	33	11[b]	Chan et al. 1983
	33	85	8	
Lard	33[c]	63	9	
Beef tallow	33[c]	50	10	
Coconut oil	33[c]	43	13	
Lard	5[c]	52	16[b]	Rogers et al. 1985
	24[c]	80	12	
	24[c, d]	70	13	
Beef tallow	5[c]	83	22[b]	Lee and Rogers 1983
	20[c]	80	19	
Rapeseed oil	5[c]	71	16	
	20[c]	66	17	
Corn oil	5[e]	66	17[b]	Cohen et al. 1986
	23[e]	87	11	
Safflower oil	5[e]	63	17	
	23[e]	87	12	
Olive oil	23[e]	63	21	
Coconut oil	3[c]	53	-	Kritchevsky et al. 1984
	18[c]	53	-	
Corn oil	5	47	12[b]	Sylvester et al. 1986b
	20[f]	56	10	
Lard	20[f]	78	10	
Palm oil	20[f]	50	10	

DMBA, 7,12-dimethylbenz[a]anthracene; MNU, N-methyl-N-nitrosourea.
[a] Fed throughout experiment unless otherwise noted.
[b] Body weight not significantly different between groups, not correlated with tumor end points.
[c] Including 1% corn oil.
[d] Diet fed only before carcinogen exposure; 5% fat after exposure.
[e] Natural ingredient diet fed before carcinogen exposure.
[f] Diet fed before and 1 week after carcinogen exposure; 5% corn oil fed thereafter.

tumor directly but decrease the interval between initiation and appearance of palpable tumors, apparently by increasing the proportion of malignant tumors which grow faster than benign tumors.

Effects of dietary fat on MNU-induced tumorigenesis, reported primarily in Fischer 344 rather than Sprague-Dawley rats, are similar to those with DMBA. Corn oil is highly effective; lard has a similar but somewhat lesser effect; beef tallow has little if any effect (Chan and Dao 1983; Dao and Chan 1983).

The timing and duration of the enhancing effect of high dietary fat have been investigated. The predominant effect is exerted after exposure to the carcinogen, and it is increased by feeding the high-fat diet longer and decreased by lengthening the time between exposure to the carcinogen and introduction of the high-fat diet (Dao and Chan 1983). However, corn oil and lard fed only before exposure to DMBA also enhance tumorigenesis (Rogers et al. 1982; Rogers et al. 1986; Sylvester et al. 1986b; Clinton et al. 1986).

The mechanisms of the effect of high dietary fat are not known. Those that have been examined include effects on circulating hormones, tissue hormone receptors, growth, differentiation, and metabolism of mammary gland and binding of DMBA (Welsch 1986, 1987). General hypotheses about effects of fat on cancer in mammary gland and other sites include effects on caloric balance, tissue peroxide content, immunological responses, prostaglandin metabolism, cell membrane composition, and response to growth factors.

The importance of active DNA synthesis in the gland in governing its age-related susceptibility to carcinogenesis led to examination of DNA synthesis in mammary glands of rats fed high lard or control diets prior to DMBA administration. DNA synthesis, evaluated by isolation and counting of DNA from terminal duct lobular units (TDLU) and by counting labeled cells in TDLU in autoradiographs, was not influenced by dietary fat at the time of DMBA administration (age 55 days) or later, until the period at which tumors began to appear. At that time [^{3}H]thymidine incorporation was greater in nontumorous glands from rats fed high lard than from control rats (Lee et al. 1988). Little or no effect of dietary fat on mammary gland differentiation and DNA synthesis was reported in mice fed diets that contained at least 5% fat; low or no fat diets retarded gland development (Welsch et al. 1985).

The search for hormonal mechanisms to explain the effect of fat has yielded negative results (Welsch 1987; Wetsel and Rogers 1984; Wetsel et al. 1984). In studies in which rats bore atrial cannulas for blood sampling throughout the estrous cycle, no effect of high dietary corn oil on serum prolactin, estrogen, or progesterone was found (Aylsworth et al. 1984; Wetsel et al. 1984). A high corn oil diet enhanced development of both hormone-dependent and hormone-independent tumors induced by DMBA and did not influence the hormone responsiveness of the tumors (Sylvester et al. 1986a).

An additional factor that makes it unlikely that certain dietary fats enhance mammary tumorigenesis by altering estrogen or prolactin secretion is the fact that similar high-fat diets increase tumorigenesis in other organs and tissues, including pancreas, liver, skin, and possibly other sites (Welsch 1987; Birt and Pour 1986; Birt et al. 1987; Rogers and Longnecker 1988).

Hormone responsiveness of receptors in mammary glands and in nontarget tissues and mammary tumors has been measured in rats fed control or high-fat diets. Receptors were found not to be affected except when extremely low fat, 0.5%, was fed (Ip and Ip 1981; Cave and Erickson-Lucas 1982; Cave and Jurkowski 1984; Wetsel and Rogers 1984).

The question of the relative importance of fat and of the calories it provides is relevant to all tissues in which tumorigenesis is enhanced by high-fat diets (Klurfeld et al. 1987; Kritchevsky et al. 1984; Kritchevsky and Klurfeld 1987). The marked effect of certain fats, such as corn oil and lard, on mammary tumorigenesis and the lower or absent effects of other, equally well-utilized fats, such as essential fatty acids (EFA)-supplemented beef tallow or olive oil, indicates that the effective fats have an activity aside from their caloric contributions. Pair-feeding studies in mammary tumor and pancreatic tumor models have also given evidence of a specific effect of fat (Rogers et al. 1985; Birt et al. 1987).

Effect of Other Nutrients and Selected Chemicals on Mammary Tumorigenesis

Selenium fed at levels in the toxic or near-toxic range inhibits mammary tumorigenesis, particularly in rats fed diets high in polyunsaturated fats. The effect is exerted both at initiation and during promotion of tumorigenesis and is increased by supplementation with vitamin E, a nutrient that is not effective by itself (Ip 1986 a, b; Thompson et al. 1984 a, b).

Reduction of DMBA- or MNU-induced mammary tumorigenesis by feeding high levels of vitamin A (retinyl acetate, RA) or synthetic retinoids has been demonstrated repeatedly. Long-term administration is effective, and inhibition by short periods of feeding occurs also. Tumors may appear rapidly after retinoid administration is stopped (Aylsworth et al. 1986; Welsch 1985; Moon et al. 1976; Moon and Mehta 1986). The stage of mammary tumor development or the means by which the retinoids act are not known. The retinoids retard growth and development of the normal mammary gland when fed at tumor-inhibiting doses. A retinoid-supplemented diet containing approximately 300 times the required amount of RA fed beginning 1 or 4 weeks after administration of MNU significantly inhibited cancer induction. The RA supplement started at 8 weeks was not effective. Lower doses of MNU permitted RA to be effective even if feeding was started as late as 16 weeks after administration of MNU, a time at which tumors were already appearing. The inhibition of tumorigenesis may have been partially due to the 4%–8% reduction in body weight as a result of RA toxicity (McCormick and Moon 1982). A lower dose of vitamin A, approximately 10 times the requirement, did not reduce tumorigenesis by MNU (Beth et al. 1987 b).

Other substances added to foods, such as antioxidants, and other chemicals, such as B-naphthoflavone and cysteamine, preparations of cruciferous vegetables, and green coffee beans, reduce DMBA tumorigenesis (Welsch 1985). Butylated hydroxyanisole (BHA) and butylated hydroxytoluene (BHT) are effective when fed at high doses (0.3%–0.6% of the diet) (McCormick et al. 1984). BHA fed at the maximum level permitted in foods (0.025%) had no detectable effect (Rogers et al. 1986). Recently, the effects of antioxidants on mammary gland carcinogenesis induced by DMBA were studied in female Sprague-Dawley rats. The antioxidants used were BHA, BHT, sodium L-ascorbate, alpha-tocopherol, ethoxyquin, and p,p-diaminodiphenylmethane (DDPM). The antioxidants were fed beginning 1 week after DMBA exposure. BHA and ethoxyquin inhibited the induction of all types of mammary tumors. The other antioxidants increased tumor latency somewhat; BHT and DDPM reduced the number of benign but not malignant tumors. The body weights of antioxidant-treated rats were 8%–22% less than weights of controls, a factor that may have contributed to the reduction of tumors. However, body weights were equivalent in groups that did or did not show inhibition of tumorigenesis (Hirose et al. 1986).

Genetics

Rat strains vary in susceptibility to chemical carcinogenesis in the mammary gland and in incidence of spontaneous tumors. Sprague-Dawley females are significantly more susceptible to mammary carcinogenesis by DMBA or N-2-fluorenylacetamide (AAF) than Fischer 344 females and are also more likely to develop spontaneous mammary tumors (Rogers et al. 1982; Chan and Dao 1981; Isaacs 1986). The differences are smaller when MNU is the carcinogen, but they are still present (Cohen et al. 1984; Isaacs 1986). Fischer 344 and other strains of rats that are relatively resistant to AAF mammary tumorigenesis tend to develop a higher incidence of liver tumors in response to AAF than rats that are susceptible (Rogers et al. 1982; Isaacs 1986). Tumor induction by estrogens has been less extensively studied but appears to follow similar patterns of strain sensitivity (Isaacs 1986). Female Copenhagen rats are the most highly resistant to AAF, DMBA, MNU, or estrogen tumorigenesis of the strains tested and do not develop mammary tumors spontaneously (Isaacs 1986). Analysis of carcinogenesis in F1 and F3 hybrids between susceptible and resistant rats gave results consistent with the view that resistance of the gland to DMBA or MNU is controlled by a single dominant autosomal allele (Isaacs 1986). Gould (1986) studied DMBA-susceptible Wistar-Furth rats and determined that susceptibility was due to a series of codominant autosomal alleles. Mammary epithelial and stromal cells from resistant and susceptible strains do not differ in capacity for activation of DMBA to a mutagen (Moore et al. 1983).

References

Aylsworth CF, VanVugt DA, Sylvester PW, Meites J (1984) Failure of high dietary fat to influence serum prolactin levels during the estrous cycle in female Sprague-Dawley rats. Proc Soc Exp Biol Med 175: 25–29

Aylsworth CF, Cullum ME, Zile MH, Welsch CW (1986) Influence of dietary retinyl acetate on normal rat mammary gland development and on the enhancement of

7,12-dimethylbenz[a]anthracene-induced rat mammary tumorigenesis by high levels of dietary fat. JNCI 76: 339–345

Beth M, Berger MR, Aksoy M, Schmähl D (1987a) Comparison between the effects of dietary fat level and of caloric intake on methylnitrosourea-induced mammary carcinogenesis in female SD rats. Int J Cancer 39: 737–744

Beth M, Berger MR, Aksoy M, Schmähl D (1987b) Effects of vitamin A and E supplementation to diets containing two different fat levels on methylnitrosourea-induced mammary carcinogenesis in female SD-rats. Br J Cancer 56: 445–449

Birt DF, Pour PM (1986) Pancreatic cancer enhancement in the hamster model by diets high in fat and/or protein. In: Scarpelli DG, Reddy JK, Longnecker DS (eds) Experimental pancreatic carcinogenesis. CRC, Boca Raton, pp 175–186

Birt DF, Julius AD, White LT, Pour PM (1987) Enhancement of pancreatic carcinogenesis in hamsters fed a high fat diet at a restricted intake. Proc Am Assoc Cancer Res 28: 153

Braun RJ, Pezzuto JM, Beattie CW (1987) Estrous cycle status at the time of n-methyl-n-nitrosourea (NMU) exposure influences rat mammary tumor growth and ovariectomy-induced tumor regression. Proc Am Assoc Cancer Res 28: 90

Carroll KK, Khor HT (1971) Effects of level and type of dietary fat on incidence of mammary tumors induced in female Sprague-Dawley rats by 7,12-dimethylbenz[a]anthracene. Lipids 6: 415–420

Carter CA, Milholland RJ, Shea W, Ip MM (1983) Effect of the prostaglandin synthetase inhibitor indomethacin on 7,12-dimethylbenz[a]anthracene-induced mammary tumorigenesis in rats fed different levels of fat. Cancer Res 43: 3559–3562

Cave WT Jr, Erickson-Lucas MJ (1982) Effects of dietary lipids on lactogenic hormone receptor binding in rat mammary tumors. JNCI 68: 319–324

Cave WT Jr, Jurkowski JJ (1984) Dietary lipid effects on the growth, membrane composition, and prolactin-binding capacity of rat mammary tumors. JNCI 73: 185–191

Chan PC, Dao TL (1981) Enhancement of mammary carcinogenesis by a high-fat diet in Fischer, Long-Evans, and Sprague-Dawley rats. Cancer Res 41: 164–167

Chan PC, Dao TL (1983) Effects of dietary fat on age-dependent sensitivity to mammary carcinogenesis. Cancer Lett 18: 245–249

Chan PC, Ferguson KA, Dao TL (1983) Effects of different dietary fats on mammary carcinogenesis. Cancer Res 43: 1079–1083

Clinton SK, Imrey PB, Alster JM, Simon J, Truex CR, Visek WJ (1984) The combined effects of dietary protein and fat on 7,12-dimethylbenz[a]anthracene-induced breast cancer in rats. J Nutr 114: 1213–1223

Clinton SK, Alster JM, Imrey PB, Nandkumar S, Truex CR, Visek WJ (1986) Effects of dietary protein, fat and energy intake during an initiation phase study of 7,12-dimethylbenz[a]anthracene-induced breast cancer in rats. J Nutr 116: 2290–2302

Cohen LA (1987) The fat effect on n-nitrosomethylurea (NMU)-induced rat mammary carcinogenesis: inhibition by (A) voluntary energy expenditure and (B) caloric restriction. Proc Am Assoc Cancer Res 28: 155

Cohen LA, Thompson DO, Maeura Y, Weisburger JH (1984) Influence of dietary medium-chain triglycerides on the development of n-methylnitrosourea-induced rat mammary tumors. Cancer Res 44: 5023–5028

Cohen LA, Thompson DO, Maeura Y, Choi K, Blank ME, Rose DP (1986) Dietary fat and mammary cancer. I. Promoting effects of different dietary fats on N-nitrosomethylurea-induced rat mammary tumorigenesis. JNCI 77: 33–42

Dao TL, Chan PC (1983) Effect of duration of high fat intake on enhancement of mammary carcinogenesis in rats. JNCI 71: 201–205

Gould MN (1986) Inheritance and site of expression of genes controlling susceptibility to mammary cancer in an inbred rat model. Cancer Res 46: 1199–1202

Grubbs CJ, Peckham JC, Cato KD (1983a) Mammary carcinogenesis in rats in relation to age at time of N-nitroso-n-methylurea administration. JNCI 70: 209–212

Grubbs CJ, Hill DL, McDonough KC, Peckham JC (1983b) N-nitroso-n-methylurea-induced mammary carcinogenesis: effect of pregnancy on preneoplastic cells. JNCI 71: 625–628

Grubbs CJ, Farnell DR, Hill DL, McDonough KC (1985) Chemoprevention of n-nitroso-n-methylurea-induced mammary cancers by pretreatment with 17 β-estradiol and progesterone. JNCI 74: 927–931

Grubbs CJ, Juliana MM, Hill DL, Whitaker LM (1986) Suppression by pregnancy of chemically induced preneoplastic cells of the rat mammary gland. Anticancer Res 6: 1395–1400

Heuson JC, Legros N (1972) Influence of insulin deprivation on growth of the 7,12-dimethylbenz[a]anthracene-induced mammary carcinoma in rats subjected to alloxan diabetes and food restriction. Cancer Res 32: 226–232

Hilf R, Bell C, Goldenberg H, Michel I (1971) Effect of fluphenazine HCl on R3230AC mammary carcinoma and mammary glands of the rat. Cancer Res 31: 1111–1117

Hirose M, Masuda A, Inoue T, Fukushima S, Ito N (1986) Modification by antioxidants and p,p-diaminodiphenylmethane of 7,12-dimethylbenz(a)anthracene-induced carcinogenesis of the mammary gland and ear duct in CD rats. Carcinogenesis 7: 1155–1159

Hopkins GJ, Carrol KK (1979) Relationship between amount and type of dietary fat in promotion of mammary carcinogenesis induced by 7,12-dimethylbenz[a]anthracene. JNCI 62: 1009–1012

Ip C (1986a) Interaction of vitamin C and selenium supplementation in the modification of mammary carcinogenesis in rats. JNCI 77: 299–303

Ip C (1986b) The chemopreventive role of selenium in carcinogenesis. In: Poirier LA, Newberne PM, Pariza MW (eds) Essential nutrients in carcinogenesis. Plenum, New York, pp 431–448

Ip C, Ip MM (1981) Serum estrogens and estrogen responsiveness in 7,12-dimethylbenz(a)anthracene-induced mammary tumors as influenced by dietary fat. JNCI 66: 291–295

Ip C, Sinha DK (1981) Enhancement of mammary tumorigenesis by dietary selenium deficiency in rats with a high polyunsaturated fat intake. Cancer Res 41: 31–34

Ip C, Carter CA, Ip MM (1985) Requirement of essential fatty acid for mammary tumorigenesis in the rat. Cancer Res 45: 1997–2001

Isaacs JT (1985) Determination of the number of events required for mammary carcinogenesis in the Sprague-Dawley female rat. Cancer Res 45: 4827–4832

Isaacs JT (1986) Genetic control of resistance to chemically induced mammary adenocarcinogenesis in the rat. Cancer Res 46: 3958–3963

Janss DH, Ben TL (1978) Age-related modification of 7,12-dimethylbenz[a]anthracene binding to rat mammary gland DNA. JNCI 60: 173–177

Klurfeld DM, Weber MM, Kritchevsky D (1987) Inhibition of chemically induced mammary and colon tumor promotion by caloric restriction in rats fed increased dietary fat. Cancer Res 47: 2759–2762

Knazek RA, Liu SC, Bodwin JS, Vonderhaar BK (1980) Requirement of essential fatty acids in the diet for development of the mouse mammary gland. JNCI 64: 377–382

Kritchevsky D, Klurfeld DM (1986) Influence of caloric intake on experimental carcinogenesis: a review. In: Poirier LA, Newberne PM, Pariza MW (eds) Essential nutrients in carcinogenesis. Plenum, New York, pp 55–68

Kritchevsky D, Klurfeld DM (1987) Caloric effects in experimental mammary tumorigenesis. Am J Clin Nutr 45: 236–242

Kritchevsky D, Weber MM, Klurfeld DM (1984) Dietary fat versus calorio content in initiation and promotion of 7,12-dimethylbenz(a)anthracene-induced mammary tumorigenesis in rats. Cancer Res 44: 3174–3177

Lee SY, Rogers AE (1983) Dimethylbenzathracene mammary tumorigenesis in Sprague-Dawley rats fed diets differing in content of beef tallow or rapeseed oil. Nutr Res 3: 361–371

Lee SY, NG SF, Busby WF, Rogers AE (1988) Mammary gland DNA synthesis in rats fed high lard or control diets. J Nutr Growth Cancer 4: (in press)

Lindsey WF, Das Gupta TK, Beattie CW (1981) Influence of the estrous cycle during carcinogen exposure on nitrosomethylurea-induced rat mammary carcinoma. Cancer Res 41: 3857–3862

McCormick DL, Moon RC (1982) Influence of delayed administration of retinyl acetate on mammary carcinogenesis. Cancer Res 42: 2639–2643

McCormick DL, Adamowski CB, Fiks A, Moon RC (1981) Lifetime dose-response relationships for mammary tumor induction by a single administration of n-methyl-n-nitrosurea. Cancer Res 41: 1690–1694

McCormick DL, Mehta RG, Thompson CA, Dinger N, Caldwell JA, Moon RC (1982) Enhanced inhibition of mammary carcinogenesis by combined treatment with n-(4-hydroxyphenyl)retinamide and ovariectomy. Cancer Res 42: 508–512

McCormick DL, Major N, Moon RC (1984) Inhibition of 7,12-dimethylbenz(a)anthracene-induced rat mammary carcinogenesis by concomitant or postcarcinogen antioxidant exposure. Cancer Res 44: 2858–2863

Minton JP, Abou-Issa H, Foecking MK, Sriram MG (1983) Caffeine and unsaturated fat diet significantly promotes DMBA-induced breast cancer in rats. Cancer 51: 1249–1253

Moon RC, Mehta RG (1986) Anticarcinogenic effects of retinoids in animals. In: Poirier LA, Newberne PM, Pariza MW (eds) Essential nutrients in carcinogenesis. Plenum, New York, pp 399–412

Moon RC, Grubbs CJ, Sporn MB (1976) Inhibition of 7,12-dimethylbenz(a)anthracene-induced mammary carcinogenesis by retinyl acetate. Cancer Res 36: 2626–2630

Moore CJ, Bachhuber AJ, Gould MN (1983) Relationship of mammary tumor susceptibility, mammary cell-mediated mutagenesis, and metabolism of polycyclic aromatic hydrocarbons in four types of rats. JNCI 70: 777–784

Ratko TA, Beattie CW (1985) Estrous cycle modification of rat mammary tumor induction by a single dose of n-methyl-n-nitrosourea. Cancer Res 45: 3042–3047

Rogers AE, Lee SY (1986) Chemically induced mammary gland tumors in rats: modulation by dietary rat. In: Ip C, Birt DF, Rogers AE, Mettlin C (eds) Dietary fat and cancer. Liss, New York, pp 255–282

Rogers AE, Longnecker MP (1988) Dietary and nutritional influences on cancer: a review of epidemiologic and experimental data. Lab Invest 59: 729–759

Rogers AE, Fernstrom JD, Ge K, McConnell RG, Leavitt WW, Wetsel WC, Yang SO, Camelio EA (1982) Endocrine interactions in the nutritional modulation of mammary carcinogenesis in rats. In: Arnott MS, Van Eys J, Wang YM (eds) Molecular interrelations of nutrition and cancer. Raven, New York, pp 381–399

Rogers AE, Conner BH, Boulanger CL, Lee SY, Carr FA, Dumouchel WH (1985) Enhancement of 7,12-dimethylbenz(a)anthracene mammary carcinogenesis by a high lard diet. In: Vahouny GV, Kritchevsky D (eds) Dietary fiber: basic and chemical aspects. Plenum, New York, pp 449–455

Rogers AE, Conner B, Boulanger C, Lee S (1986) Mammary tumorigenesis in rats fed diets high in lard. Lipids 21: 275–280

Rose DP, Pruitt B, Stauber P, Ertürk E, Bryan GT (1980) Influence of dosage schedule on the biological characteristics of n-nitrosomethylurea-induced rat mammary tumors. Cancer Res 40: 235–239

Russo J, Russo IH (1987) Biology of disease. Biological and molecular bases of mammary carcinogenesis. Lab Invest 57: 112–137

Silverman J, Shellabarger CJ, Holtzman S, Stone JP, Weisburger JH (1980) Effect of dietary fat on x-ray-induced mammary cancer in Sprague-Dawley rats. JNCI 64: 631–634

Sinha DK, Pazik JE, Dao TL (1983) Progression of rat mammary development with age and its relationship to carcinogenesis by a chemical carcinogen. Int J Cancer 31: 321–327

Sylvester PW, Aylsworth CF, Van Vugt DA, Meites J (1983) Effects of alterations in early hormonal environment on development and hormone dependency of carcinogen-induced mammary tumors in rats. Cancer Res 43: 5342–5346

Sylvester PW, Ip C, Ip MM (1986a) Effects of high dietary fat on the growth and development of ovarian-independent carcinogen-induced mammary tumors in rats. Cancer Res 46: 763–769

Sylvester PW, Russell M, Ip MM, Ip C (1986b) Comparative effects of different animal and vegetable fats fed before and during carcinogen administration on mammary tumorigenesis, sexual maturation, and endocrine function in rats. Cancer Res 46: 757–762

Tay LK, Russo J (1981) 7,12-dimethylbenz(a)anthracene-induced DNA binding and repair synthesis in susceptible and nonsusceptible mammary epithelial cells in culture. JNCI 67: 155–161

Thompson HJ, Meeker DL (1983) Induction of mammary gland carcinomas by the subcutaneous injection of 1-Methyl-1-nitrosourea. Cancer Res 43: 1628–1629

Thompson HJ, Meeker LD, Tagliaferro AR, Becci PJ (1982) Effect of retinyl acetate on the occurrence of ovarian hormone-responsive and nonresponsive mammary cancers in the rat. Cancer Res 42: 903–905

Thompson HJ, Chasteen ND, Meeker LD (1984a) Dietary vanadyl (IV) sulfate inhibits chemically induced mammary carcinogenesis. Carcinogenesis 5: 849–851

Thompson HJ, Meeker LD, Kokoska S (1984b) Effect of an inorganic and organic form of dietary selenium on the promotional stage of mammary carcinogenesis in the rat. Cancer Res 44: 2803–2806

Thompson HJ, Meeker LD, Herbst EJ, Ronan AM, Minocha R (1985) Effect of concentration of D,L-2-difluoromethylornithine on murine mammary carcinogenesis. Cancer Res 45: 1170–1173

Wei HJ, Luo X-M, Yang SP (1985) Effects of molybdenum and tungsten on mammary carcinogenesis in SD rats. JNCI 74: 469–473

Welsch CW (1985) Host factors affecting the growth of carcinogen-induced rat mammary carcinomas: a review and tribute to Charles Brenton Huggins. Cancer Res 45: 3415–3443

Welsch CW (1986) Interrelationship between dietary fat and endocrine processes in mammary gland tumorigenesis. In: Ip C, Birt DF, Rogers AE, Mettlin C (eds) Dietary fat and cancer. Liss, New York, pp 623–654

Welsch CW (1987) Enhancement of mammary tumorigenesis by dietary fat: review of potential mechanisms. Am J Clin Nutr 45: 192–202

Welsch CW, DeHoog JV (1983) Retinoid feeding, hormone inhibition, and/or immune stimulation and the genesis of carcinogen-induced rat mammary carcinomas. Cancer Res 43: 585–591

Welsch CW, Brown CK, Goodrich-Smith M, Chiusano J, Moon RC (1980) Synergistic effect of chronic prolactin suppression and retinoid treatment in the prophylaxis of N-methyl-N-nitrosourea-induced mammary tumorigenesis in female Sprague-Dawley rats. Cancer Res 40: 3095–3098

Welsch CW, DeHoog JV, O'Connor DH, Sheffield LG (1985) Influence of dietary fat levels on development and hormone responsiveness of the mouse mammary gland. Cancer Res 45: 6147–6154

Wetsel WC, Rogers AE (1984) Hepatic prolactin binding in female Sprague-Dawley rats fed a diet high in corn oil. JNCI 75: 531–536

Wetsel WC, Rogers AE, Newberne PM (1981) Dietary fat and DMBA mammary carcinogenesis in rats. Cancer Detect Prev 4: 535–543

Wetsel WC, Rogers AE, Rutledge A, Leavitt WW (1984) Absence of an effect of dietary corn oil content on plasma prolactin, progesterone, and 17 β-estradiol in female Sprague-Dawley rats. Cancer Res 44: 1420–1425

Markers in Chemically Induced Tumors, Mammary Gland, Rat

Michael J. Warburton and Barry A. Gusterson

Gross Appearance

Chemically induced rat mammary tumors are usually firm and well-circumscribed by a connective tissue capsule. The tumors are macroscopically nodular. Larger tumors are usually ulcerated.

Microscopic Features

The tumors that we have studied are dimethylbenzanthracene- and N-methyl-N-nitrosourea-induced rat mammary tumors which are well-circumscribed lesions with a connective tissue pseudocapsule. Connective tissue trabeculae extend from the capsule into the tumor, dividing the mass into lobules (Fig. 455). The connective tissue septa contain spindle-shaped stromal cells and a mixed mononuclear cell population with numerous mast cells. These glandular tumors exhibit various degrees of differentiation and following the classification in this monograph (p. 275) are mainly tubular adenomas which show transition to adenocarcinomas. Cribriform and comedo carcinoma patterns are also frequently seen. The epithelial cells are usually multilayered, with the basal cells often adopting a more elongated morphology. The lobules have the appearance of complex, papillary, intraductal and intralobular proliferations of cells with the formation of acinar structures and papillary folds. The acini and papillary projections are composed of one to six layers of a relatively uni-

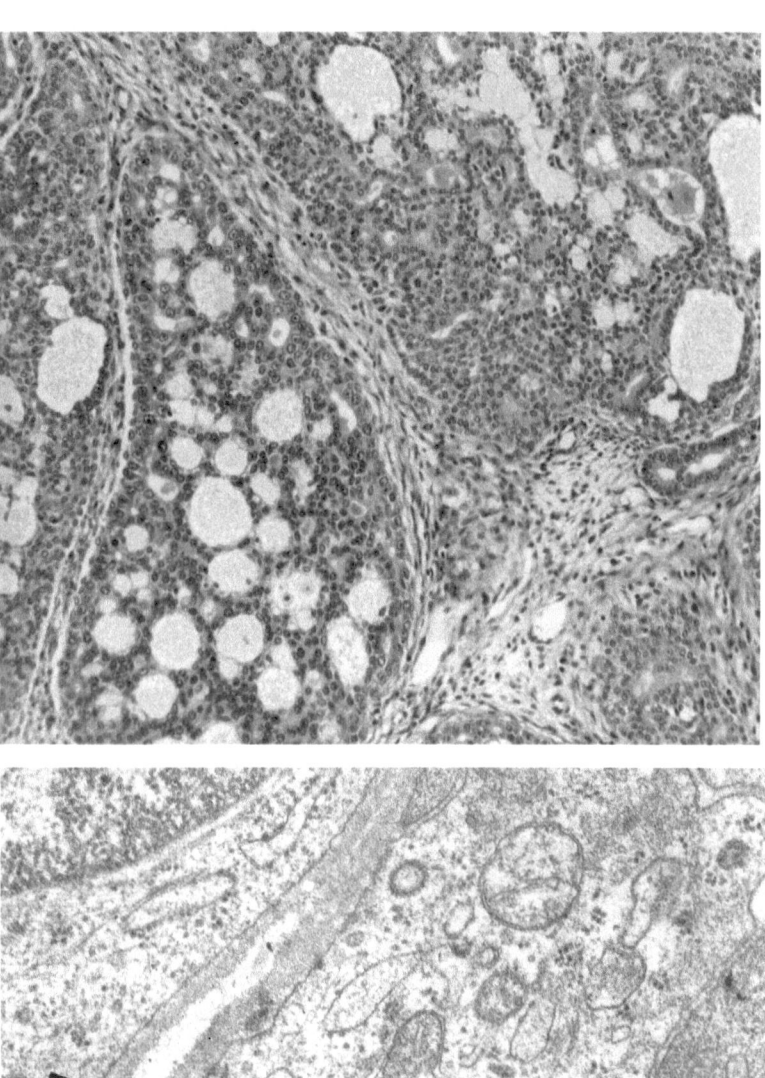

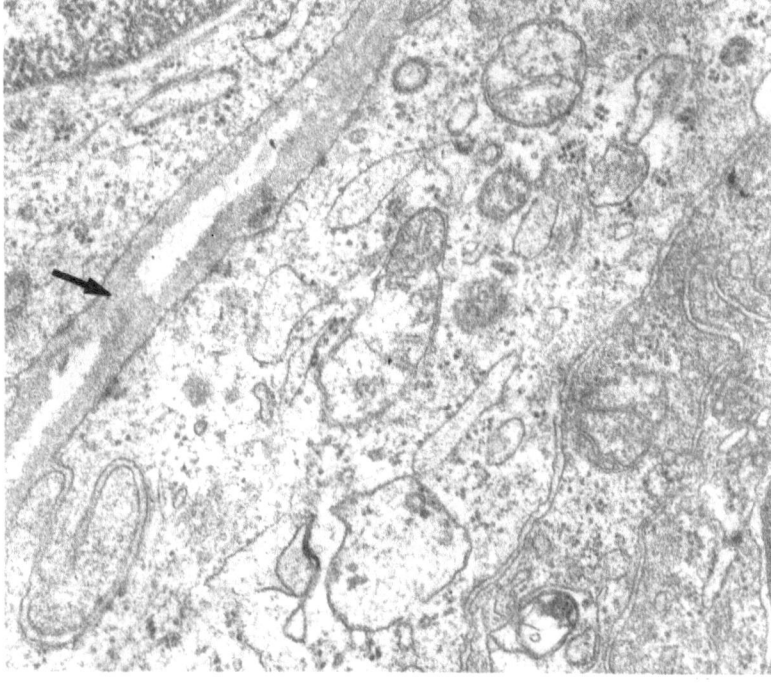

Fig. 455 *(above)*. Mammary gland, rat. Dimethylbenzan-thracene-induced tumor. Note the lobules of tumor cells, and numerous lumina. The lobules are surrounded by sheaths of connective tissue which contain numerous mast cells. H and E, × 125

Fig. 456 *(below)*. Mammary gland, rat. A dimethylbenzan-thracene-induced tumor. Note the abundant, distended rough endoplasmic reticulum and the extracellular deposits of thickened basement membrane *(arrow)*. TEM, × 35 000

form population of cells with a variable mitotic rate. Cellular pleomorphism and the presence of prominent nucleoli are variable in the lesions and are associated with transitions to carcinomas. We have found no evidence of spontaneous metastases in primary induced tumors although this is a common finding after syngeneic transplantation, indicating the malignant potential of all of these lesions including the adenomas.

Ultrastructure

The glandular regions consist of multilayers of relatively uniform, cuboidal or columnar epithelial cells with numerous junctional complexes. The basally situated cells are more irregular in shape. The more elongated basal cells contain abundant, distended rough endoplasmic reticulum and Golgi apparatus. Both intermediate filaments and microfilaments are sometimes seen in these cells. The spaces between the clusters of acini are lined with a thick layer (50–300 nm) of amorphous material which also contains striated collagen fibers (Fig. 456). Some of the basal cells form hemidesmosomes with this extracellular material. The lumina within the lobules are of two types. One type is lined with cells which bear microvilli on their luminal surface, whereas in the other type, the luminal surface of the cells is smooth and lined with an amorphous extracellular deposit which also contains occasional striated collagen fibers.

Biologic Features

The usefulness of chemically induced rat mammary tumors as models of the human disease has been questioned due to the generally benign behavior of the lesions (Young and Hallowes 1976; Russo et al. 1977). Metastases, however, have been reported to occur in 3-methylcholanthrene and N-ethyl-N-nitrosourea-induced tumors (Fisher et al. 1975; Stoica et al. 1983). Metastatic variants sometimes arise during serial transplantation of 7,12-dimethylbenz[a]anthracene-, N-methyl-N-nitrosourea-, and 3-methylcholanthrene-induced tumors (Kim 1979; Williams et al. 1982), and these workers have used epithelial markers (including keratin) to assess the degree of differentiation of the tumors and to identify metastatic deposits.

Primary tumors tend to be moderately well-differentiated, and the distribution of markers is similar to that seen in normal rat mammary glands (Dunnington et al. 1984a) (see p. 266). Antiserum to rat milk fat globule membranes (used to identify epithelial cells) stains the apical surface of those epithelial cells that line ductal structures but not those within the multilayers (Fig. 457). Many of the basal cells in the glandular structures stain with a polyclonal antiserum to human callus keratins (Fig. 458). In the normal gland, this antiserum specifically stains myoepithelial and not luminal epithelial cells. Similar staining patterns are observed with LP34, a monoclonal antibody to human callus keratins which also specifically stains myoepithelial cells in rat mammary glands (Warburton et al. 1987). However, in the tumors some of the luminal epithelial cells which are negative in the normal gland are also stained with this keratin antiserum. Antiserum to myosin, which also stains myoepithelial cells in the normal gland stains occasional basal cells. This staining pattern is in general agreement with the scarcity of myofilaments in tumor basal cells compared with normal myoepithelial cells.

The benign nature of these primary lesions is supported by the well-formed basement membrane which clearly delineates the glandular areas (Fig. 459). Antisera to laminin and type IV collagen produce a linear staining pattern at the epithelial-stromal interface with interdigitation between the lateral surfaces of the basal cells. There is occasional strong cytoplasmic staining of the epithelial cells (Fig. 460), suggesting that some of these cells are actively synthesizing basement membrane components. Staining for basement membrane proteins is also seen within the lumina in some acini (Fig. 461). Staining of serial sections with either antiserum to laminin or milk fat globule membrane reveals that lumina stain with either of the antisera but not with both. This reflects the ultrastructure of the lumina in that they are either lined with epithelial cells displaying microvilli (staining with antiserum to milk fat globule membrane) or lined with a smooth extracellular matrix (staining with antiserum to laminin). The origin of the lumina lined with basement membrane material is not entirely clear. They may simply be explained by the cutting of traverse sections of papillary ingrowths. Alternatively, the membranes of some tumor cells may become polarized to form basal surfaces with secretion of basement membrane components, whereas the surface of tumor cells in other lumina polarize to form apical surfaces (Ormerod et al. 1985). Antisera to stromal collagens and fi-

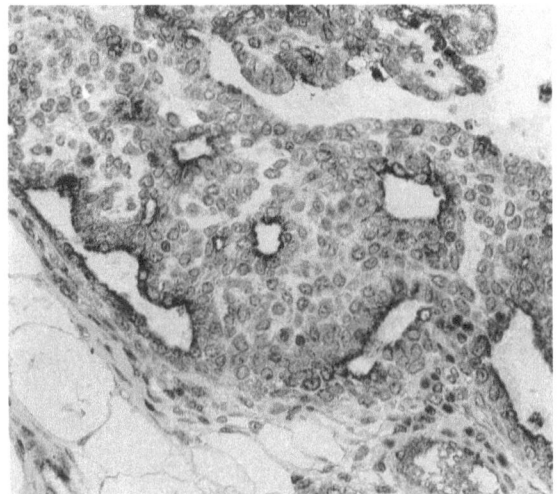

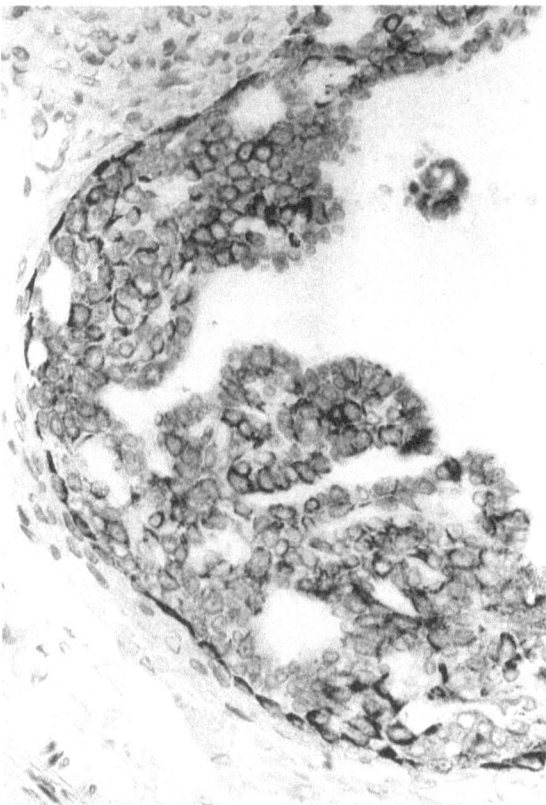

Fig. 457 *(above).* Mammary gland, rat. Section of a dimethylbenzanthracene-induced tumor stained with an antiserum to rat milk fat globule membrane. Note the staining on the apical surface of epithelial cells surrounding some of the lumina. × 360

Fig. 458 *(below).* Rat mammary tumor, induced by dimethylbenzanthracene and stained with an antiserum to human callus keratin. Note the black staining of basal cells and some of the epithelial cells within the lobules. × 450

bronectin stain connective tissue in normal glands and tumors. The only noteworthy differences are the presence of fibrillar collagens within the basement membrane and the enhanced deposition of type V collagen in the tumors (Ormerod et al. 1985).

Although primary, chemically induced, rat mammary tumors are generally considered to behave in a benign fashion and do not metastasize, a number of transplantable metastasizing tumors have been established (Kim 1979; Williams et al. 1982). The antisera mentioned above have been used to determine the degree of cellular differentiation within these tumors and also to localize metastatic deposits (Williams et al. 1985). A series of transplantable, metastasizing mammary tumors from rats treated with 3-methylcholanthrene has been established by Kim (1979). The more highly metastasizing tumors appear less well-differentiated, and the normal glandular pattern is replaced by sheets of cuboidal cells. As the number of glandular structures decreases, so does staining with antiserum to milk fat globule membrane (Dunnington et al. 1984a). The progression toward malignancy also results in the loss of basal cells staining with antisera to myosin or keratin. The disappearance of cells with myoepithelial characteristics is confirmed by ultrastructural studies, and in this respect these tumors are similar to the human disease (Gusterson et al. 1982). Another similarity to human breast tumors is the loss of tumor-derived basement membrane in malignant lesions (Siegal et al. 1981). Fragmented staining with antiserum to laminin is sometimes observed in the rat tumors, but this is probably of vascular origin.

Another approach to investigating the pathogenesis of chemically induced rat mammary tumors is to establish cell lines from the primary tumors and metastasizing variants. Dunnington et al. (1984b) and Williams et al. (1985) have established cell lines from metastasizing variants of chemically induced tumors (Williams et al. 1982). In general, the staining patterns of the tumors produced by these cell lines are similar to those described above, except that there is stronger staining of epithelial cells, both in the primaries and metastases, with antisera to milk fat globule membrane and keratin. Myoepithelial cells and basement membrane deposits are absent or greatly reduced.

In summary, the major impact of markers in chemically induced rat mammary tumors has been to demonstrate some similarities between the progression to malignancy in metastatic vari-

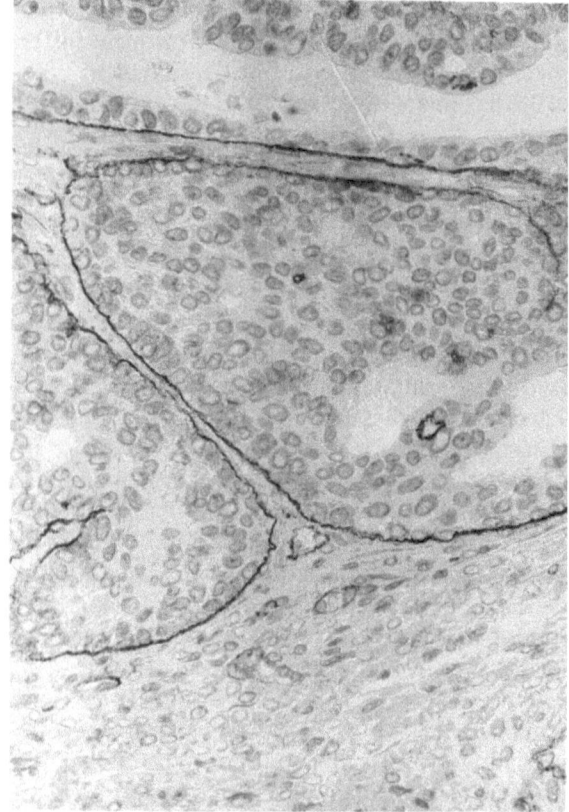

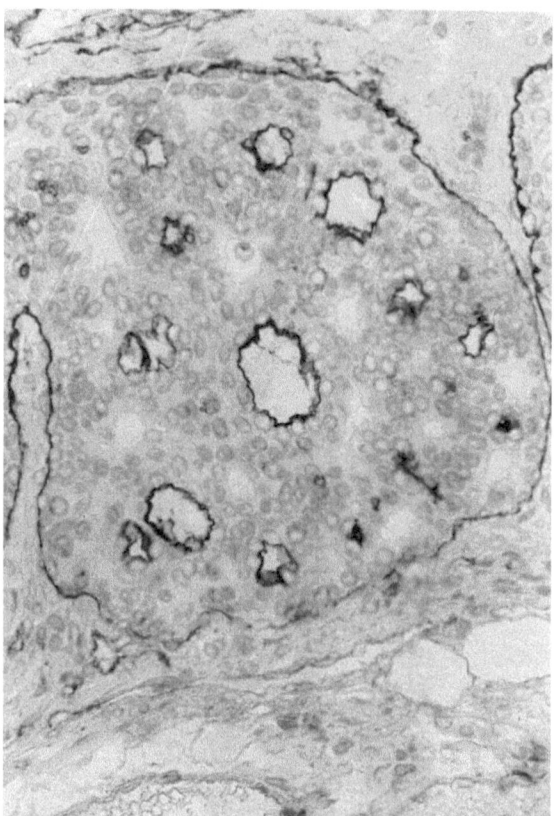

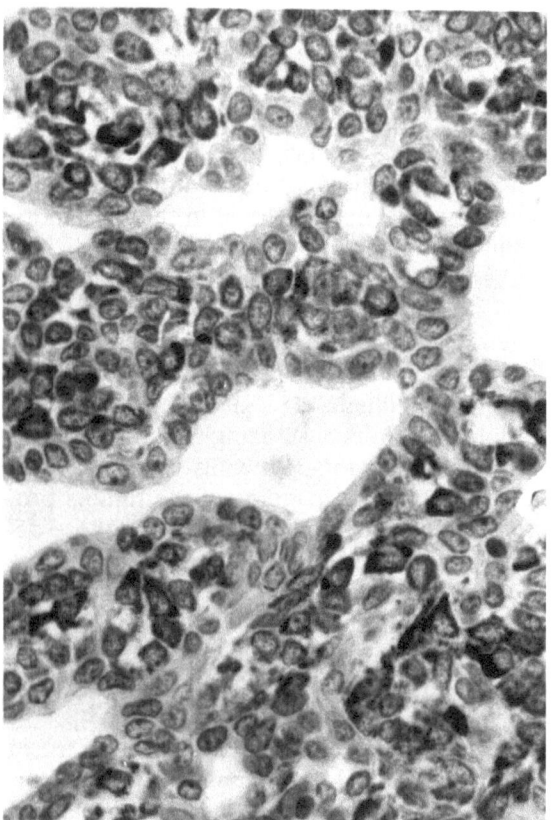

Fig. 459 *(upper left).* Tumor, mammary gland, rat, induced by dimethylbenzanthracene and stained with an antiserum to laminin. Note the linear staining at the epithelial-stromal interface. × 450

Fig. 460 *(lower left).* Tumor of mammary gland, rat, induced by dimethylbenzanthracene and stained with an antiserum to laminin. Note the strong cytoplasmic staining of some of the epithelial cells. × 600

Fig. 461 *(upper right).* Mammary gland, rat, tumor induced by dimethylbenzanthracene and stained with an antiserum to laminin. Note that some lumina are stained and others unstained. × 450

ants of these tumors and in human breast cancer. The most notable of these are loss of differentiated epithelial characteristics, loss of myoepithelial cells, and disruption of basement membrane deposition. The demonstration of other cellular components of biological interest such as growth factors, growth factor receptors, and oncogene products is outside the scope of this chapter, but may prove important in the future as markers of biological behavior.

References

Dunnington DJ, Kim U, Hughes CM, Monaghan P, Ormerod EJ, Rudland PS (1984a) Loss of myoepithelial cell characteristics in metastasizing rat mammary tumors relative to their nonmetastasizing counterparts. JNCI 72: 455-466

Dunnington DJ, Kim U, Hughes CM, Monaghan P, Rudland PS (1984b) Lack of production of myoepithelial variants by cloned epithelial cell lines derived from the TMT-081 metastasizing rat mammary tumor. Cancer Res 44: 5338-5346

Fisher ER, Shoemaker RH, Sabnis A (1975) Relationship of hyperplasia to cancer in 3-methylcholanthrene-induced mammary tumorogenesis. Lab Invest 33: 33-42

Gusterson BA, Warburton MJ, Mitchell D, Ellison M, Neville AM, Rudland PS (1982) Distribution of myoepithelial cells and basement membrane proteins in the normal breast and in benign and malignant breast diseases. Cancer Res 42: 4763-4770

Kim U (1979) Factors influencing metastasis of breast cancer. In: McGuire WL (ed) Breast cancer: advances in research and treatment, vol 3. Plenum, New York, pp 1-36

Ormerod EJ, Warburton MJ, Gusterson BA, Hughes CM, Rudland PS (1985) Abnormal deposition of basement membrane and connective tissue components in dimethylbenzanthracene-induced rat mammary tumours: an immunocytochemical and ultrastructural study. Histochem J 17: 1155-1166

Russo J, Saby J, Isenberg WM, Russo IH (1977) Pathogenesis of mammary carcinomas induced in rats by 7,12-dimethylbenz[a]anthracene. JNCI 59: 435-445

Siegal GP, Barsky SH, Terranova VP, Liotta LA (1981) Stages of neoplastic transformation of human breast tissue as monitored by dissolution of basement membrane components. An immunoperoxidase study. Invasion Metastasis 1: 54-70

Stoica G, Koestner A, Capen CC (1983) Characterization of N-ethyl-N-nitrosourea-induced mammary tumors in the rat. Am J Pathol 110: 161-169

Warburton MJ, Ferns SA, Hughes CM, Sear CHJ, Rudland PS (1987) Generation of cell types with myoepithelial and mesenchymal phenotypes during the conversion of rat mammary tumor epithelial stem cells into elongated cells. JNCI 78: 1191-1201

Williams JC, Gusterson BA, Coombes RC (1982) Spontaneously metastasising variants derived from MNU-induced rat mammary tumor. Br J Cancer 45: 588-597

Williams JC, Gusterson BA, Monaghan P, Coombes RC, Rudland PS (1985) Isolation and characterization of clonal cell lines from a transplantable metastasizing rat mammary tumor, TR2CL. JNCI 74: 415-428

Young S, Hallowes RC (1976) Tumours of the mammary gland. In: Turusov VS (ed) Pathology of tumours in laboratory animals, vol 1, pt 1. IARC, Lyon, pp 31-79

Adenoacanthoma, Mammary Gland, Mouse

Sabine Rehm

Synonyms. Adenosquamous carcinoma; mammary gland adenocarcinoma with squamous or epidermoid metaplasia; keratinizing mammary gland tumor.

Gross Appearance

Adenoacanthomas of the mouse mammary gland are grossly similar to other tumor types of this organ, i.e., they are round or coarsely nodular, well-cirumscribed, and easily separated from adjacent normal tissue. However, adenoacanthomas contain areas of yellowish or white flaky material on the cut surface in regions of extensive keratinization.

Microscopic Features

Different types of adenocarcinomas of the mouse mammary gland may include foci of squamous cell metaplasia with small horny pearls or larger areas of extensive keratinization (Van Ebbenhorst Tengbergen 1970; Sass and Dunn 1979). Dunn (1959) defined adenoacanthomas as mammary carcinomas that have keratinized squamous cell areas in 25% or more of the

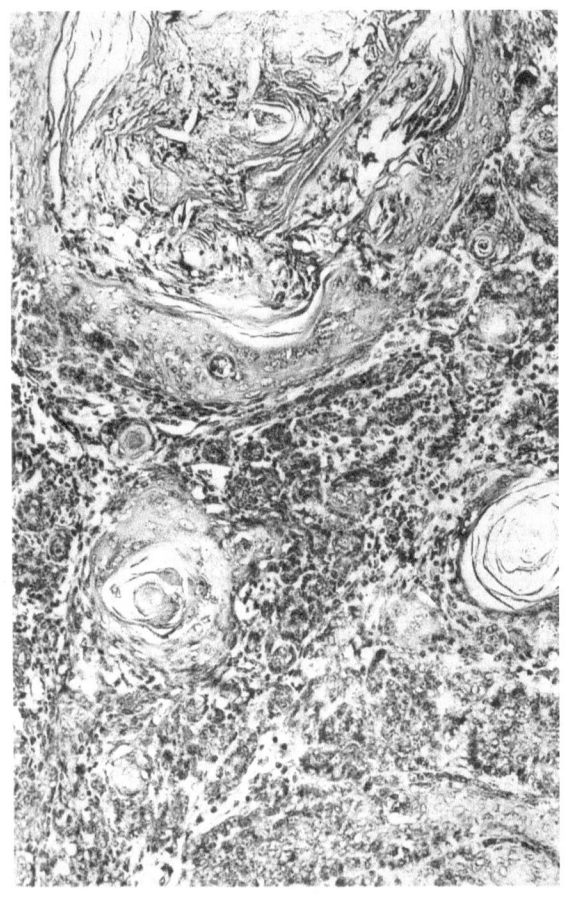

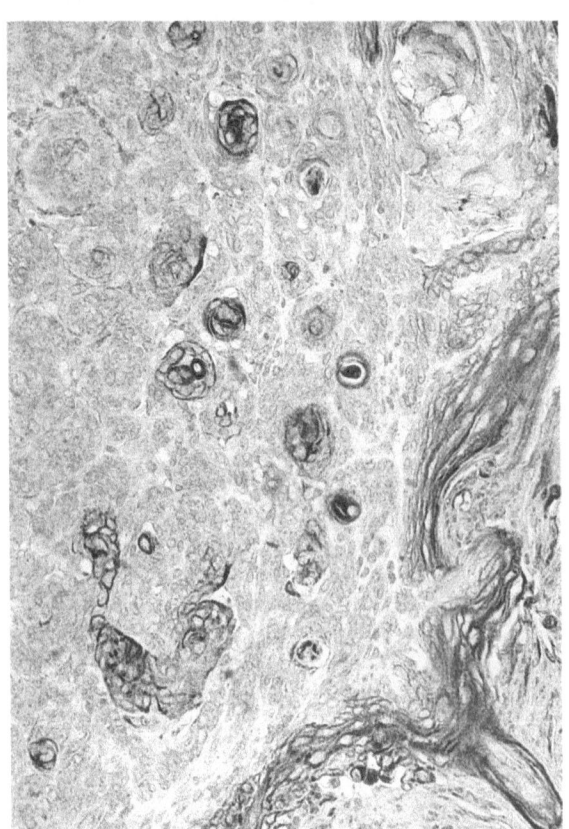

tumor (Fig. 462). This limit may vary depending on the investigator (Medina 1974), an important consideration when comparing tumor incidences in different strains or studies of identical strains. It is suggested that in cases of less than 25% squamous cell differentiation, the mammary gland tumor should be classified according to the predominant tissue type with the adjunct of "focal squamous cell metaplasia." In the metaplastic areas, a gradual change can be observed from round or polygonal mammary tumor epithelial cells to flattened squamous cells. Intracytoplasmic keratin and horny lamellae stain eosinophilic with hematoxylin and eosin stains.

The presence of abundant intracytoplasmic keratin can also be shown by immunocytochemistry using antibodies against human keratins after trypsin digestion of tissue sections (Ward et al. 1986) (Fig. 463). Specific expression of a basic keratin has been found to be characteristic for mouse mammary gland adenocarcinomas with squamous metaplasia and keratinization (Asch and Asch 1985). It must be noted, however, that mammary adenocarcinoma tumor cells without obvious squamous differentiation may also be immunoreactive for keratin, but abundant focal keratin production in adenoacanthoma is characteristic.

Differential Diagnosis

All keratinizing epithelial skin tumors such as squamous cell carcinomas and trichoepitheliomas that invade the underlying mammary gland tissue have to be considered in the differential diagnosis (see p. 275).

Biologic Features

In most cases of adenoacanthomas, squamous cell metaplasia seems to originate from neoplastic epithelial cells which form glandular elements

◀Fig. 462 *(above).* Adenoacanthoma, mouse, mammary gland. Extensive keratinization and horny pearls from squamous cell metaplasia of neoplastic epithelium from adenocarcinoma. H and E, × 100

Fig. 463 *(below).* Adenoacanthoma, mouse, mammary gland. Positive staining for keratin in metaplastic cells. Avidin-biotin immunoperoxidase complex using rabbit human-specific keratin. Counterstained with hematoxylin, × 250

or cell nests in an adenocarcinoma. These tumor cells may be of alveolar origin when produced by the MuMTV (murine mammary tumor virus) (Dunn 1959; Van Ebbenhorst Tengbergen 1970; Medina 1976) or of ductular origin when resulting from chemical carcinogenesis (Medina and Warner 1976). However, myoepithelial cells may be present in mouse mammary gland carcinomas (Asch et al. 1981) and could also be considered as the cells of origin for squamous metaplasia (Slemmer 1974; see also p.323, this volume).

Mechanisms contributing to the formation of squamous differentiation could be similar to those occurring in chronically irritated epithelia, as in major airways or the bladder. Schaefer et al. (1985) successfully induced epidermoid metaplasia in well-differentiated and anaplastic mouse mammary adenocarcinomas in tissue culture with cyclic adenine nucleotide. The formation of adenoacanthomas may further be facilitated by the hormonal milieu of the host. Mammary tumors arising in mice with pituitary isografts in one study were exclusively adenoacanthomas and were transplantable (Heston et al. 1972).

Small foci of hyperplastic, keratinized, mammary gland alveoli surrounded by lymphocytes and plasma cells (Fig.464) have been considered as preneoplastic or early neoplastic lesions of adenoacanthomas (Kirschbaum et al. 1946; Sass et al. 1982). Huseby and Bittner (1946), however, could not find a relationship between these hyperplastic foci and adenoacanthomas, since the foci appeared equally in mouse strains with high and low mammary tumor incidence and no transitional forms were observed. The frequency of these keratinized hyperplastic foci was increased by pregnancy and/or lactation. Keratotic nodules may also develop in mammary ducts of mice treated with chemical carcinogens (Kirschbaum et al. 1946; Medina 1974), particularly in mice with pituitary isografts. These nodules do not progress further when transplanted into the fat pads of syngeneic mice (Medina 1974). Squamous cell metaplasia and adenoacanthomas have been described in mouse strains with or without the mammary tumor virus (Mühlbock et al. 1952; Liebelt and Liebelt 1967; Squartini 1979). Since adenoacanthomas arise preferentially in mice aged 18 months or older (Van der Valk 1981; Rehm et al. 1985), and since mice with MuMTV which develop mammary tumors usually die before the age of 12 months (Heston et al. 1950), mice carrying the MuMTV are less likely to develop adenoacanthomas (Kirschbaum 1949). In proportion to all other mammary tumor types,

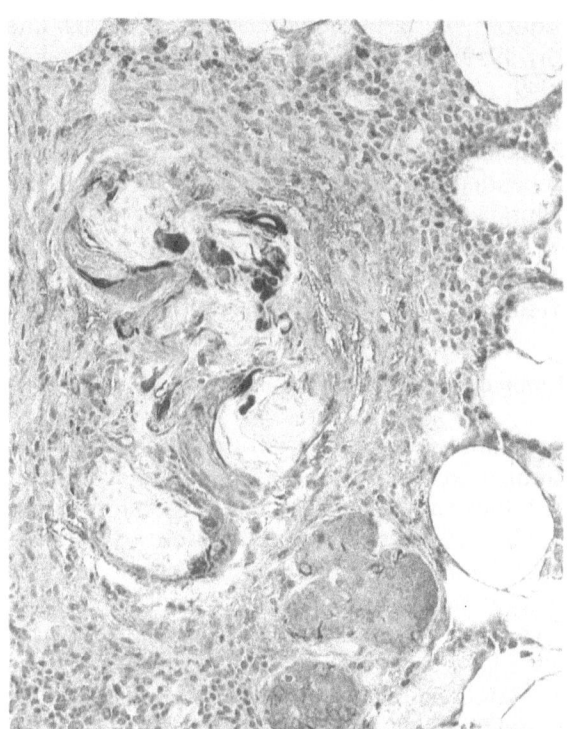

Fig.464. Hyperplastic keratotic nodule, mouse, mammary gland, surrounded by a chronic inflammatory response. Avidin-biotin immunoperoxidase complex using rabbit human-specific keratin. Counterstained with hematoxylin, × 250

Table 34. Relative incidence of adenoacanthomas in mice free of murine mammary tumor virus

Strain/stock	Incidence (%)[a]	Reference
BALB/cAnDe	58	Deringer 1965
BALB/cCr	16	Peters et al. 1972
BALB/cHeA	56	Van der Valk 1981
BALB/cCrglA	42	Van der Valk 1981
C3Hb	21	Heston et al. 1950
C3HeB	28	Deringer 1959
C3H/HeAf	16	Van der Valk 1981
RIIIeB/De	23	Deringer 1969
Han:NMRI	12	Rehm et al. 1985

[a] Refers to percentage among animals bearing mammary tumors.

adenoacanthomas, therefore, occur relatively more often in mice without MuMTV (Table 34). Squamous cell differentiation may also be related to the genetic background, i.e., be dependent on the strain of mouse. The BALB/c strain, in particular, develops a relatively high incidence of adenoacanthomas (Van der Valk 1981) (Table 34). Mammary adenocarcinomas can be induced by various hydrocarbons (Bonser and Orr 1939; Kirschbaum et al. 1946; Kirschbaum 1949; Andervont and Dunn 1950; Biancifiori and Caschera 1962; Medina 1974; Liebelt and Liebelt 1967; Medina et al. 1980) and, although dependent on the route of carcinogen administration, adenoacanthomas were observed consistently with chemical induction, arising even earlier than other adenocarcinomas (Medina 1974; Medina et al. 1980).

Comparison with Other Species

Squamous cell metaplasia or squamous cell carcinoma are rare features of human breast cancer, and these neoplasms are said to develop mainly in older patients (Scarff and Torloni 1981). Likewise, keratinized areas may be present in mammary tumors of dogs (Moulton 1978) and guinea pigs (Hoch-Ligeti et al. 1986). In rats, squamous metaplasia is commonly seen in cribriform comedocarcinomas and tubulopapillary carcinomas (Komitowski et al. 1982; Van Zwieten 1984).

References

Andervont HB, Dunn TB (1950) Response of mammary-tumor-agent-free strain DBA female mice to percutaneous application of methylcholanthrene. JNCI 10: 895–925

Asch BB, Burstein NA, Vidrich A, Sun T-T (1981) Identification of mouse mammary epithelial cells by immunofluorescence with rabbit and guinea pig antikeratin antisera. Proc Natl Acad Sci USA 78: 5643–5647

Asch HL, Asch BB (1985) Heterogeneity of keratin expression in mouse mammary hyperplastic alveolar nodules and adenocarcinomas. Cancer Res 45: 2760–2768

Biancifiori C, Caschera F (1962) The relation between pseudopregnancy and the chemical induction by four carcinogens of mammary and ovarian tumours in BALB/c mice. Br J Cancer 16: 722–730

Bonser GM, Orr JW (1939) The morphology of 160 tumours induced by carcinogenic hydrocarbons in the subcutaneous tissues of mice. J Pathol Bacteriol 49: 171–183

Deringer MK (1959) Occurrence of tumors, particularly mammary tumors, in agent-free strain C3HeB mice. JNCI 22: 995–1002

Deringer MK (1965) Occurrence of mammary tumors, reticular neoplasms, and pulmonary tumors in strain BALB/cAnDe breeding female mice. JNCI 35: 1047–1052

Deringer MK (1969) Development of tumors, particularly mammary tumors, in agent-free substrain RIIIeB/De mice. JNCI 43: 1347–1351

Dunn TB (1959) Morphology of mammary tumors in mice. In: Homburger F (ed) The physiopathology of cancer, 2nd edn. Hoeber-Harper, New York, pp 38–84

Heston WE, Deringer MK, Dunn TB, Levillain WD (1950) Factors in the development of spontaneous mammary gland tumors in agent-free strain C3Hb mice. JNCI 10: 1139–1155

Heston WE, Vlahakis G, Smith GH (1972) Mammary gland tumors in substrains C57BL/M and C57BL/He mice. JNCI 49: 805–812

Hoch-Ligeti C, Liebelt AG, Congdon CC, Stewart HL (1986) Mammary gland tumors in irradiated and untreated guinea pigs. Toxicol Pathol 14: 289–298

Huseby RA, Bittner JJ (1946) A comparative morphological study of the mammary glands with reference to the known factors influencing the development of mammary carcinoma in mice. Cancer Res 6: 240–255

Kirschbaum A (1949) Induction of mammary cancer with methylcholanthrene. II. Histological similarity between carcinogen-induced tumors and certain mammary neoplasms occurring spontaneously. Cancer Res 9: 93–95

Kirschbaum A, Williams WL, Bittner JJ (1946) Induction of mammary cancer with methylcholanthrene. I. Histogenesis of the induced neoplasm. Cancer Res 6: 354–362

Komitowski D, Sass B, Laub W (1982) Rat mammary tumor classification: notes on comparative aspects. JNCI 68: 147–156

Liebelt AG, Liebelt RA (1967) Chemical factors in mammary tumorigenesis. In: Carcinogenesis: a broad critique. 20th annual MD Anderson Hospital and Tumor Institute symposium on fundamental cancer research, 1966. Williams and Wilkins, Baltimore, pp 315–345

Medina D (1974) Mammary tumorigenesis in chemical carcinogen-treated mice. I. Incidence in BALB/c and C57BL mice. JNCI 53: 213–221

Medina D (1976) Preneoplastic lesions in murine mammary cancer. Cancer Res 36: 2589–2595

Medina D, Warner MR (1976) Mammary tumorigenesis in chemical carcinogen-treated mice. IV. Induction of mammary ductal hyperplasias. JNCI 57: 331–337

Medina D, Butel JS, Socher SH, Miller FL (1980) Mammary tumorigenesis in 7,12-dimethylbenzanthracene-treated C57BL × DBA/2fF₁ mice. Cancer Res 40: 368–373

Moulton JE (1978) Tumors of the mammary gland. In: Moulton JE (ed) Tumors in domestic animals, 2nd edn. University of California Press, Berkeley, pp 346–371

Mühlbock O, van Ebbenhorst Tengbergen W, van Rijssel TH (1952) Studies on the development of mammary tumors in dilute-brown DBAb mice without the agent. JNCI 13: 505–531

Peters RL, Rabstein LS, Spahn GJ, Madison RM, Huebner RJ (1972) Incidence of spontaneous neoplasms in breeding and retired breeder BALB/cCr mice throughout the natural life span. Int J Cancer 10: 273–282

Rehm S, Rapp KG, Deerberg F (1985) Influence of food restriction and body fat on life span and tumour incidence in female outbred Han:NMRI mice and two sublines. Z Versuchstierkd 27: 240–283

Sass B, Dunn TB (1979) Classification of mouse mammary tumors in Dunn's miscellaneous group including recently reported types. JNCI 62: 1287–1293

Sass B, Vlahakis G, Heston WE (1982) Precursor lesions and pathogenesis of spontaneous mammary tumors in mice. Toxicol Pathol 10: 12–21

Scarff RW, Torloni H (eds) (1981) Histological typing of breast tumours. International histological classification of tumours, no 2, 2nd edn. WHO, Geneva

Schaefer FV, Custer RP, Sorof S (1985) Induction of epidermoid differentiation by cyclic adenine nucleotide in cultured mammary tumors of mice. Cancer Res 45: 1828–1833

Slemmer G (1974) Interactions of separate types of cells during normal and neoplastic mammary gland growth. J Invest Dermatol 63: 24–47

Squartini F (1979) Tumours of the mammary gland. In: Turusov VS (ed) Pathology of tumours in laboratory animals, vol II. Tumours of the mouse. IARC, Lyon, pp 43–90 (IARC Sci Publ no 23)

Van der Valk MA (1981) Survivals, tumor incidence and gross pathology in 33 mouse strains. In: Hilgers J, Sluyser M (eds) Mammary tumors in the mouse. Elsevier/North-Holland, Amsterdam, pp 45–115

Van Ebbenhorst Tengbergen WJPR (1970) Morphological classification of mammary tumours in the mouse. Pathol Eur 5: 260–272

Van Zwieten MJ (1984) The rat as an animal model in breast cancer research. Martin Nijhoff/Kluwer/Academic, Boston, p 105

Ward JM, Quander R, Devor D, Wenk ML, Spangler EF (1986) Pathology of aging female SENCAR mice used as controls in skin two-stage carcinogenesis studies. Environ Health Perspect 68: 81–89

Mixed Adenocarcinoma, Mammary Gland, Mouse

Sabine Rehm, Jerrold M. Ward, and Annabel G. Liebelt

Synonyms. Carcinosarcoma; carcinoma with spindle cell formation; mixed mammary carcinomas; anaplastic carcinoma.

Gross Appearance

The mixed adenocarcinoma is grossly indistinguishable from the majority of other adenocarcinomas of the mouse mammary gland (see p. 319).

Microscopic Features

Mixed adenocarcinomas of the mouse mammary gland typically consist of at least two different cell types in varying proportions. Firstly, cuboidal or columnar epithelial cells are present, forming nests and/or glandular or papillary structures. These tumor cells may originate from either the mammary alveoli or from the duct system (Van Ebbenhorst Tengbergen 1970; Medina and Warner 1976). Secondly, tumor components are present that may be of mesenchymal or myoepithelial differentiation. In the following, several mammary gland tumors are described, of which the second tumor component is suggested to be of myoepithelial origin or differentiation.

Three spontaneous and eight chemically induced (7,12-dimethylbenz[a]anthracene) mouse mammary tumors with mixed features of carcinoma and sarcoma were obtained from the Registry of Experimental Cancers (Bethesda, MD) and from different experiments of the Laboratory of Comparative Carcinogenesis (Frederick, MD). Neoplastic glandular structures are surrounded by predominantly spindle-shaped cells that stained distinctly eosinophilic with hematoxylin and eosin (H&E). These fusiform cells at first glance appear similar to fibroblasts; however, histochemical and immunocytochemical studies indicate that they asre most likely of myoepithelial origin (Fig. 465). Only very sparse strands of connective tissue are detected by collagen stains (Masson's trichrome) in these tumors. The cytoplasm of the elongated cells is usually immunoreactive for keratin (Figs. 466 and 467, avidin-biotin immunoperoxidase), frequently in a characteristic perinuclear localization (Fig. 467).

For comparison, the immunoreactivity of normal myoepithelial cells for cytoplasmic keratin is shown in Fig. 468. Alveolar cells of the mammary gland are negative using this antibody against basic human keratins, but the antiserum is reactive with the keratin formed by cells undergoing squamous metaplasia (Fig. 468) and some ductal cells (not shown). Among the different neoplasms studied and even within the same tumor, the cells between the glandular structures varied in morphology, glycogen contents, degree of blue staining with phosphotungstic acid-hematoxylin, and immunoreactivity for keratin. Positive immunoreactivity can also be found in the glandular portions of ductal origin in DMBA-induced carcinoma.

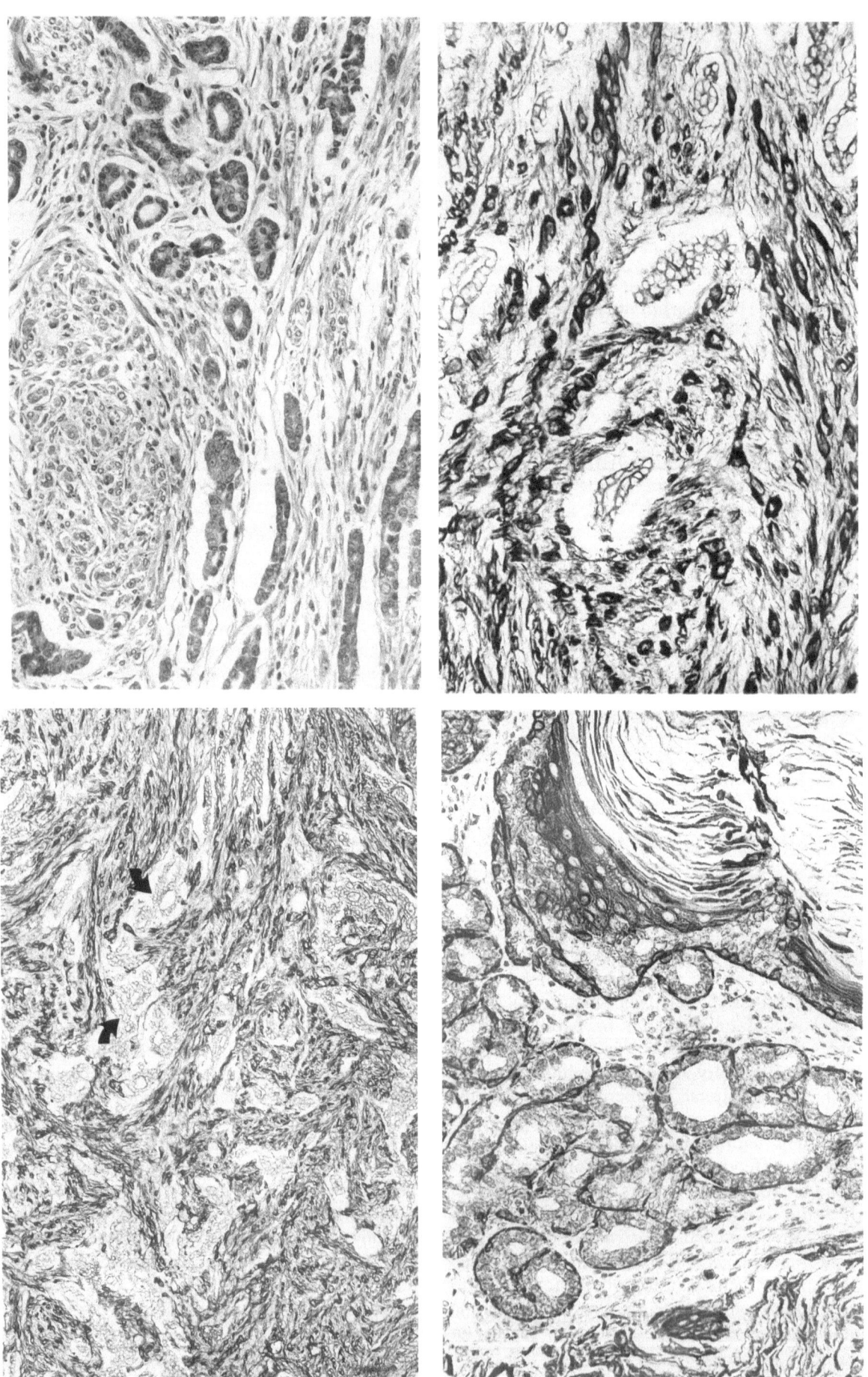

Myoepithelial cells are strongly decorated by antibodies to prekeratin and actin, and they are not specifically stained by antibodies to desmin and vimentin (Franke et al. 1980). Various keratins may be found in all epithelial cell types of the normal mammary gland at different stages of maturation and in neoplasms and single cell lines derived from mammary gland neoplasms (Krepler et al. 1981; Asch et al. 1981; Asch and Asch 1985a, b, c; Sonnenberg et al. 1986a, b). Heterogeneity of developmental markers in rat mammary tumors within the same neoplasm could be explained by differentiation of tumor cells towards adult types or dedifferentiation towards fetal cell types (Dulbecco et al. 1986a).

Ultrastructure

The only ultrastructural description on mixed mouse mammary gland tumors is given by Tarin (1969), who illustrated one case of several methylcholanthrene-induced mouse mammary gland tumors consisting of neoplastic glandular portions and areas with large numbers of fusiform cells. Ultrastructurally, these elongated cells contained fibrillar material and were therefore recognized to be neoplastic myoepithelial cells; they lay closely packed together on the epithelial side of the basement membranes. Only sparse supportive connective tissue was present.

◀ **Fig. 465** *(upper left)*. Mixed adenocarcinoma-myoepithelioma, mouse, mammary gland. Darker glandular structures of the neoplasm are separated by fusiform or polygonal neoplastic myoepithelial cells. H and E, × 250

Fig. 466 *(lower left)*. Mixed adenocarcinoma-myoepithelioma, mouse, mammary gland, same as Fig. 465. Neoplastic myoepithelial cells are immunoreactive with rabbit antibody to human keratin (DAKO, Corpintera, USA) after trypsin digestion of tissue section. Neoplastic glandular elements do not stain *(arrows)*. Avidin-biotin immunoperoxidase complex, no counter stain, × 100

Fig. 467 *(upper right)*. Higher magnification of specimen shown in Fig. 466. Artifactual tissue spaces due to fixation and processing. × 250

Fig. 468 *(lower right)*. Nonneoplastic mammary gland hyperplasia and squamous cell metaplasia, mouse. Immunoreactivity for keratin is present in cells undergoing squamous metaplasia and in flattened nonneoplastic myoepithelial cells that surround the alveolar cells. Avidin-biotin immunoperoxidase complex using rabbit human-specific keratin, counterstained with hematoxylin, × 250

Differential Diagnosis

One diagnostic alternative to mixed adenocarcinoma is that of adenocarcinoma with sarcomatous transformation. Studies have shown that cells of pure epithelial tumors change in morphology towards a simplified, elongated, sarcomatoid cell type. This change may occur naturally within the primary tumor as noted, e.g., in anaplastic squamous cell carcinoma of the mouse skin (Bogovski 1979) or in distant metastases of papillary mouse lung tumors (Stewart et al. 1970). A sarcomatous change in cell morphology can be observed particularly after successive transplantations of epithelial neoplasms (Stewart et al. 1947; Mühlbock and Van Rijssel 1954; Liebelt and Liebelt 1967) or during maintenance of cell lines in tissue culture (Sanford et al. 1961; Dexter et al. 1978; Hager et al. 1981a, b; Sonnenberg et al. 1986a).

Other diagnostic possibilities are carcinosarcomas consisting of adenocarcinomas mixed with neoplastic fibroblasts arising in the same location or in the case of differing sites of origin, fibrosarcomas and adenocarcinomas invading one another (collision tumors). Furthermore, invasion of mammary gland tissue by salivary gland myoepithelioma, fibrosarcoma, histiocytic sarcoma, rhabdomyosarcoma, or schwannoma should be considered.

Biologic Features

Mixed adenocarcinomas (adenocarcinoma-myoepitheliomas) or carcinosarcomas and pure myoepitheliomas (Squartini 1979; Sheldon and Greenman 1979; Van der Valk 1981) are very rare mouse mammary tumors. One type of carcinosarcoma was reported to have a myxoid stroma and osteoid and myoepithelial cells (Sass and Dunn 1979). Probably because of the rarity of these neoplasms, the pathogenesis of mixed malignant mouse mammary gland tumors and their possible progression from other tumors such as adenocarcinoma type C (Dunn 1959) or fibroadenomas have not been investigated. We are not aware of any previous publication describing the immunocytochemical characterization of pure or mixed myoepithelial mammary gland tumors of the mouse. Comparing photomicrographs of H&E-stained sections with material studied by us suggests that many of the carcinosarcomas presented (Dunn 1959; Heston et al. 1950; Andervont and Dunn 1950; Mühlbock et al. 1952; Squartini 1979) may be mixed adenocarcinoma-myo-epitheliomas. These tumors may arise spontaneously with a very low incidence in older mice of some strains (Van Nie and Dux 1971; Rabstein et al. 1973; Homburger et al. 1975; Sheldon and Greenman 1979). The 020 strain with a low incidence of mammary gland tumors, however, developed carcinosarcomas to a relative incidence of 30% (Mühlbock and Van Rijssel 1954). Carcinosarcomatoid features were not seen in 020 mice with murine mammary tumor virus (MuMTV); this could be an age-related phenomenon, since MuMTV carriers die early from other types of mammary gland neoplasms. On transplantation, tumors from 020 mice without the virus rapidly assumed sarcomatous features whereas no such change was seen on transplantation of mammary gland tumors from mice with MuMTV.

Chemical induction of carcinosarcomatoid mammary gland tumors in the mouse was primarily achieved with methylcholanthrene and only in mice free of MuMTV (Bonser and Orr 1939; Andervont and Dunn 1950, 1953; Tarin 1969). It has been hypothesized that secretory, ductal, and myoepithelial cells of the mammary gland are derived from one or more common stem cells (Radnor 1972; Bennet et al. 1978; Dulbecco et al. 1986b). Therefore, differing cell lines obtained from a single tumor or from metaplastic changes (squamous or sarcomatous) within an original or transplanted tumor represent expressions of inherent stem cell properties (Slemmer 1974; Dulbecco et al. 1979, 1986b; Sonnenberg et al. 1986a). Mixed adenocarcinoma-myoepitheliomas could be the result of a neoplastic transformation of two separate cell types (glandular epithelial and myoepithelial) or represent an adenocarcinoma with myoepithelial differentiation.

Comparison with Other Species

Mixed mammary gland tumors with myoepithelial components occur frequently in dogs and have been well-characterized (Moulton 1978; Jubb et al. 1985). Other tissue elements present in these mixed carcinomas are bone, cartilage, and connective tissue, and it has been suggested that these tumors are metaplastic variants originating from the myoepithelial component. Mixed mammary gland tumors with proliferating myoepithelial cells and carcinosarcomas are rare neoplasms in humans (Hamperl 1970; Zarbo and Oberman 1983), guinea pigs, (Hoch-Ligeti et al.

1986) and rats (Komitowski et al. 1982; Van Zwieten 1984).

In humans, a rare group of mammary gland neoplasms are classified under special types of carcinomas with spindle-cell metaplasia (Scarff and Torloni 1981; Linell and Ljungberg 1984) or as sarcomatoid carcinomas (pseudosarcoma; Millis 1984). These neoplasms, as in mice, also consist of two morphologically different cell types (cuboidal and fusiform). The histogenetic origin of the fusiform cell type has yet to be established. Pure myoepitheliomas of the human mammary gland are extremely rare, but some have been well-characterized by immunocytochemistry and ultrastructural studies (Schürch et al. 1985; Thorner et al. 1986; Bigotti and Giorgio 1986).

References

Andervont HB, Dunn TB (1950) Response of mammary-tumor-agent-free strain DBA female mice to percutaneous application of methylcholanthrene. JNCI 10: 895–925

Andervont HB, Dunn TB (1953) Responses of strain DBAf/2 mice, without the mammary tumor agent to oral administration of methylcholanthrene. JNCI 14: 329–339

Asch BB, Burstein NA, Vidrich A, Sun T-T (1981) Identification of mouse mammary epithelial cells by immunofluorescence with rabbit and guinea pig antikeratin antisera. Proc Natl Acad Sci USA 78: 5643–5647

Asch HL, Asch BB (1985a) Heterogeneity of keratin expression in mouse mammary hyperplastic alveolar nodules and adenocarcinomas. Cancer Res 45: 2760–2768

Asch HL, Asch BB (1985b) Expression of keratins and other cytoskeletal proteins in mouse mammary epithelium during the normal developmental cycle and primary culture. Dev Biol 107: 470–482

Asch HL, Asch BB (1985c) Expression of a 50K keratin is characteristic of mouse mammary myoepithelial cells. Ann NY Acad Sci 455: 726–728

Bogovski P (1979) Tumours of the skin. In: Turusov VS (ed) Pathology of tumours in laboratory animals, vol II. Tumours of the mouse. IARC, Lyon, pp 1–41 (IARC Sci Publ no 23)

Bennett DC, Peachey LA, Durbin H, Rudland PS (1978) A possible mammary stem cell line. Cell 15: 283–298

Bigotti G, Di Giorgio CG (1986) Myoepithelioma of the breast: histologic, immunologic, and electromicroscopic appearance. J Surg Oncol 32: 58–64

Bonser GM, Orr JW (1939) The morphology of 160 tumours induced by carcinogenic hydrocarbons in the subcutaneous tissues of mice. J Pathol Bacteriol 49: 171–183

Dexter DL, Kowalski HM, Blazar BA, Fligiel Z, Vogel R, Heppner GH (1978) Heterogeneity of tumor cells from a single mouse mammary tumor. Cancer Res 38: 3174–3181

Dulbecco R, Bologna M, Unger M (1979) Differentiation of a rat mammary cell line in vitro. Proc Natl Acad Sci USA 76: 1256–1260

Dulbecco R, Allen WR, Bologna M, Bowman M (1986a) Marker evolution during the development of the rat mammary gland: stem cells identified by markers and the role of myoepithelial cells. Cancer Res 46: 2449–2456

Dulbecco R, Armstrong B, Allen WR, Bowman M (1986b) Distribution of developmental markers in rat mammary tumors induced by N-nitrosomethylurea. Cancer Res 46: 5144–5152

Dunn TB (1959) Morphology of mammary tumors in mice. In: Homburger F (ed) The physiopathology of cancer, 2nd edn. Hoeber-Harper, New York, pp 38–84

Franke WW, Schmid E, Freudenstein C, Appelhans B, Osborn M, Weber K, Keenan TW (1980) Intermediate-sized filaments of the prekeratin type in myoepithelial cells. J Cell Biol 84: 633–654

Hager JC, Fligiel S, Stanley W, Richardson AM, Heppner GH (1981a) Characterization of a variant-producing tumor cell line from a heterogeneous strain BALB/cfC3H mouse mammary tumor. Cancer Res 41: 1293–1300

Hager JC, Russo J, Ceriani RL, Peterson JA, Fligiel S, Jolly S, Heppner GH (1981b) Epithelial characteristics of five subpopulations of a heterogeneous strain BALB/cfC3H mouse mammary tumor. Cancer Res 41: 1720–1730

Hamperl H (1970) The myothelia (myoepithelial cells). Normal state, regressive changes; hyperplasia; tumors. Curr Top Pathol 53: 162–220

Heston WE, Deringer MK, Dunn TB, Levillain WD (1950) Factors in the development of spontaneous mammary gland tumors in agent-free strain C3Hb mice. JNCI 10: 1139–1151

Hoch-Ligeti C, Liebelt AG, Congdon CC, Stewart HL (1986) Mammary gland tumors in irradiated and untreated guinea pigs. Toxicol Pathol 14: 289–298

Homburger F, Russfield AB, Weisburger JH, Lim S, Chak SP, Weisburger EK (1975) Aging changes in CD®-1 HaM/ICR mice reared under standard laboratory conditions. JNCI 55: 37–45

Jubb KVF, Kennedy PC, Palmer N (1985) The female genital system. Mammary glands. In: Pathology of domestic animals, vol 3, 3rd edn. Academic, Orlando, p 393

Komitowski D, Sass B, Laub W (1982) Rat mammary tumor classification: notes on comparative aspects. JNCI 68: 147–156

Krepler R, Denk H, Weirich E, Schmid E, Franke WW (1981) Keratin-like proteins in normal and neoplastic cells of human and rat mammary gland as revealed by immunofluorescence microscopy. Differentiation 20: 242–252

Liebelt AG, Liebelt RA (1967) Transplantation of tumors. In: Busch H (ed) Methods in cancer research, vol 1. Academic, New York, pp 143–242

Linell F, Ljungberg O (1984) Atlas of breast pathology. Lippincott, Philadelphia, p 224

Medina D, Warner MR (1976) Mammary tumorigenesis in chemical carcinogen-treated mice. IV. Induction of mammary ductal hyperplasias. JNCI 57: 331–337

Millis RR (1984) Atlas of breast pathology. MTP, Lancaster, p 95

Moulton JE (1978) Tumors of the mammary gland. In: Moulton JE (ed) Tumors in domestic animals. University of California Press, Berkeley, pp 346–371

Mühlbock O, van Rijssel TG (1954) Studies on mammary tumors in the 020 Amsterdam strain of mice. JNCI 15: 73–97

Mühlbock O, van Ebbenhorst Tengbergen W, van Rijssel TG (1952) Studies on the development of mammary tumors in dilute-brown DBAb mice without the agent. JNCI 13: 505–531

Rabstein LS, Peters RL, Spahn GJ (1973) Spontaneous tumors and pathologic lesions in SWR/J mice. JNCI 50: 751–758

Radnor CJP (1972) Myoepithelial cell differentiation in rat mammary glands. J Anat 111: 381–398

Sanford KK, Dunn TB, Westfall BB, Covalesky AB, Dupree LT, Earle WR (1961) Sarcomatous change and maintenance of differentiation in long term cultures of mouse mammary carcinoma. JNCI 26: 1139–1183

Sass B, Dunn TB (1979) Classification of mouse mammary tumors in Dunn's miscellaneous group including recently reported types. JNCI 62: 1287–1293

Scarff RW, Torloni H (eds) (1981) Histologic typing of breast tumours. International histological classification of tumours, no 2, 2nd edn. WHO, Geneva

Schürch W, Potvin C, Seemayer TA (1985) Malignant myoepithelioma (myoepithelial carcinoma) of the breast: an ultrastructural and immunocytochemical study. Ultrastruct Pathol 8: 1–11

Sheldon WG, Greenman DL (1979) Spontaneous lesions in control BALB/c female mice. J Environ Pathol Toxicol Oncol 3: 155–167

Slemmer G (1974) Interactions of separate types of cells during normal and neoplastic mammary gland growth. J Invest Dermatol 63: 27–47

Sonnenberg A, Daams H, Calafat J, Hilgers J (1986a) In vitro differentiation and progression of mouse mammary tumor cells. Cancer Res 46: 5913–5922

Sonnenberg A, Daams H, van der Valk MA, Hilkens J, Hilgers J (1986b) Development of mouse mammary gland: identification of stages in differentiation luminal and myoepithelial cells using monoclonal antibodies and polyvalent antiserum against keratin. J Histochem Cytochem 34: 1037–1046

Squartini F (1979) Tumours of the mammary gland. In: Turusov VS (ed) Pathology of tumours in laboratory animals, vol 11. Tumours of the mouse. IARC, Lyon, pp 43–90 (IARC Sci Publ no 23)

Stewart HL, Grady HG, Andervont HB (1947) Development of sarcoma at site of serial transplantation of pulmonary tumors in inbred mice. JNCI 7: 207–225

Stewart HL, Dunn TB, Snell KC (1970) Pathology of tumors and nonneoplastic proliferative lesions of the lungs of mice. In: Nettesheim P, Hanna MG, Deatherage JW (eds) Morphology of experimental respiratory carcinogenesis. USEAC Technical Information Center, Oak Ridge, pp 161–181 (AEC symposium series no 21)

Tarin D (1969) Fine structure of murine mammary tumours: the relationship between epithelium and connective tissue in neoplasms induced by various agents. Br J Cancer 23: 417–425

Thorner PS, Kahn HJ, Baumal R, Lee K, Moffat W (1986) Malignant myoepithelioma of the breast. An im-

328   Sabine Rehm, Jerrold M. Ward, and Annabel G. Liebelt

munohistochemical study by light and electron microscopy. Cancer 57: 745–750

Van Ebbenhorst Tengbergen WJPR (1970) Morphological
classification of mammary tumours in the mouse. Pathol Eur 5: 260–272

Van der Valk MA (1981) Survivals, tumor incidence and
gross pathology in 33 mouse strains. In: Hilgers J, Sluyser M (eds) Mammary tumors in the mouse. Elsevier/
North-Holland   Biomedical   Press,   Amsterdam,
pp 45–115

Van Nie R, Dux A (1971) Biological and morphological
characteristics of mammary tumors in GR mice. JNCI
46: 885–897

Van Zwieten MJ (1984) The rat as an animal model in
breast cancer research. Thesis, Martin Nijhoff Pub-
lishers, Kluwer Academic Boston, pp 1–301

Zarbo RJ, Oberman HA (1983) Cellular adenomyoepi-
thelioma of the breast. Am J Surg Pathol 7: 863–870

Subject Index*

---

* Page numbers in **boldface** indicate the principal discussion; Figures are designated by the letter "f" following the page number; Tables are found on page numbers followed by the letter "t".

346 Subject Index